Communication Development

Foundations, Processes,
and Clinical Applications

Communication Development

Foundations, Processes, and Clinical Applications

WILLIAM O. HAYNES, Ph.D.
College of Liberal Arts
Department of Communication
  Disorders
Auburn University
Auburn, Alabama

BRIAN B. SHULMAN, Ph.D.
School of Graduate Medical Education
Seton Hall University
South Orange, New Jersey

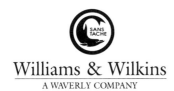

Williams & Wilkins
A WAVERLY COMPANY

BALTIMORE • PHILADELPHIA • LONDON • PARIS • BANGKOK
BUENOS AIRES • HONG KONG • MUNICH • SYDNEY • TOKYO • WROCLAW

Editor: Donna Balado
Managing Editor: Jennifer Schmidt
Marketing Manager: Christine Kushner
Production Coordinator: Carol Eckhart
Project Editor: Jeffrey S. Myers
Designer: Graphic World, Inc.
Illustration Planner: Ray Lowman
Cover Designer: Melissa Brown
Typesetter: Peirce Graphic Services, Inc.
Printer & Binder: R. R. Donnelley & Sons Company

351 West Camden Street
Baltimore, Maryland 21201-2436 USA

Rose Tree Corporate Center
1400 North Providence Road
Building II, Suite 5025
Media, Pennsylvania 19063-2043 USA

This book was previously published by Prentice-Hall, Inc.

Accurate indications, adverse reactions and dosage schedules for drugs are provided in this book, but it is possible that they may change. The reader is urged to review the package information data of the manufacturers of the medications mentioned.

Printed in the United States of America

Library of Congress Cataloging-in-Publication Data

Communication development : foundations, processes, and clinical applications / editors, William O. Haynes, Brian B. Shulman. — 2nd ed.
    p.   cm.
  Rev. ed. of: Communication development / William O. Haynes and Brian B. Shulman. c1994.
  Includes bibliographical references and indexes.
  ISBN 0-683-30278-7
  1. Language acquisition.   2. Speech disorders.   3. Speech therapy.   I. Haynes, William O.   II. Shulman, Brian B.   III. Haynes, William O. Communication development. [DNLM: 1. Language Development. 2. Language Development Disorders.   WS 105.5.C8 C7338 1998]
QP399.C65   1998
618.92′ 855—dc21
DNLM/DLC
for Library of Congress   97-33647
                                                     CIP

The publishers have made every effort to trace the copyright holders for borrowed material. If they have inadvertently overlooked any, they will be pleased to make the necessary arrangements at the first opportunity.

To purchase additional copies of this book, call our customer service department at **(800) 638-0672** or fax orders to **(800) 447-8438.** For other book services, including chapter reprints and large quantity sales, ask for the Special Sales department.

Canadian customers should call **(800) 665-1148,** or fax **(800) 665-0103.** For all other calls originating outside of the United States, please call **(410) 528-4223** or fax us at **(410) 528-8550.**

Visit Williams & Wilkins on the Internet: **http://www.wwilkins.com** or contact our customer service department at **custserv@wwilkins.com.** Williams & Wilkins customer service representatives are available from 8:30 am to 6:00 pm, EST, Monday through Friday, for telephone access.

98 99 00 01 02
1 3 4 5 6 7 8 9 10

To our children, David, Jeffrey, and Ashleigh, who showed us as we watched in wonder that communication development is far richer than any model and frankly . . . more interesting.

Foreword

How do human beings communicate with one another? For verbal communication at least, there is a sort of folk answer, suggested by a variety of metaphors in everyday use: "putting one's thoughts into words" (or) "getting one's ideas across" . . . and so on. These make it sound as if verbal communication were a matter of packing a content (yet another metaphor) into words and sending it off, to be unpacked by the recipient at the other end . . . (Thus) the study of communication raises two major questions: first what is communicated, and second, how is communication achieved?

(Sperber & Wilson, 1995, p.1)

An underlying principle of this text is that the prospective professional in child communication disorders can only achieve an integrated understanding of assessment and treatment in individual children and youth by obtaining a comprehensive grounding in normal acquisition patterns. In other words, best practices in clinical applications emerge from having a holistic knowledge base about the nature and course of developmental processes. An initial step in achieving this goal is approaching the complexity of these processes. At the same time, the future professional must also acquire skill in making this complexity transparent to be able to plan authentic communication goals and procedures for individual children.

Few human behaviors are as complex as communication. In fact, our abilities to communicate are the defining feature of being human. Spoken language and communication provide us with the power to establish social relationships with others. Through this power we are able to understand other peoples' minds and, in turn, have them understand our beliefs, values, and emotions. As we continue to learn new ways of using language and communication, we then have the capacity to discover other universes of mind—past, present, and future—accessible only by way of the written word. Because communication is so integrated with our own identities as individuals and with our memberships in a wide variety of social units from family to institutional units (e.g., school or work), we tend to think that being able to communicate is simple.

However, as Sperber and Wilson (1995) remind us, two major concerns remain to be answered completely about this most public of human behaviors. First, what kinds of knowledge do children learn to communicate? An important issue is what aspects of this learning are universal across cultures? To state this point another way, what do all children learn about language and communication regardless of differences in their social and cultural experiences?

Even if we understand the "what" of communication acquisition across cultures and the span of childhood, the "how" question still must be explained. Knowing what all children learn in common is insufficient, however, because there are significant variations in the ways that children learn to communicate their knowledge. We still must be able to interpret the facets of knowing how to communicate that arise from specific variations in the ways children are socialized through language and communication to become competent members of a variety of social units. Individual differences in the rate and manner of acquisition are the rule not the exception, a fact that can often complicate clinical decision making but also, at the same time, offer exciting challenges for knowing when a language difference is also a language disability.

The "how" question also extends into the domain of brain-behavior relationships. Is there a single neurobiological mechanism dedicated to acquiring the ability to communicate, a mechanism that allows young children to discover on their own "what counts" as communication? Or, is there a more general neurocognitive mechanism that, at least initially, is responsible for children learning how to understand, remember, and express themselves only in the social context of interactional experiences with adults? Regardless of the theoretical perspective, are there different consequences for certain types of disruptions in neural connections before birth or after birth on the subsequent course of communication acquisition? This question about cause is not a trivial one because the vast majority of children provided with language intervention services will not have a documented etiology. There are no easy answers yet; however, this text makes clear to readers the kinds of questions they will need to ask in approaching clinical planning as a problem-solving activity.

An important contribution of this text is that it provides the reader with a consistent framework for approaching the complexity of what is acquired, how it is acquired within and across cultures, and how the communication system can be disrupted. Each chapter reiterates that the parts of the language system—its forms, contents, and functions—are an integrative system whose sole purpose is always that of communication. This critical concept is also applied across chapters to the view of assessment and intervention as an interwoven process for facilitating children's real uses of communication in real social contexts.

This text offers a blueprint to future professionals in speech-language pathology and related professions. On the one hand, readers will develop an appreciation for the remarkably elegant complexity of how we learn to communicate on different topics in different ways with each other using the forms and content of language. On the other hand, readers will also find that this same blueprint offers a prism through which the many layered and interactive components of the communication system can become transparent. The journey offered by this text is discovering this transparency—being able to see, understand, and make relevant what previously was opaque and unknowable.

ELAINE R. SILLIMAN
Professor
Department of Communication
Sciences and Disorders
University of South Florida
Tampa, FL

REFERENCES

Sperber D, Wilson D. Relevance: communication and cognition. 2nd edition, Cambridge, MA: Blackwell, 1995.

Preface

There are many books dealing with the topic of language acquisition in children. For those professionals interested in meeting the educational needs of communicatively-impaired children, a knowledge of the process of communication development is essential.

Why is this knowledge required? It is necessary for professionals to have general knowledge of how communication develops to be able to determine if the acquisition process is progressing normally. Knowledge of communication development is often applied in assessment to locate a child in "developmental space." Also, the communication development progression is often applied to intervention in terms of target selection and remediation program design. Thus, for those professionals dealing with communicatively-impaired children, knowledge about communication development is basically clinical in application. For others, there is merit in studying communication development patterns solely for purposes of contributing to theoretical interpretations of how the process works, as well as to determine idiosyncratic paths taken by various children on their way to becoming competent adult communicators. Most textbooks on communication development primarily present information about the process of acquiring language, and in turn the reader is left with the sole responsibility of gleaning applications that are typically not addressed in the work.

Many instructors supplement a textbook on communication development by discussing clinical applications as they teach students about the developmental process. Our text bridges this gap between development and clinical application. Most special education or speech-language pathology students take a course in communication development prior to their exposure to assessment and treatment issues. It is crucial for students in clinical fields to study some examples of *how* the communication development research has been applied clinically. This serves to make the material relevant for a variety of reasons and impresses the student with the idea that information on communication development is not just "an interesting process to study," but is critical to clinical work as well. Too often, for exposition purposes, we fractionalize the acquisition process into discrete "boxes," and then we compound this fragmentation by separating development from assessment and intervention.

Another basic premise of this text is that language learning is *communicative* in nature. Note that most acquisition texts have the word "language" in the title. The practitioner must adopt a *holistic* (rather than fragmented) approach to studying communicative development. This approach could in turn affect the professional's approach to assessing and treating language impairment. In each chapter we emphasize the *integrative* nature of communicative development.

Certainly, a single book cannot provide an exhaustive review of the vast literature in communication development, assessment, and intervention. The primary emphasis of our text is on the research literature dealing with communication development. This is dealt with in a complete and critical manner. Overviews of how the developmental information has been applied clinically are also provided.

We would like to express our sincere appreciation to our contributors: Janet Norris, Janet Patterson, Carol Westby, and Beth Witt. These nationally renowned experts in communication development have shared our view of the importance of linking information on acquisition to the clinical process. The fact that these contributors represent diverse backgrounds, clinical experiences, and theoretical orientations has clearly strengthened this work.

We also extend thanks to those scientists and mentors who taught us to always ask questions and encouraged us to continually search for answers. We encourage you, our students and colleagues, to take the information we present here and to continue to ask clinically relevant questions that impact how we describe, assess, and treat deficits in communication development. It is important to never assume that an answer is the best or only answer; *inquiry is the key to learning, and clinical inquiry must never end in the face of the clients we service.*

WILLIAM O. HAYNES and
BRIAN B. SHULMAN

Contributors

WILLIAM O. HAYNES, Ph.D.
Department of Communication Disorders
Auburn University
Auburn, AL

JANET A. NORRIS, Ph.D.
Department of Communication Disorders
Louisiana State University
Baton, Rouge, LA

JANET L. PATTERSON, Ph.D.
Department of Communicative Disorders
University of New Mexico
Albuquerque, NM

BRIAN B. SHULMAN, Ph.D.
School of Graduate Medical Education
Seton Hall University
South Orange, NJ

CAROL E. WESTBY, Ph.D.
Department of Communicative Disorders
Wichita State University
Wichita, KS
Center for Family and Community
*   Partnership*
University of New Mexico
Albuquerque, NM

BETH WITT, M.A.
C-BARC
Goldman School Early Intervention
*   Program*
Shreveport, LA

Contents

Processes and Applications of
Communication Development

Variability and Individual Differences in
Communication Development

PART I

Foundations of Communication: Overviews and Applications

Learning about the development of communication is an immensely complex undertaking. There are several complicating factors we should mention at the outset. First, communication relies on a variety of systems. Haynes, Moran, and Pindzola (1990) characterize these systems as comprising the "BACIS" (pronounced "basis") or foundation of communication development. The acronym BACIS refers to five interlocking building blocks that are necessary for normal acquisition of communication. A child must have an intact *biologic* system to become an effective communicator. For instance, the child must have a normal speech and hearing mechanism and neurologic system to develop communication skills using the auditory-vocal channel. A child must have *access to a language model* and opportunities for relevant interactions if communication is to develop normally. *Cognitive development* is a necessity for normal communicative growth because we communicate about concepts we have about the world and language symbols require higher cortical functioning. A child must have an *intent to communicate* with others in the environment. Most of our communication serves to influence the actions and attitudes of other people. Finally, a child needs to have *social development* to develop communicatively because communication is a social event. These five areas are fundamental to the acquisition of communicative skills, and without these building blocks the communicative structure erected by a developing child will be compromised. If a child does not have the biologic prerequisites for communication, he or she will not develop normally. Without examples of normal communication, a child cannot abstract the rules of the language of his or her culture. Children with cognitive delays almost always experience problems in communication development. A child with no intent to communicate will have no reason to develop language. Finally, a child who has no interest in social interaction may have no need for play or a communication system. We can see that communication development relies on a foundation of various biologic, social, and cognitive systems. This is one reason that communication development is more complicated than it may appear at first glance.

Another reason that communication development is complex revolves around the nature of language. Language, by itself, is a multifaceted and highly complex phenomenon comprised of many components (phonology, syntax, morphology, semantics, pragmatics) and modalities (speaking, listening, reading, writing).

A third source of complexity in communication development involves the interrelatedness of the basic systems that underlie language and the linguistic systems themselves. There are complex interconnections among the areas in the BACIS of communication and further connections of the domains with the various parts of the language system.

The purpose of Part I is to introduce students to the diverse theoretical and empirical aspects of the basic areas that underlie communication development. Chapter 1 describes basic concepts in linguistics. Because language is the primary manifestation of communication development in most children, it is important to realize that linguistic systems can be examined in a variety of ways. Further, it is instructive to note that language has been viewed differently over the decades and that these views have evolved from a variety of theories in linguistics. Each era of child language research has been impacted by theoretical changes in linguistics. In turn, such impact has changed the way we examine and interpret children's utterances both in theory and in clinical activities. For each test or treatment procedure on the dusty shelves in clinics around the country, there is a theoretical basis. A chronological examination of these materials will reveal changes from syntax to semantics to pragmatics as theories changed over the years. Chapter 1 demonstrates how the thinking in linguistics has changed over time, as well as the current view that language is an interrelated system.

Chapter 2 discusses some of the neurologic underpinnings of communication both in the development of the basic neural wiring necessary for growth and in the functional aspects of using these neurologic structures.

Chapter 3 considers theories of communication development. Many experts have put forth summaries of *what* is acquired in communication development and in *what order* these milestones appear. The other questions, however, are *why* these forms are developed and *how* the development takes place. Is it the result of innate capacities, operant conditioning, social factors, cognitive inputs, or a combination of all of these? Any consideration of communication development must at least touch on classical and current theoretical views of this process.

Chapter 4 presents an overview of child development. We have said that communication develops in synchrony with cognitive, social, neurobiologic, and structural domains. This chapter attempts to provide students with a general picture of the developing child and reinforces the notion that communication does not appear independently. All areas develop together.

Chapter 5 focuses on access to the language model. Much research has been conducted on the social and linguistic environment of children learning to communicate. This chapter attempts to synthesize this information and demonstrates the importance of caretaker influences on communication development.

Chapter 6 examines how children develop cognitive skills. Various perspectives on cognitive development are presented in this chapter along with their clinical application.

Chapter 7 considers the development of play behavior. Play is a phenomenon that combines cognitive, social, and communicative domains, and an examination of a child's play behavior reveals much about each of these areas.

Part I of our text is meant to provide you with an overview of seven areas that comprise the *foundations* of communication development. No single chapter can tell us everything about areas as complex as child development, cognition, caretaker-child interactions, or linguistics. The chapters in this part can, however, provide overviews of thinking in these areas and can show students that each topic is complex and interrelated. Many terms and concepts will be defined that will be applied in Parts II and III as we address the development of communication. Some overlap or even redundancy should be noted as we move from chapter to chapter in Part I, as well as in the other parts of the book. It is our intention to show students that communication development is an *integrative* process, and the fact that some topics are discussed in multiple chapters in different ways is one way of demonstrating the basic premise. So, when the topic of cognition is discussed in chapters on linguistic theory, neurolinguistics, theories of language development, child development, caretaker-child interaction, and play, it should be clear that conceptual development either influences or is affected by a variety of areas.

Students will find early on that the material in Part I is not easy to understand, and this is for several reasons. First, whenever chapters provide overviews of topics, there is no opportunity to develop each area as thoroughly as we would like. So, students may be left with some questions about certain theories or terms. In some respects this result is good because these questions will generate discussion in classes and perhaps further inquiry. A second reason students may find this section difficult is that the material is very complex. Not even authorities in communication development fully understand all of this material, and there are often no cut-and-dry answers for questions. We do not know exactly which linguistic theories are best, the details of how the brain works, how language is developed, and all the nuances of social impacts on play and communication. This lack of exact knowledge, in some respects, makes Part I frustrating reading. It does, however, introduce students to current concepts that they will see later in the research literature and in presentations at national conventions. Interested students can seek out the bibliographic sources provided in each chapter to examine any concept further. If you read the chapters in this section carefully, we hope you will have a strong foundation for understanding the chronology of communication development and the reasons for individual variations in this process that are examined later on in the text.

REFERENCE

Haynes W, Moran M, Pindzola R. Communication disorders in the classroom. Dubuque, IA: Kendall/Hunt, 1990.

CHAPTER 1

Psycholinguistic Foundations of Communication Development

Janet A. Norris

Most people who study language development have a reason for doing so. One reason could be an interest in or curiosity about children and how they develop. Some who study language may be planning to teach children and recognize language as the most important medium for exchanging information in the classroom. Others are motivated to work with children and adults who are experiencing communication disorders, ranging from a generalized failure to learn language in a normal manner during the preschool years, to a loss of language during adulthood after having had the ability to communicate throughout ones earlier lifetime. Still others study language development to gain insights into the logical properties of language. To meet these goals, language must be consciously examined. This conscious examination provides us with an understanding of how language works and therefore with insights into what to do about it when it does not work for some individuals or ways to best facilitate it when it does. This conscious examination is not something that we ordinarily do with language.

Ordinarily, language is one of the most useful things that we possess as human beings. We use it so often and so easily that most of us take it for granted. But try to think of living even one day without language, including talking to yourself or thinking in language. How would you communicate to your friends that the reason why you could not meet them for a movie is because you had to read this chapter before tomorrow? How would you think about the existence of tomorrow or decide that reading the chapter might be important or relevant? How would you read if the words and word order had no meaning or significance to you? If you chose to go to the movie, what would the rapidly changing visual images in the movie mean to you if you did not have the accompanying language to add continuity and to create the background and plot? How would you interpret a character's emotional status since the same visual action of pounding a desk accompanied by a stern expression could mean many different things, including "I found the solution"; "Its not fair"; "I will try harder next time"; "You did something wrong"? How would you imagine abstract concepts such as "doing wrong" or "fairness," since these are value judgments created by the people in a culture rather than real world objects or actions that can be seen, smelled, or touched. The ways that we use language to make sense out of our world and to exert some control over our environment are almost endless.

WHAT IS LANGUAGE?

If it is so important and central to our lives, then what is language? This is not an easy question to answer. Language is many things, depending on the perspective from which it is viewed, the reasons for defining it, the purposes of its use, and the context in which it is embedded. Among possible answers is that language is a communication system used to share information with others (including ourselves, as we do when we think in language). Language also is an interlocking system of patterns that form words and sentences consistent with the grammar of the language. It is a process engaged in for purposes of referring to meaningful information about the world and its events and properties; it is a link between the outside world and the mind. It is a set of conventions, or arbitrarily agreed on patterns of sound, that are shared by people in a culture who know how the patterns work. It is something that exists both as a system in itself (Latin is a language whether you understand a word of it or not) and as a communication system (Latin only works to influence the beliefs and behaviors of the people who understand it). Its a tool for accomplishing goals; a method of self-expression; a system of symbols that facilitates creativity; a devise for controlling the environment; the structure underlying speaking, listening, reading, and writing; and something learned by almost all children by the time they are 2 years old.

Because it is so complex, the best that we can do in our quest to understand language is to select one perspective or one small and manageable aspect of language to examine at a time. Understanding language is very much like attempting to understand the solar system. The solar system is a vast and indivisible entity. It consists of our sun and all of the planets, asteroids, comets, and meteors that orbit around the sun. It is embedded within the even larger contexts of our galaxy and the universe. The planets within the solar system hold fixed relationships between each other, so that Mercury is always closest to the sun, Earth in the middle, and Pluto the farthest, and yet the entire system is always in motion, always in a state of transformation or change. However, the change is not random but rather systematic or patterned. Each planet rotates on its own axis with amazing regularity (23 hours 56 minutes for Earth); each revolves around the sun in a predictable orbit (Earth's occurring approximately 93,000,000 miles from the sun but elliptical so that it is nearer in January than in July) over a predictable time frame (365.2 days) at a predictable speed of 18.5 miles per second.

We can arbitrarily talk about or examine any part of the solar system in isolation from the rest such as naming the order of the planets from the sun or describing the Earth's rotation around its own axis. The mechanics of axial rotation can be examined completely independently of the results or in terms of the creation of daylight and darkness on different parts of the Earth. We can ignore asteroids, comets, or meteors in the discussion or focus on categories of similarities or differences between them. We can attend to the sun as the only star of significance in discussing our solar system or view it as only one among billions in the Milky Way galaxy. Facts about the tilt of the Earth's axis can be stated without regard to the effects on seasons and Earth's temperature. But the examination of isolated aspects of the solar system does not change the fact that it is a united, integrated, dynamic system in which predictable relationships do hold between all of the elements and the processes created and affected by them. The interactions exist whether our analysis acknowledges them or not.

The study of language is much the same and almost as vast. We can arbitrarily talk about or examine the structure of words, sentences, and conversations; the meaning that is shared through linguistic reference; or the purposes that are accomplished through language use in a context. We can talk about mental or neurologic processes involved in the generation or use of language. We can describe the stages that children advance through in their progressive mastery of adult language and the factors that influence this development. We can isolate the products from the process, the language from its user, and the use from its context of occurrence. But the examination of isolated aspects of language does not change the fact that it is a united, integrated, dynamic system in which predictable relationships hold between all of the elements and the processes created and affected by them. The interactions exist, whether our analysis acknowledges them or not. As we begin our examination of language and dissect its structures, processes, and functions, always keep the solar system in mind.

THEORIES OF LANGUAGE

Just as theories of the solar system change over time to account for new discoveries, changing perspectives, and better models, so do theories about language. Each theory contributes new dimensions and insights that help to create a more comprehensive model of language. These models help to account for what language is and how it works. Our examination of language will begin with a discussion of the most prominent theories and the contributions that they have made to our present understanding of language.

Linguistic Structuralism

Linguistic structuralism was the most dominant theory prior to the 1950s, influenced by writers such as De Saussure (1916), Sapir (1921), Bloomfield (1933), Harris (1951), and Hockett (1958) among many. Numerous important concepts resulted from this work that continue to influence theories of language and its struc-

ture today. According to the structuralists, language exists as a hierarchical organization with four main levels. Phonology, or the structure, distribution, and sequencing of speech sounds, is at the lowest level. Above this resides the morphologic level, or the internal organization of words. Syntax, or the specification of word order, sentence organization, and other elements of the sentence, comprises the third level. At the top of the hierarchy is semantics, or the meaning and content of words and word combinations. Each level is viewed as independent for purposes of analysis, so that sentence structure analysis is conducted independently of the meaning of the words within the sentence, and the sound sequences and distributions are separate from the grammatical part of speech or meaning of the words. Any linguistic phenomenon that cannot be neatly placed in one of these categories because of overlap is referred to with a hyphenated term such as morpho-phonemic or phono-syntactic.

At each level two formal structural relationships are assigned to each unit (a unit being a word, sentence, or form). The first type of structural relationship, termed *paradigmatic*, refers to the individual elements of the unit. At the level of phonology this refers to the individual consonants or vowels found within a word; at the level of morphology this is the minimal meaningful form such as a plural or past-tense ending. At the level of syntax, words that are grammatically classified the same, such as the class of nouns, maintain a paradigmatic relationship, while semantically this relationship exists between words that can meaningfully substitute for each other within some context, as in the words that can fill in the slot "The dog ate the ___." Words that can fit the slot should be compatible on the basis of the *semantic features* that define the word. These features are abstract markers such as [human] [male] [animate] [adult] that can be specified as either pertaining to that word, as in + human, or absent from its definition (− human) (Clark, 1973). No one has been able to determine a set of features that satisfactorily allows for all words that can logically fit a slot while eliminating those that would create anomalous sentences.

Clark (1983, 1987) revised her theory to involve a lexical contrast paradigm, rather than a feature specification approach. In lexical contrast theory, words do not exist as a dictionary entry with a list of defining features. Rather, children learn that a particular word can refer to a conceptual category. The speaker chooses the best word from all of those that refer to that conceptual category, selecting the one that best captures the intended aspects of meaning and contrasting it with aspects of meaning that are not intended. For example, a conceptual category such as "cat" may have many potential words used to establish reference such as "cat," "kitty," "feline," or "Persian." The one selected in a context of use best sets up the intended meaning. "The Persian won first prize" is generally more useful than "The kitty won first prize" in the context of a cat show. The manner in which these flexible and changing meanings and word selections are structured are not well specified in this theory. How meaning is represented in language remains unclear and one of the most difficult aspects of language for which to account.

The second type of formal structural relationship is termed *syntagmatic* and refers to the sequential organization found within units. At the level of phonology this refers to the allowable syllable structures found in a language such as CONSONANT + VOWEL or CONSONANT + VOWEL + CONSONANT. At the level of morphology the meaningful forms have to be ordered, so that /ly/, /un/, /ing/, and /know/ are sequenced to form the allowable word "unknowingly" rather than the incorrect "ingunlyknow." Similarly, allowable sentence structures are referred to syntagmatically at the level of syntax, as are allowable meaningful relationships at the level of semantics (i.e., relationships of action, causality, time, conditions, and so forth).

Structuralism has provided us with a highly useful means of describing language and allows us to make discriminations between sounds, forms, grammatical structures, and word meanings more accurately and rapidly. But while a description of the levels of language and its units is useful, just as describing the planets, comets, and other bodies in the solar system is useful, it does not really explain very much about how the system of language works to create sentences or to use them to accomplish purposes in a context of use.

Linguistic Transformationism

The publication of Noam Chomsky's *Syntactic Structures* in 1957 represented a major shift in linguistic theory that has been the single most influential school of analysis ever since. Structuralism took the approach of observing the data, or the words and sentences found in a language and describing their paradigmatic and syntagmatic structure. *Transformationalism*, in contrast, seeks to find the underlying grammar or system of rules that allows for all of these words and sentences to be generated. It is an attempt to define the mechanism that generates language, rather than describing the finished product. There are tens of thousands of words in a language that potentially have an infinite number of possible word-order combinations. However, speakers of a language do not randomly order words, but instead follow patterns that are consistent with the grammar of their language. They can indicate when a sentence is ungrammatical (as in "She were not happy"), when there are two potential interpretations of the same sentence (as in "The old man's hat blew away"—is it the man or the hat that is old?), or when the sentence is grammatical but does not make sense (as in "The spoon ate all day"). Furthermore, speakers can accurately produce and understand sentences that they have never heard before and could not possibly have learned from someone else.

Chomsky (1957) argued that there must

be some sort of underlying mechanism that is very generative or creative to account for all of these linguistic abilities and that this mechanism is used to interpret and produce all of the utterances to which it is exposed. Not only that, but the mechanism should have infinite capacity, capable of describing the speaker's knowledge of all allowable utterances that can be imagined, or linguistic *competence*, and not just the ones that the speaker is actually exposed to and uses, or *performance*. The mechanism that Chomsky proposed to account for these abilities is a grammar that he termed transformational-generative grammar (TGG).

Generative Rules

The transformational-generative grammar was not intended to describe the sentences that had already been formed, as structuralism had done, but rather to define the knowledge that the speaker possessed about how to generate such sentences. In other words, it focused on the hypothetical speaker rather than the sentences. The sentences were just used as data to provide evidence or insights into what type of knowledge the speaker must possess to generate these sentences. Chomsky believed that the knowledge existed in the form of a set of rules. A person who had knowledge of a fairly limited set of rules (most sentences can be accounted for with fewer than 150 rules) could understand and produce an infinite number of sentences, including all of those found in this book or in all of the books in a university library, or all of the utterances ever spoken in a language since the language evolved, and all that ever will be spoken in that language, or imagined in that language, and more. It is similar to the notion that there are a fairly limited number of laws of physics, and yet these laws can account for all of the dynamic motions and the stable positions of all of the bodies in the solar system now, in the past, and in the future.

The sentence as it is actually spoken or written is referred to as the *surface-structure* representation. It is the data or the outcome that results from applying generative rules. The underlying set of rules that actually generated that particular sentence at that particular moment of use is called the *deep-structure* representation. In our earlier example, "The old man's hat blew away," it is unclear from the surface-structure representation what meaning is intended. At the level of deep structure, there is no ambiguity. The rules that generated the sentence specify either Det + {(Adj) + N + Poss} + N + VP or Det + (Adj) + {(Adj) + N} + VP. Notice that the deep structure does not contain the actual words at all, but only abstract grammatical representations like "adjective" or "determiner." In this way it is very much like mathematical formulas, which do not care whether you are talking about planets or ducklings; $2 + 2$ is still 4, and $(X + Y) \times Z$ is different from $X + (Y \times Z)$.

Base Component

In the TGG model the most basic or foundation-level rules reside in what is called the base component. These include *phrase-structure* rules and *lexical-insertion* rules. Attached to them are a lexicon and a semantic component that assign a meaning to whatever the phrase structure and lexical insertion rules generate. The phrase structure rules do very much what they sound like—they specify what can occur in a phrase, such as a noun phrase (NP) or a verb phrase (VP). For example, a NP has to have a noun and a VP has to have a verb; when combined they form a very simple sentence such as "Cats eat." Other things within the phrases are optional, so that in the NP you also can have forms such as a determiner (*The* cats), an adjective (The *yellow* cat), or a quantifier (*Two* cats), or any combination (The two yellow cats). Of course, the phrase structure does not contain the words, only the rules such as NP → (det) + N; Det → (predet) (preart) {art/dem} (postdet). Similarly, the VP can optionally include adverbs (eat *quickly*), entire phrases like prepositional phrases (eat *under the table*) or noun phrases (eat *mice*), or any combination (eat mice quickly under the table), generated by the rules VP ➔ V (NP) (S) (PP). Elements such as prepositional phrases themselves are defined by phrase structure rules that specify what must and can be present within these units.

Lexical Insertion   The lexical-insertion rules function to insert a word selected from the lexicon (i.e., dictionary) into the phrase structure rules. For this to work, the lexicon entry must include a specification of whether the word is a noun, verb, preposition, or other grammatical form. The entry also must be marked for features such as whether the referent is +human or +concrete to prevent nonsensical utterances like "The house eats books under the grass." Finally, the morphologic structure of the word is specified in the lexicon.

Morphology   Morphology refers to elements of meaning at the level of the word. A morpheme is the smallest unit of meaning in a language. This concept roughly translates to root words and the prefixes and suffixes that can be used with them. Linguistically, the root word is referred to as an unbound or *free morpheme* because it can stand alone as a meaningful unit, while affixes are called *bound morphemes* because they cannot be meaningfully produced unless they are attached to a free morpheme. A word minimally will consist of one morpheme, as in "define," but it can consist of several morphemes, as in undefinably, which has four (i.e., / un/ /define/ /able/ /ly/). Each morpheme modifies the interpretation of the word, while maintaining the same semantic base.

Morphology adds considerable flexibility and efficiency to a language. If morphology was not used, many more words would be required in our vocabularies. Without plural markers, for example, either two completely different words would be required to refer to one versus more than one of the same object or an entire string of words would need to be used, as in "More than one X" every time we wanted to specify plurality. Morphologic forms such as plurals, past-tense endings, present-progressive -ing mark-ers, and possessives are referred to as *inflectional morphemes*. This type of morpheme modulates the meaning of the word to express a change in the time or status of an action or the number of objects referred to. However, the interpretation of the word does not change, in that action words remain as action words or verbs even after the morpheme has been added.

Morphology also functions to maintain the relationships of meaning held between variations of the same concept. For example, the word "run" is a verb and refers to action, while "runner" is a noun referring to a person. Because they share the same root word, the meaningful relationship held between them is more obvious than it would be if they were expressed through different vocabulary words. This type of morpheme is referred to as a *derivational morpheme*, because one part of speech such as a noun is derived from another part of speech such as a verb. The morpheme *-ly* may be added to most adjectives to form an adverb (quiet ➔ quietly), *-ness* to adjectives to create a noun (happy ➔ happiness), or *-ment* to verbs to create a noun (enjoy ➔ enjoyment). Because morphemes operate within the syntactic constraints of sentences, information regarding the morphologic status of the word is important to the base component in TGG.

Transformation Component

The utterances generated by the base component using phrase-structure rules are all declarative sentences that contain only one verb. But the *surface structures* of many sentences, including almost every one written in this book, are more complex than this basic form. Something happens between the deep structure of the base component where the underlying representation operates and the actual utterance that surfaces. This change occurs through the operation of another set of rules, called *transformational rules*, that convert deep structures into surface ones. Transformational rules can (1) add sentences or elements of sentences together, using strategies such as a conjunction (The cat eats *because* she is hungry) or embedding (The cat *that is hungry* eats); (2) delete parts of the underlying structure at the surface level (The cat *that* I own eats mice ➜ The cat (-) I own eats mice; or (3) reorder parts of the sentence to create very different structures such as passive constructions (The cat eats mice ➜ The mice are eaten by the cat) or questions (The cat *is* eating a mouse ➜ *Is* the cat eating a mouse?).

Phonologic Component

Both the base component and the transformational component of Chomsky's model consist of abstractions such as mathematical-like rules of grammar and abstract features within lexical entries. But the surface structure representation contains recognizable words that can actually be spoken, heard, or read. This means that the words must be converted to a form that is capable of being pronounced or spelled. Thus, a third component, called the *phonologic component*, takes the output from the transformational component and assigns a phonetic interpretation. Once again, this assignment is done by rules.

The phonetic interpretation works somewhat like an instruction manual for your lips, tongue, palate, and vocal folds, or those physical structures involved in speech production. For example, try making the two consonant sounds /s/ and /t/. You will notice that they are both made with the tongue positioned high in the mouth and near the front. The abstract features used to describe these characteristics are + consonantal, + coronal (tongue tip), + anterior (front). If you feel your throat as you produce these sounds, there will be no vibration, or voicing, and so both /s/ and /t/ are also marked—voice. So far, nothing distinguishes these two sounds as being different from each other, and many features indicate that they are highly similar. The difference is in the manner of their production. The /t/ is produced by actually touching the tongue tip to the roof of the mouth and letting air

pressure build up, followed by a quick release or mini-explosion. This does not happen at all when the /s/ is produced. Instead, the tongue is positioned slightly below the roof of the mouth so that the air flows continuously in a noisy turbulance. The /t/ is therefore marked—continuant while /s/ is marked + continuant.

All of the sounds in every language can be similarly described in accordance with patterns of presence or absence of distinctive phonetic features (Chomsky & Halle, 1968). Only fourteen features are needed to describe and distinguish between all of the consonant sounds of English. Sounds that are very similar to each other such as /b/ and /p/ differ from each other on the basis of only one feature, that is, the presence or absence of voicing. Sounds that are very different from each other in their production such as /m/ and /k/ will differ on almost all feature contrasts.

The features within the phonetic interpretation correspond to actual speech production in a very abstract or indirect way. Remember that Chomsky's goal was to define the rules that a hypothetical speaker possesses about the grammar of the language and not the mechanisms that actually produce physical speech. What is important to understand, however, is that this phonologic component is integrally connected to and part of transformational-generative grammar. Too often this interconnection is forgotten in applied situations such as intervention for children with articulation disorders, and the problem is treated in a manner that ignores the integral relationship between speech and language.

Alternatives and Revisions to the Standard Theory of TGG

Transformational-generative grammar in its standard-theory form has strongly influenced the work in fields such as linguistics, psychology, education, and speech-language pathology over the past 35 years. Much of the research in child language development has been conducted in a manner consistent with the principles and corresponding predictions made by this model about language and its learning and use. Numerous tests and evaluation procedures have been developed, based on TGG theory, to assess the language development of children and to determine if delays or disorders in acquisition exist. Intervention strategies designed to help the child discover an underlying principle or rule of grammar have been implemented. Many exercises found in language-arts curricula in schools have been designed to foster grammatical understanding and use in accord with this theory, as well as the language used in the textbooks for many reading series. Programs for language learning have been developed for specific populations, such as individuals with hearing impairments, mental retardation, and the socially/economically disadvantaged, based on TGG. Many programs for teaching articulation, or the correct pronunciation of speech, are based on the phonetic feature systems inherent in this theory.

While the influence of transformational-generative grammar has been far reaching and useful, the theory does not answer all of the questions about language or account for all linguistic data. It allows sentences to be generated that speakers of the language would not produce; fails to explain how some types of sentences are generated; allows words to occur in the same sentence that are peculiar together at the level of semantics, or meaning; and cannot designate a finite set of features that would be included in the lexical entry of a word, which would distinguish it from all other words but enable it to be appropriately inserted in the phrase structure. The standard theory itself has undergone significant changes in recent years, and many alternative theories are being proposed.

The first significant modification of the standard theory occurred because of the difficulties at the semantic level. The *extended-standard theory* (Chomsky, 1980) allowed for some aspects of semantic interpretation to be imposed at the surface structure, after transformations have occurred, instead of all interpretation occurring at the beginning, or base component level. Other transformationalists such as McCawley (1968) have proposed an alternative model to TGG, called *generative semantics*. This model relates the surface structure to semantic interpretations without the deep-structure component through transformations. Chomsky's latest revision, referred to as Government-Binding theory, incorporates some characteristics or features from generative semantics.

Government and Binding

Government-Binding theory, a major revision of the standard theory, was published by Chomsky in 1981. This model was proposed to eliminate the difficulties of ungrammatical, peculiar, or unaccounted for sentences presented by the earlier transformational grammars. In this model it is assumed that the language learner has an innate, biologically determined set of constraints about the structure of language. These constraints are part of a universal grammar that is biologically specific to humans. The universal grammar contains abstract rules or constraints that designate what is allowable in a grammar such as a method for referring to action (in English, the use of verbs) or objects (in English, nouns). The way that the universal is expressed can be different for various languages so that a word at the beginning of the sentence may refer to action, rather than a verb in the middle of the sentence as in English, or a morpheme attached to a root word or a change in vocal intonation can be used. The universal is merely a biologic placeholder that is designed to recognize the relevant form when exposed to a specific language and to fill that slot with the strategy used by that language.

This innate knowledge of language principles and constraints is proposed to be a biologically determined mechanism that is specific to language and not part of a general logical ability, such as a mental capacity to form categories or organize information according to rules. It theoretically allows the learner to construct the grammar of a specific language without exposure to all of the possible sentences. From a rather limited amount of data, children as young as 2 years of age begin to comprehend and use the grammar that they hear, and by 4 years of age they have constructed a system very much like that used by the adults in the culture. The innate universal grammar is proposed as being one of the primary reasons that they are able to accomplish such a vast feat in such a short period.

Deep Structure The deep structure still exists in Government-Binding theory but with differences. For example, in the lexicon the grammatical category of a word is specified (i.e., whether its a noun, verb, etc.), but also included is the context or "frame" that it can fit into. For the word "eat," the lexicon specifies that it is a verb, but also indicates that it can be followed by a noun phrase (eat:V ___:NP). This frame is a level of syntax that functions as an intermediary between the grammatical part of speech of the word and the phrase-structure rules that generate the sentence.

Phrase-structure rules still exist in Government-Binding theory but with differences. Instead of assuming that all sentences consist of a noun phrase + a verb phrase (S → NP + VP), it is assumed that all sentences begin with a complementizer (i.e., "that" or "what") that does not show up in the surface structure. The inclusion of a complementizer was necessary to account for many sentences whose generation could not be explained using TTG, resulting in the rule that all sentences start from the underlying structure S → COMP S, S → NP + INFL + VP. The inclusion of inflection (INFL) into the rule allows for easier movement of auxiliary verbs such as present progressive (is + ing), perfect aspect (has + been), or verb tense when transformations are applied.

Phonologic Component At the level of the phonologic component, the features attaching abstract characteristics of the sound and its production still operate, but, in addition, abstract characteristics of interpretation also can operate. This allows aspects of semantics, or the meaning, to be assigned at this level instead of only at the level of the lexicon and is needed to handle the possibility of ambiguous reference in the surface structure.

Subtheories The major addition to the earlier transformational theories in Government-Binding is the inclusion of six subtheories, referred to as bounding, government, case, binding, theta, and control theories. These place constraints on representations at each level to reduce the number of options available. Chomsky argues that without these constraints language could not be learned as fast as it is acquired in normal development and that too many ungrammatical sentences would be allowed.

Bounding theory restricts the movements of constituents such as a grammatical form or phrase within sentences. It basically states that it is not allowable to move a constituent more than one NP or Sentence in any single-rule application. Thus it is a constraint, or something that limits what can be done, rather than a specification of what can be done. *Government theory* states that there is a hierarchical relationship between grammatical structures found within the same phrase—all words in the phrase are not equal. For example, in a prepositional phrase, the preposition is primary over the attached noun phrase (ex: *under* the table). "The table" belongs to the preposition, rather than being of equal status. *Binding theory* constrains the conditions under which an NP (a words or phrase) can refer to the same referent. Pronouns are an example of this. In the sentence "The duck flew out of the pond, but the hunter had already seen it," the /it/ has to be understood to refer to the duck and not the pond or the hunter. The binding condition or constraint must be met for words to co-refer. *Control theory* involves constraints on words that can take their reference from another NP, but also can refer independently.

Two subtheories incorporate elements

from semantic theories. *Case theory* assigns an abstract case such as whether the NP is nominative (the noun that does something) or objective (the noun that receives the action), as in "The dog (nominative) chased the ball (objective)." *Theta theory* assigns roles such as "agent of action" or "goal of action" to all words or phrases that have semantic content. Proponents of Government-Binding theory suggest that the theory offers a multitude of testable hypotheses regarding language development, language disorders, and intervention strategies. The new elements of this theory provide different ways of thinking about language and exploring the data in ways that may provide new insights and solutions to both theoretical and applied problems.

Semantic Theory   While they have been highly influential, transformational grammars have not been accepted as the best description of language by all theorists. Some of the criticisms are that they are models of competence but not performance, that they ignore how people use language in a real-life situation, and that they place too little emphasis on purpose and meaning. They also point out that language is reduced to a series of states or rules that have not actually been shown to exist anywhere. Many argue that language is a meaning-making process and that it would not exist if its only purpose was for generating grammatical sentences. There would be no reason to produce grammatical strings unless they helped to convey meaning more successfully.

Case Grammar

One generative system that focuses on the influence of semantics, or meaning, on the syntactic structure of language was proposed by Fillmore (1968) and is called *case grammar.* According to Fillmore there is a level of representation more abstract or separated from the surface structure than grammatical rules. This representation is based on the speaker's distinction between sense and nonsense, rather than grammatical versus ungrammatical. Representations at this level consist of a set of universal semantic concepts, but unlike Chomsky's universals, which are thought to be biologically determined innate rules, the semantic concepts are universal because they refer to events and relationships found in the environment or within the human organism. Since all humans possess a similar sensory system with which they perceive a similar world of actions that can be performed on objects, or changes in the states of events, the general features of experience will be the same for all people even though the specifics objects or events may be different.

In grammatical models, words are categorized into only very broad concepts such as subjects versus objects of a sentence. But not all subjects are the same. In the sentence "The boy played the drums," the subject (boy) is an "agent" or person who performs an action. But in the sentence "The boy heard the drums," the subject (boy) is an "experiencer" who did not perform the action, but rather underwent an experience. The relationship between *the boy* and *the drums* is very different in the two sentences. Similarly, in the sentence "The drums interested the boy," the boy experiences a passive condition or "state" relative to the drums. Other roles for persons or objects also are possible. These distinct semantic roles are called *cases.*

Propositions   Because the semantic roles of noun phrases are defined, case grammar is able to more precisely specify the relationships of nouns to verbs. These are specified in a unit called the *proposition* of a sentence. The proposition consists of the verb and the set of noun phrases that relate to it. Particular verbs require different sets of cases, representing various sentence types or propositional structures. For example, in the three sentences (1) The boy played the drum, (2) The drum played loudly, and (3) The boy played the drum with a stick, the verb "played" requires the object (i.e., the drum) affected by the verb to be specified. But as sentence 2 demonstrates, the agent (or person playing the drum) does not have to be specified, nor does the instrument (i.e., a stick) used (compare sentence 1 and 3). The specification of those roles is optional.

Universal Cases Fillmore specifies the seven major universal cases to be *agentive* (instigator of the action), *dative* (person or animal affected by the action of the verb), *experiencer* (one who experiences an event, action, or mental state), *factitive* (the object or entity resulting from the action), *instrumental* (instrument used to cause an action), *locative* (place or spatial location), and *objective* (a neutral case, dependent on the meaning of the verb). A case consists of a case marker plus the associated noun phrase. In some languages the case marker is a morphologic form attached to the noun, so that the same word has a different ending depending on how it is used (e.g., as an agent, an object, etc.). In English, word order, prepositions, and the meaning of the verb serve to accomplish these distinctions. For example, the agent case is marked by the preposition "by" (The drum was played by the boy), while the instrumental is marked by "with" (The boy played the drum with the stick).

Modality In addition to the proposition, each sentence has a second constituent, or *modality*, which expresses other aspects of the sentence like tense, negation, mood, interrogation, and so on. The rules of case grammar include a rule for specifying a sentence (Sentence ➔ modality + proposition), and the sentence constituents (Modality ➔ {tense} + {negation} + {mood} + . . . ; Proposition ➔ Verb + {agentive} + {instrumental} + {dative} + {experiencer} + {locative} + {factitive} + {objective}). Within the proposition, the cases can be arranged in any order for purposes of emphasis or other reasons, expressed through strategies such as word order. Thus case grammar is not viewed to be independent of syntactic structure, but rather a level of representation more abstract than grammatical rules and therefore underlying those levels.

Case Grammar in Child Language

Semantic theories, including case grammar, have been highly influential in the study of child language development. During the late 1960s, Lois Bloom attempted to examine the utterances produced by young children using syntactic rules. She found that the syntactic analyses were not able to capture the meaning of many of the children's utterances, even though the meaning was clear in context. For example, the utterance "Mommy sock" was produced in two different contexts, once to refer to her mother's stocking as the child picked it up, and the other to refer to her own sock as her mother put it on the child's foot. She concluded that semantic relationships, such as "agent + action" (cat sleep) or "action + recipient + object" (give puppy the ball) were more consistent with the structure of child language than were syntactic rules.

Researchers in child language found that the cases described by Fillmore in adult language also are descriptive of children's utterances. For example, the most common cases produced in the utterances of children between 19 and 26 months of age are the agentive, objective, locative, dative, experiencer, and a case more specific to children termed essive (as in words like "doggie"). However, unlike adult case grammars where the same semantic relationships are expressed in many syntactic forms, the case grammars used to represent children's utterances exhibit a direct relationship between the case and the word produced. Children use simple word-order strategies to express many of the same cases that Fillmore proposed underlie adult sentences, but they lack the adult's more sophisticated means for expressing them. The child might say "Doggie bone" to express what the adult would communicate using a morphologic marker (The dog**'s** bone) or a preposition (The bone is owned *by* the dog). Applications of semantic theories, including case grammars, have been highly productive in the study of child language. This topic will be explored in greater depth by Haynes in Chapter 10.

LANGUAGE IN CONTEXT

The theories discussed so far in this chapter have been generated by scientists in the field of linguistics. The linguist's goal is to derive a theory that can account for a hypothetical speaker's linguistic competence, or knowledge of a language, in the most parsimonious manner. Such an account theoretically should be able to generate all of the allowable sentences, while eliminating all of the ungrammatical sentences found in a language with as few rules or procedures as possible. However, language as a communicative system that is learned and used in the real world has more dimensions involved in its use than are accounted for in linguistic theories. The speaker does not merely generate sentences, but rather produces utterances that are meaningfully related to the events ongoing in the environment or to the ideas or thoughts held by the individual at that moment. The utterances are generally produced for some purpose such as attempting to influence the behavior or beliefs of another person so they will do something for you ("Could you hand me that book?"), attend to something significant ("Look at that picture on the wall"), or adopt some information or attitude ("I think they should have used a different color").

This larger perspective on language and its development has been investigated by two interdisciplinary points of view, referred to as *psycholinguistics* and *sociolinguistics*. Psycholingistics developed as the merger between the interests of psychology and linguistics. Psychology focuses study on actual human behavior, rather than on abstract hypothetical speakers. The psychologist is interested in what motivates behavior and what processes allow for the behavior to occur. The phycholinguist therefore studies the acquisition of language by children and the processes that are used by children and adults in both the development and use of language. Many psycholinguists study the relationship of language to thought, including the question of which comes first, and whether they are separate or completely integrated processes of the mind. Other psycholinguists are interested in the psychologic processes that allow for language learning and use to occur, in-

cluding factors such as attention, memory, storage, retrieval, and perception. This point of view is closely related to that of *neurolinguistics*, or the study of brain structures and processes in relationship to language. Each of these domains of psycholinguistics include a study of language pathology, both as a method of gaining insights into normal processes by contrasting them with disordered processes and for gaining a greater understanding of the language pathology itself.

Sociolinguistics merges the interests of sociology with that of linguistics. Sociology focuses study on social roles and mores, social class, and other social variables that affect human behavior. The sociolinguist therefore studies the influence of cultural and situational variables on language development and use. Differences in language style and use related to social class and ethnic group dialects, situational variables that influence language development and use within individuals, effects of social and cultural roles on acquisition and use, and the interactions that occur between parents or other caregivers and children are all of interest to the sociolinguist. The sociologic influences on language pathology also are examined, including differences in the caregiver-child interaction patterns when the child has a disorder that limits or changes the cues and responses presented in a communicative situation, and the social factors that serve to either facilitate or inhibit the development and functioning of a child with a different learning system.

While the speech-language pathologist concentrates on disordered communication, including the causes of the disorder, evaluation of the child's communication system, and strategies that can be used to provide intervention and facilitate development, much of the work in this field falls within the domains of either psycholinguistics or sociolinguistics. The overlap between and among disciplines is a very good thing. Only through this overlap will we eventually develop a multifaceted theory that can account for the many aspects of language as it functions as an integrated system. One step in this direction is Speech Act theory.

Speech Act Theory

The study of child language and its development is inextricably embedded within a context of use. Children lack sophisticated strategies such as word order or morphologic forms to communicate ideas about agents, actions, objects, states, and all of the relationships between them. It is apparent from context, however, that they are aware of many of these relationships of meaning and are expressing them using less sophisticated means. Theories that ignore the influence of context underrepresent what children know or are able to perform in a context of use (Antinucci & Parisi, 1973; Bloom, 1970). As researchers in the area of child language development searched for a broader model to provide for a systematic account of language used in context, the theory of Speech Acts, initially proposed by a philosopher of language named Austin (1962) and elaborated on by Searle (1969), held attraction.

Speech acts are viewed as the basic unit of communication between a speaker and a hearer. The emphasis is on the word *acts* in this theory, because uttering words in an appropriate context actually accomplishes action. It is not the form or structure of the speech act that is the unit of communication, but rather the actual production of the speech act in a context of use. When a speaker says, "I don't like exercise," the words function to perform the act of disliking something. By saying, "Would you get me a cookie?" the speech functions to command someone to do something. Speech acts serve as mechanisms for maintaining power and control within the environment when the appropriate conditions for a speech act are met. This ability to control the environment serves as a powerful motivator for both the development and use of language.

Components of the Speech Act

Searle (1969) indicated that for the speech act to function, the words pro-

duced have to relate to the world, the speaker has to mean something when words are produced, and the hearer has to understand what is meant by the speaker and the words. Four different components were proposed to occur in the process of uttering a speech act to account for the interrelationships between the speaker and the hearer. The first part, or the *proposition* of the speech act, consists of the underlying meaning or content of the utterance. Propositions are the abstract meanings that exist before words are attached—we have all had the experience of trying to put our thoughts into language but groping for the words even though the thought was clear. It is the information that is referred to and the relationships between the ideas or elements, such as temporal (X then Y), causal (X because Y), spatial (X locative Y), or conditional (if X then Y) links.

In addition to meanings, speech acts also code intentions, or *illocutions.* This is the function of the utterance, whether that be to convey a belief, make a demand or command, commit to some future action, declare a psychologic state, or express other goals or intentions. The illocution is not tied to any particular grammatical representation, and the same illocution can in fact be expressed using a variety of different utterances. If the proposition is something like "I want that cookie," the speaker could choose to say "My, that cookie looks good"; "May I have that cookie?"; or more directly, "Give me that cookie." These utterances differ in their level of politeness and directness. The utterance chosen is the one believed by the speaker to be most appropriate to the context or situation, but they all could have the same underlying intention or illocution.

As a process ongoing between speakers and hearers, speech acts have *perlocutions,* or effects on the listener based on that person's interpretation. This interpretation may or may not be the same as that intended by the speaker. In general, children understand and use direct speech acts during early development and miss the underlying intention behind the more polite forms. When hearing "My, that cookie looks good," a young child is likely to agree with the speaker and eat the cookie. Perlocutionary acts can have effects such as persuading, angering, convincing, misleading, or informing the listener.

To maximize the probability that the speech act will be interpreted as intended, the speaker must produce an *utterance act* that is appropriate to the listener and the situation. Many elements are involved in the utterance act, both linguistic and non-linguistic. Certainly, word choice and word order are important, as we have seen above. But also important are elements such as vocal intonation ("*I* want that cookie" versus "I want *that* cookie"), vocal intensity and quality, fluency of expression, facial expressions, gestures, body posture, physical proximity, eye gaze, and other cues to interpretation. The utterance act is critical to the meaning of the message as it is interpreted by the listener. We have all heard the expression, "It is not what you say, but how you say it."

Conditions of the Speech Act

Certain conditions of the speech act have to be met for it to have an effect on the listener's actions or beliefs (Searle, 1969). There has to be some content or information that the speaker intends to impart to the listener (propositional content). The speaker has to believe that the listener is capable of doing the action or meeting the intent of the speech act (preparatory rule). Speakers have to say what they believe to be the truth, and they have to impart that they sincerely want the listener to respond as implied (sincerity). Purposeful violation of this condition occurs when speakers produce puns, jokes, sarcasm, or exaggeration. Finally, the effect or meaning of the speech act ultimately rests with the listener (essential rule). If the hearer does not understand any component of the speech act, then it will either have no interpretation or will have an interpretation different from that intended by the speaker. No matter what

the speaker's intention, the message interpreted by the listener is the one that is actually communicated. We have all had the painful experience of having our messages interpreted completely differently from what we intended.

These conditions have important implications for language development and for applied situations such as classroom teaching or language intervention. The information provided to children has to be comprehensible. Young children or those with language pathologies require conversation to be directed at things that are concrete or occurring in the immediate environment. Demands must be within the range of what the child is capable of understanding and performing. Direct statements may have to be used rather than more polite forms. Language that is too abstract, too complex, or that requires too many inferences will result in misinterpretations of failure to respond. Many children labeled as "behavioral problems" are really children who are not capable of responding to the speech acts that are used within the school or home environment.

Contexts for Speech Acts

The speech act is the basic unit of communication within a larger context of use such as a conversation or monologue. *Pragmatics* refers to a set of sociolinguistic rules related to language use within the communicative context. These rules entail the speech act, but also govern the discourse structures in which speech acts are embedded.

Conversational Discourse One discourse structure that has received considerable attention is the *conversation*. Conversations can be examined in units, or *sequences*, defined as a series of speaking turns that share a topic and where the participants are responsive to each other's intentions (Dore, 1986). Three primary functions can be identified within conversational sequences. Each of these can be accomplished through a number of specific *conversational acts*. The first type of function is the *initiation of interaction* with another person or the initiation of the topic of the sequence. This function requires that the speaker establish joint attention to an object or event, participation in a joint activity, or joint reference to some idea or thought. This function can be accomplished either through nonlinguistic conversational acts such as points, gestures, or actions (handing someone an object) or linguistically through conversational acts such as greetings or statements that solicit attention ("Hey, you know what?"; "Look at this"; "Hi, how is it going?").

The second function is to extend or maintain an interaction or topic once it has begun. There are many different types of conversational acts that are used to sustain dialogue, including acknowledging or confirming what the previous speaker stated, adding topic-relevant comments that extend the content beyond what the previous speaker provided, directly attempting to shift or refocus the topic, resuming the topic when the focus is lost, asking for clarifications when the previous speaker's comment is not understood, or providing a clarification when asked. Clarifications can take the form of repeating the message exactly as it was stated, indicating the speaker believes the listener did not hear it; revising the message semantically or syntactically, usually by choosing simpler words or reducing the syntactic complexity of the utterance; or paraphrasing the message.

The third function identified within a conversational sequence is the termination of the interaction or the topic. Any act that leads to the end of attention to the focus of the conversation can serve to terminate it, including nonverbal acts such as walking or looking away or linguistic acts consisting of ritualized codas such as "See you later" or "That's all."

Cooperative Principles   Within a conversation, principles of cooperation must be adhered to by the participants for turn-taking, topic maintenance, and exchange of information to occur. Grice (1975) provided a framework for examining the success of communicative ex-

changes within conversations by postulating four cooperative principles or maxims that participants must adhere to. The first principle is the *Quantity Maxim* and refers to the amount of information that each participant should contribute to the conversation. According to this maxim the participants should give enough information to ensure that the content is informative to the listener, but should not give information that is already shared knowledge between them or that is in unnecessary detail for purposes of the exchange.

The second principle, or *Quality Maxim*, requires that you believe that the information you are providing is truthful. Individuals who violate this maxim soon find that their credibility is questioned by others and that they lose some of the power associated with speech acts. The third maxim is that of *Relevance*. This principle states that the comments made by a participant must be responsive to the topic or content of the preceding utterances or speaker. A participant who does not answer questions with an appropriate response, who changes topics, or who makes off-topic comments at inappropriate times would be in violation of this maxim.

The final principle is the *Manner Maxim*. Speakers are expected to present their information or take their turns in a manner that is comprehensible to the listener. Long pauses before responding, false starts in sentence generation, events reported in an incorrect temporal sequence, and unintelligible utterances are all examples of manner violations. Language analysis procedures based on Grice's maxims have been successfully used to evaluate the conversational abilities of young children and those with communication disorders (Damico, 1985, 1992).

Narrative Discourse   Not all speech acts take place in a conversational context. Other discourse types include narration, or storytelling. Narration is quite different in both structure and function from conversation. A narrative is a specific type of monologue, or a discourse structure that requires the speaker to talk for an extended time on a topic rather than sharing the interaction with another participant (Britton, 1982). Monologues, including narratives, are a much more difficult form of discourse than conversation. They require the speaker to stay focused on a topic, adhere to a culturally determined format for telling a story, generate sentences that conform to all speech act principles, use language that specifically establishes the characters, events, and all of the sequences across changes in time and location (Westby, 1985, 1992).

A complete narrative has a specific structure consisting of the establishment of a *setting*, or "ordinary existence." In this part of a story, the speaker needs to specify a character's ordinary appearance, actions, location, or state. This is followed by an *initiating event*, or something that happens to change the ordinary state of affairs. The *response state* and *response plan* are then provided, and they include the character's emotional or cognitive response to the change and set up the character's resulting goal and plans to meet the goal. This is succeeded by one or more episodes of *attempts* to reach the goal and the *consequences* of these attempts. The story is completed by a *resolution* or final act and an *ending* that may provide a moral or a conclusion (Stein & Glenn, 1979).

Other forms of discourse are produced by speakers of a language, including a variety of expository types. Their structure has been less examined and thus less defined than that of conversation and narration. Certainly, our understanding of discourse structure and theory is just beginning to be explored.

STATUS OF PSYCHOLINGUISTIC AND SOCIOLINGUISTIC THEORIES

Psycholinguistic and sociolinguistic perspectives have provided a much broader basis from which to view language than those provided by grammatical models. It is like having an astronaut's view of the solar system, where the size, shape, and color of the planets can be viewed while they are in motion, and the effects and changes initiated in one location of the system can be observed on other entities within the system. But while these broader theories have provided us a more comprehensive and integrated view of language, it has not been without costs. Grammar is about forms and structures, and these can be defined, described, and justified according to logical principles and analysis procedures. But meaning, intention, and context are far more elusive. While the theories to date have provided us with descriptions of structures and processes related to discourse and context, they do not present a coherent model of language or how it develops and functions. A new theoretical perspective that integrates knowledge from the fields of psycholinguistics, neurolinguistics, and artificial intelligence, referred to as *connectionism*, shows promise of taking us one step closer to this goal.

Connectionism

Connectionism is a term used to refer to a variety of different models that have as a common denominator a view that cognitive processes are not carried out as a series of stages or rule applications, but rather that all processes of the mind occur simultaneously. Models that fit within this general scheme include parallel distributed processing (Rumelhart & McClelland, 1986), interactive activation (McClelland & Rumelhart, 1981), cooperative computation (Arbib, Conklin, & Hill, 1987), competition (Bates & MacWhinney, 1992), schema theory (Arbib, Conklin, & Hill, 1987), and associationist models.

Connectionism as a concept is not new, but rather dates back to the earliest scientific work on the relationship between language capacities and the brain. Researchers such as Broca (1861) and Wernicke (1874) observed the performance of adults who had suffered brain damage in locations affecting language, referred to as *aphasics*. From these observations they made judgments about the relative disruption of and qualitative changes in the processes of comprehending and producing speech. Their work established an argument for an interaction between components of the neural system underlying language performance. They found that a disruption in one area of the brain did not just affect the processes of that area, but rather had an effect on the functions associated with a second, undamaged area. Furthermore, the second area was affected in a manner that was distinguishable from the way it would function if the primary damage had occurred in the second area itself (Wernicke, 1874). These findings suggested the interconnectedness of the entire brain and also supported the view that one process is not performed as a discrete step in a series since disruptions occur in the functioning of undamaged areas.

Artificial Intelligence Framework

Much of the current work in connectionism is occurring in the field of artificial intelligence. Instead of using the traditional type of computer that operates by programming the computer with a set of rules that are activated one at a time in serial order, connectionists use a type of computer in which there are anywhere from dozens to thousands of processors, all of which are interconnected and that function in parallel or simultaneously. Rules are not programmed into the computer; instead data is provided to the system, and it undergoes a sorting and organizational process in which patterns or regularities of the data are discovered.

Connectionist computers work by computing *connections* among simple processing *units*. Units can be representations for any level of processing, including phonetic or semantic features, phonemes, words, concepts, or abstract elements. No single unit contains a representation, but rather representations are distributed across a whole cluster or pattern of units. Whenever that particular pattern is activated, the corresponding concept or meaningful element is represented or

present within the system. The moment that pattern is no longer activated, the concept is "out of mind." This occurs because the same units are used in an infinite array of different patterns or clusters—as soon as they have completed their activation for one concept, they are reactivated for use in a new pattern. This multipurpose use of the same units is much like the use of receivers and transmitters of a telephone line that may connect thousands of different phones from different parts of the country in the course of a day. They do not belong to any one phone number, but rather are used repeatedly to process different patterns and sequences of numbers.

The units receive input from the environment and from other units, much like the neuron of the brain receives input from the sensory system and from other neurons. The units take on activation values, based on the sum of the inputs that they receive from all sources. If the sum of inputs is great enough, they pass activation on to other units; if the sum is not great enough, then they inhibit or terminate further connections. The connections between units are continuously undergoing changes in connection weights or strengths. Each time the same pattern of activation occurs, the connection weights between the composite units are strengthened and are therefore much more likely to activate each other in that same pattern in the future. In other words, the system "learns" by forming predictable and stable patterns that represent meaningful concepts or elements of language. The principles of this learning are very similar to those known to occur neurologically in the human brain.

Researchers have examined the ability of connectionist systems to generate the structures of language by exposing the system to data, or sentences, and letting it sort and organize the data into patterns. To date, the results have been very promising, although not without problems or detractors. Rumelhart and McClelland (1987) presented the system with examples of regular (jump**ed**, want**ed**) and irregular (felt, ate) past-tense verbs. The system learned to use the correct past-tense marker with the 460 verbs that it was exposed to, but also generalized and transferred this learning to novel verbs that it had never been exposed to during training. During its "learning" period it produced many of the error types that are exhibited by young children, such as overregularizing irregular forms, as in "eated." Preliminary models to account for other aspects of language, including phonologic processing (McClelland & Elman, 1986), determiners in noun phrase constructions (MacWhinney, 1991), and syntactic processing (Mac-Whinney, 1987), have been tested with good initial results.

Connectionist models are very new, and much of the ability of the model to deal with language in a manner that parallels learning and use in children and adults is speculative at this time. Connectionist models differ from more traditional models in many ways such as the notion of rule learning. While traditional linguistic models postulate that the rules are an innate feature of a biologically determined mechanism, connectionist models generate the rules or the patterns from the data to which the system is exposed. The system thus operates according to patterns or "rules," but does not contain rules of language any more than the planets in the solar system rotate on their axes or revolve around the sun in predictable patterns because the have an innate, biologically determined knowledge of the rules of physics. Furthermore, rather than postulating a language-specific device for learning grammar, connectionist models demonstrate the ability to learn a wide variety of linguistic and nonlinguistic information in a general way using the same basic mechanism and processes. However, Fodor and Pylyshyn (1988) view the connectionist networks as mere mechanisms whereby linguistic rules are expressed, but not as a model of theoretical insight or interest.

To date the models have shown promise in learning and handling simple data such as single words and morphemes. They have not dealt efficiently with complex input that arrives sequentially, such as the word order of a sentence, and how this information is processed within the network. Many of the studies have examined the learning of the form of language and not how the connections within the network result in a meaningful interpretation of the message. Much more research needs to be conducted before we have answers to these questions and understand the potential of connectionist models.

Perhaps even more promising than the present ability of the models to learn and generate some aspects of morphology and phonology is the theoretical consistency that the models share with current psycholinguistic and neurolinguistic theories. One of these theories is that of event representations.

Event Representations

Nelson (1985, 1991, 1996) has suggested that the basic structure of a child's knowledge, as well as the language used to express that knowledge, is organized around events such as eating or dressing. Learning is viewed as a whole-to-part process from this perspective, with the child initially participating in the event as a whole unit. The parts, or specific objects and actions inherent to the event only gradually separate from this whole to form conceptual representations. This is in direct contrast to more traditional models that view the child's knowledge of objects and object categories to be the basic foundational units of knowledge and language (Gentner, 1982).

The child's mental representations of events are organized as a sequence of actions or changes in states, or *syntagmatic* structures (recall this concept from the discussion of linguistic structuralism). Elements within events or routines that are very different from each other, such as a spoon, applesauce, and a chair, are linked conceptually because of their spatial, temporal, causal, or other associations within the event. These relationships become strengthened in the child's mental repre-

sentation as they are encountered repeatedly within the same routine occurring across days or weeks. These elements form a network that unifies the event into a single entity such as "the eating routine."

At the same time, different objects or people that play the same role within an event also are becoming organized. For example, cereal, mashed potatoes, or pudding can be eaten with the spoon, as can the applesauce. Those elements that can fulfill a similar role within the event become mentally organized according to *paradigmatic* structures. The functional roles fulfilled by objects within a routine help a child to form a concept of that object. The paradigmatic concept (i.e., part) depends on the existence of the syntagmatic structure (i.e., whole). Because of this dependence, the paradigmatic concepts are initially situationally specific, so that the spoon is understood only in relationship to the eating routine and not as a more generalized concept.

However, as the same objects or elements are encountered within a variety of contexts, they become less tightly bound to any one context of use. The chair is an important element within the eating routine, but it also is important to the storybook reading, dressing, drawing, t.v. watching, and other events. The representations for these objects that occur in disparate contexts gradually form concepts that are more abstract, more separate from any one event because they overlap across several events. They remain connected syntagmatically and paradigmatically to the original events, but they acquire a status that allows them to exist separately from any of these event representations in the child's thought. Nelson (1985, 1996) describes six levels of representation of concepts that correspond to different phases of development, with a purely symbolic and hierarchically organized level of semantic structures forming the most abstract level of concept formation.

Nelson (1985) talks about the social role that caregivers play in facilitating

conceptual structures in children. By engaging the child as an active participant within complex routines such as eating or dressing, the child has the opportunity to experience and mentally organize the temporal, spatial, causal, and other links that form the syntagmatic aspects of the event representation. Similarly, by acting on and talking about the objects and other elements within the event, the caregiver helps the child to parse the concept out of the whole event and to see the paradigmatic relationship between elements that can fulfill the same function. The importance of adults and other caregivers to language development and language intervention is evident within this theory, as is the view that children need to be active participants within complex and frequently repeated meaningful events for language and learning to occur.

FUTURE INTEGRATIONS

The theories of connectionism and event representations share a focus on mental structures that underlie language development and processing. Connectionism closely parallels models of neurology and neurologic processes that result in the creation of networks of associations. These networks of associated elements result in the formation of patterned and recognizable concepts and linguistic structures through repeated exposure to meaningful data. Event representations are psychologic constructs that seek to explain the nature of concepts and linguistic structures that are formed through repeated exposure to meaningful experiences or events. These representations are proposed to result from the formation of networks of associated elements that are patterned and recognizable as both integrated structures and separable concepts.

Conceptually, it is easy to see how these two views of language and language development can merge. For example, it can be proposed that connection weights are established between elements within a routine in much the same way that they have been shown to form for smaller units of meaning such as morphemes or sentences. As the same elements are used in the same roles in the same sequence within events, strong connection weights for these syntagmatic relationships form. Similarly, when the same objects or elements occur in different roles within and across events, then the units that represent the object itself will form strong connection weights, or paradigmatic structure, but the associations to any one event or sequence will weaken. This dual process can account for both the development of a lexicon and the sentence and discourse structures that establish relationships between the words (Norris & Hoffman, 1994).

The simultaneous processing of multiple levels of information within the connectionist model makes the conceptualization of such a model an exciting possibility. In reality, however, we are still a long way from understanding and explaining all of the structures and processes involved in a model that can account for the universe that is language.

REFERENCES

Antinucci F, Parisi D. Early language acquisition: a model and some data. In: Ferguson C, Slobin D, eds. Studies of child language development. New York: Holt, Rinehart, & Winston, 1973.

Arbib MA, Conklin EJ, Hill J. From schema theory to language. New York: Oxford University Press, 1987.

Austin J. How to do things with words. Cambridge, MA: Harvard University Press, 1962.

Bates E, MacWhinney B. Functionalism and the competition model. In: MacWhinney B, Bates E, eds. The crosslinguistic study of language processing. New York: Cambridge University Press, 1992.

Bloom L. Language development: form and function of emerging grammars. Cambridge, MA: MIT Press, 1970.

Bloomfield L. Language. New York: Holt, Rinehart & Winston, 1933.

Britton J. Prospect and retrospect: selected essays of James Britton. London: Heinemann Educational Books, 1982.

Broca PP. Remarques sur le siege de la faculte du langage articule, suivies d'une observation d'aphemie. Bulletins de la Societe Anatomique de Paris 1861; 6:330–357.

Chomsky N. Syntactic structures. The Hague: Mouton, 1957.

Chomsky N. Rules and representations. New York: Columbia University Press, 1980.

Chomsky N. Lectures on government and binding. Dordrecht, Holland: Foris, 1981.

Chomsky N, Halle M. The sound pattern of English. New York: Harper & Row, 1968.

Clark EV. What's in a word? On the child's acquisition of semantics in his first language. In: Moore TE, ed. Cognitive development and the acquisition of language. New York: Academic Press, 1973; pp. 65–110.

Clark EV. Meaning and concepts. In: Mussen P, ed. Handbook of child psychology. Vol. 3. New York: Wiley, 1983.

Clark EV. The principle of contrast: a constraint on language acquisition. In: MacWhinney B, ed. Mechanisms of language acquisition. Hillsdale, NJ: Lawrence Erlbaum, 1987.

Damico JS. Clinical discourse analysis: a functional language assessment technique. In: Simon CS, ed. Communication skills and classroom success: assessment of language-learning disabled students. San Diego: College-Hill, 1985; pp. 157–217.

Damico JS. Systematic observation of communicative interaction: a valid and practical descriptive assessment technique. In: Secord WA, Damico JS, eds. Best practices in school speech-language pathology: descriptive/nonstandardized language assessment. New York: The Psychological Corporation, 1992; pp. 133–144.

De Saussure F. Cours de linguistique generale. Paris: Pagot, 1916.

Dore J. The development of conversational competence. In: Scheifelbusch R, ed. Language competence: assessment and intervention. San Diego, CA: College-Hill, 1986; pp. 3–60.

Fillmore CJ. A case for case. In: Bach E, Harms ET, eds. Universals in linguistic theory. New York: Holt, Rinehart & Winston, 1968.

Gentner D. Why nouns are learned before verbs: linguistic relativity versus natural partitioning. In: Kuczaj S, ed. Language development. Vol. 2. Language, thought and culture. Hillsdale, NJ: Erlbaum, 1982.

Grice HP. Logic and conversation. In: Cole P, Morgan J, eds. Syntax and semantics: speech acts. Vol. 3. New York: Academic Press, 1975; pp. 41–59.

Harris ZS. Methods in structural linguistics. Chicago: University of Chicago Press, 1951.

Hockett CF. A course in modern linguistics. New York: Macmillan, 1958.

MacWhinney B. The competition model. In: MacWhinney B, ed. Mechanisms of language acquisition. Hillsdale, NJ: Erlbaum, 1987.

MacWhinney B. Connectionism as a framework for language acquisition theory. In: Miller J, ed. Research on child language disorders: a decade of progress. Austin, TX: Pro-ed, 1991; pp. 73–104.

McCawley JD. The role of semantics in grammar. In: Bach E, Harms E, eds. Universals in linguistic theory. New York: Holt, Rinehart, & Winston, 1968; pp. 124–169.

McClelland JL, Elman J. Interactive processes in

speech perception: the TRACE model. In: Mc-Clelland J, Rumelhart D, eds. Parallel distributed processing. Vol. 2. Psychological and biological models. Cambridge, MA: MIT Press, 1986.

McClelland JL, Rumelhart DE. An interactive activation model of the effects of context on perception. I. Psychol Rev 1981;88:375–407.

Nelson K. Making sense: the acquisition of shared meaning. New York: Academic Press, 1985.

Nelson K. Event knowledge and the development of language functions. In: Miller J, ed. Research on child language disorders: a decade of progress. Austin, TX: Pro-ed, 1991; pp. 125–142.

Nelson K. Language in cognitive development: emergence of the mediated mind. New York: Cambridge University Press, 1996.

Norris JA, Hoffman PR. Whole language and representational theories: helping children to build a network of associations. J Child Commun Disord 1994;16:5–12.

Rumelhart DE, McClelland JL. On learning the past tenses of English verbs: implicit rules or parallel distributed processing? In: MacWhinney B, ed. Mechanisms of language acquisition. Hillsdale, NJ: Earlbaum, 1986.

Sapir E. Language: an introduction to the study of speech. New York: Harcourt, Brace & World, 1921.

Searle J. Speech acts. Cambridge: Cambridge University Press, 1969.

Stein N, Glenn C. An analysis of story comprehension in elementary school children. In: Freedle R, ed. New directions in discourse processing. Vol 2. Norwood, NJ: Ablex, 1979; pp. 53–120.

Werncke C. Der aphasische symptomencomplex. Breslau: Cohn & Weigert, 1874.

Westby CE. Learning to talk—talking to learn: oral-literate language differences. In: Simon C, ed. Communication skills and classroom success: therapy methodologies for language-learning disabled students. San Diego: College-Hill, 1985; pp. 181–218.

Westby C. Narrative analysis. In: Secord WA, Damico JS, eds. Best practices in school speech-language pathology: descriptive/nonstandardized language assessment. New York: The Psychological Corporation, 1992; pp. 53–64.

CHAPTER 2

Concepts in Neurolinguistics and Information Processing

William O. Haynes

"**B**ABY SPEAKS IN DELIV-ERY ROOM!" was the headline that screamed at me from the front page of the tabloid purchased at a local grocery store by one of my more aggressive students. She was sitting smugly in the front row of my class on communication development holding up the newspaper. The student said, "I thought you told us that there was a lower limit on the age at which a child could learn to talk!" On examining the article I was not surprised to find that the headline referred to a woman who was allegedly burned as a witch in the 15th century and was speaking from the past through the body of the newborn child. The article went on to say that after the "witch" was through talking, the infant reverted to the typical cry heard at birth, and, of course, there was no more talking by the child thereafter. In class we had been discussing the fact that many parents are pushing their children to learn developmental skills earlier and earlier and that there is a limit as to how soon an infant can communicate, primarily due to the neurologic and structural maturation that must take place prior to communication development. Laymen, however, often believe that there is no limit to precocity. For instance, one quarter a student brought a clipping from the newspaper that carried Ann Landers' column (Montgomery Advertiser, March 10, 1986). The following is a quote from one letter:

> I was a psychology major and a great believer in prenatal influence. When I was pregnant I read aloud to my unborn child being careful to pronounce all the words slowly and distinctly. I often patted my belly and asked "are you listening?" After the seventh month the baby responded in the form of a hard kick. I am convinced that mothers can communicate with their unborn babies and that a fetus can learn while in the womb.

There is no question that the fetus can hear and respond to sound prenatally. We know that sensory end organs and the cochlea are sufficiently developed to receive sound by the 24th week after conception (Ormerod, 1960) and 4 weeks later the fetus can hear its mothers' internal bodily sounds such as heartbeat and voice (Liley, 1972; Wedenberg & Johansson, 1970). Hearing, however, is not the same as understanding, and the appreciation of concepts, language, and communication must await the development of much neural wiring, socialization, and experience in the outside world. As there are myths about developing communication before we have the neural structures to learn a language, there are also misconceptions about how the brain processes language. Often students are heard to say that "the left side of the brain is for language," implying that the right side is not used in linguistic processing. This statement might be disconcerting to a person who speaks relatively normally after undergoing a left hemispherectomy (removal of the left hemisphere). Of course, the effects of removing the left half of the cerebral cortex are largely a function of age, and adults would show severe language impairment. When done in children, however, there are reports of near normal language development (Springer & Deutsch, 1985). Thus the right hemisphere must have *some* capacity to deal with language.

In recent decades, advances in the use of invasive and noninvasive techniques for studying the structure and function of the brain in normal and clinical groups have increased our knowledge in the areas of normal brain function during language use and have given us glimpses of potential important differences in those who have difficulty acquiring communication or lose it as a result of nervous system damage. This chapter has several goals. First, we want to show students of communication development that there are certain neurologic structural prerequisites to both cognitive and language acquisitions. This is not a recent notion, since Eric Lenneberg wrote his classic book *The Biological Foundations of Language* in 1967. We want to show that the brain develops in a relatively orderly fashion and that the maturation of the areas of the brain and their interconnections is important as it enables us to view the world cohesively and process information for learning concepts or languages. A second goal of this chapter is to review some literature on the functioning of the brain with regard to language. Most students of anatomy and physiology know all too well that there may or may not be a relationship between certain structural components and their participation in certain functions.

For instance, just because a muscle is in an ideal position to assist in elevating the rib cage, electromyographic studies may reveal that the muscle, in fact, does not participate in inhalation (Zemlin, 1968). So it can be with neurologic structures as well, since a portion of the brain or a tract can be in a perfect position anatomically to participate in a function, yet it may not (or we have no proof that it does). We will provide an overview of some of the techniques that have been used to determine the participation of portions of the brain during linguistic tasks in children and adults. Also, there are several theories about the onset of hemispheric asymmetry for language that will be discussed. We will also report the results of studies dealing with functional asymmetry in normally developing children processing linguistic material. A third goal of this chapter is to provide a cursory overview of some components of information processing that are necessary for communication development. A final goal is to report generally on how some of the neurolinguistic and information-processing research has been applied to children who are language-impaired.

STRUCTURAL ASPECTS OF DEVELOPMENTAL NEUROLINGUISTICS

There is a paucity of information on the development of the nervous system in humans between birth and age 4. Much of the histologic research was done decades ago. The present chapter owes much to the excellent existing work of Lenneberg (1967) and Selnes and Whitaker (1977). We will begin with a sketch of some of the important structural developments in the nervous system directly related to language acquisition. Later we will consider functional issues in the nervous system.

The human brain has greater size and structural complexity compared with most other species. Besides just its weight and size superiorities it has an internal structure that is significantly more complex. The convoluted surface of the cerebral cortex results in a greater area and, presumably, increased storage and processing capacity. Not only does the human brain have more nerve cells, but these neurons are interconnected in a very complex network. Fibers connect the two cerebral hemispheres, and intrahemispheric tracts allow for communication among a variety of subcortical and cortical centers within each hemisphere. When considering language function, the areas of the cortex that are most frequently cited are the posterior frontal lobe (Broca's area) and the motor cortex located in the precentral gyrus. An equally important area is in the posterior-superior temporal lobe (Wernicke's area) and its' surrounding tissue in the parietal and occipital lobes. Very generally, Broca's area in concert with the motor cortex has been implicated primarily in the organization of expressive speech and writing. Wernicke's area, on the other hand, has been associated with organization of language, linguistic comprehension, and grammatical rule structures. Figure 2.1 shows these general areas, as well as some important tracts (fasciculi) that connect

the various cortical areas. As can be seen in the figure, the area near the angular gyrus and supramarginal gyrus is in an ideal position to coordinate information from the temporal, occipital and parietal lobes and may be involved in cross-modal associations. One can easily observe the system of interconnections between the various cortical areas. The occipitofrontal fasciculus is in a position to connect the supramarginal and angular gyri with the frontal cortex. The arcuate fasciculus joins the superior temporal lobe with Broca's area. The uncinate fasciculus is in a position to play a role in transmitting information between temporal and frontal areas; however, little is known about its actual function. The observer can readily see that each of the "primary" cortical areas and their surrounding association areas can communicate with each other via these fasciculi. There are also tracts such as the corticospinal and corticothalamic that allow cortical areas to communicate with subcortical structures such as the thalamus, as well as commissural fibers such as the corpus callosum that allow

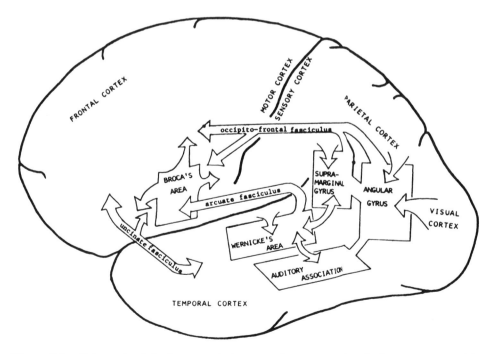

Figure 2.1.   Schematic of the long association tracts interconnecting the language areas of the left hemisphere. (Modified from Whitaker H. On the Representation of Language in the Human Brain. Edmonton: Linguistic Research, Inc., 1971.)

connection between the two cerebral hemispheres. Researchers report language disturbance in cases where damage has occurred to these tracts and also linguistic difficulties when lesions occur subcortically as in the pulvinar of the thalamus (Selnes & Whitaker, 1977). The discovery of this vast system of interconnections makes the notion of isolated functioning of certain brain structures difficult to believe. If anything, the brain functions holistically, not in isolated units. Goldman-Rakic (1987, p.616) emphasizes " . . . the integrated nature of behavior and the fact that few functions of the organism, however simple, are carried out by one part of the brain in isolation from all other parts."

When approaching this portion of the present chapter, an attempt was made to concentrate on the neurologic development that takes place in the postnatal period between birth and age 4. Although our knowledge of this area remains incomplete, some classical studies completed in the first half of this century provide insight into the "wiring" necessary for the development of thought and language.

At the outset of this section we want to be certain to indicate that we know of no evidence that shows *specific* relationships between particular neurologic structures and the development of certain language forms (e.g., nouns, verbs). Much of the available data come from damaged organisms (lesion data, etc.), and we are not sure how important a particular area of the brain is for a specific function. This type of connection is even more difficult to prove when one considers that portions of the brain may serve similar or dissimilar functions. In addition, contralateral hemispheric activity may participate in a certain function, and subcortical activity may be important in specific activities. If there is one thing that is increasingly apparent it is that the brain functions as a total interconnected unit. In electroencephalography (EEG), for instance, there is consistent activity in most areas of the brain, and what people in research are re-

ally observing are differences in the levels of participation among areas. This section suggests that a child has to undergo some basic structural changes and developments prior to acquiring thought and language. What would prevent a developing human organism from learning language and concepts at birth or soon thereafter? Developmental neurologists would suggest that prior to birth the child cannot even organize or coordinate sensory information since the interconnections between various parts of the brain are not yet developed and even the multiple layers of the cortex are not fully formed. Many of the nerve tracts that *are* present, however, are not myelinated and thus not functioning optimally. Thus the brain has a lot of developing to do between prenatal life and the acquisition of communication. Even if we observe the behavior of neonates, we can see that they are neurologically immature; as they develop neuromaturationally they are able to make advances in motor, cognitive, and linguistic areas. But, we are getting ahead of our story.

In 1967 Eric Lenneberg reviewed a series of neuroanatomic studies of the developing nervous system between birth and age 2, noting the following:

Brain Weight

During the first 2 years of life there is approximately a 350% increase in the weight of the brain. This is to be compared with only a 35% increase in the next 10 years of development. We assume that this increase in weight reflects structural growth on some level and that it is not just coincidental that the growth spurt occurs in concert with major cognitive, communicative, motor, and social acquisitions.

Neuronal Growth

In development there is not necessarily a major change in the number of neurons available, but their volume increases. It is interesting that the higher a species is on the phylogenetic scale, the lower the number of nerve cells in relation to the brain volume. Thus man has a lower cell-packing

density compared with lower animals. It is not, however, within neurons that major changes take place but in the spaces between them. Lenneberg (1967, p. 163) suggests that the increase in the distance between cell bodies results in lower cell density and provides a "histological prerequisite for the increase in dendritic arborization." Lenneberg (1967, p. 162) further states: "The major change that evidently occurs during the period of expansion of the brain is the interconnection of cells. Processes grow out from the cell body (axons and dendrites) and eventually form a dense net of interconnecting branches." Neural maturation involves the development of dendrites, which transmit and receive messages from a vast array of other cells. The number of dendrites and the development of their spines allegedly influences the information-processing capability of the cell (Maxwell, 1984).

Figure 2.2 shows examples of the development of neurologic and neuroglial processes (neuropil) between 3 and 24 months of age. Dendritic spines, as well as the extent of arborization, appear to be influenced by sensory stimulation in early development (Mollgaard, Diamond, Bennett, et al., 1971; Volkmar & Greenough, 1972; Greenough, 1976; Rosenzweig & Bennett, 1977). Sensory deprivation and malnutrition have even been thought to cause underdevelopment of dendritic spines (Maxwell, 1984). One can only speculate on the importance of the development of these interconnections to cognitive and language development, but clearly a critical minimal level is required for optimal functioning. Brain maturation research is continuing (Scheibel, 1991), and with improved technology, relations between brain maturation and language development should become clearer in the future.

Chemical Composition

As the brain matures between the ages of birth and 2 years, the cortical tissue itself, when analyzed, shows some chemical differences in the form of increases in cholesterol, cerebrosides, lipids, and phosphatides (Lenneberg, 1967). Since the brain is an electrochemical engine, these changes in composition may have an important small role in allowing the development of higher functions like communication.

Electrophysiologic Changes

Many studies report changes in the energy of brain-wave frequencies as a child matures. The lower frequencies tend to lose amplitude, while the higher ones gain (Lenneberg, 1967). These changes in brain activity probably result from the massive structural and chemical developments occurring in the first 2 years of life.

Myelinization

Myelinization, the production of the lipid and protein sheath surrounding axons, has been shown to occur at different rates throughout the nervous system. This is important since the neural conduction of myelinated fibers is said to be faster, and perhaps more efficient, than unmyelinated nerves.

We can also see a general relationship between myelinization and certain bodily functions. For instance, there is a general trend toward myelinization of pathways dedicated to performing basic physiologic processes occurring first and myelinization of fibers more associated with more complicated mental and motor activities occurring later. Some myelinization is not complete until adolescence and beyond. The corpus callosum is composed of bundles of several million fibers that connect the cerebral hemispheres. The corpus callosum has been said to facilitate interhemispheric transfer of information. Developmentally, the corpus callosum is myelinated later than other fiber tracts and is not complete until about the twentieth month at the earliest and as late as 6 years of age at the latest (Selnes, 1974). We can only speculate about the significance of myelinization of nerve fibers, but as Maxwell (1984, p. 46) states: "It is reasonable to assume that neural fibers do not function at optimal levels until myelination is completed."

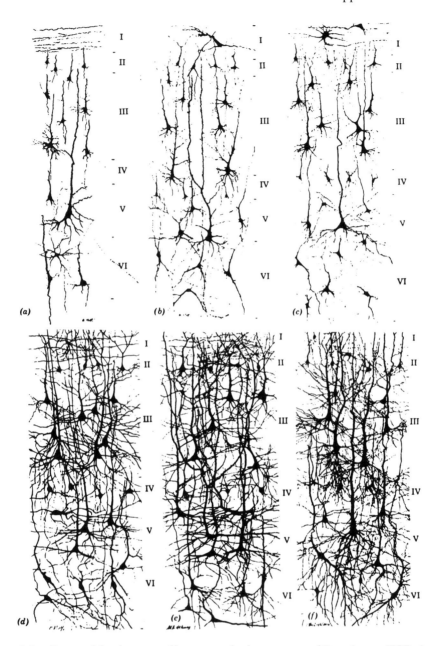

Figure 2.2. Postnatal development of human cerebral cortex around Broca's area (FCBm); camera lucida drawings from Golgi-Cox preparations; *a*, newborn; *b*, 1 month; *c*, 3 months; *d*, 6 months; *e*, 15 months; *f*, 24 months. Inspection of original sections shows an even more dramatic increase in density of neuropil between 15 and 24 months. The Roman numerals represent the six layers of the cerebral cortex. (From Conel JL. The postnatal development of the human cerebral cortex. Volumes I through VI. Cambridge, MA: Harvard University Press, 1939–1959.)

The development of the nervous system progresses in a cephalic direction beginning with lower centers such as the brainstem and culminating with the cortex, which as we have seen, may not reach total maturity until late adolescence. Developmentally, large neurons with long axons mature initially in embryology and typically form the basic primary sensory and motor pathways. These have been called by some Type I neurons (Jacobson, 1970). Other types of neurons (II and III), which are typically smaller, mature later and depend on adequate sensory stimulation for optimal development. Selnes and Whitaker (1977, p. 29) discuss the maturation of neurons and their connections as follows:

> Maturation within a cortical area starts with the innermost layers (VI and V) and progresses toward the outer layers (II and I). This implies that the first major connections to be established are those between the periphery and primary cortical areas (sensory-motor, visual, and auditory cortices). The next connections to develop are those between these primary areas and their respective association areas. The last pathways to become fully developed are the ones between the different association areas. These long association tracts, including the arcuate fasciculus and the corpus callosum, do not become fully myelinated until about the age of puberty.

Thus it can be seen that many structural changes take place within the developing nervous system between birth and 2 years of age. The above information makes clearer the observation that infants appear to be able to perform some basic functions (seeing, hearing, moving, feeling) and yet cannot coordinate these senses in a cohesive way. When a young child is holding an object and it goes out of his visual field, he "forgets" about it. Then when it comes back into view, he is surprised by the object. The interconnections between cortical areas allow the world to be cohesive and promote coordination of sensory and motor schemes.

These neurologic developments will clearly relate to our later chapters on child development and cognitive maturation. As many authors indicate, we do not presently know how certain neural developments relate to specific cognitive or linguistic acquisitions. We can only assume that neural growth is to some extent reflected in cognitive and linguistic development. Lenneberg (1967, p. 168) states the following:

> The infant's obvious incapacity to learn all but the most primitive beginnings of language during his first fifteen months is, at least intuitively, attributable to a general state of cerebral immaturity . . . we are,

therefore, suggesting as a working hypothesis that the general nonspecific states of maturation of the brain constitute prerequisites and limiting factors for language development. They are not its specific cause.

Fischer, however, (1987, p.623) states the following:

> Obviously brain development relates to cognitive development . . . Yet it has proved to be difficult to establish specific developmental relations. Global correlations exist, of course: myelination occurs progressively throughout infancy, childhood and even adolescence. . . . Both dendritic branching and synaptic density change systematically during infancy . . . To be meaningful, a relation must be specified more precisely. For example, what particular changes in the brain relate to what specific new capacities emerging in children?

It is just this type of information that is on the horizon according to some authorities (Goldman-Rakic, 1987). Some preliminary research on rhesus monkeys shows that concurrent synaptogenesis (synapse formation) in the frontal lobe is correlated closely with the ability to do the delayed-response task, an analog to the object permanence tasks of Jean Piaget (1954). Bell and Fox (1992) have used EEG techniques to monitor frontal lobe involvement in specific cognitive tasks in 7- to 12-month-old infants confirming some work on nonhuman primates in this area. Only future research can illuminate this potentially intriguing area.

FUNCTIONAL ASPECTS OF NEUROLINGUISTICS

For decades researchers and theorists have talked about lateralization of various functions in the human nervous system. Language has been a primary topic in the lateralization literature and most laymen accept the old adage that "the left side of the brain is for speech and language." We know that it is common for human beings and some species of animals to exhibit contralateral control of certain functions. For instance, the left side of the brain controls the right side of the body for motor movements and vice versa. It is not as common, however, for one side of the brain to take over a disproportionate amount of control over a particular function as compared with the contralateral hemisphere. A primary example is the left side of the brain being "dominant" for language activities and the right side for visual-spatial functions. Perhaps we should not be surprised at functional asymmetries for language and visual-spatial tasks since there are actually anatomic asymmetries in the cerebral cortex. Most people think of the brain as bilaterally symmetric, but differences between the left and right hemispheres have been noted by many researchers, especially in the area of the temporal lobe. Specifically, the left hemisphere has a larger plenum temporale (about one-third larger) as compared with the right, and the left hemisphere is typically larger at birth (Geschwind & Levitsky, 1968). These differences are seen in fetuses and neonates, and they tend to increase with age. We must, of course, be mindful of the fact that anatomic asymmetries are, at present, uninterpretable for specific functions of the brain, just as there is no invariant correlation between topographic landmarks on the brain surface and brain volume (Kinsbourne, 1981).

There are at least two major points of view about the onset of hemispheric asymmetry for language in children. These two perspectives are still debated in the literature and some have even made attempts to combine the theories within a neurodevelopmental context (Satz, Strauss, & Whitaker, 1990). One view is that at birth the cerebral hemispheres are relatively equal or "equipotential" in their ability to develop language and that, as a child matures, a gradual asymmetry develops between the hemispheres with one (usually the left) becoming dominant for language functions (Lenneberg, 1967). Proponents of this equipotentiality theory sometimes cite the data that show the youthful nervous system to possess a large degree of plasticity or ability to change as a result of damage. It is true that the right hemisphere has

been suspected to take over functions of language when the left has been damaged or removed surgically. This does suggest that both hemispheres do have the capacity to deal with language, but more current researchers have pointed out that the plasticity argument is not necessarily incompatible with the point of view that there is early asymmetry of function in the nervous system (Witelson, 1987). There has been little research support for the notion of gradual asymmetry developing in children for language functions. Most studies have used dichotic listening or lateral motor tasks (tapping), and these investigations have difficulty separating real asymmetry differences from increased learning abilities associated with advances in chronologic age (Witelson, 1987).

Another theory suggests that neonates possess early asymmetries of function from birth and that these asymmetries change little during maturation. Some of the support for the early asymmetry point of view comes from examining early infant turning preferences (Turkewitz & Birch, 1971) in which they turn to the right significantly more often than the left. Provins (1992), however, suspects that these preferences may not reflect cerebral organization per se, but other variables such as prenatal and postnatal experience. Also, many Auditory Evoked Potential (AEP) investigations show asymmetric evoked potential responses for speech stimuli and nonspeech stimuli in neonates (Molfese, 1977; Molfese & Molfese, 1980, 1985).

Additionally, EEG asymmetries have been reported for speech in children as young as 3 months of age (Davis & Wada, 1977; Gardiner & Walter, 1977). When children are older and can participate in inferential tasks such as dichotic listening, the bulk of studies show that asymmetries exist as young as age 2 to 3 years (Witelson, 1977). Recently, Witelson (1987, p. 667), after an exhaustive review of the asymmetry literature, states the following:

> In summary, on the basis of the neuropsychological studies with normal children, regions in the left hemisphere appear

to be specialized for mediating speech and language processes and possibly also for the programming of voluntary sequential motor behavior from the first few months of life, probably from birth. Although there are large gaps in the empirical record, the available evidence indicates that hemisphere specialization is functionally present in the neural system from the beginning. In addition, the evidence indicates that the magnitude of functional asymmetry does not increase but rather remains constant or invariant over chronological development.

A General Review of Techniques Used in Exploring Hemispheric Asymmetry

Basically, the methods used to gain insight into functional asymmetry of the hemispheres can be viewed in a variety of ways. Some of the methods used are invasive and require injection/inhalation of substances, surgery, or examination of lesioned areas of the cortex. Other methods rely on behavioral responses and then "infer" greater processing in one hemisphere as compared with the other. These techniques are not typically invasive since they require only behavioral responses to specially produced stimulus items.   Each procedure has its advantages and disadvantages. The following is a general review of techniques used in neurolinguistic research. By far, most neurolinguistic research has been done on adults because they are more capable of responding to experimental tasks and because risks are involved in some of the procedures.

Invasive Procedures

Lesion Data   For decades scientists have gathered data on the speech and language characteristics of a brain-damaged patient and then performed an autopsy to determine the site of lesion. Presumably, the damaged area of the cortex played a role in mediating the linguistic, motor, or perceptual function that was impaired prior to the patient's death. We have known for years that patients with damage to the left hemisphere display more speech and language deficits than do those with damage to their right hemisphere. Lesions in Broca's area result in

slow, effortful speech and writing and in general more difficulty in language production. Lesions in Wernicke's area show more fluent speech and writing with less effort, but there may be significant deficits in the way sentences are formulated and in language comprehension. Even damage to the major interconnections between the language areas may result in language problems. Lesions of subcortical structures also may result in aphasia. Thus lesion data suggest that the left hemisphere and subcortical structures are important to language and that damage to areas on the left side of the brain interrupts language processing. A potential difficulty with relying on lesion data, however, lies in the fact that we are dealing with a damaged organism. We do not know if the brain operates in the same manner when damaged as when it is undamaged. For instance, other portions of the brain can compensate for lesioned areas. Thus it is difficult to infer the operation of an intact brain by studying subjects that are suffering from cortical lesions. Most researchers, however, would say that the lesion data in adults support the idea that the left hemisphere plays a greater role in language production and comprehension as compared with the right side of the brain. The problems are compounded when using lesion data on child subjects. It is often difficult to specifically know about the onset of the lesion, and a child may have developed compensatory anatomic connections. In addition, researchers often cannot do premorbid evaluation of functions, and handedness may not be known.

Split-Brain Studies   Certain patients with severe epilepsy have undergone severing of the corpus callosum (commissurotomy) in an attempt to reduce the severity of seizures. This procedure is not done routinely and indeed is done rarely in present times. The patients that have undergone section of the cerebral commissures, however, have been interesting subjects for research because, in essence, the two sides of the brain are relatively isolated and independent of each other.

Some have said it is like having two separate systems. However, in actuality the two hemispheres have ways of sharing information on the subcortical level so the person can operate normally in daily life situations. It is mainly in experimental tasks that a commissurized person shows deficits (Springer & Deutsch, 1985). Normal subjects can transfer information between the hemispheres and rely on this hemispheric communication to solve problems. If a researcher sends a linguistic stimulus to the right hemisphere of a split-brained subject via the visual system, for instance, it can be determined what capabilities the right side of the brain has with regard to generating or comprehending language. Most studies of split-brained individuals have shown that the left hemisphere has a significant advantage over the right in language production. The right hemisphere, however, may not be as alinguistic as has been previously thought. Some studies have shown that the right hemisphere has a substantial lexical capability and can understand language. Gazzaniga (1970), for instance, found that the right hemisphere in split-brained subjects is able to "understand" simple nouns, but it performed poorly on verbs. Zaidel (1978) reported even greater comprehension by the right hemisphere implementing a "Z lens" procedure that uses a contact lens to ensure presentation of stimuli to only one visual field at a time, while allowing patients considerable time to visually study stimulus items. Gazzaniga (1983) has argued that the right hemisphere in normal, non-split-brained subjects may well have less linguistic ability and that perhaps the brain-damaged subjects used in split-brain research also had damaged left hemispheres, which resulted in reorganization of language functions to the right hemisphere. We must remember that, as with the lesion data, the split-brained subject is not functioning normally, and thus it is not totally valid to infer normal processing of information from these experiments; however, interesting insights have been gained from this research. Overall,

this research indicates that the left hemisphere is more adapted to dealing with language and that the right is better at visual-spatial activities.

Sodium Amytal Injection   Some researchers (Wada, 1949) have injected sodium amytal into the internal carotid artery on either the right or left side, thus inhibiting the function of the cerebral hemisphere on the injected side. When one hemisphere is incapacitated, language functions may be tested for a 2- or 3-minute period. This procedure typically results in a transient aphasia if the hemisphere that specializes in language (usually the left) is temporarily anesthetized. Relatively little language interruption is seen when the right hemisphere is injected. More recently, Loring, et al. (1990, p.831) found that 79 of 103 subjects displayed "exclusive left hemisphere language representation, and 22 patients had language represented in each hemisphere. In the 22 patients with bilateral language, an asymmetry was present in 17 cases (13 L>R, 4 R>L)." These findings suggest that exclusive right hemispheric language specialization is rare and that most subjects exhibit either left or bilateral language representation. Again, this would support the notion that the left hemisphere is more specialized for language.

Regional Cerebral Blood Flow (rCBF)
This is a method of brain imaging in which a subject inhales a low-level gas that is radioactive and a computerized display shows the level of blood-flow activity in various brain regions during the performance of certain tasks. Increased cortical blood flow has been observed in the left hemisphere during linguistic tasks and in the right hemisphere when the subject is engaged in the perception of music (Carmon, Lavy, Gordon, & Portnoy, 1975). Wallesch, Henriksen, Kornhuber, and Paulson (1985) documented increased blood flow in left cortical and subcortical areas for a linguistic task especially related to Broca's area in the frontal lobe, caudate nuclei, and left thalamic/pallidal areas. This type of result

would suggest that the left hemisphere is more active in language processing and the right in dealing with certain types of music. Another technique that obtains similar imaging is Positron Emission Tomography (PET); however, it involves injection of radioactive material into the arterial system. Both of these procedures may have some interpretive ambiguities according to Witelson (1987). More research using PET and magnetic resonance imaging (MRI) technology (Shaywitz, Shaywitz, Pugh, et al., 1995) will no doubt verify prior research with other techniques and add new dimensions to our understanding of brain/language relationships (Mazziotta & Metter, 1988).

Noninvasive Techniques

The noninvasive techniques are largely inferential in nature and rely on the subject reporting what was seen or heard in a series of stimulus presentations. Other noninvasive methods examine the electrical activity of the brain and infer relative hemispheric participation during a variety of tasks.

Dichotic Listening   When two stimuli are presented simultaneously to both ears (CV syllables or words), most normal, right-handed subjects will evidence a preference for or an advantage of one ear over the other. In essence, they will have more correct reports in one ear than the other. Theoretically, the reason for this is that most auditory stimuli are processed via contralateral fibers so that stimuli entering the right ear will go primarily to the left hemisphere and vice versa and functionally override ipsilateral processing. Most normal, right-handed subjects demonstrate a right ear advantage (REA) for linguistic material and even for CV syllables (Berlin & Lowe, 1972; Kimura, 1961a, 1961b, 1963). Some studies show a left ear advantage (LEA) for nonspeech stimuli (Knox & Kimura, 1970; Kimura, 1973). Sidtis, Sadler, and Nass (1987) also studied 7- to 12-year-old children and found a REA for speech and a LEA for pitch discrimination. These general findings suggest that the right ear would have

an advantage for linguistic material because it goes directly to the left hemisphere, which is more adept at language processing. Material going to the left ear goes to the right hemisphere, which might then "consult" the left hemisphere via the commissural fibers.

Overall, the dichotic findings would support the notion that the left hemisphere is more involved in language activities as compared with the right. Some problems with the dichotic listening paradigm are reported by several authorities. Ipsilateral fibers exist in addition to the contralateral fibers, and there may be some "ipsilateral leakage" of information. Dichotic listening is also affected by attention. If subjects pay attention to the emotional tone of a stimulus, a LEA is found, but if they pay attention to linguistic factors, a REA is evidenced (Haggard & Parkinson, 1971). Even instructions to attend to a particular ear over the other may influence the direction of ear advantage (Obrzut, Hynd, Obrzut, & Pirozzolo, 1981). Also, the magnitude and direction of the asymmetry between ears is not stable from day to day in individual subjects, but is fairly stable in groups of subjects.

Tachistoscopic Tasks   The visual system is also arranged in a primarily contralateral fashion and has no ipsilateral fibers like the auditory system. If a stimulus is presented to the right or left visual field of each eye, this information travels to the contralateral hemisphere. Thus, if a vertically arranged word (to prevent left to right scanning) is presented in a short enough time epoch < 200 milliseconds), the linguistic stimulus will be viewed only by the right or left visual field and therefore will go to the contralateral hemisphere. The major purpose of the tachistoscope is to present the material rapidly enough to prevent eye movement and thus avoid "leakage" from one visual field into another.

Some more recent studies use a specially constructed contact lens to control the subject's viewing (Zaidel, 1978), but most investigations have used a tachistoscope, and the subject merely looks through a binocular eyepiece. Most of the tachistoscopic studies have found, as in the dichotic listening studies, that subjects can more accurately report stimulus items presented to one of the visual fields. Typically, in normal, right-handed subjects a right visual-field preference (RVFP) is found, suggesting that information presented to the right visual fields goes directly to the left hemisphere and is processed more effectively than information going to the right side of the brain (McKeever & Huling, 1971). There have also been studies of visual-spatial processing of faces, dots, and geometric forms for which a LVFP is often demonstrated (Kimura, 1969). This is supportive of the idea that the left hemisphere is more adapted to language processing than the right. An obvious shortcoming of tachistoscopic tasks is that they cannot be administered to very young children who are not able to read, and thus this research is largely limited to school-age children and adults.

Lateral Motor Tasks Some studies have investigated finger tapping and the decrement in performance that occurs when a subject attempts to engage in tapping and speaking simultaneously. One relevant report (Kinsbourne & Hiscock, 1983) found that there was a decrement in the tapping performance of the right hand when the subject is talking, but there was no decrement in the left-hand tapping ability while talking. This is presumably because of a "time sharing" phenomenon where the left hemisphere is controlling the right hand, but it is also engaged in the primary role of language/speech production, so the tapping is affected only in the right hand but not in the left. This provides indirect support for the idea that the left hemisphere is more responsible for language than the right.

Electroencephalography Some studies have used electroencephalic (EEG) recordings of certain brain-wave frequencies as an index of hemispheric processing of a variety of stimuli (Robbins & McAdam, 1974; Dumas & Morgan, 1975;

Galin & Ellis, 1975). The most common brain rhythms used in research are alpha waves, which are between 8 and 13 Hz. Early research indicated that alpha was incompatible with organized thought, and thus an attenuation or suppression of alpha wave amplitude over one hemisphere or the other has been interpreted as an indication of "processing." The presence of high-amplitude alpha over one hemisphere and low amplitude over the other suggests that one side of the brain is processing material to a greater degree than the other. Most studies using the EEG paradigm have shown that alpha suppression occurs for language material more over the left hemisphere than the right and vice versa for most visual spatial material. This again shows the left hemisphere to be superior to the right in language processing.

Evoked Potentials The monitoring of Averaged Evoked Responses (AER) during visual and auditory stimulation also has been used as an index of hemispheric asymmetry. McAdam and Whitaker (1971) and Callaway and Harris (1974) have shown that AER amplitude is increased over the left hemisphere as compared with the right during verbal tasks. As mentioned previously, many recent investigations of neonates show early asymmetries for linguistic material. These findings again support the notion that the left hemisphere is more adapted to the processing of linguistic material as compared with the right.

So, what does all this research tell us when taken as a whole? Basically, if one were to take the results at face value, the conclusion would be that the left hemisphere is better adapted for language, and the right is better suited for visual-spatial and intonational processing. Many of the techniques described above utilize tasks that lack ecologic validity, and thus we must be cautious in making broad statements about what the brain typically does based on brief and highly artificial sampling conditions. In the natural language-processing situations one encounters in daily life the brain may behave quite differently. There is a big difference between listening to dichotically presented syllables or words and listening to a lecture. Likewise, subjects who sit in darkened rooms staring into the binocular eyepiece of a tachistoscope may process those rapidly flashed, vertical-letter arrangements differently than they would when reading a book. The EEG and rCBF techniques provide an opportunity for more naturalistic tasks since connected speech can be used as stimuli. It seems from our review of the research that the more naturalistic the language processing task, the more likely investigators are to see individual strategies in dealing with information because there are fewer experimental constraints. We do know, however, that it is not completely accurate to say that the left hemisphere is the "language hemisphere" and the right is a "nonlanguage hemisphere." This is because certain variables have been shown to affect hemispheric processing of information, and any general characterization of one hemisphere as performing a specific function is soon shown to have multiple exceptions.

VARIABLES AFFECTING HEMISPHERIC PROCESSING OF INFORMATION

The following are some general areas that according to available research may affect a subject's way of dealing with information. In some of the areas there is controversy, and in others there appears to be fairly strong agreement among researchers.

Handedness

Human beings are predominantly right-handed (about 93%). In the right-handed population approximately 95% are left-hemisphere "dominant" for language on the measures described in the previous section. This means about 5% of right-handed people show right hemispheric or bilateral processing of language material (Rasmussen & Milner, 1977). Hugdahl and Anderson (1989) studied the

dichotic listening performance of 126 left-handed children and found approximately two-thirds of this population to have left-hemisphere dominance for language as revealed by the REA. This certainly would suggest that a statement indicating that the right hemisphere is a "nonlanguage" part of the brain would be erroneous. Indeed, there are a number of people who have sustained damage to the left hemisphere in childhood and subsequently developed language using the right hemisphere. In fact, there are even children who have undergone left hemispherectomy who clearly have used the right hemisphere to develop language. Recall also that tachistoscopic studies in split-brained subjects showed that the right hemisphere was capable of some linguistic processing. Getting back to handedness, in the sinistral or left-handed population, only about 70% exhibit a left hemisphere preference for language and the remaining 30% are equally divided between right hemispheric and bilateral representation. Some studies have even shown that familial handedness may affect processing of information. For instance, a person may be left-handed, but if there are left-handed siblings or parents in the family information may be processed differently from another left-hander who had no sinistral relatives (Springer & Deutsch, 1985). Hand preference studies suggest that handedness may be established quite early, by 18 months of age (Archer, Campbell, & Segalowitz, 1988). Some authorities have reported motor asymmetries (e.g., turning preferences) well before this time, but it is controversial if these motor tendencies reflect cerebral organization (Povins, 1992). The handedness of research subjects is a critical variable to control in hemispheric-processing research since an investigator would not want results biased by a group with mixed handedness. For instance, if an experimenter were studying sex differences between males and females in hemispheric processing of language, the researcher would not want more left-handers in the male group as compared with the female group. This could cause the groups to perform differently and have nothing to do with their sex, but everything to do with their handedness. Researchers do not presently know why there is a general relationship between handedness and language processing; however, there are several intriguing theories.

Sex

Some researchers have attempted to show differences between the sexes in processing information. Society has many unfortunate stereotypes about women "thinking" differently than men and vice versa. There are many studies that have shown females to exhibit superiority over males on tasks involving language. On the other hand, males appear to be more adept than females on visual-spatial and mechanical tasks (McGlone, 1980; McGee, 1979). Some evidence from clinical studies of right-handers also shows that subsequent to left-hemisphere damage, males are three times more likely to exhibit language impairment than females (McGlone, 1978). The most popular thinking is that females have more bilateral representation of language compared with males. Hiscock, Inch, Jacek, et al. (1994) reviewed extensive neuropsychologic literature on auditory laterality and found support for a "weak population level sex difference" in hemispheric specialization, mostly supporting the notion of greater specialization in males compared with females. The research taken as a whole, however, appears to be contradictory since some studies have shown males to be more lateralized than females (with females being more bilateral), while many other investigations have shown no differences between the sexes on processing tasks (Springer & Deusch, 1985). A recent study using magnetic resonance imaging (MRI) supported the notion that females tend to be more bilateral in processing language, while males were more lateralized to the left hemisphere (Shaywitz, et al., 1995). It is difficult to reconcile these findings, and some authorities cite the differences in methodologies among the studies as being the cause of the disparity in the literature. Other scientists indicate that studies with significant sex differences would tend to be accepted for publication more often than those showing nonsignificant findings, thus making the sex difference more "imagined" than real. Even in light of the above, most researchers "control" for the sex factor in their experiments, and the gender research continues using more sophisticated technologies.

Stimulus

The type of stimulus to be processed has shown differences in subjects' performance. For instance, most studies have shown language material to be processed significantly more left-hemispherically in most subjects using a variety of techniques. Conversely, visual-spatial stimuli (faces, geometric forms, etc.) tend to be lateralized more to the right hemisphere. Some studies have even shown a difference in the processing of high-imagery (concrete) and low-imagery (abstract) types of words (Hines, 1976, 1977; Ellis & Shepard, 1974; Day, 1977). An example might be that a word like "boy" is highly concrete and imaginable, while a word like "honesty" is abstract and difficult to mentally imagine. Some studies have shown more right-hemispheric processing of concrete words and more left-hemispheric processing of abstract words. This is supposedly due to the greater visual-spatial (imagery) capability of the right hemisphere and the necessity to define an abstract word using language, which is more of a left-hemispheric task. Some studies have also shown that music tends to be processed more in the right hemisphere by most right-handed nonmusicians (Gates & Bradshaw, 1977). Some studies disagree with the stimulus effects cited above, and more research needs to be done on this issue.

Task

Some studies have shown that processing may differ depending on what a subject is asked to do with a stimulus item. Some studies report greater left hemispheric activation during and preceding motor-speech tasks (Zimmerman & Knott, 1974). Thus a response mode involving motor behaviors may influence the way information is processed. For instance, would a person process information for a test differently if it were a multiple-choice examination (recognition) or an essay examination (recall)? That is, would you listen to the material differently or store it differently depending on what you had to do with it? There is controversy on whether hemispheric activity changes in these two types of tasks (Haynes & Moore, 1981). Haynes (1980) in a preliminary report noted that subjects exhibited significantly more left-hemispheric activation when listening to linguistic stimuli they were instructed to imitate than when listening to the same stimulus items under instructions not to imitate and simply attend to the syntactic structure. The task-demand requirements on the subject's use of information may influence the way it is processed or coded for storage.

Idiosyncratic Processing Strategies in Individual Subjects

Perhaps the most elusive of effects on hemispheric activation is the use of idiosyncratic approaches to dealing with information. We have already suggested that most laypersons tend to process music more with the right hemisphere than the left. Some studies have shown, however, that musicians or conductors are more left hemispheric in their processing of musical stimuli (Gates & Bradshaw, 1977). Thus individuals possess unique characteristics and can deal with information on a variety of levels, focusing on it in a number of different ways.

Robbins and McAdam (1974) had subjects examine picture postcards in three conditions and use covert imagery. In one condition the subjects were given instructions to focus on shapes and colors in the cards using a visualization/imagery strategy, while in another condition they were told to recall the cards in words. The conditions differed on the hemispheric activation as revealed by EEG procedures with more left-hemisphere processing for the word rehearsal and more right-hemisphere activation for the color/shape rehearsal. Thus a particular individual can choose to process information in a variety of ways.

Haynes and Hannay (1983) performed an EEG study in which right-handed children between the ages of 4 and 10 years listened to and watched stories under two conditions: an auditory-only condition, where the child heard a tape recording of a story with no visual stimulus relating to the story, and an audio-visual condition, which included a tape recording and accompanying film strip of a story. The children were told that they would have to answer some simple questions about the story after it was presented. It was thought while planning the study that the auditory-only presentation would result in more left-hemispheric processing and that the audiovisual would result in more right-hemispheric processing. As often happens, the data did not cooperate with our predictions. At each age group it was found that about half of the children processed the material with the left hemisphere primarily and that the other half used the right hemisphere primarily no matter which stimulus condition they were exposed to. It may be helpful to state that the subjects were given no specific instructions regarding *how* to process the material. It may well be that in the audiovisual condition some may have attended more to the pictures, others to the story line from the tape recording. In the auditory-only condition some children may have mentally "visualized" the story happening even though we provided no pictures, while others listened intently to the language from the tape recording. At any rate, this may be a good example of individual processing strategies since we controlled for age, intelligence, handedness, and most other pertinent variables. A "loosely structured" task as described above will probably not be as likely to demonstrate differences between groups as compared with highly structured tasks such as those used in dichotic listening and tachistoscopic studies. Cognitive researchers know that there are different problem-solving strategies in children and adults and that probably a host of variables come into play in deciding how to deal with a specific problem. Most current authorities agree that a subjects' "psychological set" is a significant determiner of the way information is dealt with in the brain (Carey & Lockhart, 1973; Hall, Grossman, & Elwood, 1976).

THE HEMISPHERES AS PROCESSORS

It has become popular to view the cerebral hemispheres as possessing two different processing styles that are not necessarily confined exclusively to a particular hemisphere, but are characteristic of the way each side of the brain is most adapted to dealing with information (Witelson, 1987). Clearly, if the right hemisphere can take over language functions after damage to the left hemisphere, it is capable of processing segmental information. Instead of saying that the left and right sides of the brain are best at dealing with specific types of stimuli like language or visual stimuli, it is now popular to describe more general processing characteristics. The left hemisphere appears better at dealing with segmental, analytic, time-dependent stimuli and tasks. Segmental implies segments or sections of something. Analytic implies analysis in which elements are compared with each other and sequences are examined. Time-dependent implies segments related to each other in the stream of time like events or movements or words.

Much of language is segmental since it can be divided into phonemes, syllables, words, phrases, clauses, sentences, and paragraphs. To deal with language processing, we need to analyze these segments in relation to one another in both production and comprehension. One can readily see that learning a language requires the attention to segments in the stream of speech and analysis of relationships between segments for the abstrac-

tion of linguistic rules. Thus, the left hemisphere, being a segmental processor, is best adapted to dealing with the structural aspects of language learning and processing. The right hemisphere has been characterized as nonsegmental, holistic, gestalt, and time-independent. Things with no segments like faces or geometric forms must usually be dealt with as wholes, not parts. An intonation contour or a gradual change in pitch in a musical passage may be dealt with nonsegmentally. One can easily see how a musician could deal with music either segmentally or nonsegmentally, since music is composed of many segments such as rhythms, several notes that make up a chord (that may be perceived as a whole), and arpeggios. Depending on a person's strategy, music may be processed either right or left hemispherically. It is interesting that in language acquisition an early characteristic of children's speech production is the imitation of parental intonation contours and the exaggeration of these suprasegmental characteristics by caretakers (Garnica, 1974). Perhaps the right hemisphere plays an important role in early language acquisition.

So, what have we learned thus far? First, we have learned that there are structural developments that must take place in the first few years of life that permit cognitive and linguistic development. The formation of the primary areas, association areas, and massive interconnections are an important part of our ability to process information. A second important point concerns the functional aspects of the way the brain handles information. Our current research suggests that the brain is capable of different types of processing, and two of these types are segmental and nonsegmental. The left hemisphere apparently is best adapted to segmental processing in most normal, right-handed people, and the right is better at nonsegmental processing. Language has both segmental, as well as nonsegmental, components, and it is most likely that both hemispheres play a role in the production and interpretation of linguistic elements. We must not forget, however, the way information processing is heavily influenced by subject, stimulus, task, and idiosyncratic psychologic variables. As in most matters, when one attempts to make a general statement about how all people do anything, the statement is most likely to be in error.

OTHER IMPORTANT INFORMATION-PROCESSING CAPACITIES IN COMMUNICATION DEVELOPMENT

Once the hardware and software of the neurologic system are developed to a functional point, the human organism is capable of processing large amounts of information. Many models of this process exist, none of which has been universally accepted, and we will deal here only with aspects that are included in the majority of models. Specifically, to learn to communicate we must (1) have an intact sensory system; (2) pay attention to linguistic, nonlinguistic, and contextual stimuli; and (3) somehow commit to memory our experiences. We know that early in the first year of life the child develops attentional skills and recognition memory as revealed by studies using Event Related Potentials (ERP) (Nelson & deRegnier, 1992). Many books and articles have been written about each of these three processes, and we will touch on them only generally here.

Sensory Apparatus

Imagine the difficulty a child who is deaf and blind would have in acquiring the language of his culture. A person needs auditory ability to hear the language spoken by others, and the visual system allows one to see the referents that are talked about in conversations. In a person with normal abilities the sensory organs transduce environmental stimuli into nervous impulses and transmit them to cortical centers for integration and interpretation. Since communication and cognitive development depend to such a great extent on sensory information, al-

most any sensory impairment can result in a developmental delay. The reader should recall from the prior section on the development of the nervous system that the basic wiring for sensation develops first and then the connections for integrating different types of sensory data.

Attentional Mechanisms

Hubbell (1981) presents an interesting discussion of attention. He indicates that levels of attention range from a general "set" to attend to concentrating on specific aspects of an event. For instance, a child may choose to look at pictures with an adult (general) but may fail to examine specific things in the pictures that the adult desires. Attention is affected by a variety of factors, the two most potent being energy and change. We tend to pay attention to stimuli with more energy (loud, bright, etc.) or those that fluctuate. Advertisers capitalize on these factors as evidenced by the large, bright, blinking signs placed in front of stores. Another highly individual factor that affects attention is the relevance of a stimulus to solving a certain problem. If, for instance, I told a class that I would pay a dollar for each time a student caught me saying an adjective, the attention of the more materialistic members of the group probably would shift from the main point of the lecture to scanning for parts of speech. Thus, energy, change, and relevance affect the salience of stimuli. Think of a child learning to communicate. The communication behaviors of caretakers are certainly of high energy since the human voice is distinctive and louder than most stimuli in an interaction. As mentioned previously, caretakers typically exaggerate intonation patterns and intersperse their speech with whispering, which serves to increase the fluctuating nature of the verbal model. Attention is also heightened by the use of gestures and exaggerated facial expressions. Finally, relevance is clearly present in communication. The child is listening to a person who provides all necessities of life and social interactions. Also, the parent is providing names for the very stimulus items in which the child is currently interested. Thus attention plays a large role in communication development, and children are able to attend generally and specifically during the time they are learning language. This is a major change from the first month of life when the neonate cannot even track a moving object in a 180° arc. We must also add that attention can be influenced by operant conditioning and instructions from significant others.

Memory

The area of memory is large and complex. We mention it here because communication development requires several different types of memory. We are not implying that language is learned through rote memory, like a parrot would learn to talk. Certainly, some aspects of language are learned through rote memory, but for the most part, sentences are constructed in a generative manner using general algorithms or rules. This is how we can construct sentences that we have never heard anyone say (The spotted elephant was incensed by his tax return.) Hubbell (1981, p.28) has distinguished between *episodic memory* and *semantic memory*:

> In episodic memory an item is remembered as a whole, with little analysis of its component parts or structure . . . because the material is not analyzed, this type of memory does not include inference or generalization, but is rather a copy of the event involved. . . . Semantic memory, on the other hand, is independent of any specific event. . . . A reproduction from semantic memory is a reconstruction of the event, focusing on the gist of that event, rather than a holistic copy.

Adults, for instance, might not remember the exact sentences in a story, but they can remember what happened to the characters (the gist). We can memorize sentences if we so desire, but there is simply too much language to learn it in an episodic manner. We tend to learn language and its rules largely through semantic memory.

Another way to think of memory is the length of time information is to be remembered. Most models of information processing include a short-term memory component in which data that have been sensed are temporarily stored prior to being shuttled to long-term memory or simply forgotten. The most common example of short-term memory is attempting to remember a telephone number between the time you look it up and when you dial it. Some telephone numbers you will want to rehearse and retain in long-term memory. This brings up the important point that memory is dynamic and influenced significantly by a person's psychologic set (Muma, 1978). Miller (1956) talked about the famous "magic number seven," which was supposed to be the number of items an adult could hold in short-term memory (plus or minus two items). As Muma correctly points out, many educators and psychologists misinterpreted this as being seven digits and thus the "digit span" has been used and abused in educational assessment. Actually, Miller meant that the seven items could be defined individually by a person's psychologic set and strategy for "chunking" the information. For instance, one person may try to remember a series of items one at a time, while another may memorize many more items in seven chunks of three items each. Because language has structure (phrases, clauses, etc.), it can easily be "chunked" by a person in a memory task. While a person may only be able to remember seven digits, he may be able to remember a long sentence that has seven chunks in it. (The boy went to town, bought a shirt, washed the car, paid a bill, walked the dog, called his mom, and got dressed for the dance.) This sentence actually included 26 words, which could be chunked in seven "items." Again, the strategies used by children and adults for short-term memory depend largely on individual psychologic processes, as do the rehearsal techniques for episodic memory. Some use imagery, while others may use alternate association techniques. Language rules, it would seem, are relegated to long-term memory.

To acquire communication, a child must be able to sense it, attend to important aspects of it, and remember both specific linguistic elements, as well as abstract language rules. If a deficit exists in any of these areas, communication development may be delayed.

NEUROLINGUISTIC CLINICAL APPLICATIONS

By this point the reader should be highly aware that neurologic structures and processes underlie every human activity from those as simple as moving a finger, to those as complex as using thought and language. It would be beyond the scope of a single chapter to discuss all the clinical implications of neurolinguistics for language-impaired children. Some of the reasons for this are explained in the following sections.

Heterogeneity of the Language-Impaired Population

One obvious application of the neurolinguistic information reviewed above would be to consider if language-impaired children have any structural differences in their neurologic makeup as compared with normal-language children. An important point to consider at the outset is that the population exhibiting language impairment is a highly heterogeneous one. There are many subgroups of language-impaired children that exhibit obvious neurologic differences, and some youngsters with language disorders have no demonstrable neurologic deficits. For example, some language-impaired children have neurologic damage from experiences after birth (e.g., victims of trauma or acquired brain damage). Other children experience brain injury prior to or during the birth process (e.g., intraventricular hemorrhage, cerebral palsy). There are also those in whom we infer neurologic differences, but we may not be able to specifically demonstrate them (e.g., mentally retarded, learning disabled, reading disabled, autistic). Finally, there are children with language impairment who apparently have perfectly normal nervous systems. Thus at present we cannot say that language impairment is specifically caused by a particular neurologic deficit in *all* children with delayed communication development. Certainly, if one were to examine the nervous system in detail, some subtle differences might be found between children who are language-impaired and those with normal communicative development; but at present we are left with fairly gross measures that show no consistent differences. We only know that the nervous system has to mature to a certain degree before communication will develop, and we are not equipped to state what specific neurologic failures are responsible for imperfect communication development in all cases.

The Multitude of Processes Subserved by the Nervous System

The nervous system mediates all sensory, motor, thought, and language processes in the human organism. One can easily see that a breakdown in oral language acquisition could be due to deficits in information processing or in cognitive, sensory, or even motor processes. The list of possible assessment techniques to probe all aspects of even one of these areas is extensive. The neuropsychologic literature abounds with evaluation tasks calculated to probe different parts of the neurologic, cognitive, and linguistic processes (Rourke, Bakker, Fisk, & Strang, 1983; Tramontana & Hooper, 1988; Spreen, Tupper, Risser, et al., 1984). Even a general introduction to neuropsychologic assessment is beyond the scope of this portion of the present chapter. It is enough to appreciate that any child with known neurologic damage should have a thorough neuropsychologic evaluation to determine strengths and concerns in neurolinguistic abilities. Such evaluation procedures are also used in cases where there is no known brain injury to determine how the language-impaired child processes linguistic material in a variety of tasks; these procedures vary in difficulty, input modality (auditory, visual), and types of output (speech, gestures, writing).

The Possibility of Functional Differences in the Absence of Structural Differences

A number of studies have examined language-disordered and learning-disabled children with linguistic problems to determine if they process information differently than normal youngsters. Specifically, these studies endeavored to find if language-impaired children process language stimuli more right-hemispherically as compared with normal language subjects. If language-impaired children are using the right hemisphere to process segmental material, then they may be using the side of the brain that is less well adapted to dealing with linguistic information. Most of the studies done have used the dichotic listening paradigm.

Studies concerning children strictly defined as "learning-disabled" show conflicting results with some supporting the notion of incomplete or weaker lateralization (Obrzut, Obrzut, Bryden, & Bartles, 1985; Guyer & Friedman, 1975; Obrzut, Hynd, Obrzut, & Pirozzolo, 1981) and with others showing no significant lateralization differences as compared with normally achieving subjects (Hynd, Obrzut, Weed, & Hynd, 1979; Obrzut, Hynd, Obrzut, & Leitgeb, 1980). The research in the area of reading difficulties shows disagreement with some studies demonstrating less or reversed lateralization in dyslexics as compared with normal readers (Fried, Tanguay, & Boder, 1981; Thompson, 1976; Zurif & Carson, 1970; Bakker, Smink, & Reitsma, 1973; Garren, 1980) and with other reports demonstrating no appreciable difference (Yeni-Komshian, Isenberg, & Goldberg, 1975; Caplan & Kinsbourne, 1982; Vellutino, Bentley, & Phillips, 1978). Finally, in children with specific language disorders the literature has also shown some studies suggesting reversed or reduced laterality for language (Pettit & Helms, 1974; Rosenblum & Dorman, 1978; Sommers & Taylor, 1972), and some studies have found no difference between normal language subjects and those with language disorders (Springer &

Eisenson, 1977; Sommers & Taylor, 1972; Isaacs & Haynes, 1984).

From the above brief review it can be seen that language-impaired children as a group cannot be said to exhibit hemispheric-processing differences. The disparity in the literature may be a product of differing groups of language-impaired subjects, different stimuli, and different tasks used in the various experiments. There may be a subgroup of children who do, in fact, exhibit right hemispheric processing of language, which makes learning the code more difficult. Even in studies cited above that found no processing differences in language-impaired children, it is entirely possible that they did exhibit right-hemispheric processing strategies during the earlier language-learning period. Most of the studies of language-impaired children were done on subjects over the age of 5 years.

Another aspect of research on children with language disorders has dealt with their rapid auditory processing. Many studies have shown that children with language impairments have difficulty processing rapid, sequenced auditory stimuli (Stark & Tallal, 1981; Tallal & Stark, 1981; Anderson, Brown, & Tallal, 1993). Tallal and Merzenich (1996) presented data on computer-generated treatment programs designed to improve temporal processing by presenting a slower, more salient version of rapidly changing acoustic elements of speech and then gradually decreasing the processing time. While this method has shown language gains for some children with language impairments, more research must confirm these findings, and a determination must be made as to the type of language impairment that is best suited to this mode of treatment. Also, work needs to be done on the extent of generalization to spontaneous conversation.

Treatment Differs Dramatically From Case to Case

Some children with certain neurologic disorders such as seizures or hydrocephaly can benefit from medical intervention. In many cases the medical treatment coupled with therapy can dramatically improve the child's chances of learning language. On the other hand, if a child has widespread damage to the nervous system, there is most often little that can be done to alleviate the structural anomaly. For instance, if a child is mentally retarded, there is little hope for medication or neurosurgery to cure him. This is frustrating to parents and clinicians alike. Equally frustrating, however, are the many cases of language impairment in which the neurologist will probably indicate that there is no abnormality in the nervous system. Language disorders are more easily explainable when some neurologic deficit can be demonstrated.

However, even in some cases of mental retardation, where there is a high probability of cognitive damage somewhere in the child's nervous system, the neurologic examination may turn out to be normal. Perhaps a detailed study of the development of the brain and a histologic study of the interconnections would reveal differences, but this is not typically possible except in autopsy. In summary, if the child has not developed the basic wiring necessary for communication or if there is damage to the nervous system, little can be done to repair the abnormality. The child must learn to compensate for the damage or inadequate development through extensive treatment.

There are many ways that speech-language pathologists teach children to compensate for neurologic deficits. The child's ability to learn strategies for effective language learning depends to a great degree on the site and extent of brain injury. Some children require work on basic processes of attention, memory, and discrimination. Others require specific training on strategies for information retrieval, organization, or processing of information in specific modalities (reading, writing, listening). Children who are nonverbal require specific language training to learn vocabulary words and the concepts that underlie them. These children then need to learn word combinations

and the rules for generating syntactically correct sentences. Thus the treatment of language-impaired children may involve more than just training linguistic symbols but also the mechanisms that we use for information processing. Each case will have different strengths and limitations, and the speech-language pathologist must be prepared to design treatment programs to fit the unique needs of the language-impaired individual.

REFERENCES

Anderson K, Brown C, Tallal P. Developmental language disorders: evidence for a basic processing deficit. Curr Opin Neurol Neurosurg 1993; 6:98–106.

Archer L, Campbell D, Segalowitz S. A prospective study of hand preference and language development in 18- to 30-month olds. I. Hand preference. Dev Neuropsychol 1988;4(2):85–92.

Bakker L, Smink T, Reitsman P. Ear dominance and reading ability. Cortex 1973;9:301–312.

Bell M, Fox N. The relations between frontal brain electrical activity and cognitive development during infancy. Child Dev 1992;63:1142–1163.

Berlin C, Lowe S. Temporal and dichotic factors in central auditory testing. In: Katz J, ed. Handbook of clinical audiology. Baltimore: Williams & Wilkins, 1972.

Callaway E, Harris P. Coupling between cortical potentials from different areas. Science 1974;183:873–875.

Caplan B, Kinsbourne M. Cognitive style and dichotic asymmetries of disabled readers. Cortex 1982;18:357–366.

Carey S, Lockhart R. Encoding differences in recognition and recall. Memory and Cognition 1975;1:297–300.

Carmon A, Lavy S, Gordon H, Portnoy Z. Hemispheric differences in CBF during verbal and nonverbal tasks: brain work. Munksgaard: Alfred Benzon Symposium IV, 1975.

Davis A, Wada J. Hemispheric asymmetries in human infants: spectral analysis of flash and clicked evoked potentials. Brain and Language 1977; 4:23–31.

Day J. Right hemisphere language processing in normal right handers. J Exp Psychol [Hum Percept] 1977;3:518–528.

Dumas R, Morgan A. EEG asymmetry as a function of occupation, task and task difficulty. Neuropsychologia 1975;13:219–228.

Ellis H, Shepherd J. Recognition of abstract and concrete words presented in left and right visual fields. J Exp Psychol 1974;193:1035–1036.

Fischer K. Relations between brain and cognitive development. Child Dev 1987;58:623–632.

Fokes J. Fokes' sentence builder. New York: Teaching Resources, 1976.

Fried I, Tanguay P, Boder E, et al. Developmental dyslexia: electrophysiological evidence of clinical subgroups. Brain and Language 1981;12:14–22.

Galin D, Ellis R. Asymmetry in evoked potentials as an index of lateralized cognitive processes: relation to EEG asymmetry. Neuropsychologia 1975;13:45–50.

Gardiner M, Walter D. Evidence of hemispheric specialization from infant EEG. In: Harnad S, et al., eds. Lateralization in the nervous system. New York: Academic Press, 1977.

Garnica O. Some characteristics of prosodic input to young children. Paper presented at the SSRC Conference on Language Input and Acquisition, Boston, 1974.

Garren R. Hemispheric laterality differences among four levels of reading achievement. Percept Mot Skills 1980;50:119–123.

Gates A, Bradshaw J. The role of the cerebral hemispheres in music. Brain and Language 1977;9403–431.

Gazzaniga M. The bisected brain. New York: Appleton-Century-Crofts, 1970.

Gazzaniga M. Right hemisphere language following brain bisection: a 20 year perspective. Am Psychol 1983;38:525–537.

Geschwind N, Levitsky W. Human brain: left-right asymmetries in temporal speech region. Science 1968;161:186–187.

Goldman-Rakic P. Development of cortical circuitry and cognitive function. Child Dev 1987;58:601–622.

Greenough W. Enduring brain effects of differential experience and training. In: Rosenzweig M, Bennett E, eds. Neurological mechanisms of learning and memory. Cambridge, MA: MIT Press, 1976.

Guyer B, Friedman M. Hemispheric processing and cognitive styles in learning disabled and normal children. Child Dev 1975;46:658–668.

Hall J, Grossman L, Elwood K. Differences in encoding for free recall versus recognition. Memory and Cognition 1976;4:507–513.

Haynes W. Task effect and EEG alpha asymmetry: an analysis of linguistic processing in two response modes. Cortex 1980;16:95–102.

Haynes W, Hannay J. Alpha asymmetry for audiovisual and auditory processing of continuous linguisitc information by children. Aust J Hum Commun Disord 1983;11(2):15–24.

Haynes W, Moore W. Recognition and recall: an electroencephalographic investigation of hemispheric alpha asymmetries for males and females on perceptual and retrieval tasks. Percept Mot Skills 1981;53:283–290.

Hines D. Recognition of verbs, abstract nouns, and concrete nouns from the left and right visual halffields. Neuropsychologia 1976;14:211–216.

Hines D. Differences in tachistoscopic recognition between abstract and concrete words as a function of visual half-field and frequency. Cortex 1977;13:66–73.

Hiscock M, Inch R, Jacek C, et al. Is there a sex difference in human laterality? I. An exaustive survey of auditory laterality studies from six neuropsychology journals. J Clin Exp Neuropsychol 1994;16(3):423–435.

Hubbell R. Children's language disorders: an integrated approach. Englewood-Cliffs, NJ: Prentice-Hall, 1981.

Hugdahl K, Andersson B. Dichotic listening in 126 left-handed children: ear advantages, familial sinistrality and sex differences. Neuropsychologia 1989;27(7):999–1006.

Hynd G, Obrzut J, Weed W, Hynd C. Development of cerebral dominance: dichotic listening asymmetry in normal and learning disabled children. J Exp Child Psychol 1979;28:445–454.

Isaacs L, Haynes W. Linguistic processing and performance in articulation-disordered subgroups of language-impaired children. J Commun Disord 1984;17:109–120.

Jacobson M. Developmental neurobiology. New York: Holt, 1970.

Kimura D. Cerebral dominance and the perception of verbal stimuli. Can J Psychol 1961a;15:166–171.

Kimura D. Some effects of temporal lobe damage in auditory perception. Can J Psychol 1961b; 14:156–165.

Kimura D. Speech lateralization in young children as determined by an auditory test. J Comp Physiol Psychol 1963;56:899–902.

Kimura D. Spatial localization in left and right visual fields. Can J Psychol 1969;23:445–458.

Kimura D. The asymmetry of the human brain. Sci Am 1973;228:70–78.

Kinsbourne M. The development of cerebral dominance. In: Filskov C, Boll T, eds. Handbook of clinical neuropsychology. New York: Wiley, 1981.

Kinsbourne M, Hiscock M. The normal and deviant development of functional lateralization of the brain. In: Haith M, Campos J, eds. Handbook of child psychology. Vol. 2. Infancy and developmental psychobiology. New York: Wiley, 1983.

Kirk S, McCarthy J, Kirk W. Illinois test of psycholinguistic abilities. Urbana, IL: University of Illinois Press, 1968.

Knox C, Kimura D. Cerebral processing of nonverbal sounds in boys and girls. Neuropsychologia 1970;8:227–237.

Lasky E, Cox L. Auditory processing and language interaction: evaluation and intervention strategies. In: Lasky E, Katz J, eds. Central auditory processing disorders: problems of speech, language and learning. Baltimore: University Park Press, 1983.

Lenneberg E. Biological foundations of language. New York: Wiley, 1967.

Liley A. The fetus as a personality. Aust N Z J Psychiatry 1972;6:99–105.

Loring D, Meador K, Lee G, et al. Cerebral language lateralization: evidence from intracarotid amobarbital testing. Neuropsychologia 1990; 28(8):831–838.

Maxwell D. The neurology of learning and language disabilities: developmental considerations. In: Wallach G, Butler K, eds. Language learning disabilities in school-age children. Baltimore: Williams & Wilkins, 1984.

Mazziotta J, Metter E. Brain cerebral metabolic mapping of normal and abnormal language and its acquisition during development. In: Plum F, ed. Language, communication and the brain. New York: Raven Press, 1988.

McAdam D, Whitaker H. Language production: electroencephalographic localization in the normal human brain. Sci Am 1971;222:66–78.

McGee M. Human spatial abilities: psychometric studies and environmental, genetic, hormonal and neurological influences. Psychol Bull 1979; 86:889–918.

McGlone J. Sex difference in functional brain asymmetry. Cortex 1978;14:122–128.

McGlone J. Sex differences in human brain asymmetry: a critical survey. Behav Brain Sci 1980; 3:215–263.

McKeever W, Huling M. Lateral dominance in tachistoscopic word recognition as a function of hemisphere stimulation and interhemispheric transfer time. Neuropsychologia 1971;9:291–299.

Menyuk P. Linguistic problems in children with developmental dysphasia. In: Wyke M, ed. Developmental dysphasia. New York: Academic Press, 1978.

Miller G. The magical number seven, plus or minus two: some limits on our capacity for processing information. Psychol Rev 1956;63:81–96.

Molfese D. Infant cerebral asymmetry. In: Segalowitz S, Gruber F, eds. Language development and neurological theory. New York: Academic Press, 1977.

Molfese D, Molfese V. Cortical responses of preterm infants to phonetic and nonphonetic speech stimuli. Dev Psychol 1980;16:574–581.

Molfese D, Molfese V. Electrophysiological indices of auditory discrimination in newborn infants: the bases for predicting later language development? Infant Behav Dev 1985;8:197–211.

Mollgaard K, Diamond M, Bennett L, et al. Qualitative synaptic changes with differential experience in rat brain. Int J Neurosci 1971;2:113–128.

Nelson C, deRegnier R. Neural correlates of attention and memory in the first year of life. Dev Neuropsychol 1992;8:119–134.

Obrzut J, Hynd G, Obrzut A, Letigeb J. Time sharing and dichotic listening asymmetry in normal and learning disabled children. Brain and Language 1980;11:181–194.

Obrzut J, Hynd G, Obrzut A, Pirozzolo F. Effect of directed attention on cerebral asymmetries in normal and learning disabled children. Dev Psychol 1981;17(1):118–125.

Obrzut J, Obrzut A, Bryden M, Bartels S. Information processing and speech lateralization in learning disabled children. Brain and Language 1985;25:87–101.

Omerod F. The pathology of congenital deafness in the child. In: Ewing A, ed. The modern educational treatment of deafness. Manchester, England: Manchester University Press, 1960.

Pettit J, Helms S. Cerebral dominance and language and articulation disordered children as measured by dichotic listening tasks. Paper presented at the American Speech and Hearing Association Convention, Las Vegas, 1974.

Provins K. Early infant motor asymmetries and handedness: a critical evaluation of the evidence. Dev Neuropsychol 1992;8(4):325–365.

Rasmussen T, Milner B. The role of early left brain injury in determining lateralization of cerebral speech functions. In: Dimond S, Blizzard D, eds. Evolution and lateralization of the brain. New York: New York Academy of Sciences, 1977.

Robbins K, McAdam D. Interhemispheric alpha asymmetry and imagery mode. Brain and Language 1974;1:189–193.

Rosenblum D, Dorman M. Hemispheric specialization for speech perception in language deficient kindergarten children. Brain and Language 1978;6:378–389.

Rosenzweig M, Bennett E. Effects of environmental enrichment or impoverishment on learning and on brain values in rodents. In: Oliverio A, ed. Genetics, environment and intelligence. Amsterdam: Elsevier-North Holland, 1977.

Rourke B, Bakker D, Fisk J, Strang J. Child neuropsychology: an introduction to theory, research and clinical practice. New York: Guilford Press, 1983.

Satz P, Strauss E, Whitaker H. The ontogeny of hemispheric specialization: some old hypotheses revisited. Brain and Language 1990;38:596–614.

Selnes O. The corpus callosum: some anatomical and functional considerations with special reference to language. Brain and Language 1974;1:111–139.

Selnes O, Whitaker H. Neurological substrates of language and speech production. In: Rosenberg S, ed. Sentence production: developments in research and theory. Hillsdale, NJ: Lawrence Erlbaum Associates, 1977.

Shaywitz B, Shaywitz S, Pugh K, et al. Sex differences in the functional organization of the brain for language. Nature 1995;6515:607–610.

Sheibel A. Some structural and developmental correlates of human speech. In: Gibson K, Peterson A, eds. Brain maturation and cognitive development: comparative and cross-cultural perspectives. New York: Aldine De Gruyter, 1991.

Sidtis J, Sadler A, Nass R. Dichotic complex-pitch and speech discrimination in 7 to 12 year old children. Dev Neuropsychol 1987;3(4):227–238.

Sommers R, Taylor M. Cerebral speech dominance in language disordered and normal children. Cortex 1972;8:224–232.

Spreen O, Tupper D, Risser A, et al. Human developmental neuropsychology. New York: Oxford University Press, 1984.

Springer S, Deutsch G. Left brain, right brain. New York: W. H. Freeman, 1985.

Springer S, Eisenson J. Hemispheric specialization

for speech in language disordered children. Neuropsychologia 1977;16:287–293.

Stark R, Tallal P. Perceptual and motor deficits in language impaired children. In: Keith R, ed. Central auditory and language disorders in children. San Diego: College-Hill, 1981.

Tallal P, Merzenich M. New treatments for language-impaired children: integrating basic and clinical research. Invited session presented at the annual convention of the American Speech-Language-Hearing Association, Seattle, WA, 1996.

Talla P, Stark R. Speech acoustic cue discrimination abilities of normally developing and language impaired children. J Acoust Soc Am 1981;69:568–574.

Thomson M. Laterality and reading attainment. Br J Educ Psychol 1976;46:317–321.

Tramontana M, Hooper S, eds. Assessment issues in child neuropsychology. New York: Plenum Press, 1988.

Turkewitz G, Birch G. Neurobehavioral organization of the human newborn. In: Hellmuth J, ed. Exceptional infant. II. Studies in abnormalities. New York: Brunner/Mazel, 1971.

Vellutino F, Bentley W, Phillips F. Inter- versus intra-hemispheric learning in dyslexic and normal readers. Dev Med Child Neurol 1978;20:71–80.

Volkmar F, Greenough W. Rearing complexity affects branching of dendrites in the visual cortex of the rat. Science 1972;76:1445–1447.

Wada J. A new method for the determination of the side of cerebral speech dominance. Med Biol 1949;14:221–222.

Wallesch C, Henriksen L, Kornhuber H, Paulson O. Observations on regional cerebral blood flow in cortical and subcortical structures during language production in normal man. Brain and Language 1985;25:224–233.

Witelson S. Early hemisphere specialization and interhemisphere plasticity: an empirical and theoretical review. In: Segalowitz S, Gruber F, eds. Language development and neurological theory. New York: Academic Press, 1977.

Witelson S. Neurobiological aspects of language in children. Child Dev 1987;58:653–688.

Yeni-Komshian G, Isenberg D, Goldberg H. Cerebral dominance and reading disability: left visual field deficit in poor readers. Neuropsychologia 1975;14:83–93.

Zaidel E. Auditory language comprehension in the right hemisphere following cerebral commissurotomy and hemispherectomy: a comparison with child language and aphasia. In: Caramazza A, Zurif E, eds. Language acquisition and language breakdown. Baltimore: Johns Hopkins University Press, 1978.

Zemlin W. Speech and hearing science. Englewood-Cliffs, NJ: Prentice-Hall, 1968.

Zimmerman G, Knott J. Slow potentials of the brain related to speech processing in normal speakers and stutterers. Electroencephalogr Clin Neurophysiol 1974;37:599–607.

Zurif E, Carson G. Cerebral dominance and reading disability: left visual field deficit in poor readers. Neuropsychologia 1970;8:351–361.

CHAPTER 3

Theories of Communication Development

Brian B. Shulman

ow do children acquire *communication skills?* This is certainly an easy question to pose, yet quite a difficult one to answer. This question has been asked for thousands of years, dating back to the days of historic Greece. Knowledge about how children develop communication skills is never-ending. That is to say, research into communication development is a continuous process. Researchers all over the world are conducting studies to further our understanding of these very complex phenomena called language and communication. Moreover, the role of innate processes and the environment (i.e., nature versus nurture) in children's language acquisition continues to be argued by many theorists. Over the years, however, four theoretical perspectives on language development have surfaced: the *Behavioral*, *Psycholinguistic-Syntactic*, *Semantic-Cognitive*, and *Social-Pragmatic*. The purpose of this chapter is to describe each perspective, offering both limitations and contributions and to extend the discussion into making inferences about how each theoretical perspective may impact clinical assessment and treatment for children who exhibit deficits in communication development.

THE BEHAVIORAL PERSPECTIVE

World-renowned psychologist B.F. Skinner (1957) and others (Mowrer, 1954; Osgood, 1963; Staats, 1963) have proposed a behavioral or *empiricist* perspective on language acquisition. Language is, therefore, learned or conditioned through experience and by an association between a stimulus and the subsequent response. It is thought to be a set of associations between meaning and word, word and phoneme, statement and response (Owens, 1988).

Behaviorists assert that language is a set of verbal behaviors learned through *operant conditioning*, a method of changing behavior in which one waits for the response to be conditioned to occur spontaneously, immediately after which the child is provided a reinforcer (i.e., *selective reinforcement*). James provides a linguistic example to illustrate this concept:

A child says *mama* as his mother starts to pick him up. The mother, who is delighted that the child knows her name, gives him a big hug and kiss and says, *Mama, that's right—I'm mama!* The affectionate physical response from the mother is undoubtedly pleasurable and is likely, therefore, to increase the probability that the child will say *mama* again. In other words, the mother's response to the child's behavior was a reinforcer (1990, p. 165).

In addition to selective reinforcement, the behaviorists believe that language is learned or mastered by *imitation* and *practice*. Imitation is behavior that copies, almost exactly, the behavior of another. More specifically, the behaviorist perspective notes that when the parent says a word, the child, in learning the word, imitates the adult's production. The parent may accept an approximation of the desired word imitation (e.g., "ba" for "bottle") from the child at a young age. This is termed *shaping*, a technique for obtaining responses that are not in the child's (linguistic) repertoire (Nicolosi, Harryman, & Kresheck, 1989). Such will not be the case, however, when the child gets older. The child will be given numerous opportunities to *practice* the correct production. As he matures, responses that approximate the adult model will be reinforced. By reinforcing correct productions, the parent shapes the child's utterances until they are grammatical and acceptable (Bernstein & Tiegerman, 1985). It is thought that imitation plays a major role, not only in the child's acquisition of single words but also in acquiring more advanced strings of word combinations.

Limitation

Like any theoretical orientation, aspects of the behavioral perspective have been criticized by many (Brown & Hanlon, 1970; Chomsky, 1957, 1959; McNeill, 1970; Moerk, 1974; Bloom, Lightbown, & Hood, 1975). Specific points of criticism include the following:

1. Parents of young language-learning children reinforce only a small percentage of their children's utterances. They tend to ignore grammatical errors and reinforce for truthfulness of utterances; parents rarely, if ever, correct or punish children's grammatical errors (Brown & Hanlon, 1970).

2. Chomsky makes the following two statements:

> I have been able to find no support whatsoever for the doctrine that slow and careful shaping of verbal behavior through differential reinforcement is an absolute necessity (1959, p. 42).

> There is little point in speculating about the process of acquisition without a much better understanding of what is acquired (1959, p. 55).

3. Imitation is infrequently used by children above the age of 2 years (Moerk, 1974; Nelson, 1973; Owens & MacDonald, 1982; Bloom, Lightbown, & Hood, 1975; Chomsky, 1957; McNeill, 1970).

Contributions/Clinical Applications

While the Behavioral perspective has been criticized over the years, it has recently received greater attention and importance relative to communication development. Researchers (Fitzgerald & Karnes, 1987; McDade & Varnedoe, 1987; Newport, 1976; Snow, 1972) have reaffirmed the role of parental linguistic input in communication development. Carrow-Woolfolk (1988) stated the following:

> The essence of assessment, according to behavioral theory, is the clinician's judgment of the inadequacy of a child's language ability based on *performance* (what the child does), compared with what the child should be doing. The basic approach of this theory to intervention is that of *teaching* the nonlanguage child (using a basic stimulus-response [S-R] paradigm) to produce adequate language structure (1988, p.9).

Furthermore, Bernstein & Tiegerman (1985) note that systematic training designs and their applications to nonspeaking individuals have been a direct outgrowth of the behavioral perspective. Such structured assessment and intervention programs are described by Schiefelbusch and Bricker (1981) and McCormick and Schiefelbusch (1990).

THE PSYCHOLINGUISTIC-SYNTACTIC PERSPECTIVE

The Psycholinguistic-Syntactic perspective is also referred to as the *Innatist* or *Nativist* perspective. Regardless of the name used, the belief here is that the acquisition of language is an innate, physiologically determined, genetically transmitted phenomenon.

During the late 1950s and into the early 1960s, psycholinguist Noam Chomsky stressed the role of language form (or syntax) and its underlying mental processes (or "electronic circuitry") in describing language acquisition. He stated the following:

> The problem for the linguist, as well as for the child learning the language, is to determine from the data of performance the underlying system of rules that has been mastered by the speaker-hearer and that he puts to use in actual performance. Hence, in the technical sense, linguistic theory is mentalistic, since it is concerned with discovering a mental reality underlying actual behavior (Chomsky, 1965, p. 4).

Chomsky tried to describe language from a scientific perspective and, in turn, create a theoretical explanation for the manner by which humans create and make judgments about language (Owens, 1988). He notes further that children have an innate predisposition or capacity to apply linguistic rules. Moreover, Chomsky asserts that the newborn is "pre-wired" for language acquisition and is born with a *Language Acquisition Device (LAD)*, an innate linguistic mechanism that is activated by exposure to linguistic stimuli. The LAD is assumed to contain two parts: a set of rules or general principles for forming sentences, and the procedures for discovering how these principles are to be applied to the child's particular language (Bernstein & Tiegerman, 1985).

The original focus of this perspective was on grammatical development, and the description of language was in the form of characterizing specific syntactic components (i.e., parts of speech). "Subsequent movement from an emphasis on syntax

and the theory of innateness in development to an emphasis on semantics and the consequent concern with the cognitive role in language learning was a movement from a purely linguistic interpretation of language to a psycholinguistic one" (Carrow-Woolfolk, 1988, p. 14).

Limitations

Like the Behavioral perspective, the Psycholinguistic-Syntactic perspective has also been criticized (Bowerman, 1976; Brown, 1973; Fillmore, 1968; Nelson, 1973; Newport, 1976; Owens, 1988; Phillips, 1973; Schlesinger, 1977; Sinclair-deZwart, 1973; Snow, 1972). Specific points of criticism include the following:

1. Chomsky treats language learning as if it occurred independently of cognitive development (Schlesinger, 1977; Sinclair-deZwart, 1973).

2. Language depends more on underlying semantic knowledge than on grammatical rules (Fillmore, 1968). Furthermore, a theory based solely on a syntactic orientation cannot explain why the sentence, "Lively tables leap narrowly under the ceiling" does not make any sense (Owens, 1988).

3. Parental input enhances language learning (Nelson, 1973; Newport, 1976; Phillips, 1973; Snow, 1972).

4. "The issue of innateness is the weakest aspect of Chomsky's theory. The notion of a language acquisition device is too simplified and provides an inadequate explanation. To assume the ability to use language is innate does little to facilitate our understanding of the actual process of language development" (Owens, 1988, p. 41).

Contributions/Clinical Applications

The model of language proposed by Bloom and Lahey (1978) and presented in Figure 3.1 describes language as the integration of *form* (language structure), *content* (language meaning), and *use* (purpose of language is a particular communicative context).

Such a model may be viewed as an out-

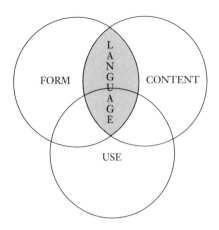

Figure 3.1. Model of language. (From Bloom L, Lahey M. Language development and language disorders. New York: John Wiley, 1978; p. 22. Reprinted with the permission of Macmillan Publishing Company.)

growth of the Psycholinguistic-Syntactic perspective. From a clinical standpoint, this model has been used by speech-language pathologists to determine the extent to which the child applies rules of language form (syntax), content (semantics), and use (pragmatics). The language the child needs to learn is determined by comparing the child's language performance with normative data, and not by judging adequacy related to underlying emotional, intellectual, or physiological factors (Carrow-Woolfolk, 1988).

THE SEMANTIC-COGNITIVE PERSPECTIVE

The Semantic-Cognitive perspective on language acquisition focused on the meanings conveyed by the child's productions and not on the syntactic complexity of the utterances. Beginning in the late 1960s and early 1970s, Lois Bloom studied children's language at the multiword or combinatory stage. In examining the utterances used by one child, she noted that the child used the utterance "mommy sock" on two different occasions to convey two different meanings. She used this two-word utterance to describe her mother putting on her (i.e., the child's) sock and also when describing that the sock she was picking up belonged to her

mother. After further analysis, Bloom concluded that children's language extends meaning and that meaning relationships or **semantic relations** are coded by children as they reach this multiword, combinatory stage in language acquisition (see Chapter 10 for a detailed discussion of early multiword language development). Bloom further postulated that children express meanings long before they know anything about syntax, and the meanings they convey are based on prior cognitive knowledge (Bernstein & Tiegerman, 1985).

As a result of Bloom's (1970) pioneering work, greater emphasis was placed on cognitive development and its impact on the language-learning process. A move from a less structural-syntactic approach to a more meaning-based approach (i.e., "a semantic revolution") predominated this period (Schlesinger, 1971; Slobin, 1973). Bernstein and Tiegerman (1985) noted Norma Rees' (1980) comment as best describing the Semantic-Cognitive perspective on language acquisition. Rees states that "children say only what they know how to mean" (1980, p. 21).

Limitations

Limitations of the Semantic-Cognitive perspective have been described in the literature (Bowerman, 1978; Cromer, 1974; McLean & Snyder-McLean, 1978; Schlesinger, 1977). Specific points of criticism include the following:

1. This approach does not explain why some children are behind in language development yet have normal cognitive skills (Cromer, 1974).

2. This theory ignores the role of linguistic input in the language-learning process (Schlesinger, 1977).

3. Such an approach does not answer the question of how children acquire language, nor does it explain the relationship between later cognitive abilities and subsequent linguistic development (Bowerman, 1978).

4. McLean and Snyder-McLean (1978) argue that any theory of language acquisition "must also include the basic nature and purpose of children's communicative trans-actions within the social context in which they reside or function" (p. 41).

Contributions/Clinical Applications

The Semantic-Cognitive perspective has attempted to stress the interrelation-ship between language learning and cogni-tion. In assessing a potential language problem, the speech-language pathologist should include some description about the child's cognitive knowledge (i.e., the strate-gies he uses to acquire new information). In describing the impact this theoretical per-spective has had on intervention, Carrow-Woolfolk (1988) stated the following:

> The emphasis on intervention is three-fold: increasing the child's quality and quantity of internal relations, improving the child's strategies of learning and dis-covering, and increasing the accuracy and speed of using the skill (e.g., language). In-tervention involves making input available so that analysis and learning can take place (p. 21).

THE SOCIAL-PRAGMATIC PERSPECTIVE

The Social-Pragmatic perspective is the most contemporary of the four theo-retical perspectives on language acquisi-tion. Its major thrust has been described quite eloquently by Searle (1965) who stated the following:

> The purpose of language is communica-tion. The unit of communication in lan-guage is the speech act, of the type called il-locutionary act. The problem (or at least an important problem) of the theory of lan-guage is to describe how we get from the sounds to the illocutionary acts . . . The rules enable us to get from the brute facts of the making of noises to the institutional facts of the performance of illocutionary acts of human communication (p. 38).

The Social-Pragmatic perspective con-siders *communication* to be the basic func-tion of language, quite different from the basic tenets of the three other theoretical orientations previously discussed.

According to this perspective, the *speech act* is the basic primitive commu-nicative unit used by the child within a particular setting or *context* (Austin, 1962; Bates, 1976; Coggins & Carpenter, 1981; Dore, 1974, 1975, 1986; Halliday, 1975; Muma, 1978; Searle, 1965). This perspec-tive is viewed not only within a *communi-cation* framework, but within a *social* framework as well.

Within this model, language learning is first observed within mother/caretaker-child interactions. As caretakers respond to infants' early reflexive behaviors and gestures, the infant learns to communi-cate intentions (see Chapter 5 for a com-plete discussion on caretaker-child inter-action).

Limitations

The Social-Pragmatic perspective, as with the other theoretical orientations presented here, does not satisfactorily ex-plain language acquisition. Specific criti-cisms include the following:

1. Bernstein & Tiegerman (1985) cite two major questions that remain unan-swered by this theoretical perspective: *How do communicative intentions get linked to linguistic structures?* and *How do children acquire symbols for referents?*

2. The newness of this theoretical per-spective has resulted in researchers unable to agree on a common system for classify-ing communicative intentions (see Bates, 1976; Dore, 1975; Halliday, 1975; Roth & Spekman, 1984).

Contributions/Clinical Applications

This perspective emphasizes the *socio-communicative* aspect of language. McLean and McLean (1978) delineate five major points specific to understand-ing the "social dynamics which affect and effect the language acquisition process" (p. 78). These are as follows:

1. Language is acquired because, and only if, the child has a reason to talk. This, in turn, means that he has become "so-cialized" . . . and has learned that he can affect his environments through the process of communication.

2. Language is first acquired as a means of achieving already existing communicative functions. These preverbal communicative functions seem to be directly related to the functional or pragmatic aspect of later language.

3. Linguistic structure is initially acquired through the process of decoding and comprehending incoming linguistic stimuli. At later stages of development, the processes of imitation and expansion may serve to help the child refine his emerging language system.

4. Language is learned in dynamic social interactions involving the child and the mature language users in the environment. The mature language users facilitate this process through their tendency to segment and mark the components of the interaction and to provide appropriate linguistic models.

5. The child is an active participant in this transactional process and must contribute to it a set of behaviors which allow him to benefit from the adult's facilitating behaviors (p.78).

From a clinical standpoint, knowledge provided by this theoretical perspective has facilitated the design of procedures that assess and treat the child's language impairment from a sociocommunicative and contextual perspective. Based on this perspective, Arwood (1991) states that the major goal of assessment is to study the effectiveness of the child's interactions and success in using linguistic skills to manipulate the environment. Furthermore, assessment involves the description of the child's pragmatic skills observed in naturalistic contexts. Specific assessment instruments have been designed that evaluate young children's pragmatic skills (Bray & Wiig, 1987; Coggins & Carpenter, 1981; Shulman, 1986), as well as more advanced conversational skills in school-age children (Damico, 1985; Simon, 1986; Semel & Wiig, 1982; Wiig, 1982a, 1982b, 1987, 1990).

In turn, the goal of intervention is *social communicative competence*. Intervention provided in naturalistic, language-learning settings will facilitate the development of socially appropriate, pragmatic (communicative) behaviors. Intervention procedures and activities based on the tenets of the Social-Pragmatic perspective have also evolved (Glaser, Johnston, & Weinrich, 1984, 1986, 1987; Hoskins, 1987; Marquis, 1985, 1988a, 1988b, 1990a, 1990b; Simon, 1981; Wiig, 1982).

It is important to remember that as theoretical perspectives emerge, we acquire an expanded knowledge base about the ways in which we can answer the question, *How do children acquire communication skills?* Each perspective presented in this chapter has, in some way, impacted the assessment and intervention procedures currently used by speech-language pathologists. Owens (1988) stated the following:

> We must also face the possibility that none of the descriptive units used within the four theoretical models has any reality for children. In each case, linguists have imposed adult classification models upon child language. Children may be organizing their worlds in very nonadult ways as they play and explore, as they fantasize and create, and as they think and speak (p. 61).

In summary, the question posed at the beginning of the chapter remains unanswered. However, numerous attempts have been made to bring us closer to answering this very important question. Our knowledge about language acquisition has extended from a purely structural orientation to one that is more interactive, social, and communicative.

REFERENCES

Arwood EL. Semantic and pragmatic language disorders. 2nd ed. Gaithersburg, MD: Aspen Publishers, 1991.

Austin JL. How to do things with words. Cambridge, England: Oxford University Press, 1962.

Bates E. Language and context: the acquisition of pragmatics. New York: Academic Press, 1976.

Bernstein DK, Tiegerman E. Language and communication disorders in children. Columbus, OH: Charles E. Merrill Publishing, 1985.

Bloom L. Language development: form and function of emerging grammars. Cambridge, MA: MIT Press, 1970.

Bloom L, Lahey M. Language development and language disorders. New York: John Wiley, 1978.

Bloom L, Lightbown P, Hood L. Structure and variation in child language. Monogr Soc Res Child Dev 1975;40:1–97.

Bowerman M. Semantic factors in the acquisition of rules for word use and sentence construction. In: Morehead D, Morehead A, eds. Normal and deficient child language. Baltimore, MD: University Park Press, 1976.

Bowerman M. The acquisition of word meaning: an investigation in some current conflicts. In: Waterson N, Snow C, eds. The development of communication. New York: John Wiley, 1978.

Bray CM, Wiig EH. Let's talk inventory for children. San Antonio, TX: The Psychological Corporation, 1987.

Brown R. A first language: the early stages. Cambridge, MA: Harvard University Press, 1973.

Brown RJ, Hanlon C. Derivational complexity and order of acquisition. In: Hayes J, ed. Cognition and the development of language. New York: John Wiley, 1970.

Carrow-Woolfolk E. Theory, assessment and intervention in language disorders: an integrative approach. Philadelphia: Grune & Stratton, 1988.

Chomsky N. Syntactic structures. The Hague: Houston, 1957.

Chomsky N. A review of Skinner's "Verbal Behavior." Language 1959;35:26–58.

Chomsky N. Aspects of the theory of syntax. Cambridge, MA: MIT Press, 1965.

Coggins TE, Carpenter RL. The communicative intention inventory: a system for coding children's early intentional communication. Appl Psycholinguist 1981;2:235–252.

Cromer R. The development of language and cognition: the cognitive hypothesis. In: Foss D, ed. New perspectives in child development. New York: Penguin Education, 1974.

Damico JS. (1985). Clinical discourse analysis: a functional language assessment technique. In: Simon CS, ed. Communication skills and classroom success: assessment of language-learning disabled students. San Diego: College-Hill, 1985; pp. 152–217.

Dore J. A pragmatic description of early language development. J Psycholinguist Res 1974;3:343–350.

Dore J. Holophrases, speech acts, and language universals. J Child Language 1975;2:21–40.

Dore J. The development of conversational competence. In: Schiefelbusch R, ed. Language competence: assessment and intervention. San Diego, CA: College-Hill Press, 1986.

Fillmore C. The case for case. In: Bach E, Harmes R, eds. Universals in linguistic theory. New York: Holt, Rinehart & Winston, 1968.

Fitzgerald MT, Karnes DE. A parent-implemented language model for at-risk and developmentally delayed preschool children. Top Lang Disord 1987;7(3):31–46.

Glaser AJ, Johnston EB, Weinrich BD. A sourcebook of pragmatic activities: theory and intervention for language therapy. Tucson, AZ: Communication Skill Builders, 1984.

Glaser AJ, Johnston EB, Weinrich BD. A sourcebook of adolescent pragmatic activities: theory and intervention for language therapy. Tucson, AZ: Communication Skill Builders, 1986.

Glaser AJ, Johnston EB, Weinrich BD. A sourcebook for remediating language: lesson plans for developing communication within the cognitive-experience frame. Tucson, AZ: Communication Skill Builders, 1987.

Halliday MAK. Learning how to mean: explorations in the development of language. New York: Elsevier-North Holland Publishing, 1975.

Hoskins B. Conversations: language intervention for adolescents. Allen, TX: DLM Teaching Resources, 1987.

James SL. Normal language acquisition. Boston, MA: Little, Brown, 1990.

Marquis MA. Pragmatic-language trivia. Tucson, AZ: Communication Skill Builders, 1985.

Marquis MA. More pragmatic-language trivia: games for promoting effective communication in older children and adolescents. Tucson, AZ: Communication Skill Builders, 1988a.

Marquis MA. The question collection: teaching questioning strategies: a pragmatic approach. Tucson, AZ: Communication Skill Builders, 1988b.

Marquis MA. Pragmatic-language trivia for thinking skills: a game for promoting effective communication in older children and adolescents. Tucson, AZ: Communication Skill Builders, 1990a.

Marquis MA. Pragmatic-language trivia junior: a game for promoting effective communication in children ages 7–10. Tucson, AZ: Communication Skill Builders, 1990b.

McConnell NL, Blagden CM. RAPP! Resource of activities for peer pragmatics. Moline, IL: LinguiSystems, 1986.

McCormick L, Schiefelbusch RL. Early language intervention. 2nd ed. Columbus, OH: Merrill Publishing, 1990.

McDade HL, Varnedoe DR. Training parents to be language facilitators. Top Lang Disord 1987;7(3):19–30.

McLean JE, Snyder-McLean LK. A transactional approach to early language training. Columbus, OH: Charles E. Merrill Publishing, 1978.

McNeill D. The acquisition of language: the study of developmental psycholinguistics. New York: Harper & Row, 1970.

Moerk E. Changes in verbal mother-child interaction with increasing language skills of the child. J Psycholinguist Res 1974;3:101–116.

Mowrer O. The psychologist looks at language. Am Psychol 1954;9:660–694.

Muma J. Language handbook: concepts, assessment, intervention. Englewood Cliffs, NJ: Prentice-Hall, 1978.

Nelson K. Structure and strategy in learning to talk. Monogr Soc Res Child Dev 1973;38:136.

Newport E. Motherese: the speech of mothers to young children. In: Castellan J, Pisoni D, Potts G, eds. Cognitive theory. Vol. 2. Hillsdale, NJ: Lawrence Erlbaum Associates, 1976.

Nicolosi L, Harryman E, Krescheck J. Terminology of communication disorders: speech-language-hearing. 3rd ed. Baltimore, MD: Williams & Wilkins, 1989.

Osgood C. On understanding and creating sentences. Am Psychol 1963;18:735–751.

Owens RE. Language development: an introduction. 2nd ed. Columbus, OH: Merrill Publishing, 1988.

Owens R, MacDonald, J. Communicative uses of early speech of nondelayed and Down syndrome children. Am J Ment Defic 1982;86:503–511.

Phillips J. Syntax and vocabulary of mothers' speech to young children: age and sex comparisons. Child Dev 1973;44:182–185.

Rees N. Learning to talk and understand. In: Hixon TJ, Shriberg LD, Saxon JH, eds. Introduction to communication disorders. Englewood Cliffs, NJ: Prentice-Hall, 1980.

Roth FP, Spekman NJ. Assessing the pragmatic abilities of children. J Speech Hear Disord 1984;49:2–17.

Schiefelbusch RL, Bricker DD, eds. Early language: acquisition and intervention. Baltimore, MD: University Park Press, 1981.

Schlesinger I. The role of cognitive development and linguistic input in language acquisition. J Child Lang 1977;4:153–169.

Searle J. What is a speech act? In: Black M, ed. Philosophy in America. New York: Cornell University Press, 1965.

Semel E, Wiig EH. Clinical language intervention program (CLIP). San Antonio, TX: The Psychological Corporation, 1982.

Shulman BB. Test of pragmatic skills—revised. Tucson, AZ: Communication Skill Builders, 1986.

Simon CS. Communicative competence: a functional-pragmatic approach to language therapy. Tucson, AZ: Communication Skill Builders, 1981.

Simon CS. Evaluating communicative competence: a functional pragmatic procedure. Tucson, AZ: Communication Skill Builders, 1986.

Sinclair-deZwart H. Language acquisition and cognitive development. In: Moore TE, ed. Cognitive development and the acquisition of language. New York: Academic Press, 1973.

Skinner BF. Verbal behavior. New York: Appleton-Century-Crofts, 1957.

Slobin D. Cognitive prerequisites for the development of grammar. In: Ferguson C, Slobin D, eds. Studies of child language development. New York: Holt, Rinehart & Winston, 1973.

Snow C. Mother's speech to children learning language. Child Dev 1972;43:549–566.

Staats AW. Complex human behavior. New York: Holt, Rinehart & Winston, 1963.

Wiig EH. Let's talk: developing prosocial communication skills. San Antonio, TX: The Psychological Corporation, 1982a.

Wiig EH. Let's talk inventory for adolescents (LTI-A). San Antonio, TX: The Psychological Corporation, 1982b.

Wiig EH. Wiig criterion referenced inventory of language (CRIL). San Antonio, TX: The Psychological Corporation, 1990.

CHAPTER 4

Child Development

Brian B. Shulman

Communication development is a part of human development. As children develop the ability to communicate effectively in the real world, they develop other skills relating to their ability to think (i.e., cognitive development), their ability to move about the environment and manipulate objects (i.e., motor development), and their ability to interact appropriately with others (i.e., social development).

Owens (1988) states that "development is more than a cumulative list of changes and accomplishments" (p. 63). It is a predictable, orderly, and sequential process. In describing the developing child, Owens (1988) delineates the following five general principles:

- *Development is predictable.*
- *Developmental milestones are attained at about the same age in most children.*
- *Developmental opportunity is needed.*
- *Children go through developmental phases or periods.*
- *Individuals differ greatly.*

Child development is a continuous sequence that establishes a regular pattern, which, in turn, should result in steady refinement as it progresses. Within a particular developmental process, children proceed through various developmental phases or stages that are not linear in fashion, but rather are orderly and predictable. Emphasis here is placed on specific developmental areas. In physical development, for example, we note two phases of rapid growth: a period from the prenatal months to 6 months and, again, a period from 10 or 12 months to 15 or 16 months. During these periods the infant's nutritional needs are greatest and during other periods, growth is decelerated. Such physical stages of development do not necessarily coincide with the stages of cognitive or social development; each area is represented by its own *developmental cycle.*

As the child matures, specific developmental milestones are attained at roughly the same chronologic age in most children. Certain skills and behaviors are developed at predictable ages. It is important to note that heredity, learning, and maturation play a major role in child development. Developmental milestones alone cannot entirely account for a child's overall growth and development. Maturation, for example, allows for some skills to become refined that are also preprogrammed functions such as biologic growth and anatomic growth (Bourne & Ekstrand, 1979).

Numerous skills do, however, develop at roughly the same time in most children independent of any specific training. Skills such as eye focus and movement, walking, and talking develop as the result of optical and vocal muscle development, as well as general muscular development. While specific training may not be required to develop such skills, Owens (1988) does note that for these abilities to develop, the *opportunity* for learning must be evident. Walking, for example, will not take place unless the child receives the opportunity to practice such prerequisite skills as kicking, crawling, or pulling oneself up. Such developmental opportunities play a significant role in how well or how poorly the child's overall development progresses over time. A child must grow up in an environment that is *stimulating;* one which offers opportunity for cognitive, motor, social, and communication development. Children who grow up in environments that are not stimulating are at risk for developmental disabilities.

The purposes of this chapter are to provide a general overview of cognitive, motor, social, and communicative development from birth through school-age; to describe the importance and relationships of each area to communication development; and in turn, to describe how knowledge about child development impacts the clinical assessment process.

A DEVELOPMENTAL OVERVIEW

To provide a general description of cognitive, motor, social, and communication development from birth through the school-age years, tables adapted from those contained in Nicolosi, Harryman, and Kresheck (1989, pp. 305–308, 315–317, 319–320) are used throughout this section to illustrate the various milestones achieved by the child within each developmental domain. Each table further describes the skill (i.e., cognitive, motor, social, communicative) based on the age levels of *Infancy I* (birth to 6 months), *Infancy II* (6- to 12 months), *Early Childhood* (12 to 24 months),

Preschool (2 to 5 years), and *School-Age* (5 years and older).

Cognitive Development

Cognitive development refers to the progressive and continuous growth of perception, memory, imagination, conception, judgment, and reason; it is the intellectual counterpart of one's biologic adaptation to the environment (Nicolosi, Harryman, & Kresheck, 1989). Cognitive development also involves the methods a child uses to organize, store, and retrieve information for problem solving and generalization (Owens, 1988). Cognitive development is based primarily on four factors: *maturation, physical experience, social interaction,* and *a general progression toward equilibrium* (Piaget, 1950, 1952, 1954, 1974; Piaget & Inhelder, 1958, 1969; Pulaski, 1980). For Piaget, intellectual development is the process of restructuring knowledge. The process starts with a structure or a way of thinking. Some external disturbance or intrusion on an ordinary way of thinking creates a conflict or *disequilibrium.* The child compensates for the disturbance and solves the conflict by means of his own intellectual activity. The final state is a new way of thinking and structuring things, a way that provides new understanding and satisfaction, a state of *new equilibrium.* No single factor can account for intellectual development by itself. It is a combination of maturation, physical experience, social interaction, and equilibrium and the interactions between and among them that influence this development.

Moreover, the study of cognitive development, namely, the child's intellectual growth, has been based on some theoretical orientations, including *faculty psychologies, Piagetian theory,* and *schema theories.* For the purpose of this chapter, however, the Piagetian perspective will be addressed as it relates to the child's progression through a series of developmental stages described in the literature (Labinowicz, 1980; Piaget, 1950, 1952, 1954, 1974; Pulaski, 1980; Rosenblith & Sims-Knight, 1985).

In observing children Piaget noticed patterns in their responses to intellectual tasks. Children of similar ages responded in ways that were at the same time remarkably similar and yet remarkably different from adult responses and expectations. Likewise, children at different ages had their own characteristic way of responding (Labinowicz, 1980). Table 4.1 illustrates the four cognitive developmental stages categorized by Piaget.

The first two stages of development, the sensorimotor and preoperational periods, are collectively termed the *preparatory, prelogical stages*. Likewise, the concrete and formal operational stages are collectively called the *advanced, logical thinking stages*. Each individual stage, however, is characterized by specific developmental milestones.

Beginning at birth and extending to age 2 years, the child coordinates his physical actions. His behavior, while primarily motoric, is described as *prerepresentational* and *preverbal*; there is no conceptual thought, although the infant's reflexive behavior emerges into intellectual behavior. During the preoperational stage, ranging from 2 to 7 years, the child is able to represent action through thought and language. His intellectual development at this stage is called *prelogical*.

As the child matures and enters the advanced, logical thinking stages, he develops the ability to apply logical thought to concrete problems such as *reversibility* (i.e., the ability to follow a line of reasoning back to where it began), *seriation* (i.e., the ability to mentally arrange elements in a series according to value, size, or any other criterion), and *classification* (i.e., the act of grouping objects according to their similarities). As the child enters Piaget's formal operations stage of cognitive development, he begins to develop an ability to solve both verbal and scientific problems. Abstract thought and logical reasoning predominate the intellectual growth of the child at this final stage of cognitive development. Table 4.2 illustrates milestones achieved by the child from birth through 11 years of age across the four major Piagetian stages of cognitive development.

Morehead and Morehead (1974), in describing important aspects of Piaget's theory, delineate some relationships between cognitive development and communication development. Chapter 6 offers detailed discussions of cognitive development and its relationship to the acquisition of communication skills, respectively.

Motor Development

When describing a child's motor development, it is important to differentiate between *fine motor* and *gross motor* skills. According to Nicolosi, Harryman, and Kresheck, these terms are defined as follows:

Table 4.1 *Piaget's Stages of Cognitive Development*	Stage	Age Range	Characteristics
Preparatory, prelogical stages	Sensorimotor	Birth–2 years	Coordination of physical actions; prerepresentational + preverbal
	Preoperational	2–7 years	Ability to represent action through thought + language; prelogical
Advanced logical-thinking stages	Concrete operational	7–11 years	Logical thinking, but limited to physical reality
	Formal operational	11–15 years	Logical thinking, abstract and unlimited

Used with permission from Labinowicz E. *The Piaget primer: teaching, learning, teaching.* Menlo Park, CA: Addison-Wesley, 1980, p. 60.

Category	Age Range	Piagetian Stage/Substage	Milestones/ Concept
Infancy I	0–6 months	*Sensorimotor:* Reflexive	Total absence of control over movement
		Primary circular reactions	Reflexes change as a result of experience
		Secondary circular reactions	First habits: if by accident a movement has an interesting result, that's fun—so do it again
Infancy II	6–12 months	Secondary circular reactions (cont'd)	Intention begins
		Coordination of early schemes	
Early childhood	12–24 months	Tertiary circular reactions	Repetition with variation Active experimentation with objects
		Invent new means-end	New means through mental combination
			Cause-effect
Preschool	2–4 years	*Preoperational:* Preconceptual	Language learning Begins developing awareness of space, time, and quantity relationships
School-age	4–7 years	Intuitive	Develops concepts of classification, seriation, and conservation
	7–11 years	*Concrete operations*	Develops logical thinking about concrete/physical entities
	11–15 year	*Formal operations*	Develops logical abstract thought

Table 4.2 *Cognitive Development Milestones:Infancy Through School-Age*

Adapted from Nicolosi L, Harryman E, Kresheck J. Terminology of communication disorders: speech-language-hearing. 3rd ed. Baltimore, MD: Williams & Wilkins, 1989.

Fine motor

Pertaining to skillful, discrete, spatially oriented movements requiring use of small muscle sets, as in speech and the grasping and use of small objects.

Gross motor

Pertaining to movements of large, refined muscles for activities such as locomotion and balance (1989, p. 167).

During the first 6 months of life, the infant achieves a variety of fine-motor and gross-motor milestones, ranging from a se-ries of involuntary and automatic reflexes to the purposeful grasping and holding of two objects. As the child approaches the second half of the first year of life, he is able to move about the environment, first by creeping at around 7 months of age and later by walking when one hand is held (around 12 months). Likewise, fine-motor skills develop concurrently with these gross-motor behaviors. Specifically, at around 8 months of age the child is able to reach and grasp for toys with the palm of his hand, at around 10 months attempts to build a block tower and scribble imitatively, and at approximately 12 months of age can finally grasp objects with his fingers.

As the child approaches his second year of life, he begins to walk alone, removes his socks and shoes, learns to feed himself, and begins to demonstrate hand preference, among other significant behaviors. Table 4.3 illustrates these and other developmental sequences of fine-motor and gross-motor behaviors spanning the period from 1 month through 6 years of age.

The development of communication skills very closely parallels the development of motor abilities. For example, by 4 months of age, the child exhibits cooing behavior and, at around the same age, is typically able to self-support his head. Further-

Table 4.3 *Fine-Motor and Gross-Motor Developmental Milestones: Infancy Through School-Age*

Category	Age Range	Gross Motor	Fine Motor
		Milestones/Concepts	
Infancy I	0–6 months	Tonic neck reflex; Head droops; Lifts head and shoulders	Hand clenches Reflex grasp; Visual localization
		Legs thrust in play; Head erect in vertical position; Waves arms when lying on back	Gains control of 12 oculo-motor muscles Eyes follow pencil or moving person
		Neurologic maturation sufficient to control vocal mechanism; Reaches for objects; Holds head steady; Lifts head and chest when on stomach	Watches play with hands; Pulls at clothing; Puts objects to mouth;
		When prone, elevates self by arms; Sits with support; Holds self erect when pulled to sitting position Turns from side to side; Sits with slight support Sits leaning forward; Gains control of trunk; Tries to creep or roll toward objects	Plays with hands and fingers; Eyes help with reaching action Uses hands for support Can grasp and hold 2 objects; Gains control of hands; Can transfer and manipulate objects
Infancy II	6–12 months	Moves self by creeping; Maintains standing position briefly Can roll from back to stomach; Sits easily without support Creeps and crawls; Pushes from stomach to sitting position easily Moves from sitting to prone position;	Bilateral reaching, but with some spatial error Reaches unilaterally and persistently for toys; Grasps with palm of hand Begins to use index finger more; Rotates wrist and tries to throw objects Attempts to build block tower;

cont'd

Table 4.3 *Fine-Motor and Gross-Motor Developmental Milestones: Infancy Through School-Age (continued)*

Category	Age Range	Milestones/Concepts	
		Gross Motor	Fine Motor
		Creeps and pulls self up;	Attempts to scribble imitatively
		Takes stepping movements; Takes side steps while holding on Takes first independent step Walks when one hand is held	Holds crayon adaptively; Extends toys, but will not release them; Begins to drink from cup; Grasps with fingers
Early child-hood	12–24 months	Begins walking alone; Can open a closed door; Removes socks and shoes; Seats self in chair; Walks well with feet slightly apart; Walks up stairs unassisted; Crawls down stairs backwards; Walks down stairs with hand held; Jumps in place; Pedals tricycle	Learns to feed self; Picks up small objects with precision; Smooth reaching movements; Uses push-pull toys; Builds tower of 3–4 blocks; Scribbles but marks go off page; Turns pages of book 2 or 3 at a time; Begins to show hand preference
Preschool	2–4 years	Runs on whole foot; Climbs on furniture; Walks on tiptoes: Tries to stand on one foot; Walks on line; Swings in swings; Squats to play on floor; Catches bounced ball; Sits with feet crossed at ankles; Runs easily and smoothly	Strings beads; Makes circular scribbles; Takes things apart and puts them back together; Begins to match like objects; Builds tower of 7–16 blocks Cuts with scissors; Good hand and finger coordination; Folds paper; Copies circle, cross and square; Uses spoon well; Puts on shoes; Prints a few capital letters
School-age	4–7 years	Climbs ladder; Skips on one foot; Stands on one foot 8–10 seconds; Dances to music; Is able to sit longer; Skips using alternating feet	Hold paper with other hand in writing; Prints simple words; Copies star; Draws very simple house; Draws man with 2–3 parts and then adds about 7 parts; Frequently reverses letters; Prints first name and numbers 1–5 unevenly; Laces shoes; Draws triangle

Adapted from Nicolosi L, Harryman E, Krescheck J. Terminology of communication disorders: speech-language-hearing. 3rd ed. Baltimore, MD: Williams & Wilkins, 1989.

more, at about the same time that the child babbles and produces reduplicated sounds (i.e., 6 to 9 months), he is able to sit alone, pull himself to a standing position, and make initial attempts to reach for an object. While additional parallel relationships can be drawn between communicative and motor development, *exact ages for the emergence of specific behaviors is not important. What is important to remember is the fact that, for example, at about the same time the child coos, he will also be able to hold up his head.* As Hopper and Naremore state "all normal children learn to talk in similar ways and along similar schedules, with practice apparently having little importance. The only conclusion possible is that communicative development is closely tied to the general biological development of the human animal" (1978, p. 15).

Social Development

Social development typically begins with the development of the infant's attachment to his mother and extends to mother-infant and father-infant interactions (Ainsworth & Bell, 1969; Belsky, 1979; Brazelton, Tronick, Adamson, Als, & Wise, 1975; Clarke-Stewart, 1973, 1978, 1980; Earls & Yogman, 1978; Lamb, 1977, 1981; Yogman, 1982).

The process by which the infant establishes parental attachment is developmental in nature (Ainsworth, 1972, 1973, 1974; Ainsworth & Bell, 1969; Bowlby, 1958, 1969; Carr, Dabbs, & Carr, 1975). The literature documents a developmental process consisting of three phases. At birth, the infant cannot recognize his mother nor can he exhibit different emotional responses to her. However, he does exhibit *undiscriminating social responsiveness* during the first 2 or 3 months of life. During this initial phase, the infant is able to orient to salient features of the environment, exhibiting such behaviors as *visual fixation, visual tracking, listening, rooting,* and *postural adjustments* when they are held. The infant can also gain or maintain human contact in a limited way through sucking, grasping, smiling, crying, and/or vocalizing, although not exhibited to maintain social

contact (Rosenblith & Sims-Knight, 1985). At approximately 3 or 4 months of age, infants learn to discriminate one human from another based on observable and similar facial expressions, vocal characteristics, and vocal imitations made by the parent. The second phase in the development of attachment is called *discriminating social responsiveness.* Here the infant responds differently to one or a few familiar figures than he would to a stranger. At about 7 months of age the third and final stage emerges, termed *active initiative in seeking proximity and contact.* Ainsworth (1973) notes a striking increase in the infant's initiative in promoting proximity and contact. The infant's signals are intentional and elicit a response from the mother. *Goal-corrected* sequences of behavior also emerge during this stage and coincide with the emergence of Piaget's fourth substage of sensorimotor development, *Coordination of Secondary Schemes,* in which *object permanence* (i.e., the awareness that an object is relatively permanent and is not destroyed if removed from the visual field) is observed (Ainsworth, 1967, 1973; Bowlby, 1969).

During the first 6 months of life, the infant is also able to establish eye contact with his mother, smile spontaneously, get excited when familiar faces are seen, visually discriminate between different people and objects, explore the face of the person holding him, and plays social games such as "Peek-a-Boo." As the child experiences the second half of his first year of life (i.e., Infancy II), he or she verbalizes for attention, is very attached to his mother, and exhibits different moods and emotions. During the Early Childhood stage, the child enjoys music and dancing, exhibits pretend play behavior, tests the adult's limits, orders people around, and communicates feelings and needs. When reaching the Preschool stage, the child takes turns and plays cooperatively with others, calls attention to his or her own performance, and displays affection for younger siblings. As the school-age years approach, we can observe general changes in the child's overall behavior and affect, as well as in play behavior.

Table 4.4 illustrates developmental

Table 4.4   *Social Development Milestones: Infancy Through School-Age*

Category	Age Range	Milestones/Concepts
Infancy I	0–6 months	Follows moving light with eyes; Pupils dilate and constrict; Eyes turn toward direction of body part touched; Body reacts to loud sounds; Smiles when talked to; Regards faces and voices; Perceives objects in three dimensions; Responds by turning head to voice; Gives spontaneous social smile; Responds to angry tone by crying; Responds to pleasant speech by smiling and laughing; Vocalizes to own image in mirror and to toys
Infancy II	6–12 months	Smiles at onlookers; Plays "Pat-a-Cake" and other such games; Feeds self crackers, cookies, etc. Differentiates between family and strangers; Adjusts to simple commands; Cooperates in dressing
Early childhood	12–24 months	Indicates wants and responses by gestures and vocalizing; Indicates wet pants; Resistant to change in routine;
Preschool	2–5 years	Repeats actions laughed at; Pretends to read; Explores environment energetically; Engages in parallel play; Initiates own play activities; Engages in simple make-believe activities; Constantly demands mother's attention; Has tantrums when frustrated, but attention is easily distracted; Has no concept of sharing; Defends own possessions with determination; Is active, restless, and rebellious; Looks for missing toys; Insists on being independent; Has more disputes with others than at any other age; Shows affection with younger siblings; Plays interactive games such as tag, playing house (replaces parallel play); Cooperates with other children and takes turns; Shows off dramatically; Calls attention to own performance
School-age	5+ years	Asks meanings of words; Behaves in a more sensible, controlled, and independent manner;

cont'd

Table 4.4	*Social Development Milestones: Infancy Through School-Age (continued)*	
Category	Age Range	Milestones/Concepts
		Protects younger playmates; Plays with 2–5 children in a group; Chooses own friends; Plays with imaginary playmates; Is socially comfortable; Conforms to adult ideas; Asks adult help as needed

Adapted from Nicolosi L, Harryman E, Krescheck J. Terminology of communication disorders: speech-language-hearing. 3rd ed. Baltimore, MD: Williams & Wilkins, 1989.

sequences in the social development of the child beginning at 1 month of age through 6 years and additionally provides specific examples of social milestones achieved. Chapter 5 describes in greater detail care-taker-child interaction and its impact on the communication development process.

Language/Communication Development

Although crying is the most frequent vocalization used by infants in the first 6 months of life, it is important to note that infants engage in both crying and noncry-ing vocalizations from birth. Early crying vocalizations are primarily indications of the infant's physical state (i.e., comfort or discomfort). Truby, Bosma, & Lind (1965) attribute this to the infant's achieve-ment in expending air and in moving parts of the vocal mechanism during vocaliza-tion. Ostwald & Peltzman (1974) state that "crying is one of the first ways in which the infant is able to communicate with the world at large" (p. 85). As the infant gains greater control over the respiratory and vo-cal mechanisms, patterned vowel-like pro-ductions such as "ah" and "ee" are observed around 3 months of age. Furthermore, "conversations" between the infant and caregiver are noted in which the adult vo-calizes, waits for a response from the infant, and then vocalizes again, either in response to the infant's vocalization or to elicit a re-sponse from the infant (Lewis & Freedle, 1973). These dyadic interchanges have been termed *conversational turn-taking*.

Conversational turn-taking begins when the infant indicates readiness by the nature of the vocalizations produced and by being quietly alert for longer periods of time (Rosenblith & Sims-Knight, 1985). In addition to conversational turn-taking ability, infants communicate needs and feelings through gazing, touching, smil-ing, laughing, vocalizing, grasping ob-jects, and sucking.

Other linguistic milestones achieved during this developmental period include cooing and babbling behavior. Cooing is described as early infantile sounds that are produced by the infant usually in response to the caregiver's smiles or vocalizations. Such vocalizations are primarily vowel-like; however, some consonantal elements may appear around 8 weeks of age.

Unlike cooing, babbling has been ob-served as early as 3 to 4 months and can ex-tend into the second half of the first year of life. It is characterized by deliberate, voli-tional play and experimentation with sound (Nicolosi, Harryman, & Kresheck, 1989). There are two types of babbling be-havior: *reduplicated* and *nonreduplicated* babbling. Reduplicated babbling occurs when the infant, usually between 6 and 8 months of age, produces a series of conso-nant-vowel syllables such as "baba." Nonreduplicated babbling is usually ob-served in children between the ages of 9 and 18 months in which the consonants and vowels used in one syllable may be dif-ferent from those used in a subsequent syl-lable, for example, as in "bagu."

In addition to nonreduplicated babbling behavior, the child uses his first true word during the second half of the first year of life (see Chapter 9 for specifics). As the child learns new words to add to his *lexicon* (or vocabulary), language assumes a greater communicative role in that words produced typically relate to the child's communicative needs. Words are, therefore, produced by the child to signify *communicative intent*. The child uses words to *label* objects (e.g., "cookie"), *answer* questions (e.g., shaking head to indicate "yes"), *request* an object (e.g., "want car"), *greet* (e.g., "hi"), or to *protest* (e.g., "no!"), among others. Such *illocutionary* acts are typically observed between 9 and 18 months of age. Chapter 8 provides a detailed discussion of these and other *pragmatic language behaviors*. As the child enters his second year of life, utterances expand from single word to combinatory productions (e.g., "mommy go," "eat cookie," "book [in] chair"). Such multiword utterances mark the beginnings of early grammatical development. The child exhibits the awareness and knowledge that, for example, in the utterance "mommy go," the meaning conveyed is "Mommy is going to the store." Furthermore, in the utterance "eat cookie," the child voluntarily selects the words "eat" and "cookie," and orders them in such a way to denote the meaning generated by the sentence, "Mommy is eating a cookie." These utterances illustrate quite clearly the child's further development of the *semantic relations* (or meaning relationships) that can be conveyed by word order. Such relationships are observed in the linguistic repertoires of 2- and 3-year-old children. From a pragmatic perspective, the child's conversational skills are developing to the extent that he begins to adopt *conversationalist roles*. The child begins to understand that dialogue involves conversational partners that function in different discourse roles—the speaker and the listener (or respondent). Consequently, the child's language behavior during dyadic verbal interaction is operationally different when he functions as a speaker rather than a respondent, or vice versa. Furthermore, on entering the preschool years (i.e., 2 to 4 years), the child asks a greater number of questions and his conversations are more organized and thematic (i.e., topically controlled) than they were before. While far from being characterized as adultlike,

the types of words and sentences used by the child at this stage of communicative development are more sophisticated as evidenced by the increased use of morphologic word endings such as "-ing" as in "eat-*ing*" (to denote the present progressive tense), "-s" as in "dog*s*" (to denote plural), and "-ed" as in "jump*ed*" (to denote regular past tense), among many others (Chapter 11 provides an extensive discussion of morphologic development).

On entering school the child *begins* to develop more complex sentence forms characterized by conjoining and embedding behavior (see Chapter 12 for specifics) along with the rapid expansion of vocabulary to include not only more concrete words but also abstract words. Throughout the school-age years the child refines his syntactic, semantic, and pragmatic language repertoires in an attempt to match more adult forms. Table 4.5 displays language/communication developmental milestones typically observed from infancy through school-age.

It is quite obvious that the child develops many skills and abilities beginning at birth and extending into the school-age years. It is important, therefore, to have a general working knowledge of developmental milestones specific to the developmental domains of cognitive, motor, and social development to appreciate the potential impact these developmental areas have on communication development. In doing so, knowledge about the total child can be attained. While there are professionals who may be more knowledgeable about cognitive, motor, and social development (e.g., clinical psychologists, physical therapists, occupational therapists), it behooves the speech-language pathologist to make every attempt possible to secure the expertise of such professionals during the clinical assessment and treatment processes.

CLINICAL APPLICATIONS

In addition to teaming with those colleagues who also possess expertise in the areas of child development, the speech-language pathologist may choose to use various types of developmental scales, check-

Table 4.5 *Language/Communication Development Milestones: Infancy Through School-Age*

Category	Age Range	Milestones/Concepts
Infancy I	0–6 months	Birth cry;
Infancy II	6–12 months	*Perlocutionary acts:* Gazing, crying, touching, smiling, laughing, vocalizing, grasping, sucking; Cooing Babbling First word (e.g., mama, dada) Single word production (i.e, names of objects and actions *Illocutionary acts:* Labeling Answering Requesting Calling Greeting Protesting Repeating Practicing
Early childhood	12–24 months	Use of two-word combinations and emergence of grammatical morphemes *Locutionary acts:* Dialogue Adoption of conversational roles: Speaker 　　　　　　Listener
Preschool	2–4 years	Further development and expansion of word combinations and meanings; Expansion of grammatical morpheme use; Rapid growth in vocabulary; Rapid growth in grammatical development; Beginnings of stylistic variations in language use; Role playing
School-age	5+ years	Complex grammatical development (i.e., embedding and conjoining); Vocabulary expands to include abstract words and their meanings; Pragmatic language competence extends to other discourse behaviors (e.g., topic introduction/maintenance/change /extension, etc) Development of narrative and metalinguistic abilities

Adapted from Nicolosi L, Harryman E, Krescheck J. Terminology of communication disorders: speech-language-hearing. 3rd ed. Baltimore, MD: Williams & Wilkins, 1989.

lists, and other instruments to assess the child's overall level of developmental functioning. This section will offer a discussion of eight developmental assessments available for use by speech-language pathologists and other professionals.

Brigance Diagnostic Inventory of Early Development (Brigance, 1978)

This instrument is intended for use with children below 7 years of age. Specific developmental areas assessed include, among others, the following: fine-motor and gross-motor skills, self-help skills, prespeech behaviors, speech and language skills, general knowledge and comprehension, basic reading skills, and mathematics.

Early Language Milestone Scale-2 (ELM-2) (Coplan, 1987, 1993)

The *ELM-2* is a standardized screening instrument that primarily assesses speech and language development during infancy and early childhood. It is organized into three sections: Auditory Expressive (examines behaviors such as cooing and babbling), Auditory Receptive (examines execution of specific commands, sound recognition, and localization), and Visual (examines visual fixation, tracking, and recognition of parents and other familiar persons; also response to or initiation of various gestures).

Vineland Adaptive Behavior Scales (VABS) (Sparrow, Balla, & Cicchetti, 1984)

The *VABS* is a revision of the *Vineland Social Maturity Scale* (Doll, 1965). It assesses "personal and social sufficiency of individuals from birth to adulthood" (Sparrow et al., 1984, p. 1). This revised, norm-referenced, adaptive-behavior scale consists of three versions, each measuring four developmental domains: communication, daily living skills, socialization, and motor skills.

Cognitive, Linguistic, and Social Communicative Scales (CLASS) (Tanner & Lamb, 1984)

The *CLASS* is an instrument that assesses language development through pre-

sentation of developmental milestones for the cognitive, linguistic, and social-communicative systems. A sequence of eleven developmental levels extending from birth through age 6 years is presented.

Birth to Three Checklist of Learning and Language Behavior (Bangs, 1986)

This instrument is not norm-referenced, but rather is *criterion-referenced*, meaning that it was designed to accompany and measure a set of skill-mastery criteria rather than the performance of a group of individuals (Overton, 1992). This checklist evaluates five developmental categories in children ranging in chronologic age from birth through 36 months. Specific categories are (1) language comprehension, (2) language expression, (3) avenues to learning (i.e., problem solving), (4) social/personal behaviors, and (5) motor behaviors. Data are collected based on direct observation of the child's behavior in response to specific probes designed to elicit the developmental information.

Battelle Developmental Inventory (BDI) (Newborg, Stock, Wnek, Guidubaldi, & Svinicki, 1988)

The *BDI* is a standardized instrument that assesses five developmental domains in children ranging in chronologic age from birth to 8 years. The domains assessed are *Personal-Social* (measures adult interaction, expression of feelings/affect, self-concept, peer interaction, coping, and social role), *Adaptive* (measures attention, eating, dressing, personal responsibility, and toileting), *Motor* (measures muscle control, body coordination, locomotion/movement, fine-motor skills, and perceptual motor development), *Communication* (measures language comprehension and production), and *Cognitive* (measures perceptual discrimination, memory, reasoning, and conceptual development).

Denver II (Frankenburg, Dodds, Archer, Bresnick, Maschka, Edelman, & Shapiro, 1990)

The *Denver II*, based on the original Denver Developmental Screening Test

(DDST) (Frankenburg, Dodds, Fandal, Kazuk, & Cohrs, 1973), is an individually administered, norm-referenced, screening instrument designed for the early identification of children with developmental and behavioral problems. It was standardized on over 2000 children and is intended to provide a gross estimate of delayed development. Intended for use with children from birth to 6 years of age, the *Denver II* consists of 125 items presented across four developmental areas: personal-social development, fine-motor adaptive development, language development, and gross-motor development.

AGS Early Screening Profiles (ESP) (Harrison, Kaufman, Kaufman, Bruininks, Rynders, Ilmer, Sparrow, & Cicchetti, 1990)

The *ESP* is a screening instrument for children ages 2 years 0 months through 6 years 11 months, which identifies children who may be at risk for subsequent learning problems and those who may be gifted. It consists of seven parts, three of which measure major areas of development—the *Cognitive/Language Profile*, the *Motor Profile*, and the *Self-Help/Social Profile*. The remaining four parts (i.e., the Articulation, Home, Health History, and Behavior Surveys) supplement the Profiles and are typically completed by the parent, teacher, or examiner. This instrument was standardized on over 1100 children.

Pediatric Language Acquisition Screening Tool for Early Referral—Revised (PLASTER-R) (Shulman & Sherman, 1996)

This is a new screening instrument that is parent administered and does not rely on the direct cooperation of infants and toddlers. It is comprised of a series of questions that address developmental milestones of children ranging in chronologic age from 3 through 60 months. Its purpose is to identity *potential* speech, language, and/or hearing problems. See Sherman, Shulman, Trimm, and Hoff (1996)

for a discussion of its use with high-risk infants and toddlers.

Data obtained from administering any of these developmental assessment instruments along with a general working knowledge of developmental milestones can assist the speech-language pathologist and other professionals in describing the child's level of developmental functioning. Furthermore, such data are extremely helpful in determining whether specific developmental deficits are interfering with the child's ability to develop age-appropriate communication skills. It is important to remember that the development of cognitive, motor, and social skills has a direct impact on the child's ability to develop communicative competence. The development and use of linguistic symbols depends on attaining certain cognitive, social, and motor skills (Owens, 1988). If we make every attempt possible to understand child development, we can then fully appreciate those behavioral changes associated with communication development.

REFERENCES

Ainsworth MDS. Infancy in Uganda: infant care and growth in love. Baltimore, MD: Johns Hopkins University Press, 1967.

Ainsworth MDS. Attachment and dependency: a comparison. In: Gewirtz JL, ed. Attachment and dependency. Washington, DC: Winston, 1972; pp. 97–137.

Ainsworth MDS. The development of infant-mother attachment. In: Caldwell BM, Ricciuti HN, eds. Review of child development research. Vol. 3. Chicago, IL: University of Chicago Press, 1973; pp. 1–94.

Ainsworth MDS. Infant-mother attachment and social development: socialization as a product of reciprocal responsiveness to signals. In: Edwards M, ed. The integration of the child into the social world. Cambridge, England: Cambridge University Press, 1974.

Ainsworth MDS, Bell SMV. Some contemporary patterns of mother-infant interaction in the feeding situation. In: Ambrose JA, ed. Stimulation in early infancy. London: Academic, 1969; pp. 133–170.

Bangs TE. Birth to three assessment and intervention system: checklist for learning and language behavior. Allen, TX: DLM Teaching Resources, 1986.

Belsky J. Mother-father-infant interaction: a naturalistic observational study. Dev Psychol 1979; 17:3–23.

Bourne LE, Ekstrand BR. Psychology. 3rd ed. New York: Holt, Rhinehart, & Winston, 1979.

Bowlby J. The nature of the child's tie to his mother. Int J Psychoanal 1958;39:350–373.

Bowlby J. Attachment and loss: Vol. 1. Attachment. New York: Basic Books, 1969.

Brazelton TB, Tronick E, Adamson L, et al. Early mother-infant reciprocity. In: Hofer MA, ed. Parent-infant interaction. London: Ciba, 1975.

Brigance AH. BRIGANCE Diagnostic Inventory of Early Development. North Billerica, MA: Curriculum Associates, 1978.

Carr S, Dabbs J, Carr T. Mother-infant attachment: the importance of the mother's visual field. Child Dev 1975;46:331–338.

Clarke-Stewart K. Interactions between mothers and their young children: characteristics and consequences. Monogr Soc Res Child Dev 1973;38:6(Serial No. 153).

Clarke-Stewart K. And daddy makes three: the father's impact on mother and child. Child Dev 1978;49:466–478.

Coplan J. The Early Language Milestone Scale-2. Austin, TX: Pro-Ed, 1993.

Coplan J. The Early Language Milestone Scale. Revised edition. Austin, TX: Pro-Ed, 1987.

Doll EA. Vineland Social Maturity Scale. Circle Pines, MN: American Guidance Service, 1965.

Earls F, Yogman M. The father-infant relationship. In: Howells J, ed. Modern perspectives in the psychiatry of infancy. New York: Bruner/Mazel, 1978.

Frankenburg WK, Dodds J, Fandal A, et al. Denver Developmental Screening Test: reference manual. Revised edition. Denver, CO: LA-DOCA Project and Publishing Foundation, 1975.

Frankenburg WK, Dodds J, Archer P, et al. Denver II: screening manual. Denver, CO: Denver Developmental Materials, 1990.

Harrison PL, Kaufman AS, Kaufman NL, et al. AGS Early Screening Profiles. Circle Pines, MN: American Guidance Service, 1990.

Hopper R, Naremore RJ. Children's speech: a practical introduction to communication development. 2nd ed. New York: Harper & Row, 1978.

Labinowicz E. The Piaget primer: teaching, learning, teaching. Menlo Park, CA: Addison-Wesley Publishing,1980.

Lamb ME. Father-infant and mother-infant interaction in the first year of life. Child Dev 1977; 48:167–181.

Lamb ME, ed. The role of the father in child development. New York: John Wiley, 1981.

Lewis M, Freedle R. Mother-infant dyad: the cradle of meaning. In: Pilner P, Kranes L, Alloway T, eds. Communication and affect: language and thought. New York: Academic Press, 1973.

Morehead D, Morehead A. From signal to sign: a Piagetian view of thought and language during the first two years. In: Schiefelbusch RL, Lloyd LL, eds. Language perspectives—acquisition, retardation, and intervention. Baltimore, MD: University Park Press, 1974; pp. 153–190.

Newborg J, Stock JR, Wnek L, et al. Battelle developmental inventory. Allen, TX: DLM Teaching Resources, 1988.

Nicolosi L, Harryman E, Kresheck J. Terminology of communication disorders: speech-language-hearing. 3rd ed. Baltimore, MD: Williams & Wilkins, 1989.

Ostwald R, Peltzman P. The cry of the newborn. Sci Am 1974;230:84–90.

Overton T. Assessment in special education: an applied approach. New York: Merrill, 1992.

Owens RE. Language development: an introduction. 2nd ed. Columbus, OH: Merrill Publishing, 1988.

Piaget J. The psychology of intelligence. London: Routledge & Kegan Paul, 1950.

Piaget J. The origins of intelligence in children. New York: International Universities Press, 1952.

Piaget J. The construction of reality in the child. New York: Basic Books, 1954.

Piaget J. The language and thought of the child. New York: The New American Library, 1974.

Piaget J, Inhelder B. The growth of logical thinking from childhood to adolescence. New York: Basic Books, 1958.

Piaget J, Inhelder B. The psychology of the child. New York: Basic Books, 1969.

Pulaski MAS. Understanding Piaget: an introduction to children's cognitive development. New York: Harper & Row, 1980.

Rosenblith JF, Sims-Knight JE. In the beginning: development in the first two years. Monterey, CA: Brookes/Cole Publishing, 1985.

Sherman T, Shulman BB, Trimm RF, Hoff C. PLASTER: Predicting communication impairments in an NICU follow-up population. Infant-Toddler Intervention: The Transdisciplin J 1996;6(3): 183–195.

Shulman BB, Sherman T. The Pediatric Language Acquisition Screening Tool for Early Referral-Revised (PLASTER-R): experimental edition. Unpublished manuscript, 1996.

Sparrow S, Balla DA, Cicchetti DV. Vineland Adaptive Behavior Scales. Circle Pines, MN: American Guidance Service, 1984.

Tanner DC, Lamb WM. CLASS: The cognitive, linguistic and social-communicative scales. Tulsa, OK: Modern Education Corporation, 1984.

Truby H, Bosma J, Lind J. Newborn infant cry. Acta Paediatr Scand Suppl 1965;163:7–59.

Yogman MW. Development of the father-infant relationship. In: Fitzgerald HE, Lester BM, Yogman MW, eds. Theory and research in behavioral pediatrics. Vol. 1. New York: Plenum, 1982; pp. 221–279.

CHAPTER 5

Caretaker-Child Interaction[1]

William O. Haynes

There was once an anecdote in the language development literature that told of a deaf couple who had a son with normal hearing. The parents wanted the boy to speak normally, and since they could not provide him with a good speech model, they decided to leave the television playing throughout the day so that the child could have language stimulation. Needless to say, the child mercifully did not learn the language of "the tube" and ended up developing sign language. Why is this so? We know that to develop a language we must be exposed to a model of the system we hope to acquire, and, certainly, the television provided such an example from many different speakers on a variety of topics. The

reason, of course, that the child did not learn language from the television was that the model of language must be presented in *relevant interactions*, not just played as ambient noise in the child's environment. There are those who would argue that much of television is irrelevant, even when we understand language, but that is another issue. The main point to be understood here is that to acquire language one must be exposed to a consistent model in meaningful interactions. Since language is a code and a tool used to influence the attitudes, attention, and acts of other people, it only makes sense that it is acquired in meaningful activities. Up to this point, we have only talked about the effects of caretaker-child interaction on language development, but many more areas of acquisition are facilitated by the everyday activities of parents and children. For instance, the caretaker and child jointly develop social skills, emotional attachments, concepts, games, motor skills, and a host of other important attainments. Since the focus of this book is on communication development, and communication is much more than just language, we will spend some time talking about these other areas in addition to the

---

[1] The research in this area uses a variety of terms to refer to the people most involved in raising a child. Among these are: parent, mother, father, primary caregiver, caregiver, caretaker and adult. There are more terms we could mention, but the point is fairly clear. Because children grow up in differing circumstances, they could be raised by parents, live in institutional settings or reside in the homes of relatives, foster parents or others. We have decided to primarily use the term "caretaker" because we could find no consensus in the literature on a particular term, and this terminology could conceivably encompass a wide variety of people.

linguistic code. There are literally hundreds of investigations and book chapters written on the topic of caretaker-child interaction, and the present chapter can only serve to skim the surface. This is especially true when we take the point of view that the parent-child interaction provides more than just a language model, but an important impetus to social, affective, and cognitive development as well. We will cite some specific studies in this chapter to reinforce relevant points, but the reader should be aware that many other investigations could have also been quoted.

OVERVIEW OF THE RESEARCH ON CARETAKER-CHILD INTERACTION

Snow (1986), a pioneer in caretaker-child interaction research, has noted a trend in the evolution of studies in this area. In the early 1960s she found that much of the research was on the structural aspects of language addressed to children and indicated that language models were well-formed, simple, and redundant. There were studies of the length, complexity, pausing, and other measures of the form of language used in talking to children. A second stage in this research began in the 1970s, and the focus was on what mothers talked about with their children. Analyses were done on the semantic content and the various semantic relations used by caretakers, and it was found that they largely talked about the "here and now," coding aspects of the child's environment that were currently relevant and meaningful. In the late portion of the 1970s and early part of the next decade the research began to consider conversational aspects of interactions between mothers and children and variables like contingency, topic manipulation, and the relatedness of a mother's utterance to a prior child utterance. Also, specific "teaching" procedures used by caretakers when faced with an incomplete or unelaborated child verbalization were studied. Basically, this progression from syntax to semantics to pragmatics mirrors the direction taken in all areas of child language research. When this information is assembled, it is clear that we know quite a lot about the language addressed to children during communication development. If this information about the language model is coupled with other data on mother-child interactions that concern nonverbal communication and cognitive and social development, we can begin to see a picture of a very complex and fascinating relationship. To untangle the complexity of this interaction, we will divide our consideration of the literature into several sections that build on one another. The relationship is considered chronologically across the social, cognitive, and communicative domain, so we begin with the initial interactions of neonates and their mothers and progress to interactions between parents and toddlers. The intricacy and fine-tuning of the interactions is present from the beginning with both the mother and child learning to take the other into account. One more point should be made here. The bulk of the studies done on interactions with children have primarily or exclusively used mothers as subjects. This in no way is intended to minimize the importance of fathers and other caretakers in influencing the development of communication. Indeed, we will review some research suggesting that *any* interactant who communicates with children provides a simpler and less complex language model and has the potential of facilitating communication development.

CARETAKER CONTRIBUTIONS TO DEVELOPMENT OF COMMUNICATIVE FOUNDATIONS

The first impact of caretaker-child interaction that comes to mind is typically its effect on the development of language structures (semantics, syntax, etc.). However, caretaker-child interaction has many significant effects on communication development even before a child begins to speak. Several areas are logically considered to be prerequisite to the development of language for communication. First, a child must have an available caretaker who is in close physical proximity because the infant's sensory system cannot deal with stimuli that are distant. Early on, the child's immature visual system does not operate effectively for distance. The child also cannot coordinate turning of the head to visually track a stimulus or localize a sound. Thus it is important that a caretaker is in close physical proximity. Also, the caretaker must provide the child with physical assistance, both in feeding/changing activities and in exploring the environment. A second major area has to do with the relationship that develops between an infant and caretaker. The child develops an attachment to specific people, and this relationship facilitates interaction, familiarity, and the drive to "identify" with the behavior of the caretaker. Third, the caretaker and child develop the ability to joint reference, or attend to the same objects and actions during their interactions. This joint attending behavior appears to be critical in communication development. Finally, the caretaker and child engage in reciprocity or turn-taking in both nonverbal and vocal behaviors. This turn-taking is later seen in language use. Each of these four areas potentially have a great deal to do with later language development and also cognitive, social, and affective acquisitions. Each area will be discussed in more detail.

Proxemics and Physical Assistance

Human infants, compared with many other species, are remarkably dependent on a caretaker for survival. Whether this person is the mother, a foster parent, a day care provider or a relative, the infant must rely on close and frequent interactions for feeding, changing, bathing, comforting, and general companionship. This necessity for recurring contact provides a plethora of opportunities to learn about the world. Early on, the caretaker attempts to modify the child's wake-sleep cycle to be similar to her own so that a greater number of interactions can conve-

niently take place. Studies have shown that during feeding, the caretaker's face is about 8 inches from the infant, and this distance is near the optimal focusing range of the neonate (Robson, 1967; Stern, 1977). Even more interesting is the finding that infants tend to focus on areas of contrast and the human face is an excellent subject, with many areas of demarcation such as the eyes, hairline, mouth, and nostrils (Fantz, 1964). Some studies suggest that infants have a special attraction to the caretaker's eyes (Wolff, 1963). As if this were not enough, caretakers have been shown to exaggerate facial expressions and speak in expanded intonation patterns to infants, all of which make an even more fascinating display. We also know from studies of early low-level speech perception that infants under 6 months of age are sensitive to auditory stimuli that differ in frequency, intensity, duration, and location (Morse, 1974). There is even some evidence that infants have a preference for human voices as compared with nonspeech stimuli (Eisenberg, 1976). Morse (1974) cites several studies that show infants are able to discriminate their mother's voice from that of an unrelated female. Papousek, Bornstein, Nuzzo, et al. (1990) found that 4-month-old infants could discriminate "approving" from "disapproving" intonation contours and hypothesized that these discriminations "may function as didactic caregiving messages for infants" (p. 539). Thus it can be seen that the infant and its caretaker are evidently "preprogrammed" in some manner to attend to one another and begin a long series of repeated interactions.

Between birth and about 6 months of age a child's interactions seem to be more "person centered" than "object centered." After 6 months a child appears to have a significant interest in objects, so the interactions become more "triadic" among the infant, caretaker, and object (Owens, 1996).

In interactions involving objects, the mothers are also quite forgiving. They try to set up successful opportunities for their infants to explore novel objects and succeed in motor skills. Schaffer (1977) lists characteristic behaviors that caretakers engage in that facilitate infant success in learning about the world. For instance, the caretaker "phases" or times behavior so that the infant is attending when presented with an object to view. Behavior is adapted so that the child can fully appreciate it as in slowing down a movement to facilitate infant visual tracking. The caretaker "facilitates" infant participation, perhaps by holding an object for the child to manipulate because simultaneous holding and exploring are too difficult. The caretaker "elaborates" uses of objects, showing the child other functions for objects he has manipulated in only one manner. The mother "initiates" by directing the child's attention to specific stimuli or aspects of stimuli. Finally, caretakers "control" interactions that the infant has with persons and objects by forcing object manipulation or by telling the child what to do with specific items. All of these characteristics of caretaker's interactions with infants not only facilitate social development and turn-taking, but also help the child develop cognitively through sensorimotor exploration, imitation, and functional object use. During each interaction the mother is "coding" or talking about salient aspects of the object or event so that the child can hear the linguistic label for an object or the action being performed. Thus we can see that the caretaker not only is assisting the child communicatively, but also with regard to concepts and socialization.

Attachment Theory and Interaction During Early Communication Development

The relationship between a caretaker and a child is the basis for all of their social interactions. Bowlby (1969) has postulated that enduring relationships between one or several individuals and a child form the basis of attachment. McLean and Snyder-McLean (1978) suggest that there is some evidence that frequency of contact between the person(s)

and the child is a variable contributing to the formation of attachment. Attachment bonds that are stable tend to be associated with certain maternal behaviors such as sensitivity, acceptance, cooperation, and accessibility (McLean & Snyder-McLean, 1978). The opposites of these characteristics may lead to unstable attachments. McLean and Snyder-McLean (1978, p.58) stated the following:

> Overall then, the theory and data on attachment formation suggest that the consistent presence and accessibility of one or a few adults who are sensitive to and accepting of the infant's own behavioral tendencies—rather than being intrusive and insisting upon controlling all of the child's behavior—are critical environmental requirements if the child is to form successfully the attachment bonds which will serve as the basis for social interactions with the world of adults. Ironically, the environmental factors described here are precisely those which are most typically lacking in institutional settings.

There have been some specific studies dealing with attachment and communication development. Some of these investigations have focused on play interactions, which are the contexts for learning about communication, as well as cognitive development. For instance, Roggman, Langlois, and Hubbs-Tait (1987) studied groups of securely attached and "anxiously" attached children at age 14 months in a free-play situation. They found that the securely attached group exchanged toys with mothers more frequently, had fewer maternal play demonstrations, had more "positively toned" maternal vocalizations, and fewer "nonpositively toned" infant vocalizations. They found no difference in the cognitive quality of the toy play. Slade (1987a) studied secure and anxiously attached 11/2 to 21/2 year olds and found secure children to have the longest episodes of symbolic play and that in the latter part of this age range they spent more time in symbolic play than anxious peers. Further, mothers of securely attached children reported enjoying active play interaction, and mothers of anxiously attached children preferred more passive play involvement. There have also been some interesting studies done on "unavailable" mothers during interactions with their own infants. Field, Vega-Lahr, Scafide, and Goldstein (1986) studied the effects of physical, as well as emotional, unavailability. In one situation the mother physically leaves a child in a room, and the infant becomes obviously distressed. In another condition the mother remains in the room and becomes emotionally unavailable by assuming a "still face" posture and being unresponsive. The investigators found that the "still face" condition was even more stressful to the child than the physical absence of the mother. This brings up some provocative, related research on depressed mothers. These mothers may often be emotionally unavailable to their children and thus affect attachment. Brezhitz and Sherman (1987) examined discourse between depressed and nondepressed mothers and their 3-year-old children. They found depressed mothers to vocalize less frequently and respond less quickly to cessation of their children's speech. They stated the following (p. 395):

> Children of the depressed mothers spoke less than children of healthy women . . . The groups of children are exposed to very different patterns of socialization. The offspring of depressed women are being taught both to keep social interaction to a minimum and to be overreactive to even mild stresses.

More research needs to be done in the area of attachment theory and communication development, but the logic of the relationship is clear. A supportive caretaker who responds to the child's communications and play preferences would be ideal for supplying a language model in relevant contexts.

Joint Reference: An Important Precondition for Communication Development

From a very early age it has been shown that infants and caretakers follow each other's line of visual regard (Bruner, 1975; Collis & Schaffer, 1975). This joint focus on a particular entity or event is called joint reference. The child will generally look at an object or event the mother is interested in, and the mother will joint reference with the child as he examines something of interest to him. Just from a logical point of view alone, joint reference would clearly be crucial to cognitive, social, and communicative development. A child participates in social games by sharing joint attention to objects and events. How could the child learn to be social without joint attention? In the development of concepts, parents often demonstrate functional object use and stimulate sensorimotor exploration of objects. This too would be difficult without joint reference. Communication development, perhaps even more than the cognitive and social areas, depends on jointly attending to a referent while the caretaker provides a model of the language used to name or describe it. If a caretaker modeled language for one event while the child attended to another, the communication development process would be arduous indeed. Thus joint reference is necessarily related to a host of developmental acquisitions, and its importance cannot be overemphasized.

Many empirical demonstrations of the importance of joint reference to communication development exist, and several examples are discussed below. Tomasello and Farrar (1986) examined natural play interactions between mothers and their children at ages 15 and 21 months. In analyzing their data, they isolated episodes of joint attentional focus between mother and child. The researchers found that, within the joint attention episodes, mothers produced more utterances, used shorter utterances, and made more comments and that the dyads engaged in longer conversations than in episodes that did not involve joint attention. They discovered that mother's references to objects already in the child's attentional focus were positively correlated with the child's vocabulary at 21 months of age, while no behaviors outside joint referencing episodes related to language development. They also did an experimental study in which new words were taught to 17-month-old children. They found that the words relating to objects already in the child's focus were learned more easily than words presented in an attempt to redirect the child's attention. This clearly emphasizes the importance of joint referencing in communication development. The initiation of joint attention appears to change with age. Cohn and Tronick (1987) point out the complex interplay between mothers and children in dyadic face-to-face interactions at different age levels. At 6 and 9 months many interactions begin with the mother positively eliciting the infant's attention. At 3 and 6 months the mother's positive expression (smiling, exaggerated facial expression, etc.) precedes the onset of the infant's positive expression, and at 9 months the reverse may be true with the infant becoming positive prior to the mother. This shows how joint attention and affective variables interact as mother and child take turns in initiating their exchanges. Bakeman and Adamson (1986) studied mother-child interaction in children at ages 9, 12, and 15 months. They examined gestural and verbal responses and joint referencing patterns. They indicated that children's productions of communicative words and gestures is facilitated because "Adults often provide aid in the form of 'scaffolds' or 'standard action formats' which help the infant maintain joint attention to a referent as well as time their communicative acts appropriately" (p. 216). These researchers found that the early words and gestures were indeed facilitated by "availability of an attentive, comprehending partner, joint attention toward an object with this partner and enactment of an action format" (p. 216). The infants gestured and spoke more when mothers paid attention to them. Specifically, when mothers and children joint referenced on objects, the children produced the most gestures and words, especially in the 15-month-old age group. Slade (1987b) found that the level of com-

plexity of symbolic play in children between 20 and 28 months was enhanced by maternal involvement and active interaction as compared with conditions when the mother was less available for interaction. This suggests that, in addition to the communicative benefits mentioned above in other studies, children benefit from the joint interaction and increase their play level as a result.

Some reports in the literature indicate that preterm infants may differ from full-term infants in some social interaction behaviors such as early face-to-face (Field, 1977) and feeding interactions (Bakeman & Brown, 1980). Landry (1986), however, found similar joint attention behaviors in toy-centered interactions with mothers of preterm and full-term children who were 6 months of age. The only difference was that the preterm babies moved their attention away from joint engagement more often than full-term babies. Maternal joint referencing behaviors did not differ between the groups. Harris, Jones, Brookes, and Grant (1986) studied one group of children who were acquiring language at a normal rate and another group developing language more slowly. The children were all less than 24 months of age. The investigators were especially interested in the maternal behaviors during interactions of mothers and children in the two groups. They found that there was a significant difference between the mothers of normally developing and slower developing children in their references to objects. Specifically, they noted the following:

> . . . there was a difference in the *timing* of mothers' utterances in the two groups. Whereas mothers in the normal development group talked about things the child was attending to, mothers in the slower development group often talked about an object before or after the child was attending to it (p.268).

This clearly has a direct bearing on the mother's sensitivity to joint referencing. Of course, this behavioral difference between mothers could be either the cause or the effect of slowly developing language. We will address this issue more fully in a later section. It is evident from this brief review, that joint reference is extremely important to communication development.

Social Games and Activities for Joint Referencing

Early in development, caretakers engage children in social games during which there are circumscribed roles, predictable events, and redundant utterances. In the beginning, games like "Peek-a-boo," "I'm gonna get you," tickle games, and other routines provide a source of joint reference (Owens, 1996). Most interactions take place in the "here and now," where caretaker and child share the focus of an object or event and the parent codes salient aspects of the stimulus. Often the interactions are recurring and repetitive in which a particular toy is a cue for the parent and child to engage in a certain routine with predictable accompanying verbalizations. As the child becomes older, book-reading routines are often incorporated as part of the daily schedule. Even before the child can appreciate the language being read by the parent, he often attends to pictures and seems to delight in the caretaker's narration of depicted events.

Snow (1981) has discussed the importance of social games that are played between parents and children. These games appear to be universal across cultures and are of similar types. First, mothers "fine-tune" the timing of their behavior with the child's behavior in reciprocal interchanges. This allows the infant a "turn" and facilitates the concept of reciprocity so integral in later conversation. Second, well-rehearsed routines such as social games provide a predictable framework in which to code linguistic elements. Since the game routine is relatively circumscribed, the child can focus on the language used in the exchange, and this language stimulation even becomes redundant after a time when the routine is used frequently. Snow estimates that the average infant experiences more than 1000 episodes of game-playing routines in the first 6 months of life and that only about five different games are played frequently, which makes the routines even more powerful. Mothers whose children are 4 to 6 months old tend to engage in games that stimulate the child's attention and produce excitement. As the child gets older, the games include more conventional roles, as well as turn taking, and the child's role becomes more active as opposed to passive (Crawley, Rogers, Friedman, et al., 1978; Gustafson, Green, & West, 1979). Camaioni and Laicardi (1985), in a study of mother-child dyads, enumerated the types of games played in Table 5.1. They found that between 6 and 12 months of age is an important time for the growth of social games and that the variety and level of these routines increased during this period. Interestingly, all of their subjects produced their first linguistic utterances only within the conventional games.

Several studies have documented the phenomenon of joint book reading between parents and language-learning

Table 5.1   *Types of Caretaker-Child Games Played*

Nonconventional Games		Conventional Games	
Tactile and/or motoric stimulation	Give and take Peek-a-boo	Build/knock-down No	Question/answer Linguistic imitation
Perceptual stimulation (visual/auditory)	Horsie Pat-a-cake	Point and name Put on/take off	
Vocal imitation	Bye-bye	Open/shut	
Gestural imitation	Ball	Joint book reading	

children (Ninio & Bruner, 1978; Ninio, 1980, 1983). Lemish and Rice (1986, p.252) indicated the following:

> Two features of book reading contribute to children's language acquisition: routinization of the book reading situation and predictability of adult utterances. Parents tend to "read" a child's favorite picture books to the child many times, discussing the same pictures with the same labels or phrases. Children recall the reading situations and accompanying utterances, and eventually learn the repeated parental utterances.

Some other research has found that children's verbalizations with parents while watching television is highly similar to the utterance productivity in joint book reading (Wells, 1985). Lemish and Rice (1986) have also documented the consistent occurrence of language interactions between parents and children while viewing television. Usually, these interactions are joint attention activities accomplished while performing another task and are not focused television watching. For instance, the child or parent calls attention to the television, and then joint reference and conversation occur before returning to the original activity in which they were engaged. Thus social games and shared interactions form a basis from which linguistic and communicative behaviors can emerge.

O'Brien and Nagle (1987) reported parent-child interaction differences as a product of play context, which was defined by the types of toys used in the sessions (O'Brien & Nagle, 1987). The interactions were divided into three sections, which included doll play, play with vehicles, and play with a shape sorter. The two former activities were said to reflect sex role play stereotypes for boys and girls. The children had a mean age of 1 year 9 months. The language used by parents was analyzed during the three play conditions. Interestingly, the play with dolls showed the most parental language directed to the children, and the play with vehicles involved little language. They found few differences attributable to either parent or

child gender, while the play context had a significant effect. The researchers hypothesized about the possible effects of sex-stereotyped play on child-directed language and its possible contribution to sex differences in language acquisition.

Early Turn-Taking Behavior

Even from the beginning, the caretaker treats the infant as a "communicator." Petrovich-Bartell, Cowan, and Morse (1982) found that mothers can identify and respond to infant cries, and most mothers will indicate that they know the significance of different cries. Some of their knowledge may be based on contextual cues, since some parents have difficulty identifying the causes of cries (hunger, pain, etc.) when tapes are played at a later time (Muller, Hollien, & Murry, 1974). Some more recent evidence suggests that there are parents who evidently do not require strong contextual cues and can identify types of cries after a period of 3 weeks (Petrovich-Bartell, Cowan, & Morse, 1982). The fact that mothers treat these cries as having meaning attests to the early onset of caretaker-child communication. Research has shown that mothers take turns communicating with children as young as 1 to 3 months old (Snow, 1977). The infants' "turns," however, are biologic activities (burping, coughing, smiling, laughing, etc.), but the caretaker responds to them as if they were communicative. When the child smiles, the caretaker might say "oh, you like that don't you?" Then the child smiles even more broadly, which is another turn, and the caretaker responds to this behavior with more communication. Caretakers even answer for a child when they are very young ("you don't want that, do you?. . . . .no"). As a child becomes older, the turns are more and more well formed and linguistically correct, but the basic idea of interacting and taking turns can be traced back to early mother-child communication. In this case, the mother is compensating for the child's inability to take a meaningful turn. She waits for the child to do something and then responds as if it were communicative. The behaviors exhibited by mothers are more those that "pass turns" rather than those that "grab turns." That is, the mother sets up an opportunity for the child to take a turn and waits for the turn expectantly, rather than snatching the chance for herself and dominating the interaction.

CARETAKER CONTRIBUTION TO DEVELOPING LANGUAGE FORM AND USE

In early writings it was not unusual to find references to children's language learning as an amazing process because the child is born into a world of confusion. The child, however, ended up acquiring language in spite of these confusing models with no direct instruction and perhaps a good deal of interference. Reference was also made to the abstract nature of adult speech and the many retrials and disfluencies in the language, thus making it even more difficult to learn linguistic conventions. If one were to couple the immature nervous system of the child with the less than ideal language model, it is indeed amazing that language was learned at all. In the 1960s, however, studies began to emerge that closely examined the speech directed to children, and the above scenario was not supported. It turned out that caretakers significantly modify the language they use in talking to children as compared with the speech used in talking with adults, and it was not confusing at all. It was more like a model that was ideal for teaching language. This section endeavors to describe the caretaker model from a linguistic point of view.

Length

A number of studies have shown that caretakers modify the length of utterance when talking to children. Adult verbalizations typically become shorter in Mean Length of Utterance (MLU) and number of words (Phillips, 1973; Snow, 1972). Adult's use shorter noun phrases in the subjects of sentences (Snow, 1972; Broen, 1972). It appears that on the average the caretaker uses sentences that are about 2.4 morphemes longer than the child's MLU between ages 1 and 2 (Chapman, 1981). This length constraint has a predictable effect on the complexity of sentences since the shorter utterances do not have as many relations as longer ones. The picture that emerges is one in which the parent and child are on a staircase and the caretaker is several steps above the child. As the child increases length of utterance, the parent also increases the number of words per sentence. It almost appears to be a process of the caretaker "helping the child" up the staircase. This, of course, does not mean that *all* of a parent's utterances are short. As with all of these structural parameters, we are referring to a model set of behaviors. Indeed, there are frequent reports of long and complex utterances directed at children (Gelman & Shatz, 1977).

Complexity

As mentioned above, the shorter utterances contribute to the effect of lessening sentence complexity. Newport, Gleitman, and Gleitman (1977) and Broen (1972) report that less than 10% of mothers' speech to children between ages 1 and 2 is composed of complex sentences involving embedding or conjoining of propositions. There is controversy in saying that mothers do not address some complex language to children since most adult conversations are mainly declarative sentences and speech to children contains a high percentage of question forms that could be construed as more complex than declaratives (Newport, Gleitman, & Gleitman, 1977). With this exception noted, however, we believe that caretaker speech to children is clearly less complex overall than speech addressed to adults. Also, the speech addressed to children is highly grammatical, and most ungrammatical utterances are typically single words, partial repetitions, and omitted beginnings of yes/no questions. Many authorities believe that the complexity level of the caretaker model is attuned to the child's perceived level of language comprehension by the parent.

Disfluency

Another possibly confusing aspect in speech heard by children could be disfluencies or false starts and repetitions of words, phrases and sounds that are present in 10% of adult speech (Chapman, 1981). In speech to children, however, disfluency rates have been less than 1%, showing an extremely fluent model that is relatively free of these retrials, which could be confusing to the language-learning child (Newport, Gleitman, & Gleitman, 1977).

Semantics

Studies of the types of words used by caretakers to children have shown less diversity in vocabulary (Broen, 1972; Phillips, 1973; Rondal, 1978). This means that a small core of lexical items is being used over and over in talking to the child, which can clearly aid in language learning since the child can concentrate on a limited set of frequently recycled words. The types of words that are included in this limited vocabulary are typically high in frequency of occurrence in the language (Longhurst & Stepanich, 1975). Predictably, these words are concrete in nature (e.g., ball) and are more imaginable than abstract words (e.g., honesty) used in adult conversation (Phillips, 1973). There are even certain words uniquely used in talk to children that are not used in conversations with adults. Many of these words are simplifications of adult terms involving reduplication or use of the diminutive (e.g., tummy, tee tee, jammies, etc.). Additionally, pronoun use has been reported as different in speech to children (Gleason & Weintraub, 1978). Parents often use kin terms instead of pronouns ("Where is Daddy's nose?") or use a name where a third-person pronoun "you" might be used ("Where is Jeffrey's eye?").

Semantic Relations

Chapman (1981) provides an impressive summary of the specific types of semantic relations used by mothers to their 2-year-old children. Interestingly, the types of word combinations used by mothers are, for the most part, the same kinds as those reported by Brown (1973) in the speech of early language children. These two-, three-, and four-term semantic relations are comprised of the roles found in Stage I of language acquisition: agent, action, object, nomination, locative, entity, possessor, attribute, and state. Thus mothers are modeling many of the same types of utterances that children will later produce.

Suprasegmentals

Garnica (1977) has some interesting data on prosodic characteristics that quantify ubiquitous behaviors that almost all adults use when talking to children. As mentioned previously, we tend to exaggerate suprasegmentals and facial expressions when addressing youngsters. Garnica compared adult talk to 2 year olds, 5 year olds, and other adults to determine prosodic alterations in addressing the various groups. As one would predict, the mothers used a higher fundamental frequency (pitch) when talking to 2 year olds (267 Hz) than when talking to adults (about 200 Hz). The adults also used a wider pitch range in talking to 2-year-old children (19 semitones) than when talking to adults (10.5 semitones). The combined picture is a high-pitched, variable, vocal model that is likely to be salient and interesting to children learning language. The high pitch is also nearer the pitch of the child's own voice than a typical adult model. Garnica also noted that there were alterations in durations of certain words (colors and verbs) addressed to children that were not present in speech to adults ("Hit the greeeeeen ball" or "Thrrrrrrow the ball"). More recently, Swanson and Leonard (1994) found mothers' speech to children evidenced significantly longer vowel durations in the phrase's final position than when they talked to adults. These lengthened durations may also serve to hold the child's attention. The parents also often placed stress on more than one element in a sentence when addressing 2 year olds, while talk to adults may only have one stressed element. One of Garnica's examples is "*Push* the *green* square." Other elements noted in Garnica's work are the slower rate used by caretakers speaking to children and the use of whispering in some utterances. The speech rate to children is almost half that used in talking to adults (Gleason & Weintraub, 1978). Parents have also been observed to whisper more in talking to children than when addressing older listeners. Although the use of occasional whispering might be initially construed as a way to *de-emphasize* the parents' language model, further consideration suggests that whispered utterances interspersed in a stream of highly exaggerated verbalizations actually makes these soft models even more salient because they are different than typical stimuli. Finally, Broen (1972) has pointed out that parents tend to pause at utterance boundaries between single words or sentences when talking to children. In adult speech, pauses occur in a variety of places within an utterance for purposes of planning the rest of the verbalization. This adult pattern would be confusing in terms of letting a child know utterance boundaries.

Phonology

Several phonological changes have been noted in speech addressed to children by adults. First, some phonetic units are present in speech to children that may not be observed in adult-adult conversation (Ferguson, 1974). Also, some phonologic simplifications such as consonant cluster reduction (e.g., "top" for "stop") and reduplication (e.g., "wawa" for "water") have been reported in caretaker speech models (Gleason & Weintraub, 1978).

Cognitive Complexity

There is a difference between cognitive and linguistic complexity. For instance, it is conceptually less difficult to understand or answer a question like "What is this?" than a cognitively complex question such as "Why is the faucet leaking?" One involves the "here and now" and has perceptual support. The other question is more abstract and involves reasoning about cause-and-effect relationships. Not many studies have specifically investigated the cognitive complexity of language directed to children. Conti-Ramsden and Friel-Patti (1986) used a scale developed by Blank and Franklin (1980) that ranks the cognitive complexity of utterances on a scale of 1 to 4 with 1 being cognitively simple and 4 being complex. These researchers studied children between 12 and 24 months of age in conversations with their mothers. It was found that mothers most often used level-1 utterances (simple) and only occasionally the higher complexity levels. Interestingly, the children used level-1 utterances as well, and it was concluded that mothers either matched their child's cognitive complexity or were one step ahead of their child's complexity level. This would appear to be ideal for cognitive and language-learning purposes. More research is needed in this area, but these findings support the notion of reduction of cognitive complexity, in addition to linguistic simplifications.

Pragmatic/Interactional Features

These alterations in the speech of caretakers revolve around turn taking, the management of conversations, the types of speech acts, and the use of context in communicating to children. First, Chapman (1981) has noted that the speech acts used by caretakers most often are requests for information, statements, descriptions, and requests for action. There are other speech acts as well, but the ones listed above constitute over 80% of the utterances addressed to 2 year olds by mothers. Thus the developing child is hearing a variety of speech acts that represent declarative, imperative, and interrogative functions. A second pragmatic characteristic that has been observed is the increased amount of repetition in caretakers' speech to children. These repetitions are most frequent in speech to younger children (below age 2) and decline with age. Studies report mothers' self-repetitions of utterances addressed to younger groups to be as high as

43%, leveling off to about 25% in groups of 2 year olds (Newport, Gleitman, & Gleitman, 1977; Cross, 1977). With regard to the actual topic of conversation between mothers and children, Cross (1977) reports that 48% of the subjects focus on child events and 16% concern mother events, while only 9% deal with the events of other participants. Snow (1977b) also found that a large percentage of mothers' utterances were directly related to the child's nonverbal, vocal, or verbal behaviors. This suggests that mothers typically talk about the "here and now" and that topics concerning events removed in time and space are largely avoided. From both a linguistic and cognitive point of view, this is an ideal situation for the child learning language.

The area of turn taking has been a productive research area in caretaker-child interaction. Keller and Scholmerich (1987) studied infant vocalizations and parental reactions during the first 4 months of life, the infants being from 2 to 14 weeks of age. They found that the infants performed a variety of vocalizations and that these can be interpreted as affective states when the child is as young as 2 weeks of age. Positive vocalizations occurred most frequently in conditions of mutual attentiveness with eye contact. These positive vocalizations were responded to with increased verbal/vocal behaviors by the parent more than the negative, affective vocalizations, which were typically perceived as expressing affect or behavioral states and evoked tactile/vestibular behaviors from the parent. The authors speculate that infants who produce positive affective vocalizations will receive more language stimulation from parents during joint referencing. Thus, as mentioned earlier, parents and children are "communicating" from the outset, and infant vocalizations are treated as messages by parents. Many findings are available that indicate parents and infants engage in smoothly coordinated sequences involving both gaze and vocalizations during the first year of life (Richards, 1971, 1974; Kaye, 1982; Kaye & Fogel, 1980; Trevarthen, 1979). Rutter and Durkin

(1987) bring up the important point that we do not presently know whether the child plays a role in perpetuating these early interactions or if the reciprocity is merely an illusion because the mother simply follows the child's lead and makes the turn taking happen. Rutter and Durkin (1987) report some interesting data that suggest that up to 24 months the child simply behaves in a particular way and the mother simply follows, making the reciprocity occur. After 24 months, however, the child begins to play a more important role in the sequencing and controlling of the interaction. They stated the following (p.60):

> By the end of the second year, in other words, children were patterning their looks in exactly the way one would expect if they were using gaze in the same way as adults: looking up at the ends of their own turns to signal that they were finishing, and looking up at the end of the other's turns to confirm when the floor was about to be offered.

Thus we can see that caretakers make a host of segmental, cognitive, and suprasegmental changes in their speech to children. As mentioned previously, most studies on caretaker-child interaction have focused almost exclusively on mothers. It is only recently that fathers have been investigated at all. The next section reviews some research on fathers.

Research on Mothers and Fathers During Interactions With Children

Recently, many changes have occurred in societal attitudes toward parenting. As a result, fathers have begun to break away from the traditional stereotype where mothers did most of the work raising children, while fathers acted as breadwinners who went to work, came home, read the paper, and waited for dinner to be served to them. In this traditional stereotype the father would kind of "dabble" in his interaction with the infant and was not really in his element until the child was able to walk, talk, and take an interest in sports. This traditional stereotype is unfortunate on many levels, perhaps the most significant one being that it is accurate in many cases. Some research indicates that mothers show greater overall levels of involvement with infants, devote a greater percentage of their time to caregiving, and engage in nonphysical, verbal play, while fathers exhibit less overall involvement with the infant, but play more, and this play generally involves physical stimulation rather than verbal-social interactions (Power, 1985). We once met a father who bragged that he had never changed a diaper and had only fed his child three times. The sad aspect of this statement is that fathers who are not involved in the early development of their children miss out on a host of satisfying experiences. Keller, Hildebrandt, and Richards (1985) studied the effects of extended father-infant contact during the newborn period. They found that the fathers who had extensive postpartum contact with their children engaged in greater amounts of *en face* behavior and vocalization with their infants and were also more involved in the caretaking responsibilities 6 weeks after birth. They also had higher self-esteem scores than fathers who had traditional amounts of postpartum contact. Currently, many fathers take a significant interest in their children, even prenatally. More men are participating in the birth of their children than ever before and are forgoing the wasted time in the waiting room passing out cigars. There are many books for new parents that mention both mothers and fathers, and there are even texts directed just at new fathers. Although times have changed significantly, we suspect that even in families where both parents are involved, mothers still do a disproportionate amount of the child-rearing in the early years. This is, unfortunately, true even in double-income families, which currently comprise over 50% of American households.

The traditional mother-father stereotypes fostered many myths about parents. One, of course, is that mothers have some special sense about dealing with children that fathers cannot possess. Fathers were often characterized as inept with babies and were better equipped to deal with older youngsters. Also, fathers were sometimes portrayed as disinterested in babies and as a result did not spend time with neonates unless forced into the compromising position of having to substitute for mother while she had to be away for short periods. This then became "crisis management" because the father had few skills and felt awkward caring for a baby. Rebelsky and Hanks (1971) did an early study of father's verbal interactions with infants. They attached a microphone to babies clothing, and used a voice-operated relay to record interactions with the child 24 hours a day during samples over a 3-month period. They found that fathers spent little time interacting with their infants. The mean number of interactions was 2.7, which took place largely in the morning and the evening. The shocking thing about this study was that these fathers had an average length of interaction of only 37.7 seconds. Even the longest interaction by a father was less than 11 minutes. This study, of course, represents only a single data point and is certainly not enough to indict fathers as being poor models for language development due to unavailability. There have not been many studies, however, of the frequency of interaction of either mothers or fathers. Other studies during this period concentrated on the quality of the language models presented by fathers.

Kriedberg (In: Gleason & Weintraub, 1978) studied mothers' and fathers' speech to young children and found that the models were similar in terms of length for both parents. However, fathers' speech differed from the mothers' in some subtle ways. When analyzed, the fathers' speech contained more imperatives (commands), more threats, more negative name-calling (e.g., "ding-a-ling", etc.), and more low-frequency lexical items (e.g., "aggravating"). Gleason (1975) studied male and female attendants at a day care center and also found that the sexes had highly similar speech samples on structural grounds in length and complexity. One reported difference, however, aligned well with the

Kriedberg study in that the male attendants used more imperatives than the females. In another study Weintraub (1976) found some differences between fathers and mothers in questioning behavior. The fathers asked more WH questions, while the mothers asked more yes/no questions. Clearly, the former place more of a burden on the child in conversation, because specific material must be retrieved for the answer. However, when mothers asked WH questions and the child did not respond correctly, they "linguistically downshifted" and asked a yes/no question to help the child. For instance, they might ask "What's this?" and if the child did not answer they would say, "Is it a truck?" This suggests that the mothers were more sensitive to the child's communicative development level and provided additional cues so that an appropriate response could be made to maintain the interaction. Giattino and Hogan (1975) reported that the father they studied did not imitate or expand the child's utterances as mothers typically do, and this father used complete and grammatically correct sentences that were not redundant. Subjectively, the father seemed to be trying to carry on a conversation, while the mother seemed to be trying to facilitate language acquisition.

Some more recent studies of parents have also been conducted. Hladik and Edwards (1984) examined ten dyads of mothers, fathers, and their 2 year olds. They found similar mean lengths of utterance and total numbers of responses in mothers and fathers with no differences in sentence types used while engaged in triadic interactions (mother-child-father). Some significant differences in terms of total verbal output occurred when mothers and fathers interacted separately with the child. Also, fathers used more instances of ungrammatical utterances than mothers, but these were largely simplifications of the adult model (e.g., "You want to go to bed?"). This study supports the notion that the speech of mothers and fathers is more similar than different. Brachfeld-Child (1986) studied mothers and fathers of 8 month olds during a task

where they taught the infants to place cubes into a cup. They found many similarities between the parents, but the fathers spent more time talking to the babies and prohibiting infant activity. This suggests that fathers are more prone to control the training situation, which may be related to the studies cited earlier where fathers used more commands in dealing with their children. Power (1985) studied mothers and fathers play interactions with infants at 7, 10, and 13 months of age. He found that the parents were highly similar in terms of the kinds of play and general types of play encouragements that they engaged in. The analysis of play "style," however, showed significant differences between fathers and mothers. First, mothers tended to follow the child's lead more in choosing toys, while fathers tended to disregard the child's line of interest and even interfere with infant behavior. At age 13 months the infants were more likely to respond to the mother's direction rather than the fathers. In fact, with age, mothers of girls were more directive and mothers of boys were less directive. Other studies have shown sex differences in directiveness, with parents of boys being less directing and facilitative of exploration and parents of girls being more directive (Power, 1981; Fagot, 1978; Power & Parke, 1985; Smith & Danglish, 1977).

Bernstein-Ratner and Corazza (1985) studied mothers' and fathers' lexical specificity in speech to young children to determine if fathers used more semantically demanding language than mothers. They studied children between 18 and 24 months of age and found that, although not statistically significant, the trends suggested that fathers used more demanding lexical items. They report specific phrases like "Made in Taiwan" or "classic father-son film" as being produced by fathers, although these were the exception rather than the rule. Overall, there appeared to be many more similarities than differences between the parents. Girolametto and Tannock (1994) found both similarities and differences between mothers and fathers in their directiveness when interacting with young children who have developmental delay. Fathers tended to demand more responses from the children and changed topics more often than mothers.

Thus a general picture emerges from the literature comparing mothers and fathers during interactions with language-learning children. Basically, most research has shown that mothers and fathers do make structural changes in their language by reducing length and complexity of utterances. If any differences exist they are probably in style of play, use of imperatives, and subtle differences in lexical items and tone of the interaction. The model presented by both mothers and fathers is certainly a "learnable" one from a structural point of view, and a child exposed to language from either parent could surely use it to acquire communicative skills. The fact that there are few sex differences in the model suggests that perhaps it is not the sex factor that is important. The most significant factor may simply be that whenever *any* interactant is placed in a communicative situation with a child, he/she makes an effort to tailor communications to the level of the other member of the dyad. Therefore, if either a mother or father is trying to communicate with a child that has few communicative skills, it becomes important to compensate for this naive communicator by simplifying the language model.

This pragmatic skill of taking into account the perspective of an interactant develops early and is even seen in young children. Some studies (Sachs & Devin, 1976; Shatz & Gelman, 1973) have shown that children as young as age 4 simplify their language when talking to babies (ages 1.5 to 2.5) and dolls as compared with when they address peers and adults. Thus, rather than indicate that mothers and fathers have some special sense of how to talk to children, it is more parsimonious to suggest that communicators want to be understood and take into account the level of their listener when talking. This is seen even in young children who are not par-

ents, and the same phenomenon is observed when adults and children talk to pets. The above studies do not imply, however, that the model provided by a 4 year old to an infant is as ideal as parental models for language learning. In fact, Bates (1975) reviewed research focusing on peer language and came to the strong conclusion that children who learn communication from peers are at a disadvantage when compared with children who learn from adults. Young children may simplify some structural components of language when they talk to babies, but they are not equipped to really understand the cognitive level of an early developing child and may also not talk about situationally relevant topics. Also, little is known about their joint referencing ability as it relates to linguistic stimulation. For instance, more recent studies (Vandell & Wilson, 1987) have found that siblings of children aged 6 to 9 months were not as able to respond contingently to the infants' interests and actions and that they spent less time in turn-taking exchanges. Tomasello and Mannle (1985) found that, although preschool siblings did make some structural simplifications in their language model when talking to an infant, the changes were not as great as parents typically make. Also, the preschoolers did not use as many conversational devices to maintain dialogue and "teach" language to the infants. Andersen and Johnson (1973) found that by age 8 children have distinctly different ways of talking to 1, 3, and 5 year olds, much the same as adults do.

Communication Models in Day Care Settings

With the bulk of American families earning double incomes, a significant increase in concern about adequate day care facilities has arisen. Also, increased divorce rates over the last few decades have resulted in a significant rise in the number of single parents who need someone to care for their child while at work. Some industries and governmental institutions have begun to establish day care programs for employees, and there is increasing federal and state regulation on child care facilities. This is a trend that will only increase, and experts in the acquisition of communication are interested in the potential impact of day care environments on language development. Clearly, there are salient differences between the "traditional" home environment and a day care facility. An obvious difference involves the numbers of children who are vying for the attention of day care professionals for language stimulation. With less individual attention, one might expect that cognitive and linguistic development might occur more slowly in a day care environment. Some reviews of the literature on the effects of day care (Belsky & Steinberg, 1978) suggest that there is no significant effect, either positive or negative, on intellectual development.

On the other hand, some of the studies of day care environments have methodologic problems either in the matching of subjects studied or in the fact that only high-quality facilities were investigated. Other studies suggest that the quality of the language stimulation in day care settings may be important instead of just quantity of communications (Tizard, Cooperman, Joseph, & Tizard, 1972). Schindler, Moely, and Frank (1987) found day care experience to be positively related to increased social participation and associative peer interaction. McCartney (1984) examined the effect of quality of day care facilities on language development in 166 families whose children attended child care facilities in Bermuda. She used the *Early Childhood Environment Rating Scale* (Harms & Clifford, 1980) to rate each center for quality. The scale evaluates personal care, furnishings, language, reasoning, fine- and gross-motor activities, creative activities, and social development. McCartney found that overall quality of the day care center was predictive of intelligence measures and language development in her subjects, while statistically controlling for family background and day care provider experience. Additionally, it was learned that children from centers that had high levels of caretaker interaction, as opposed to high occurrences of peer speech, had higher scores on language tests. Jacobson and Owen (1987) found considerable variability in day care caregivers in terms of initiation of interaction, stimulation of infant play, and use of affect in 28 day care centers studied. Much more research needs to be done on day care environments and their effects on a host of child development parameters.

The Use of Specific "Teaching Strategies" by Caretakers

Over the years, certain interactional behaviors used by caretakers have been perceived as particularly "instructional." This is because these behaviors resemble what teachers would logically do if they had to overtly foster the development of communication in a child. We will consider several categories of "teaching strategies" with the cautions in mind that (1) not all parents do the full range of these behaviors; (2) research is lacking in some areas to provide actual proof of the facilitative effect of the behaviors; and (3) authorities label the specific behaviors using diverse terms.

Parallel Talk

This is when the parent talks about what the child is doing, such as describing actions or objects that the child is interacting with. The parent might say to a child who is pushing a car: "You're pushing the car." Essentially, the parent "codes" linguistically what the child is feeling or doing (Van Riper & Emerick, 1984).

Self Talk

In self talk the parent performs an action or attends to an object while providing the linguistic code to describe it (Van Riper & Emerick, 1984). For instance, a parent might be putting a cake in the oven and say "I'm putting the cake in the oven." In both parallel-talk and self-talk situations the child is presented with a model that provides linguistic tags for ongoing events, feelings, and objects for which there is joint reference between parent and child. Either context could conceivably assist in language development.

Repetition

As mentioned earlier, the frequent repetition of parents (almost one-third of utterances) in early interactions could facilitate language learning. Often an utterance is broken down into portions and then combined again (e.g., "Throw the ball over here. . . . throw it . . . over here. . . . throw it to me . . . give me that ball"). Recycling the message in many different ways, some of which are slightly discrepant, can logically aid in acquiring a language.

Expansion

One of the earliest mechanisms thought to be important in language stimulation is expansion. This involves taking a child's incomplete or telegraphic utterance (e.g., "read book") and making it into a complete, adult-like sentence (e.g., "Mommy will read the book"). This obviously gives the child the opportunity to see how an utterance would be said by an adult and helps to "fill in the blanks" of a youngster's primitive constructions. Snow, Arlman-Rupp, Hassing, et al. (1976) found that middle-class mothers expand utterances significantly more than parents who are lower socioeconomically. Some studies have found no experimental evidence that expansions aid in language development (Cazden, 1965), while other investigations do support the effect of expansions on language learning (Seitz & Stewart, 1975).

Recast Sentences

Some authorities view recast sentences as simply a variation of an expansion, but they are mentioned separately here because a body of literature is beginning to emerge on these mechanisms. A recast sentence, like an expansion, preserves the meaning of the child's sentence, but adds new syntactic information. In the expansion example listed above we stated that an expansion takes a telegraphic utterance and makes it adult-like. A recast sentence can take a child's sentence that is adult-like ("I like the dog") and change the syntactic structure to another sentence type ("you do like the dog, don't you?"). It is a subtle distinction, but perhaps a relevant one. Nelson, Carskaddon, and Bonvillian (1973) found recast sentences presented to 3 year olds increased their scores on syntactic measures in comparison to a group that did not receive intervention with recast sentences. Nelson (1976) increased complex sentences and verb forms in the spontaneous speech of 21/2 year olds by selectively using recast sentences in training sessions. Thus relevant recasts may play a role in the development of certain types of linguistic constructions.

Questioning

Howe (1980) has indicated that caretakers often ask children questions. Many of these questions (over 50% in some cases) do not really seek information because the caretaker already knows it, or the answer is obvious from the context. The purpose of these questions, then, must be either tutorial in nature or may serve to initiate specific interactions. If a parent is reading a book with a child and looks at a picture of a boy climbing a tree, he or she might say "What's the boy doing?" Another kind of question may serve as a prompt or contingent query. A child may say "I going (unintelligible)" and the parent says "You're going where?" This prompts the child to attend to a particular constituent and gives the message that communication failure has occurred.

Direct Teaching

Friedlander, Jacobs, Davis, and Wetstone (1972) report three varieties of direct instruction in language used by parents. First, there is "directed mimicry" in which the child is essentially told to imitate something (e.g., "say ball"). Second, sometimes parents tell the child that something has been said wrong (e.g., "No, that's not a dog . . . it's a cow"). Finally, prompts in the form of nonlinguistic, nonverbal, or physical cues may be given. Here they refer to physical nudges or intonational cues, such as a parent poking a child to facilitate saying "You're welcome" or "Thank you."

Early researchers (Brown & Hanlon, 1970) suggested that parents engaged in very little overt correction or teaching, but more recent studies have reported the occurrence of some direct and a greater amount of indirect feedback on the correctness of child utterances (Moerk, 1983; Hirsh-Pasek, Treiman, & Schneiderman, 1984; Demetras, Post, & Snow, 1986). Parents also engage in frequent routines that have verbal behaviors as an integral part such as politeness, trick or treat, and greetings (Gleason & Weintraub, 1978). These routines are taught most often on an elicited imitation basis, and the child is corrected if the correct utterance does not occur at the appropriate time.

Extension

Extension is sometimes known as modeling or expatiation, and it occurs when an adult responds to a child's utterance on the same topic, but the response is not simply a rephrased version of the child's utterance. For instance, if a child says "I like milk," and the parent responds "You will grow big and strong if you drink milk," an extension of the child's utterance has occurred.

All of these alleged "teaching strategies" could logically facilitate communication development in children. We do not know at present whether one, or a combination, of these techniques is the most effective in contributing to communication development. We do know that they all occur in caretaker speech to children, although they are present to a different degree in individual parents. Also, not all techniques are always used by a particular person. Nevertheless, these are the techniques that we recommend to parents and teachers when we want to "stimulate" language development in children who are delayed, or just to augment the development of children who are acquiring communication normally.

Research on the Long-Term Effects of Early Interactions

We know that there appears to be a positive relationship between caretaker verbal stimulation and children's lan-guage/cognitive development (Bing, 1963; Bradley & Caldwell, 1976; Clarke-Stewart, 1973). Some studies have longitudinally investigated children over periods ranging from several months to a number of years to determine if certain early language experiences are statistically predictive of later linguistic or cognitive abilities. For instance, Bornstein (1985) and Bornstein and Ruddy (1984) report several studies concerning the prediction of language development and intellectual attainment at 4 years of age from behaviors recorded in the first 6 months of life. Infants were observed at 4 months of age and followed longitudinally until age 4 years. Bornstein (1985, p. 7471) found the following:

> . . . the amount of maternal encouragement given to young infants to attend to properties, objects and events in the environment—i.e., caretaker didactics—was a moderately good predictor of toddlers language development over the short term as well as children's intellectual attainment over the long term. The 4-month infants whose mothers prompted them more consistently tended to possess larger expressive vocabularies at 1 year and to score higher on the WPPSI at 4 years.

In another study, Olson, Bayles, and Bates (1986) conducted longitudinal evaluations of mother-child interactions at 6, 13, and 24 months of age. They evaluated each child's language and cognitive abilities, and mothers assessed their child's vocabularies at 13 and 24 months. It was found that the children with larger, more diverse vocabularies were more developmentally advanced when compared with peers. In essence, the vocabulary size at 13 months predicted children's cognitive and linguistic competence at age 2. Interestingly, the children's vocabularies did not appear to be directly related to level of overall maternal stimulation. Instead, the vocabulary growth was related more closely to "frequent, responsive mother-child language interaction, even when family social class and maternal education were controlled" (p. 1). The variable that was important was maternal *verbal* responsiveness, involving both corrective, as well as accepting, feedback with regard to the children's utterances.

Students and researchers must be very careful in interpreting preliminary data using correlational techniques such as the studies reported above. There may be multiple variables that affect language development in addition to caretaker interactions, but these investigations provide some interesting support for the potential importance of these episodes in communication development.

Beyond Dyadic Interaction:
A Real World View

The vast majority of the hundreds of studies on caretaker-child interactions can be criticized on two major fronts. First, as mentioned previously, most studies involved only mothers and only recently have fathers been included in research. A second point, however, is that most of these studies were of dyadic communication between mothers and their children. This is a bit unrealistic since up to 80% of American children have one or more siblings (Brody & Stoneman, 1982). Although a parent usually talks to only one child at a time, the dynamics of interactions with three or more participants are altered when compared with dyadic communication. This is even changed further when one considers the age levels of the participants in conversation (i.e., a group consisting of a parent and children ages 2, 4, and 6). Wellen (1985) studied triadic interactions among mothers, a younger child, and an older child. She found generally that the mothers used fewer rephrased questions, fewer questions providing hints, fewer expansions, and fewer repetitions in triadic interactions than in dyadic ones. Generally, the younger child's responses were reduced by 50% in triadic interactions when an older child was present. Wellen and Broen (1982) have also studied interruptions by siblings of children with language impairment. They found that brothers and sisters of these children engage in interruption more than siblings of nonde-

layed children. Stoneman and Brody (1981) found that in triadic interactions of two parents and their child, both parents spoke less, and there was a striking difference especially in the verbal output of fathers, who spoke significantly less in the three-way conversations than in dyads.

Estimating the Actual Contribution of Caretaker Models on Communication Development

In virtually every model that attempts to explain how language develops in children the role of the caretaker is addressed on some level. In some theories of language acquisition the caretaker's examples of communication are pivotal to the child in learning language, and in other theories these parental models assume a less important position. Owens (1996) summarizes four major theories of communication development: behavioral, psycholinguistic-syntactic, psycholinguistic-semantic/cognitive, and sociolinguistic. In the behavioral theory, the parent serves mostly as a model of the language to be acquired and as a mediator of reinforcement or extinction. The syntactic point of view portrays the child as a possessor of innate capacities for language acquisition and, according to Owens, the input from the environment basically serves as a model that activates the child's hypothesis-testing mechanism. This point of view also assumes that adults do not necessarily simplify their utterances for children. In the Semantic/cognitive theory, universal cognitive structures allow the child to apprehend relationships on a nonlinguistic level, and these basic concepts are later expressed in semantic relations. The environment is important in this view because the child forms the cognitive basis for language through active involvement with objects and people. Caretaker language models are important because language "codes" or "maps" onto underlying cognitive structures. The parent presents these models in relevant situations so the child can learn the correspondence between concepts and the semantic relations that refer to them. Finally, in the sociolinguistic view, communication is initially established between caretaker and child on a nonlinguistic level. Then, the caretaker models language beginning with simple utterances and progressing to complex sentences. Feedback is provided to the child, and he or she learns that communication can take place on a linguistic level, as well as a nonlinguistic level. The point here is that, in all theories of language acquisition, caretaker language models have been judged as important to communication development. The importance of caretaker models, however, varies in degree and in the specific mechanism by which they contribute to communication development.

Another way to look at the contribution of caretaker models to communication development is in terms of continuity. For instance, does the prelinguistic stimulation from caretakers actually relate to linguistic development, or not? When a child is nonverbal and the parent is stimulating certain types of linguistic forms, are these the forms that are actually developed? Do nonverbal behaviors of the caretaker such as reciprocity actually relate to turn-taking behavior later seen in verbal exchanges? These questions relate to a continuity point of view (Messer, 1986). On the other hand, there may be discontinuity in the relationship between caretaker stimulation and later communication development. There is disagreement in the literature as to the importance of the continuity/discontinuity issue (Bloom, 1983; Shatz, 1983; Sugarman, 1983). Finally, there is little empirical proof of the actual contribution of preverbal communications with caretakers on linguistic development (Messer, 1986).

Some other problems exist in attributing influences from caretaker interactions directly to communication development. One problem is the considerable variation in parent's use of "motherese" with their children. Also children use many individual strategies to acquire communication (Nelson, 1981). For instance, some non-Western cultures have different caretaker-child interaction patterns from those reviewed above. The Kaluli tribe of New Guinea have been reported to interact differently with their language-learning children. Schieffelin and Ochs (1983) report that parents in this culture do not reduce the complexity of their speech to infants and that they have fewer dyadic interactions with their children. Samoans are less contingent in responding to children's utterances than members of Western cultures. The Kipsigis of Kenya and rural Blacks in Louisiana provide more directives and explanations to their children as opposed to high proportions of questions or comments about ongoing activities (Harkness, 1977; Ward, 1971). As Snow (1986) points out, it would be inaccurate to suggest that some of these cultures are not interested in language learning. Children in these cultures acquire communication at about the same time developmentally as Western youngsters. The techniques of modeling are different, however. The Kaluli and Samoan cultures use a more direct modeling approach to language teaching that involves elicited imitation where children are told what to say in conversations. Evidently, it is not important whether they comprehend the utterances or not, at least initially. The point here is that these cultural differences make one wonder about the specific importance of the modifications of caretaker speech to children, since other types of modeling appear to result in language acquisition that is seemingly as effective.

Another way of looking at caretaker language contributions to language development is to review studies that have attempted to statistically correlate certain parental linguistic behaviors with specific language acquisitions in children. Some studies have failed to find many significant relationships between structural simplifications of adult speech to children and language acquisition (Cross, 1978; Wells & Robinson, 1983; Scarborough & Wyckoff, 1986).

Some studies that have found relationships between structural aspects of adult speech and child language development have been criticized on methodologic grounds (Scarborough & Wyckoff, 1986; Schwartz & Camarata, 1985). The use of gain scores and performing multiple correlations on data are some statistical difficulties, and some problems also have been associated with types of samples used in these studies. Some authorities suggest that use of passive observation and language sampling cannot really illuminate the issue as well as experimental manipulation of caretaker model variables and examination of the effects on communication development. It is important to note that most of these studies have examined whether certain *degrees* of caretaker speech simplification aid in language acquisition and that they have not compared samples that do, and do not, modify caretaker speech to children. Scarborough and Wyckoff (1986, p. 437) state the following:

> . . . individual differences in motherese may be largely unimportant, as long as some minimum degree of adequacy is achieved . . . Just as vitamins are necessary to health, but doses in excess of daily requirements contribute little to improved health, so too may the motherese input threshold be low enough that nearly all children receive the necessary environmental stimulation for language acquisition, and observed degrees of difference among (mainly middle-class) mothers have little or no effect . . . If so, only for extreme cases of insufficient (or perhaps hyperstimulating) input would strongly supportive evidence of motherese effects be measurable.

Thus, although we do not know the specific effects of language directed to children by parents in our culture, we do know that the model is important. The communication development process is remarkably resilient, probably because it has to be "buffered" against varying types of genetic and environmental influences that could be detrimental to language acquisition. The wide variety of caretaker models in different cultures and even socioeconomic strata in Western cultures, attests to a general, rather than a specific contribution of particular styles of speaking to children. Most of them learn to communicate whether they have "exemplary" models or are exposed to imperfect models in a family of 12 children. Differences may or may not occur in rate of development. There must certainly be some very complex and multivariate interactions taking place among environmental, genetic, and behavioral factors.

APPLICATIONS TO CHILDREN WITH LANGUAGE IMPAIRMENT

Since the late 1970s study of the interaction that takes place between parents and children with delays in language development has been increasing (Wulbert, Inglis, Kriegsmann, & Millis, 1975; Cramblit & Siegel, 1977; Millet & Newhoff, 1978; Giattino, Pollack, & Silliman, 1978; Petersen & Sherrod, 1982; Price, 1983; Schodorf, 1982; Conti-Remsden, Hutcheson, & Grove, 1995; Donahue & Pearl, 1995). One motivation for this research was to determine if parents of children with language impairment present models of communication that are not conducive to language development and that therefore might play a role in causing or perpetuating the linguistic delay. Cross (1984) reviewed the literature on the interactions between children with language-delay and their parents and found several trends in the research. Most studies showed that parents of these children used fewer semantically contingent utterances than parents of normals. This suggests that they did not use "here and now" utterances to contingently respond to their children's verbal and nonverbal behaviors. This type of contingency, as stated earlier, appears to be important in normal language acquisition. Another variable found in the review was that parents of children with language impairment seemed to be less positive and accepting of their children's utterances in terms of acknowledging and reinforcing them. Other findings indicated that these parents repeated themselves more than parents of normal-language children, used more imperatives, and used more WH questions. Finally, some studies showed parents of children with language impairment to produce less speech over-all and use a faster rate than parents of normal-language children. Although some methodologic problems were found in the studies on this issue, Cross (1984, p. 12) concludes the following:

> Studies equating normal and communicatively impaired children on age or language ability repeatedly show patterns of deviation in language and conversation style for parents of impaired children . . . This survey of research into both normal and impaired language development indicates that clinicians should not only intervene with language-impaired children, but they should also recruit the parents into habilitation.

It should also be stressed that the literature is not totally in agreement on the quality of models presented to children with language impairment. Some studies have failed to find deficiencies in the linguistic environments of these children (Conti-Remsden & Friel-Patti, 1983; Rondal, 1977; Lederberg, 1980). It is possible that parents respond differently to children with communication disorders, or perhaps there are sampling differences among the various studies on this topic. Whatever the reason, clinicians should not expect all parents of children with language impairment to exhibit deficiencies in their interactions with these youngsters. The precise role of the parent model in contributing to a child's impairment is, in most cases, impossible to determine. The parent's way of communicating to a child with a language impairment may either be the cause or the effect of the child's communication delay, or neither. While it is tempting to argue that any interactive differences found in parents of youngsters with language delay may have caused the disorder, it is just as potent to argue that the way parents of such children talk is a product of the child's nonresponsiveness to their formerly ideal models. The most important point to make in this section, however, is that some fairly consistent differences have been found in the models presented to children with language impairment by

their parents, and this means some assessment and treatment implications should be considered.

ASSESSMENT APPLICATIONS OF CARETAKER-CHILD INTERACTION RESEARCH

Perhaps the biggest assumption underlying the clinical application of research on caretaker interaction with normally developing children is that this type of stimulation facilitates language development. Although it has not been demonstrated that specific aspects of caretaker interaction relate to certain linguistic acquisitions, we do know that important general relationships exist. For instance, there is agreement that the presence of a communication model in relevant interactions is required for language development. This means that the child must joint reference with an adult who uses appropriate communication during these interactions. There is also some general agreement that the adult must simplify the communication model to some degree, although the specific level of simplicity has not been determined. Even in cultures that do not have a distinct "motherese" register no evidence has been found to show that the parents present models that are overly complex, and there is even support for specific teaching routines such as imitation tasks. Thus some measure of simplification and indirect or direct tutoring seem to be associated with communication development.

Most authorities in child language disorders recommend that the caretaker-child interaction be evaluated in cases where the child is nonverbal, speaking in single words, or speaking in telegraphic speech (e.g., "push car"). The caretaker-child interaction can be analyzed either using a formal system or by informally taking note of behaviors exhibited by both parent and child. Some clinicians videotape these interactions and actually take data on certain behaviors (e.g., directiveness, requests for imitation, questioning, etc.). This evaluation typically takes place in a clinical setting where one or both of the parents are asked to accompany the child into a playroom and interact in a "typical" manner. The room usually contains a variety of toys and objects that will hopefully stimulate a diversity of interactions. It is assumed by most clinicians, that the parent's interaction will, if anything, be more facilitative of communication than it typically is because of the awareness that communication is being evaluated. During a 15- to 20-minute interaction period clinicians can get a reasonable idea about how the caretaker joint references with the child by watching behaviors such as gaze, eye contact, initiation of play routines, and reciprocity in directing activities. Special consideration is given to whether the caretaker presents models while the child is attending to objects and actions or if the model is given while the child is not paying attention. Characteristics of the language model itself are also evaluated such as vocabulary, syntactic complexity, concreteness, suprasegmentals, length of utterance, and other variables mentioned earlier in this chapter that are found to occur in models presented to children acquiring language normally.

In a more formal vein, other clinicians prefer to use some specific type of system to evaluate caretaker-child interaction (Flick & McSweeney, 1987). An area that should not be overlooked is the evaluation of other environments in which the child spends time (e.g., school, day care). Also, just because a clinician observes a parent in a clinical setting, it does not mean that the parent always behaves in a similar manner. One of the present authors once worked with a mother who stimulated language quite well in the clinic. Since she usually spent each day at home with her child, she was asked about her daily routine. She reported spending over 75% of her time either watching television or playing the stereo so loud that her dinnerware rattled in a corner china cabinet. During these times the child was encouraged to "entertain" himself, and he did so in silent, solitary play. Not much language stimulation could occur in these circumstances. The point here is that somehow the clinician will have to determine if the existing interaction patterns among family members are conducive to language development in the delayed child or if certain changes in either the family routine or the language models might increase the probability of learning.

TREATMENT APPLICATIONS OF THE CARETAKER-CHILD INTERACTION RESEARCH

As mentioned previously, it is altogether possible that a child who is delayed in communication development may experience this impairment because of insufficient stimulation, a faulty language model, or a language model that is not presented in relevant contexts. Take the extreme case of a child with psychotic parents who never talk to the child or spend time joint referencing. The child will not have the opportunity to experience a model of communication often enough to extract the rules of language. This, of course, would be a highly unusual circumstance. Let's take a less severe example. A child has parents who spend little time playing and joint referencing, and when they do talk, they do not simplify their language. Perhaps this child will be delayed in acquiring language because of lessened opportunity and exposure to difficult examples. One must say, however, that many children are from environments where the caretaker's language model is not optimal and the parents spend little time with them; yet, these youngsters manage to develop language normally. This brings up the important variable of the child's contribution to the process. Whether it is due to genetic predisposition or simply a child's information-processing strategy, some children require few relevant models and seem to learn communication skills anyway. The system of acquiring communication somehow compensates for deficiencies or variations in caretaker models in many cases.

If a child is delayed in communication development, however, the speech-language pathologist assumes that the child needs all the help possible in acquiring language, and typically the recommendation is made to train parents in presenting a heightened model of communication. This usually means that parents are asked to incorporate as many of the characteristics of normal caretaker communication models as possible (suprasegmentals, complexity, joint referencing, teaching strategies, etc.). The hope is that, with the accentuated model, the child will find it easier to abstract the language rules of the culture. This parent training is, in some cases, the only treatment applied, and some children respond to the augmented models by beginning to develop language. In other cases language therapy is required, but in most cases the parents are also trained in providing appropriate language stimulation during the time that the child is at home.

Research has clearly shown that language treatment programs directly involving parents are more effective than those that do not include significant others in the child's family (McDade & Varnedoe, 1987; Fey, 1986). This attests to the facts that (1) parents can be trained and (2) that treatment carried out in extraclinical environments can be a useful addition to clinical training. Historically, speech-language pathologists have faced several thorny problems in language training. First, the clinician sees the child for a limited number of hours during the week, and many additional opportunities occur for language learning during the time a child is at home or school. Parent training helps to extend the number of hours per week that communication is emphasized, and this would logically assist the child in learning.

A second problem has been one of generalization or carryover of skills trained in a clinical setting to more natural environments. The use of parents in treatment would naturally facilitate generalization to other environments since the parents would be stimulating language in these situations. Finally, sometimes clinical training tasks are relatively unnatural, and activities for language treatment must be contrived. Even in situations where the child is engaged in "naturalistic" play therapy, an element of unreality exists, since activities must be set up in advance and often a child is asked to talk more than in a real situation. On the other hand, in a child's "real" life outside the clinic, there are numerous opportunities to stimulate language naturally and to require a child to respond a particular way because it is the natural thing to do. Parents have access to these natural circumstances, and if properly trained, can use them for facilitating communicative development. Thus we know that parent involvement in language training is helpful, and this is especially true in cases of younger children. In fact, federal law (PL 99–457) requires speech-language pathologists to involve parents in the treatment of language impaired children and to develop a specific plan as to how they will be integrated.

Parents could be involved in language training in a variety of ways. A general method recommends use of natural situations and use of the "teaching strategies" mentioned in an earlier section to facilitate language development. The parents typically undergo a series of training sessions, but they are more general than specific. For instance, parents may first be told about the common strategies of facilitating language in normal children (e.g., self talk, parallel talk, expansion, recasts, enlargement, etc.). Then, the parents will be given several opportunities to practice these techniques with the clinician, either in role playing or with their own child. After the parents have had enough practice, they might be videotaped using the techniques with their child and jointly review the tape with the clinician. A key point here is that in any parent involvement they must be specifically trained. Most clinicians know that a short talk with parents after a therapy session and providing some handouts on language stimulation are usually not sufficient to gain the type of understanding and cooperation that will actually contribute to successful therapy.

REFERENCES

Andersen E, Johnson C. Modifications in the speech of an eight year old as a reflection of age of listener. Papers and Reports on Child Language Development, Stanford University, 1973.

Bakeman R, Adamson L. Infants' conventionalized acts: gestures and words with mothers and peers. Infant Behav Dev 1986;9:215–230.

Bakeman R, Brown J. Early interaction: consequences for social and mental development at three years. Child Dev 1980;51:437–447.

Bates E. Peer relations and the acquisition of language. In: Lewis M, Rosenblum L, eds. Friendship and peer relations: the origins of behavior. Vol. 3. Chichester: Wiley, 1975.

Belsky J, Steinberg L. The effects of day care: a critical review. Child Dev 1978;49929–949.

Bernstein-Ratner N, Corazza P. Mothers' and fathers' lexical specificity in speech to young children. Paper presented at the convention of the American Speech-Language Hearing Association, Washington, DC, 1985.

Bing E. Effect of child-rearing practices on development of differential cognitive abilities. Child Dev 1963;34:631–648.

Blank M, Franklin E. Dialogue with preschoolers: a cognitively based system of assessment. Appl Psycholinguist 1980;1:127–150.

Bloom L. Of continuity and discontinuity, and the magic of language development. In: Golinkoff R, ed. The transition from prelinguistic to linguistic communication. Hillsdale, NY: Erlbaum, 1983.

Bornstein M. How infant and mother jointly contribute to developing cognitive competence in the child. Proc Natl Acad Science USA 1985;82:-7470–7473.

Bornstein M, Ruddy M. Infant attention and maternal stimulation: prediction of cognitive and linguistic development in singletons and twins. In: Bouma H, Bouwhuis D, eds. Attention and performance X: control of language processes. London: Lawrence Erlbaum, 1984.

Bowlby J. Attachment and loss: Vol. 1. Attachment. London: Hogarth Press, 1969.

Brachfeld-Child S. Parents as teachers: comparisons of mothers' and fathers' instructional interactions with infants. Infant Behav Dev 1986;9:127–131.

Bradley R, Caldwell B. The relation of infants' home environments to mental test performance at 54 months: a follow-up study. Child Dev 1976;47:1172–1174.

Breznitz Z, Sherman T. Speech patterning of natural discourse of well and depressed mothers and their young children. Child Dev 1987;58:395–400.

Brody G, Stoneman Z. Family influences on the language and cognitive development. In: Worell J, ed. Development in the elementary years. New York: Academic Press, 1982.

Broen P. The verbal environment of the language learning child. American Speech and Hearing Association Monograph No. 17. American Speech and Hearing Association, Washington, DC, 1972.

Brown R. A first language: the early stages. Cambridge, MA: Harvard University Press, 1973.

Brown R, Hanlon C. Derivational complexity and order of acquisition in child speech. In: Hayes J, ed. Cognition and the development of language. New York: Wiley, 1970.

Bruner J. The ontogenesis of speech acts. J Child Lang 1975;2:1–19.

Camaioni L, Laicardi C. Early social games and the acquisition of language. Br J Dev Psychol 1985;3:31–39.

Cazden C. Environmental assistance to the child's acquisition of grammar. Unpublished doctoral dissertation, Harvard University, 1965.

Chapman R. Mother-child interaction in the second year of life. In: Schiefelbusch R, Bricker D, eds. Early language acquisition and intervention. Baltimore: University Park Press, 1981.

Clarke-Stewart K. Interactions between mothers and their young children: characteristics and consequences. Monogr Soc Res Child Dev 1973; 38:1–108.

Cohn J, Tronick E. Mother-infant face-to-face interaction: the sequence of dyadic states at 3, 6 and 9 months. Dev Psychol 1987;23(1):68–77.

Collis G, Schaffer H. Synchronization of visual attention in mother-infant pairs. J Child Psychol Psychiatry 1975;16:315–320.

Conti-Ramsden G, Friel-Patti S. Mothers discourse adjustments to language-impaired and non-language-impaired children. J Speech Hear Disord 1983;48(4):360–367.

Conti-Ramsden G, Hutcheson G, Grove J. Contingency and breakdown: children with SLI and their conversations with mothers and fathers. J Speech Hear Res 1995;38:1290–1302.

Conti-Ramsden G, Friel-Patti S. Mother-child dialogues: considerations of cognitive complexity for young language learning children. Br J Disord Commun 1986;21:245–255.

Cramblit N, Siegel G. The verbal environment of a language-impaired child. J Speech Hear Disord 1977;42:474–482.

Crawley S, Rogers P, Friedman S, et al. Developmental changes in the structure of mother-infant play. Dev Psychol 1978;14:30–36.

Cross T. Mothers' speech adjustments: the contribution of selected child listener variables. In: Snow C, Ferguson C, eds. Talking to children. Cambridge, England: Cambridge University Press, 1977.

Cross T. Mothers' speech and its association with rate of linguistic development in young children. In: Waterson N, Snow C, eds. The development of communication. Chichester: Wiley, 1978.

Cross T. Habilitating the language-impaired child: ideas from studies of parent-child interaction. Top Lang Disord 1984;4,(4):1–14.

Demetras M, Post K, Snow C. Feedback to first language learners: the role of repetitions and clarification questions. J Child Lang 1986;13:275–292.

Donahue M, Pearl R. Conversational interactions of mothers and their preschool children who had been born preterm. J Speech Hear Res 1995; 38:1117–1125.

Eisenberg R. Auditory competence in early life: the roots of communicative behavior. Baltimore: University Park Press, 1976.

Fagot B. The influence of sex of child on parental reactions to toddler children. Child Dev 1978; 49:459–465.

Fantz R. Visual experience in infants: decreased attention to familiar patterns relative to novel ones. Science 1964;146:668–670.

Fey M. Language intervention with young children. San Diego, CA: College-Hill Press, 1986.

Field T. Effects of early separation, interactive deficits and experimental manipulations on infant-mother and face-to-face interaction. Child Dev 1977;48:763–771.

Field T, Vega-Lahr N, Scafidi F, Goldstein S. Effects of maternal unavailability on mother-infant interactions. Infant Behav Dev 1986;9:473–478.

Flick L, McSweeney M. Measures of mother-child interaction: a comparison of three methods. Res Nurs Health 1987;10:129–137.

Friedlander B, Jacobs A, Davis B, Wetstone H. Time sampling analysis of infants' natural language environments in the home. Child Dev 1972;43:730–740.

Garnica O. Some prosodic and paralinguistic features of speech to young children. In: Snow C, Ferguson C, eds. Talking to children. Cambridge, England: Cambridge University Press, 1977.

Giattino J, Hogan J. Analysis of a fathers' speech to his language-learning child. J Speech Hear Disord 1975;40(4):524–537.

Giattino J, Pollack E, Silliman E. Adult input to language impaired children. Paper presented to the American Speech and Hearing Association Convention, San Francisco, 1978.

Girolametto L, Tannock R. Correlates of directiveness in the interactions of fathers and mothers of children with developmental delays. J Speech Hear Res 1994;37:1178–1192.

Gelman R, Shatz M. Appropriate speech adjustments: the operation of conversational constraints on talk to two year olds. In: Lewis M, Rosenblum L, eds. Interaction, conversation and the development of language. New York: Wiley, 1977.

Gleason J. Fathers and other strangers: men's speech to young children. In: Dato D, ed. Georgetown University round table on languages and linguistics. Washington, DC: Georgetown University Press, 1975.

Gleason J, Weintraub S. Input language and the acquisition of communicative competence. In: Nelson K, ed. Children's language. Vol. 1. New York: Gardner Press, 1978.

Gustafson G, Green J, West M. The infants' changing role in mother-infant games: the growth of social skills. Infant Behav Dev 1979;2:301–308.

Harkness S. Aspects of social environment and first language acquisition in rural Africa. In: Snow C, Ferguson C, eds. Talking to children. Cambridge, England: Cambridge University Press, 1977.

Harms T, Clifford R. Early childhood environment rating scale. New York: Teachers College Press, 1980.

Harris M, Jones D, Brookes S, Grant J. Relations between the nonverbal context of maternal speech and rate of language development. Br J Dev Psychol 1986;4:261–268.

Hirsh-Pasek K, Treiman R, Schneiderman M. Brown and Hanlon revisited: mothers' sensitivity to ungrammatical forms. J Child Lang 1984;11:81–88.

Hladik E, Edwards H. A comparative analysis of mother-father speech in the naturalistic home environment. J Psycholinguist Res 1984;13(5):321–332.

Howe C. Learning language from mothers' replies. First Lang 1980;1:83–97.

Jacobson A, Owen S. Infant-caregiver interactions in day care. Child Study J 1987;17:197–209.

Kaye K, Fogel A. The mental and social life of babies. Brighton, England: Harvester Press, 1980.

Kaye K, Fogel A. The temporal structure of face-to-face communication between mothers and infants. Dev Psychol 1980;16:454–464.

Keller W, Hildebrandt K, Richards M. Effects of extended father-infant contact during the newborn period. Infant Behav Dev 1985;8:337–350.

Keller H, Scholmerich A. Infant vocalizations and parental reactions during the first 4 months of life. Dev Psychol 1987;23(1):62–67.

Landry S. Preterm infants' responses in early joint attention interactions. Infant Behav Dev 1986; 9:1–14.

Lederberg A. The language environment of children with language delays. J Pediatr Psychol 1980;5:141–159.

Lemish D, Rice M. Television as a talking picture book: a prop for language acquisition. J Child Lang 1986;13:251–274.

Longhurst T, Stepanich L. Mothers' speech addressed to one, two and three year old normal children. Child Study J 1975;5:3–11.

Messer D. Adult-child relationships and language acquisition. J Soc Pers Relation 1986;18:101–119.

McCartney K. Effect of quality of daycare environment on childrens' language development. Dev Psychol 1984;20(2):244–260.

McDade H, Varnedoe D. Training parents to be language facilitators. Top Lang Disord 1987;7(3):19–30.

McLean J, Snyder-MClean L. A transactional approach to early language training. Columbus, OH: Merrill, 1978.

Millet A, Newhoff M. Language disordered children: language disordered mothers. Paper presented at the convention of the American Speech and Hearing Association, San Francisco, 1978.

Moerk E. A behavioral analysis of controversial topics in first language acquisition: reinforcements, corrections, modeling, input frequencies and three-term contingency. J Psycholinguist Res 1983;12:129–155.

Morse P. Infant speech perception: a preliminary

model and review of the literature. In: Schiefel-busch R, Lloyd L, eds. Language perspectives: acquisition, retardation and intervention. Baltimore: University Park Press, 1974.

Muller E, Hollien H, Murry T. Perceptual responses to infant crying: identification of cry types. J Child Lang 1974;1:89–95.

Nelson K. Facilitating childrens' syntax acquisition. Dev Psychol 1976;13:101–107.

Nelson K. Individual differences in language development: implications for development and language. Dev Psychol 1981;17:170–187.

Nelson K, Carskaddon G, Bonvillian J. Syntax acquisition: impact of experimental variation in adult verbal interaction with the child. Child Dev 1973;44:497–504.

Newport E, Gleitman H, Gleitman C. Mother, I'd rather do it myself: some effects and non-effects of maternal speech style. In: Snow C, Ferguson C, eds. Talking to children. Cambridge, England: Cambridge University Press, 1977.

Ninio A. Picture book reading in mother-infant dyads belonging to two subgroups in Israel. Child Dev 1980;51:587–590.

Ninio A. Joint book reading as a multiple vocabulary acquisition device. Dev Psychol 1983;19:445–451.

Ninio A, Bruner J. The achievement and antecedents of labelling. J Child Lang 1978;5:1–15.

Obrien M, Nagle K. Parents' speech to toddlers: the effect of play context. J Child Lang 1987;14:269–279.

Olson S, Bayles K, Bates J. Mother-child interaction and childrens' speech progress: a longitudinal study of the first two years. Merrill-Palmer Q 1986;32(1):1–20.

Owens R. Language development: an introduction. 4th ed. Neeham Heights, MA: Allyn and Bacon, 1996.

Papousek M, Bornstein M, Nuzzo C, et al. Infant responses to prototypical melodic contours in parental speech. Infant Behav Dev 1990;13:539–545.

Peterson G, Sherrod K. Relationship of maternal language to language development and language delay of children. Am J Ment Defic 1982;86:391–398.

Petrovich-Bartell N, Cowan N, Morse P. Mothers' perceptions of infant distress vocalizations. J Speech Hear Res 1982;25:371–376.

Phillips J. Syntax and vocabulary of mothers' speech to young children: age and sex comparisons. Child Dev 1973;44:192–195.

Power T. Sex typing in infancy: the role of the father. Infant Ment Health J 1981;2:226–241.

Power T. Mother and father infant play: a developmental analysis. Child Dev 1985;56:1514–1524.

Price P. A preliminary report on an investigation into mother-child verbal interaction strategies with mothers of young developmentally delayed children. Aust J Hum Comm Disord 1983;11:17–24.

Rebelsky F, Hanks C. Fathers' verbal interaction with infants in the first three months of life. Child Dev 1971;42:63–68.

Richards M. The development of psychological communication in the first year of life. In: Connolly K, Bruner J, eds. The growth of competence. London: Academic Press, 1974.

Richards M. A comment on the social context of mother-infant interaction. In: Schaffer H, ed. The origins of human social relations. London: Academic Press, 1971.

Robson K. The role of eye to eye contact in maternal-infant attachment. J Child Psychol Psychiatry 1967;8:13–25.

Roggman L, Langlois J, Hubbs-Tait L. Mothers, infants and toys: social play correlates of attachment. Infant Behav Dev 1987;10:233–237.

Rondal J. Maternal speech to normal and Down's syndrome children matched for mean utterance length. In: Meyers C, ed. Quality of life in severely and profoundly mentally retarded people. Washington, DC: Research Foundation for Improvement, American Association on Mental Deficiency, 1978.

Rutter D, Durkin K. Turn taking in mother-infant interaction: an examination of vocalizations and gaze. Dev Psychol 1987;23(1):54–61.

Sachs J, Devin J. Young childrens' use of age-appropriate speech styles in social interaction and role playing. J Child Lang 1976;3:81–98.

Scarborough H, Wyckoff J. Mother, I'd still rather do it myself: some further non-effects of "motherese." J Child Lang 1986;13:431–437.

Schaffer R. Mothering. Cambridge, MA: Harvard University Press, 1977.

Schindler P, Moely B, Frank A. Time in day care and social participation of young children. Dev Psychol 1987;23:255–261.

Schodorf J. A comparative analysis of parent-child interactions of language-delayed and linguistically normal children. Dissert Abstr Int 1982;-42(5):1838B.

Schwartz R, Camarata S. Examining relationships between input and language development: some statistical issues. J Child Lang 1985;12:199–207.

Seitz S, Stewart C. Limitations and expansions of some developmental aspects of mother-child communication. Dev Psychol 1975;11:763–768.

Shatz M. On transition, continuity and coupling: an alternative approach to communicative development. In: Golinkoff R, ed. The transition from prelinguistic to linguistic communication. Hillsdale, NY: Erlbaum, 1983.

Shatz M, Gelman R. The development of communication skills: modifications in the speech of young children as a function of listener. Monogr Soc Res Child Dev 1973;38(5):1–37.

Slade A. Quality of attachment and early symbolic play. Dev Psychol 1987a;23(1):78–85.

Slade A. A longitudinal study of maternal involvement and symbolic play during the toddler period. Child Dev 1987b;58:367–375.

Smith P, Danglish L. Sex differences in parent and infant behavior in the home. Child Dev 1977;48:1250–1254.

Snow C. Mothers' speech to children learning language. Child Dev 1972;43:549–565.

Snow C. The development of conversation between mothers and babies. J Child Lang 1977a;4:1–22.

Snow C. Mothers' speech research: from input to interaction. In: Snow C, Ferguson C, eds. Talking to children. Cambridge, England: Cambridge University Press, 1977b.

Snow C. Social interaction and language acquisition. In: Dale P, Ingram D, eds. Child language: an international perspective. Baltimore: University Park Press, 1981.

Snow C. Conversations with children. In: Fletcher P, Garman M, eds. Language acquisition: studies in first language development. Cambridge, England: Cambridge University Press, 1986.

Snow C, Arlman-Rupp A, Hassing J, et al. Mothers speech in three social classes. J Psycholinguist Res 1976;5:1–19.

Stern D. The first relationship. Cambridge, MA: Harvard University Press, 1977.

Stoneman Z, Brody G. Examination of mothers' and fathers speech to their young children. Child Dev 1981;52:705–707.

Sugarman S. Empirical versus logical issues in the transition from prelinguistic to linguistic communication. In: Golinkoff R, ed. The transition for prelinguistic to linguistic communication. Hillsdale, NY: Erlbaum, 1983.

Swanson L, Leonard L. Duration of function word vowels in mothers' speech to young children. J Speech Hear Res 1994;37:1394–1405.

Tizard B, Cooperman O, Joseph A, Tizard J. Environmental effects of language development: a study of young children in long-stay residential nurseries. Child Dev 1972;43:332–358.

Tomasello M, Farrar M. Joint attention and early language. Child Dev 1986;57:1454–1463.

Tomasello M, Mannle S. Pragmatics of sibling speech to one year olds. Child Dev 1985;56:911–917.

Trevarthen C. Communication and cooperation in early infancy: a description of primary intersubjectivity. In: Bullowa M, ed. Before speech: the beginning of interpersonal communication. Cambridge, England: Cambridge University Press, 1979.

Vandell D, Wilson K. Infants' interactions with mother, sibling and peer: contrasts and relations between interaction systems. Child Dev 1987;-58:176–186.

Van Riper C, Emerick L. Speech correction: an introduction to speech pathology and audiology. Englewood-Cliffs, NJ: Prentice-Hall, 1984.

Ward M. Them children: a study of language learning. New York: Holt, Rinehart & Winston, 1971.

Weintraub S. Some sex differences in the language parents address to children. Paper presented to the First Annual Boston University Conference on Language Development, Boston, 1976.

Wellen C. Effects of older siblings on the language young children hear and produce. J Speech Hear Disord 1985;50(1):84–99.

Wellen C, Broen P. The interruption of young children's responses by older siblings. J Speech Hear Disord 1982;47:204–210.

Wells G. Language development in the preschool years. Language at home and at school. Vol. 2. Cambridge, England: Cambridge University Press, 1985.

Wells C, Robinson W. The role of adult speech in language development. In: Fraser C, Scherer K, eds. The social psychology of language. Cambridge, England: Cambridge University Press, 1983.

Wolff P. Observations on the early development of smiling. In: Foss B, ed. Determinants of infant behavior II. New York: John Wiley, 1963.

Wulbert M, Inglis S, Kriegsmann E, Mills B. Language delay and associated mother-child interactions. Dev Psychol 1975;11:61–70.

Cognition and the Cognitive-Language Relationship

Beth Witt

anguage, the symbolic system used to express and understand thoughts, ideas, and feelings, is a component of the human mind. Few today dispute this statement. However, what continues to be disputed—and widely studied—is the relationship that exists between language and cognition. Also a "component" (element or part) of the mind, cognition is defined as "a general concept embracing all the various forms of knowing: perceiving, remembering, imagining, conceiving, judging, reasoning" (Nicolosi, Harryman, & Kresheck, 1989). The two are closely intertwined, so much so that one cannot talk about either cognition or language without utilizing both cognition—and language! This chapter will examine the relationship of these two higher functions of the human mind by reviewing several theories of cognition, by discussing how these theories relate to language acquisition and proficiency, and by examining clinical applications of these theories for the speech-language pathologist. In so doing, we will look at beliefs from fields such as philosophy (study of principles of knowledge), psychology (science of mental states and processes), and linguistics (science of language studies) (Stein, 1980).

EARLY VIEWS OF COGNITION

Around the 5th century bc philosophers began to consider the origins of thought or ideas, moving gradually toward explanations that were more like those for other processes noted in their natural world and away from the supernatural explanations that characterized earlier oral tradition cultures. Many of the early Greek philosophers such as Democritus separated "sense perception" from "genuine knowledge." Plato, for example, conceived of sense perception as simple ideas gained from experience. These he viewed as more "matter" or more of the body than of the mind, though entwined with the mind. True knowledge, he believed, is found in the soul-mind (the two terms were synonymous to Plato), *is present at birth*, and must gradually be recalled through a process of questioning (using language to do so). Socrates, Plato, and Aristotle all attempted to refine the questioning process or "laws of logic" in understanding the mind. Today, Plato is considered to be the original rationalist or *innatist*, believing that the mind had ideas beyond those derived from experience (Frost, 1962).

Later Greek philosophers were influenced by the beliefs of Epicurus, who postulated that all knowledge comes through the senses and that true knowledge is a result of adequate, correct observations. This school of epistemology (philosophical branch that investigates the origins, nature, methods, and limits of human knowledge) has come to be known as empirical. Essentially, rationalists held that man is born with innate, but not at first consciously realized, ideas, that are gradually drawn to a level of consciousness through response to sensory experiences. Empiricists believed that man took in information from the world through the senses, that it was imprinted in the mind, and that the mind gradually organized it into higher-level ideas. Throughout the centuries, these two theories have held sway and stood in contrast (Frost, 1962).

Early Modern Theories

Almost 2000 years later, in the 17th century, scholars were still taking sides on these issues. René Descartes ("I think, therefore I am."), considered the first psychologist of early modern times, was essentially an innatist. He took a medieval belief in three soul dimensions (the *nutritive*, responsible for nourishment and reproduction; the *sensitive*, responsible for sensory perception and locomotion; and the *rational*, seat of logical thought) and shaped the theory for his purposes. Descartes noted that all animals possessed the nutritive and sensitive aspects and that these were associated with the physical body. Only man was in possession of rational thought, Descartes believed, and this thought was seated in the mind, separate from the physical being or body (Lowry, 1982; Watson, 1968). Thus Descartes was a promoter of mind-body *dualism*. His vague explanation as to how mind and body worked together—that the two made contact at the brain's pineal gland—was vague, unsatisfactory, and inaccurate.

Descartes discussed creative language as being evidence of the rational mind of mankind, noting that only man uses language to reason and to express more than signals for survival and "passion" (in Chomsky, 1966, p. 5). Studies over the past 30 years involving attempts to teach communicative symbols and use to animals have failed to disprove Descartes' contention that language is species-specific to man. Though animals have learned to employ some symbols for communication, they have failed to create "rule systems" (such as morphology, syntax, and discourse) to govern their attempts (Premack, 1986; Terrance, Pettito, Saunder, & Bever, 1979). Descartes varied Platonic ideas by conceiving of thought as being *derived*, arising from objects in the external environment, and *innate*, not learned but emerging from consciousness alone on reflection (Watson, 1968).

John Locke, more an educator and a philosopher than a psychologist, studied "knowing" around the same period. The ultimate empiricist, Locke believed that the child is born with a mind that is like a blank slate (*tabula rasa*) on which is marked sensory impressions from the "world of matter" (Frost, 1962). Though the mind does not have inborn ideas, Locke believed it is possessed with an ability to organize impressions (simple ideas) such that it can produce consistent, logical thoughts (complex ideas). Though Locke remained a *dualist* in terms of mind and body, he moved toward *monism* as he believed each affects the other and are therefore interactant; however, he was not able to explain how. Locke was able, though, to develop his philosophy into a remarkably practical design for educating youth, a process of physical exercise and extended environmental experiences and exposure to a variety of types of people and societal roles. His aim was a sound mind in a sound body; an individual well able to care for himself within his society and natural environment. Such an educational philosophy helped extend empiricism to the "nurture" (belief in the beneficial aspect of appropriate mental, physical, and social stimulation during maturation) side of the nature-nurture controversy that has continued to occupy scholars of the 20th century.

Nineteenth-Century Brain-Mind Studies

In the early 1800s various physicians began to secretly dissect and explore the human brain, which had come to be accepted as the "organ of the mind" (Penfield & Roberts, 1966). They subdivided the brain into "little organs." Some physicians, most notably Franz Gall and his Viennese colleague Spurzheim, began to try to explain the function of the brain by assigning specific faculties: propensities, dispositions, qualities, aptitudes, and abilities to each "little organ." Included among music, art, love of children, benevolence, and criminal behavior was—language. These *phrenologists* (analyzers of mind function), as they came to be called, produced work that even today divides many in their study of mind function into two camps: those who believe function is a result of the whole brain at work and those who believe that separate functions or "faculties" are centered in separate compartments of the brain.

Further work by later 19th-century physicians such as Broca, Wernicke, Fritsch, and Hitzig pointed toward, if not autonomous separate faculties, at least localization of functions such as speech, verbal understanding, and movement control (Penfield & Roberts, 1966). The stage was set for the explosion of theories on the workings of the mind and its relationship to language ability that have developed in the 20th century.

FACULTIES OF THE MIND: CURRENT THEORIES

The concept of the mind as a package of domain-specific faculties, not a popular one among many scholars today, developed out of the nativist position that there must be a genetically endowed system ready to process sensory information from the environment. Various applications of this idea have produced interesting side-theories and work, several of which include the mind-language relationship. For example, Howard Gardner (1983) has proposed a more readily accepted version of the faculty theory in his "multiple frame model of intelligence." This theory diverges from the commonly accepted "verbal" and "performance" intelligences to conceive of a profile of intellectual strengths across seven levels of competence: musical, logico-mathematical, spatial, bodily-kinesthetic, intrapersonal, interpersonal, and linguistic (verbal). Miller (1990) described an assessment scheme based on Gardner's model, which addresses competence across five intellectual domains (Highnam, 1994). Additionally, educational approaches aimed at capitalizing on specific intellectual strengths in the Gardner model have been developed (Gardner, 1995). Theories that are quite well developed and based on the mental-faculties concept are the modular theories of Fodor (1983).

Symbol-Manipulating Devices: Modules

Fodor's (1983) theories are extremely nativist; he suggests that cognitive systems are essentially symbol-manipulating devices, part of which are composed of "modules." He defined modules as cognitive components with which an individual is born that are "hard-wired" into the neural mechanism (i.e., particular neurons perform their operations). These modules do not contain or own knowledge, *à la* Descartes, but process information in particular ways. There are two types of modules: vertical, which operate autonomously (independently) and do not interact or rely on each other for operation, and horizontal, which are self-contained but may cross content domains in their operations (Fodor, in Highnam, 1994).

Vertical Modules

Fodor (1983) describes the work of vertical faculties in a model he calls *trichotomous functional taxonomy*. There is a *transduction unit*, which conducts sensory input forward as neural energy. This energy is received by the *input system* and is transformed into representations that can be functionally acted on by the *central processor*. In other words, vertical faculties are "bottom-up," or data-providers rather than concept-expectant (top-down) computational devices. They do not routinely use information from higher, meaning-driven, cognitive levels to make inferences or conclusions. The interesting aspect of Fodor's theory is that he includes language as one of the vertical modules. He believes that language, like vision and touch, functions to prepare information from the distal (outside) environment for central processing. For example, whereas a visual module might perceive color, analyze shape, and recognize faces, auditory/language modules might recognize a voice, perceive pitch and intensity of intonation, and/or recognize a string of words as a sentence. Fodor further defines the first two levels of the modules as having various features such as rapid speed, information encapsulation, fixed neural architecture, and characteristic breakdown and growth patterns that are not shared by the central processor. Integrative in nature, the central processor can utilize information from several sources to solve problems, is not encapsulated or domain-specific, and may therefore work more slowly (Fig. 6.1). We will look further at this theory and its inclusion of language as a module.

Horizontal Modules

The difference between horizontal and vertical modules is that horizontal modules may interact or "cross content domains." Though Fodor (1983) notes that horizontal modules are highly specified in function and streamlined in operation, they may not be localized or innate and may involve several locations in the brain. Fodor says they may be a module assembled (from elementary units) for a specific purpose; communicative intent (goal-directed communicative behavior) is an example of such a specific purpose given by Bates, Bretherton, and Snyder (1988). Horizontal modules can operate top-down, as well as bottom-up, and are influenced by task familiarity. Though interactive to a de-

gree, horizontal modules fall short of the cumulative and integrative organization of current interactionist theories (Highnam, 1994). Bates and colleagues (1988) provide an orientation toward horizontal modules much akin to Fodor's: "self-contained components of mind. . . characterized in terms of the processes and/or representations needed to operate in a specific content domain. . . particularly important for the organism" (p.11).

In summarizing faculty of mind psychology, the three theories we have examined (Gardner's "multiple intelligences," 1983; Fodor's vertical and horizontal faculties, 1983) follow Descartes (i.e., they are neo-Cartesian) in the point of view that various kinds of knowledge are innate (present and functioning at birth) and species-specific. Gardner's competences and Fodor's processing modules both include language as a "kind of knowledge," though very differently: Gardner's as a type of facility or talent and Fodor's two theories as processors that ready components of language for use by a central processor. Vertical modules bring in bits of information in an independent, autonomous fashion. Horizontal modules enable operation across domains, so that language could be based in or strongly influenced by other cognitive skills (Highnam, 1994).

COGNITIVE DETERMINISM

Frequently called "the strong cognitive hypothesis," cognitive determinism is the notion that all higher-order (what the Greeks called rational) behavior, including language, is based in cognition and is controlled by it. Cognitive theorists across disciplines are concerned with the development and functioning of the mind as a whole. The influential work of Swiss Jean Piaget in explaining human cognitive development and growth is discussed as most representative of this theoretic school.

Jean Piaget

Jean Piaget, trained in biologic science and abnormal psychology, considered himself an epistemologist foremost, one

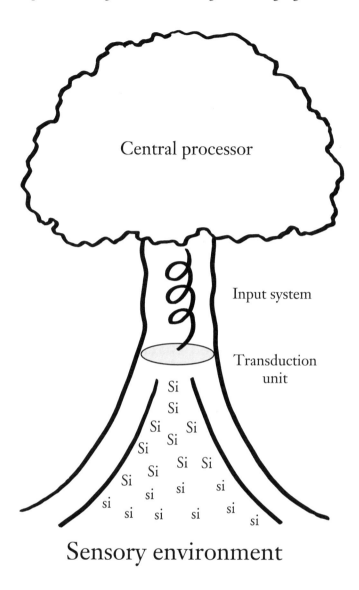

Figure 6.1. Fodor's vertical module model: trichotomous functional taxonomy. The central processor integrates/interprets; it enables "knowing" at the conscious level. The input system transforms salient sensory energy into appropriate representation for mental use. The transduction unit chooses salient sensory input and fast-forwards. *Si*, salient sensory information; *si*, sensory information.

who studies the nature of knowing. He attempted to answer three of the same questions posited over 2,000 years ago: (1) How does one come to "know" something?, (2) Does absolute truth transcend human conception of truth?, and (3) Is knowledge innate or learned? He formulated scientific hypotheses around these questions and then examined them.

Because of his biologic background,

Piaget believed children are born with (innatist view) a set of human systems (he called them sensorimotor) that allow them to actively perceive and engage with their environment. Such engagement results in the incorporation of experiences in an on-going, changing process that allows children to construct and reconstruct their representation or understanding of the world surrounding them, an empiricist view. Piaget, in other words, believed that the acquisition of knowledge is the result of both innate factors and experiential factor, or nature *and* nurture! His theories are most generally referred to as *constructivist;* the child is viewed as a constructor of knowledge through the formulation and testing of hypotheses, which grow in complexity over time (Highnam, 1994; Hoffman, Paris, Hall, & Schall, 1988).

Piaget applied his biologic principles to intellectual maturation—to features of cognitive structure (Miller, 1983):

(1) The intellect accommodates to reality and assimilates it in the way biological organisms adapt to their environments.

(2) Cognitive growth is like the growth of an embryo in which an organized structure becomes more finely differentiated over the course of its life.

To Piaget, children's mental "structures" (relationships between parts organized into a whole) change in nature and quality as children grow older. Infant-toddler mental structures (he called them *schemata*) may be viewed outwardly as gradually more organized behavior (e.g., moving from grasping to throwing objects, or from intentional reaching to communicative pointing), but indicate the mental networking of information gained from sensory and motor explorations. As the child grows, mental representation moves from symbols of the concrete, visible world to more abstract operations or reasoning with use of a network of basic information and symbolic ideas. He depicts children as "driven" biologically to adapt to their environment through mental processes of accommodation and assimilation, which result in increasingly complex cognitive organization of experience.

Piaget's Stages

Piaget , as a result of his studies, proposed four major stages of cognitive development that occur between birth and young adulthood, during which development and change may occur vertically (increasing in complexity) and horizontally (across skill areas within stages). The stages include sensorimotor period (birth to 2 years), preoperational period (2 to 7 years), concrete operational period (7 to 11 years), and formal operational period (11 to 15 years).

Sensorimotor Period

During this period the child inhibits involuntary reflexes, which constrain his movement, and learns to be an increasingly mobile being. Thus the child explores and expands horizons, and develops some organized schemas for comprehending and responding to the world. Piaget details this early stage as progressing in six substages.

Substage 1: Reflex Modification (Birth to 1 Month)   At birth the infant is bound by innate reflexes, very basic motor responses to various stimuli that appear (due to immaturity of the linkages between the peripheral and central nervous system) for such protective purposes as protection or food location. Absence or weakness of these reflexes at birth can indicate possible neurologic impairment. Repeated use of reflexes soon after birth serve to allow the child to adapt to new circumstances through modifications that occur as the child accommodates learning into the system. For example, he or she may turn and/or arouse more readily to the sight, sound, and smell of those caretakers who generally feed him. Piaget viewed both the original reflexes and the tendencies to *assimilate* (fit into and broaden existing schemas), *accommodate* (modify old schemas into new through the integration of new information), and even *practice* (repeat for automaticity or ease of retrieval or use) new actions—as innate, the product of genetic endowment. He believed these tendencies allowed the child to move forward to more volitional and differentiated behavior—controlled by the child and serving a variety of purposes—enabling him to be *adaptive*, able to respond appropriately to environmental changes and demands.

Substage 2: Primary Circular Reactions (1 to 4 Months)   Infants in this period randomly notice results of actions they do. Alerted and curious, they repeat the actions numerous times (the circularity is the series of repetitions), each time exacting a similar effect. The reactions are called *primary* in that the effects are limited to those that directly affect the child's body. Highnam (1994) gives as an example a child's accidentally scratching a bedsheet as she clenches her fingers, and repeating the action, as the sensory feedback is new and interesting. In so doing, she *assimilates* and *accommodates* new tactile, kinesthetic, and auditory information. Most primary circular reactions strongly involve tactile and kinesthetic senses and "close" receptors (skin, muscle, and joint sensors), with distance receptors such as audition and vision appearing incidental to the more primarily sensed tasks. The child has learned to imitate her own behavior by the end of this stage. Examples of skills that develop during this period are grasping, volitional kicking, and thumb sucking, each suggesting a network of expanding mental schemes.

Substage 3: Secondary Circular Reactions (4 to 8 or 10 Months)   These reactions follow the same design principle as primary reactions, as effects are noted following a random occurrence, and an action is repeated to recreate them. However, the child now focuses on acting on the outside environment, rather than maintaining stimulation for her own body. Distance receptors (vision and audition) are more utilized. The child practices a variety of action schemas with new objects and with toys that are now known for the feedback they give to the body (taste and feel) and that now are explored for the action schemas that can be enacted with them: shaking, dropping, patting, and hitting (Highnam, 1994). Given a spoon to hold and suck on, a baby in this stage can entertain itself quite well through turning and examining it, banging it on the high chair and on the table, and finally dropping it, losing interest only when it is completely out of sight. Given a spoon a week later, the child will go through the same exploratory reactions with it, as if they had never been experienced before. In other words, objects and people may be "recognized" when they reappear, but are not ac-

tively sought when they disappear, indicating movement toward but not attainment of representational *object permanence* ("knowledge" of the existence of some entity that is not physically perceivable).

Substage 4: Coordination of Secondary Schemas (8 or 10 to 12 Months)   In this stage, according to Piaget, the ability to coordinate action schemes enables a small repertoire of "complex" skills to develop; for example, combined shaking and releasing develops into a throwing gesture, which, with practice, will become further refined (Highnam, 1994). The development of object permanence enables a child to persist to find out-of-sight objects or develop behavior designed to "call" or make significant others reappear. Means-end behavior develops as the child begins to show true intentionality in his actions. The results of these two abilities and the ability to use imitation to learn result in "plan-ful" behavior, in which one can see the child has a *goal* and makes attempts to achieve it, even to the extent of using tools such as pulling strings. The child may begin to refine his gestures (a reach becomes more like a point) and his sounds (reduplicated babbles become wordlike homonyms such as *bah!* for bottle) in a coordinated effort to request objects or actions from others.

Substage 5: Tertiary Circular Reactions (12 to 18 Months)   By this stage most babies are mobile and are actively exploring an expanded environment, seeking "novel" objects and events to explore. Through trial and error, they problem-solve new situations and learn new schemas for play. Children in this stage will climb up, crawl under, and use sticks to obtain desired objects beyond their reach. They learn to activate toys by pushing and pulling parts of them instead of exploring the whole toy in a sensory manner. They can now imitate actions and sounds of *others* (touch a comb to their hair; say "bye-bye" spontaneously as someone leaves). Actions that "work for them" are repeated and refined.

Substage 6: Invention of New Means Through Mental Recombinations (18 to 24 Months)   During this final sensorimotor stage the child progresses more closely to competent representational thought. He has created for himself an impressive mental network of information that he begins to be able to manipulate for reasoning purposes. The child no longer has to reason using objects directly in front of him, but can rely on mentally stored images and words to help him problem-solve. These abilities are observable in the child's play and language use, as objects and actions are combined during play in a reenactment of the common daily routines in which he participates and in the talk that might accompany such play, for example, "eat peas!" Immediate imitation of novel models is also evident during this period (Ginsburg & Opper, 1979).

The close of the sensorimotor period finds the child ready to transition into the preoperational stage as a relatively efficient thinker, whose thought capacity is manifested in a variety of ways; symbolic play and language are the most evident at this point, and drawing, dreaming, and imagery will become more obvious in the next stage. Piaget regards language therefore as one of several mentalistic and symbolic activities, made possible by the development of representational thought (Highnam, 1994).

Preoperational Stage (2 to 7 Years)

During the preoperational stage all that the child has discovered during the sensorimotor stage about objects, people, space, time, movement, relations, and causality comes to be more competently organized and refined within mental representation. This enables three important cognitive abilities: the formation of mental symbols, the use of symbolic play, and the use of language. None of this occurs overnight, but gradually. Symbols develop from internalized imitations by the child of world elements (Ginsburg & Opper, 1979). Imitation now occurs "under cover" or mentally, rather than overtly (physically). Symbolic play moves from re-enactment of the common routines of daily living to play involving less common routines (shopping, traveling), to events seen on television or read about (Westby, 1980). Children use objects to "stand in" for other objects, like a basket for a shopping bag and begin to combine play schemes in highly creative ways.

Among cognitive characteristics that describe the thought and language of this developmental period is *egocentrism* (Miller, 1983), the child's tendency to perceive and interpret events in terms of his or her own perspective. Preoperational children have little appreciation for listener needs or the affective states of others. Communicatively, they engage in "egocentric speech," what Piaget refers to as "collective monologue." This egocentrism results in inaccurate assumptions about the amount of information needed during a conversation and difficulty in maintaining a conversational topic, behaviors that would be considered pragmatically inappropriate or immature today (Highnam, 1994).

Linguistically, the preoperational child develops a stable, functional language system consisting of perhaps 14,000 appropriately used words (Miller, 1977). The development of rule systems in the language domains of phonology, morphology, syntax, and pragmatics enable him to verbalize most intentions and frequently modify them for listener needs—by the end of the preoperational period. Prior to that, he experiences some frustrating times, with frequent communicative breakdowns and inappropriate language use, resulting in occasional angry outbursts. How such language facility develops is not addressed directly by Piaget; to him, language is simply a growing representation of changing inner mental activity and ability.

Concrete Operational Stage (7- to 11 Years)

During the concrete operational stage children begin to mentally organize information they have acquired about their physical world, as their perceptual boundedness gives way to conceptual flexibility (Pulaski, 1980). Three types of concept ability that began to develop at the latter end of the preoperational period, *classification*, *seriation*, and *conservation*, now are refined enough to enable a type of problem solving that Piaget calls concrete operations. This refers to mental manipulation of problems involving concrete materials in a real world. Pulaski (1980) refers to the nature of such tasks as "describing-thinking" (in Highnam, 1994).

Classification problem solving requires children to be able to sort or "class together" materials on the basis of both physical properties (which most can do by the latter part of the preoperational stage) and hierarchies, which involve part-whole relationships. Hierarchical class inclusion proficiency is not usually developed until the concrete operations stage. Now children can class together types of chairs as "things to sit on," *and* they can place them in a larger hierarchy of furniture (objects that furnish a home) and include a variety of items beside chairs (Pulaski, 1980).

Seriation is a more quantitative and qualitative skill, requiring children to order objects that are graduated by size, weight, or amount. To manipulate this principle, Gross (1985) notes that children must be able to have an internalized understanding of seriation, not just know how to order the real, physical objects. Then problems such as "If A>B and B>C, then A>C" may be solved.

Conservation requires the child to understand that certain properties of objects do not change, though their appearance may change. Children will come to refine their ability to use this type of information to solve problems involving number, length, volume in liquid and mass, weight, and area. By 5 or 6 years of age, children understand that a liquid amount is the same in a tall, thin glass as in a short, fat glass and that blocks spread over a larger area are the same amount. It is not until they are 12 to 14 years, however, that most children apply this principle to solid mass (Lowery, 1977a).

Internalized classification, seriation, and conservation enable children to mentally manipulate and solve many problems about their physical world. We will discuss how language skill impacts use and understanding of these concrete operations in the section on the language-cognition relationship.

Formal Operational Stage (12 years and Up)

Formal operational thinking contrasts with concrete operations in that mental application of "operations" or problem solving has moved from the concrete world to focus on cerebral ideas or hypotheses, what Piaget referred to as "second order operations" (Pulaski, 1980). Such abstract thought requires the ability to inference, or as Blank and colleagues (1978) described it, to "reason beyond perception." Highnam (1994) provides an example that a youth cannot conceptualize an imperfect mathematical correlation without first quantifying and seriating the two entities in relation to each other.

Piaget described two substages of formal operations. First, children learn how to mentally analyze all possible combinations of a proposition (idea), while gradually developing the ability to test hypotheses by manipulating one variable while mentally holding the others constant. In the second substage, children learn to organize their reasoning, deductive approach to such problems. They learn to perform operations of conjoining (solution is A and B), disjoining (solution is A *or* B), negating (solution is neither A nor B), and implication (A is true, so C is true) (Lowery, 1977b).

Piaget's position of cognitive primacy in regard to the relation of language to formal operational ability will be discussed in the section on cognition and language. Although this relationship was highly discussed by many psychologists and linguists, Piaget nevertheless maintained his position of cognitive abilities first, then language ability, in this stage, as in prior stages (Table 6.1).

INTERACTIONISM

Many factors work together to influence the development of any particular aspect or stage of cognition, according to interactionist approaches. Because these factors include maturational-biologic, along with social, linguistic, and nonlinguistic experiences, these theories would fall under the

Table 6.1 *Piaget's Stages of Cognitive Development*

Stage	Age (yr)	Major Cognitive Themes	Language	Key Terms
Sensori-motor	0–2	Growing control of movement; prerepresentational to symbolic thought. Learns to imitate, use tools as means to end, plan simple actions	Moves from nondifferentiated crying to use of a functional vocabulary to influence others to meet own needs	Object Permanence Means-end Causality Distancing
Preoperational	2–7	Mastering of relationships in physical world; thought increasingly decontextualized (space, time, quantity concepts develop)	Language develops in complexity of vocabulary, structure, and function; is used to socialize and learn	Classification Seriation Conservation Centration Irreversibility
Concrete operations	7–11	Can think logically about concrete world and its parameters	Verbal reasoning is internalized	Decentration Reversibility
Formal operations	11–15	Can reason and hypothesize about ideas	Abstract verbal thought	

rubric of nature and nurture categories, though now the perception is one of "complementary interaction between innate capacities and environmental forces" (Friel-Patti, 1994, p. 376). Interactionists believe that elements interact and thus modify each other in the course of development. Unlike "faculty psychology" approaches, components are not considered dissociable (separate and independent in action); in fact, they are so mutually dependent, dynamic, and interactant that pulling them apart for study is very difficult. There are a number of interactionist approaches to the study of cognition, some of which are discussed elsewhere in this text. Actually, Piagetian constructivism and information processing theories are frequently considered under the umbrella of interactionism. We will discuss in particular *schema theories*, as the various types are particularly relevant to language development.

Schema Theory

Rumelhart (1977) defines schemas as hierarchically arranged knowledge structures that individuals employ to represent the world. The schema view of cognition consists of general beliefs of how knowledge is mentally represented. Various psychologists use the term to represent many different types of knowledge, some of which are general and some more specific (Highnam, 1994). This approach to the study of learning and knowing has, however, proven both educationally and linguistically beneficial, as we will later discuss.

Rumelhart's (1980) "schema" is very generally used to refer to the building blocks of cognition. Rumelhart believes all mental organization is *schematic*—that is, it has some sort of framework for ease of retrieval. Such organization includes a wide range of knowledge such as object knowledge and classes of objects, events and classes of events, personality characteristics and social norms (Highnam, 1994).

Mandler (1984), in contrast, is one of several psychologists who rejects this notion of schema as overly general. She proposes several types of knowledge structures, among which only a few are schematic in nature. Among Mandler's nonschematic structures are categorical structures, matric structures, and serial structures. Class-inclusion structures such as animal taxonomies (vertebrates-primates-humans, etc.) are categorical in nature; whereas matrix structures are those in which elements are framed together according to the number of shared properties (e.g., color, size, composition). Highnam (1994) notes that we can profitably play a game like 20 questions because of well-developed matrix structures. Serial structures are linear and progress in one direction; an example would be the alphabet or counting from one to ten.

Mandler's (1984) schemas represent hierarchically organized part-whole "collections" of related units of information comprising generalized knowledge. She proposes two types: *events*, which represent temporally organized domains of experience, and *scenes*, which have spatial organization. Though these two schemas share a number of properties (particularly their hierarchical structure and part-whole relationship between units), space is the defining element in scenes and time for events, according to Mandler.

Event schemas are perhaps one of the more easily recalled structures, because of their tightly interconnected organization and two-dimensional integrity. Mandler (1984) notes these structures develop from oft-experienced routines and uses a birthday party to illustrate. Within this overall event are smaller, embedded events (opening presents, eating cake). The sequence of the various smaller events may be arbitrary (opening presents or eating cake), or determined by cause-and-effect relationships (lighting candles before blowing them out) or by tradition (making a wish before blowing out candles). The party may have vertically sequenced events (an order of time sequence), as well as horizontal relationships (seating of guests, placement of food on table).

Scene schemas, which involve internalized organization of our environment and serve as a map by which we navigate, include both inventory information and spatial information (Mandler & Johnson, 1976). As they are hierarchical part-whole collections, representations might range from a bedroom closet to a house; a dress shop to a shopping mall. Inventory information would include objects that typically appear in a scene such as clothes, hangers, rods, and shoe racks in a closet. Spatial information refers to the actual spatial arrangement, some of which is invariant (windows in a house), and some which are optional (carpets or wood floors). Like event schemas, scenes have multiple connections and are also easy to recall, according to Mandler (1984).

Nelson (1986) carries schemas a step forward with her "generalized event representations" (GERs), which she characterizes as beyond perceptual representations (such as visual images) and akin to paradigmatic abstractions, like Mandler's scene and event schemas combined. Highnam (1994) suggests as an example of a GER, framed information regarding a restaurant, which could include spatial properties (tables, kitchen, restroom, check-out counter) and temporal events (gaining seating, ordering, eating, and paying check). Much of our "what-to-do and how-to-behave" world knowledge is likely a result of such schema knowledge. Schank and Abelson (1977) extend Nelson's GER with a knowledge structure that they term *script*, sequences of actions appropriate to a particular context and organized around goals. Highnam (1994) provides an example for a script common to today's culture, knowledge framed about a supermarket. Filling script "slots" would be actors, each with their own goals (shopper, cashier, carry-out boy), and props (including inventory and arrangement of store objects). Actions would vary, according to goals; but most people today have a general "script" to guide their actions in a supermarket.

Nelson (1986) believes the development of early world knowledge is drawn from experiences encountered in repeated, routine events. Children learn information about people, objects, relationships, and appropriate and referential language use with these events. Until their horizons widen, much of this information is undergeneralized and remains contextualized to the events. Hence, the limited reference we note in much early word meaning in young children ("baby" may be used only to refer to a baby sibling and not to other babies or to dolls during first usages). With expanded experiences, children decontextualize (extend an entity's relationship to more than one context) and broaden a concept (e.g., "candles are only used on birthday cakes" and come to realize candles add ceremony to a variety of rituals, as well as serving practical functions such as light during a power outage) (Highnam, 1994).

Nelson's (1986) theories map well onto observations of the behavior and "talk" observed in even very young children. An examination of children's play or their language use reveals their growing understanding of the events of their lives. First they specify the "setting" (actors and states), then show their understanding of temporally sequencing related actions, and then demonstrate growing understanding of causality. Children with delays may progress more readily when raised with dependable caretaking routines and repeated referential language use (Bruner, 1977). In terms of schema theory, such progress appears to occur from internalized expectations or top-down operations as a result of framed events. Use of familiar events has been hypothesized to occur in two stages, as proposed by Farrar and Goodman (1991). During the first stage, the child learns to perform *schema confirmation*, during which his presently experienced event is matched to a known schema, and attention is focused on what is expected. (Therefore, a young child might expect all adults who take him to the movie to automatically buy him popcorn.) Within new events, the mental processor attempts to create a new schema based on the present event and past experiences. During the second stage of processing, *schema deployment*, inconsistent information is given more focus and time for decision-making purposes. (After an experience of not having popcorn at the movie,

the child might learn to plan ahead and take some money to buy his own.) Schema theory is a highly cognitively interactive theory and is vastly different from passive, automatic, modular views of cognition.

SUMMARY

A variety of cognitive theories have been reviewed here in preparation for a discussion on the relationship between cognition and language. Modular theories such as those of Fodor (1983) view much of cognition as innate, a hard-wired system for the selection, conduction, and interpretation of data. Language is viewed as largely independent of cognition, though the horizontal modules described by Bates and colleagues (1988) would allow at least some correlation of language with cognition. Piaget, in strong contrast, views cognition as primary and necessary to language development at all developmental levels. Cognition develops as a result of environmental experiences; language, to Piaget, is only one of several types of mental representation. Under interactionist theory, as illustrated by schema theory (Mandler, 1984), language is a product of many factors, including maturation and experience in cognitive, social, and linguistic areas, with each element affecting the growth and development of other elements. We will now examine evidence to support these theories, in their relation to language development.

COGNITIVE ASPECTS OF COMMUNICATION DEVELOPMENT

Are language and cognition related, or does one control the other? What kind of evidence exists to support any of these relationships? What do these diverse beliefs have to do with the development of language ability? These are issues to be discussed in this section of the chapter.

Innatist Theories

Language as a system is very complex, involving the integration of many types of information, and yet is acquired in an amazingly short period. For these reasons, innatists (or nativists) believe language to be a genetically based system ready (at birth) to process specific kinds of language-enabling information—and not just a part of a more general cognitive system. Chomsky (1965, 1972), for example, conceived of a *language acquisition device* (*LAD*), which he believed to act as a type of "language processor" with knowledge of linguistic "universals" (or commonalities) that prepare children to quickly organize information leading to linguistic rule induction and mastery of their language. Chomsky's original theory, *transformational grammar* (*TG*), was not sufficient to explain *how* children acquire their native tongue, and he has extended the theory specifically to account for language development.

Government-Binding Theory: Universal Grammar

Chomsky's (1986) government-binding theory consists of a formal system of rules and principles in the form of a universal grammar (UG), which he proposes as common to most of the language grammars of the world. Chomsky claims his UG to be a "language faculty—with . . . specific properties, structure, and organization, one 'module' of the mind" (p. 12) that works by placing natural restrictions or constraints on language learners. Essentially, these constraints permit children, no matter what language they are learning, to recognize and integrate the salient rules of their language system very quickly (by 4 or 5 years) because the number of informational possibilities to be considered are reduced.

Leonard and Loeb (1988), in a tutorial for speech-language pathologists, have attempted to explain Chomsky's very complex theory of universal grammar, which includes a number of subcomponents and subtheories. Two aspects of the theory are relevant here in its understanding from a cognitive-language standpoint. First, this theory consists of multiple levels, which result in "linguistic rule economy" (Stevenson, 1988). These levels include the following: *D-structures*, which represent sentences at a meaning level and contain rules for the creation of syntactic construction and the morphologic representation of words within the syntax; *S-structures*, which allow for movement of syntactic constituents to change sentence construction (as active to passive or interrogative); and a *third level*, which includes both **PF** (phonetic form—deals with sound characterization and phonologic rules) and **LF** (logical form—determines the meaning in ambiguous sentences). Another relevant element of UG is the concept of "parameter setting." Though UG principles are constant across languages, there exist structural variations that may be referred to as parameters or linguistic boundaries, which are assigned one of two values: default or marked. Linguistic information learned from experience is "marked," whereas default information is "unmarked" and becomes part of the language system of the user when no evidence to contradict it is presented.

In Highnam (1994) two examples of parameters are illustrated from Leonard and Loeb (1988): prodrop parameters and stem parameters. Prodrop parameters establish whether a specific language requires subjects to be stated in a sentence. In English, "marked" experience with sentences such as "*They* sing well," would establish a rule induction of overt subject expression as a common pattern of this language for a young user. In Italian, however, young language learners induce from lack of experiences (from default) that sentences can be expressed without subjects, as in "*Cantano bene.*" Stem parameters involve the use of inflections on word forms (addition of morphologic forms to word stems that modify their meaning, in terms of person, number, tense, etc.). English is a language that is relatively uninflected and even allows verbs to be correctly used with no inflections, that is, as a "bare stem" (i.e., "They swim fast."). Italian, on the other hand, does not permit bare stems and inflects for person: *canto* (I sing) and *canti* (you sing). Patterns from experience (or lack of experience) with a first language are extracted through the fixing of the UG's parameters, and children are able to establish a core grammar in developing language proficiency (Stevenson, 1988).

Chomsky (1980) maintains that the language faculty "computes" phonology, syntax, morphology, and selected semantic structures and that these are biologically programmed and *not subject* to control from general cognition. On the other hand, he does allow conceptual components of language, such as thematic, pragmatic, and real-world knowledge, control outside the domain of the language faculty—and, by implication, within the domain of general cognition (Highnam, 1994).

Other theories (and their theorists) that propose underlying linguistic operating principles that facilitate the acquisition of grammar (i.e., rules for the sequencing or inflection of a string of words for meaning purposes) include the following:

1. The *universal language-learning principles* of linguist Daniel Slobin (1978), who studied more than forty languages before proposing these natural linguistic "operating principles" that children utilize to decode spoken language for its meaning. Examples of these principles are "Pay attention to the ends of words," and "The use of grammatic markers should make sense."

2. Bickerton's (1984) *language bioprogram hypothesis*, which suggests that the infrastructure or underlying foundations of language involve a series of modular, task-specific devices that interact with a task-specific, processing component to enable output of appropriately structured language. Similar to Chomsky's UG (1980), this theory adds a list of "preferred settings" to grammatical parameters.

3. Pinker's (1984, 1987, 1989) *learnability theory*, which focused on the lack of evidence available to a child to directly instruct him what combinations are possible in a language. Pinker accepted the theory of universal grammar and parameter setting, but zeroed in on the "bootstrapping problem" the child faces: what does the child use to determine *how* each word in a sentence is used (subject, verb, modifier) before inducing grammatical rules about each. Pinker

(1984) settled on the "semantic bootstrapping hypothesis"; he proposed that children analyze content for semantic structures previously learned—from context and from explicit instruction on the part of parents. Because Pinker's view stresses the importance for conceptual (networking of information) components necessary for word learning, the role of cognition is elevated somewhat in this theory. His discussion of parental roles in bootstrapping is interesting, and most professionals would support his conclusion that parents typically do not instruct children on what is grammatically permissible, but are usually very helpful concerning the meaning of words (Brown & Hanlon, 1970).

Fodor and Modularity

As previously stated, Fodor proposes that within the mind's architecture are "hard-wired" mechanisms that are defined by their function, which is to represent information from the senses (through the transducers) to higher cognitive levels (a central processor) in a useful form. Fodor views language processing as one of these input mechanisms, unlike the deliberative and executive-level behavior conceptualized by many professionals. Highnam (1994) discusses some of the characteristics of Fodor's input system in considering that the perception of language is to organize data regarding communication for the brain's consideration.

Comprehending an utterance involves analyses at several levels of representation: phonetic, phonologic, semantic/lexical, and syntactic; to Fodor, domain specificity apparently means that the vertical faculty system reacts to distinct types of stimuli. For example, he believes that speech perception is very different from the perceptual analysis of nonspeech, as a result of the work of the language module. His belief appears to be supported to some degree by the research of Liberman and colleagues (1967), who observed that different computational systems appear to be active in the analysis of speech versus nonspeech sounds. Fodor proposes that rapid speed is characteristic of the system and explains that this can occur because much of the perceived information is ignored, with only salient data "fast-forwarded" to the next level. His discussion of limited central access and information encapsulation, which suggests that most of the work of the module is "bottom-up" (enabling the central processor to focus on that necessary for the extraction of meaning), does allow some "top-down" affect, though restricted. For example, in reading a rather erudite text or participating in a discussion about relatively new theory, one's central processor is able to focus on the derivation of overall meaning, until an unfamiliar concept is encountered, at which time more in-depth perceptual analysis may be necessary to extract meaning and incorporate this feedback into the on-going task. Fodor's theory permits such an analysis.

As support for his theory, Fodor (1983) points out the similarity of language growth patterns across languages and cultural groups as strongly suggesting a system that is biologically endowed and species specific. He uses illustrations such as "cloze" ability (a person's ability to supply a missing word in a sentence) and phoneme restoration (recognition of a word when only part of it was heard) as being indicative of the facility of the input mechanisms to appropriately activate the central processor. Though arguments could be made for the integration of information to achieve these skills, Fodor continues to maintain that language acquisition proceeds independently of cognitive potential.

Summary

This section has presented a number of theories that support innatist beliefs in language as a biologically endowed system of the mind, specific to man, relatively independent of general cognition and dependent on the environment only in "triggering" maturation of the system. Chomsky's (1980) universal grammar is a mental system for enabling the child to recognize patterns and establish boundaries or parameters resulting in rules for appropriate language use. Slobin (1978) suggested

principles for the pattern-recognition that children use, and Pinker (1984, 1989) focused on how children make use of specific words to get to the language regularities. Bickerton (1984) suggests that universal grammar might include "preferred settings" among the parameters, aiding children further in pattern analysis. Fodor (1983) proposes that one of the neurolinguistic modules that function to select and process certain input types is a language module that is influenced in a very limited way by general cognition.

Cognition Hypothesis

Piaget's Assumptions—"The Strong Cognition Hypothesis"

Usually associated with the theories of Piaget (1955), the "strong" cognition hypothesis insists that cognition (growing representational knowledge and thought) precedes and is necessary for the existence and development of language. Further, Piaget believes language to be part of general representational ability, even contingent on (following after and related to) other representational abilities (Piaget & Inhelder, 1969, cited in Highnam, 1994). Research has attempted to prove the theory that structure and content of language is a result of nonlanguage cognitive structures and operations. Among this literature base are findings that provide evidence of (1) parallels between early sensorimotor achievements and language, and (2) later connections between cognitive operations and associated linguistic behaviors. "Cognition-first" theorists base their ideas on the premise that cognitive shifts in the way children think enable the learning of certain language behaviors. Also, linguists studying semantic development have attempted to establish causal relationships between specific cognitive content areas and the linguistic abilities that allow their expression (Highnam,1994). Variations of the "strong" cognitive hypothesis that are currently still considered viable include the "local homology" approach associated with Bates, Benigni, Bretherton, et al. (1979) and Cromer's (1979, 1988) "weak cognitive hypothesis."

Sensorimotor Achievements and Language Skills Various areas of sensorimotor achievement (expanding representational schemas or cognitive ability) have been correlated with language acquisition milestones in the first 2 years of life. Proponents of the strong cognitive hypothesis maintain that a deep homology (deepseated cognitive capacity) exists that connects certain types of language learning to stagelike qualitative cognitive developments (Bates et al., 1979). We will examine the relationship between such Piagetian sensorimotor areas as object permanence, means-end relationships, imitation, causality, and "schemes for relating to objects."

Object permanence, as it relates to language development, may be the most widely researched sensorimotor achievement. During the period of her research that led to the "semantic revolution," Lois Bloom (1973) proposed that cognitive object permanence (mental storage or "knowledge"of an out-of-sight object) is important in developing firm semantic categories and necessary to the establishment of a "stable-meaning" noun and verb (substantive) lexicon between 18 and 24 months (Piaget's substage 6). Research conducted by Smolak and Levine (1984) provided children at this age and stage with object permanence tasks involving several "invisible displacements"(the children were not able to see the actual hiding of the objects). Most of the children already displaying representational language were able to perform these Substage 6 tasks, and none of the nonlanguage children were capable of finding the hidden objects—supporting Bloom's theory. Corrigan (1978), one of several researchers who challenged the notion that object permanence is necessary for the development of a substantive lexicon, conducted periodic probes of object permanence. Though she found no such relationship between this sensorimotor ability and substantive word acquisition, she did discover (unlike previous researchers) an increase in the use of certain function words such as the ones that mark disappearance (all gone) and recurrence (more). These unsurprising findings have been substantiated by Gopnik and Meltzoff (1986).

Perhaps because object permanence is not so much an "aha" as a continuum of discovery that involves increasing understanding and mental storage of objects and their place in the environment, many professionals, including Bates et al. (1979), have found minimal relationship between this Piagetian skill and language development. What relationship has been found is related to Stage 4 and Stage 6 - level object permanence. At Stage 4, Roger Brown (1973) has suggested that object permanence may be sufficient for the development of single words, and Jon Miller and colleagues (1980) suggest a relationship to the child's ability to comprehend the names of present persons. At Stage 6, along with the findings suggested earlier, others (Bates & Snyder, 1987; Ramsay, 1977) have posited that object permanence, perhaps because of increased memory for absent objects, may be related to the large growth of vocabulary at the end of the second year (Owens, 1996).

A sensorimotor area of achievement considered to be most important in language development is *means-end* schemes. Bates and colleagues (1975, 1977, 1979) in particular have found that the establishment of an ability to use tools ("novel means") to obtain desired objects and services correlated well with infant attempts to communicate generally and vocally, using both gestures and words. Such communication among Bates' subjects involved attempts to either secure adult attention to an object or secure adult assistance in obtaining an object; the authors called these efforts "protodeclarative" and "protoimperative." Since they did not find the acquisition order for tool use and intentional communication invariable, Bates and colleagues did not term the relationship causal. Instead, they speculated that a "homologue" or deeper sensorimotor concept (in this case, intentionality) was possibly causing the occurrence of both tool use and communication. This notion is discussed further in the section on local homology theory.

Several other sensorimotor areas have been correlated by research data, though their exact relationship has not been specified. These include imitation, causality, "schemas for relating to objects," and play. For example, from Stage 4 (8 to 12 months) on, the ability to imitate different behaviors is increasingly correlated to speech production especially but also to paralinguistic areas such as facial and prosodic imitation (Owens, 1996). Imitation at Stage 6 (deferred imitation is possible) is also correlated with the emergence of recognitory gestures and verbal labeling (Bates & Snyder, 1987). Harding and Golinkoff (1978) consider sensorimotor causality one of the necessary conditions for communication development, and Jon Miller and colleagues (1980) related causality to the understanding of semantic relations. Steckol and Leonard (1981) confirmed Bates and colleagues' theory that infant communication skills were correlated with Stage 5 "schemas for relating to objects." They found that children who received "relating-to-objects" training acquired a greater degree of gestural communication than a control group (Highnam, 1994). The relationship of language and symbolic play will be discussed briefly under Bates and local homology theory.

Cognitive Operations and Communication Skills   The relationship between developmental use and understanding of language concepts and concrete operations, such as *conservation* and *reversibility*, has also been studied to some degree. The influence of liquid conservation on certain language forms was examined by Sinclair-DeZwart (1969), who found that specific language expressions involving relative amounts were not frequently used prior to when children could demonstrate conservation of liquid in experimental tasks.

The influence of reversibility on the use of language forms was researched by Ferreiro and Sinclair (1971). Their study

found that children who could not yet mentally "reverse" could not use "before" and "after" consistently and meaningfully to order clauses and could not always correctly describe the temporal order of events. Children who *were* reversing were also able to produce adequate linguistic descriptions. Tremaine (1975) found that comprehension of syntactic forms was more proficient by first- and second-grade English-speaking students in French-speaking classrooms who had reached concrete operations. Her data also indicated that Piaget's "numeration" task was most predictive of syntactic success.

Finally, a series of studies by Beilin (1975) examined concrete operational logic and both comprehension and production of syntactic forms. Though some general relationships were revealed, Beilin found them sufficiently imperfect to rule out a cause-effect relationship (Highnam, 1994).

Cognitive Content Areas and Communication Development   Throughout the literature on language acquisition, examples abound that suggest (in support of the cognition hypothesis) that children come to language learning with a "stock of ideas onto which they learn to map the language of the environment they experience" (Highnam, 1994, p. 178). Illustrating this idea is Slobin's (1973) axiom stating that new linguistic forms first express old ideas, and new ideas are first expressed by old linguistic forms. Highnam suggests the very young child is, at first, not able to reflect on the past, being bound to the "here and now," and thus does not use past-tense markers on her verbs. When she first begins to think about the past, she is not yet able to express this in her speech appropriately, and so *new ideas* (past action) are first expressed in *old forms* (uninflected verbs). Later, she notes the "ed" ending people use when speaking of the past and begins to inflect her own verbs thus; however, by this time, these (verb +ed) are *new forms* used to express a now *old idea* (past action).

Another supporting observation for the cognition hypothesis is the fact that the order of acquisition of lexical terms emerges similarly to the order of the expressed concepts: from general to specific. Maratsos (1973) proposes this order mirrors increasing cognitive complexity, or cognitive growth, from general ideas to complex, specific concepts. Examples are spatial prepositions and quantitative concepts (Johnston, 1981). In other words, children usually express and understand "big" before more-specific "tall" or "long," and "over there" before "on the table."

In the area of semantics, Clark (1973) proposed that children's overextensions of meanings in early words was possibly a result of their cognitive organization of salient features of objects. A young child might call a moon a cookie or a ball because of the most salient feature of roundness. Highnam (1994) notes that if children learned word meaning on the basis of language input exclusively, the range of extension errors would be smaller and include more phonetically based errors than perceptually based ones. Other work has demonstrated that children are able to categorize objects before naming them (Rosch & Mervis, 1977). These findings tend to demonstrate that children do have a means of organizing world knowledge before they become language users, and they tend to suggest that language learning entails the child's mapping of semantic meanings onto cognitive categories (Highnam, 1994).

Local Homologies—"A Changing Relationship" Piaget's "strong" cognition hypothesis suggests that language develops and exists as a result of cognitive development, and this subservient relationship remains constant over time. In contrast to Piaget's notion is the local homology model of Bates and colleagues (1979), which proposes that the language-cognition relationship changes over time. The hypothesis name reveals its two primary beliefs: (1) that deep-seated cognitive abilities ("homologues") result in the formation of both language and nonlanguage ideas, and (2) within restricted windows of time ("local"), highly specific relationships occur between language and cognition (Highnam, 1994).

"Deep-seated cognitive capacities" (Bates et al., 1979) is illustrated with the homologue "symbolic representation" (the ability to represent one thing or idea with another). Within the local homologies model, the capacity of symbolic representation results in concurrent growth in nonlanguage symbolism (function, or recognitory gestures) and language symbolism (words, or verbal labels). Because these two skills (as with a number of other similarly related skills) are usually noted to emerge at approximately the same time in normal children, Bates and colleagues believe that specific underlying capacity is the causative factor.

From the "local" aspect of the theory, Bates and colleagues (1979) suggest that within specific time-frames, specific communicative elements (e.g., communicative gestures, words, word combinations) correlate (and emerge) with specific, related, nonlanguage elements (e.g., tool use, gestures, gesture combinations). The researchers go on to note that these behaviors, which are correlated because of similar structural features sharing a common underlying cognitive base, may not share such a relationship at a later time. Highnam (1994) gives examples to illustrate. Early word learning is at first correlated with recognitory gestures (ability to produce gestures that demonstrate knowledge of an object's function, as drinking from a toy cup). As children move toward combining words into multiword phrases, recognitory gestures disappear but are replaced by combinatory play gestures (relating two toys meaningfully during play, as giving a doll a drink with a cup) and then "multischeme gestural combinations" (a sequence of play actions that illustrate knowledge of steps in a daily routine, such as pretending to pour from pitcher to cup and then serving a drink) (Thal, 1991; Shore, 1986). This growth in semantics (meaning), syntax (ordering of units for meaning), and script (framed world knowledge) enactments is believed to possibly result from underlying increases in the ability to mentally represent numbers of informational units (Thal, 1991).

The local homology theory (Bates et al., 1979) found support in a 1989 study by Kelly and Dale, which examined 20 12- to 24-month-old children for a relationship between language and Piagetian cognitive areas. Their investigation of object permanence, means-ends, play, and imitation skills found that all but object permanence predicted one or more language levels. Their conclusion that "specific cognitive skills seem temporally associated with some linguistic abilities although attainment of skills can be evidenced first in language *or* cognition" (p. 645) is consistent with the hypothesis of local homology. In short, there is a good bit of evidence to support the belief of Bates and her fellow researchers (1979) that temporally and structurally related achievements in both language and nonlanguage areas may be manifestations of deeper cognitive achievements that are biased toward neither area (Highnam, 1994).

Weak Cognition Hypothesis   Proposed by Richard Cromer (1979), this hypothesis acknowledges the primacy (origin and support) of cognition for much of language learning, but argues that some of the learning process may result from the particular formalisms (forms and their organization) of a language. Cross-language studies indicate that children acquire much of the concepts of language in a particular sequence, but, because the structures for expressing some concepts differ in complexity from language to language, their emergence across languages may differ temporally. Linguist Slobin, in 1973, reported his beliefs that cognition accounted for the "lower boundary" for learning and expressing a linguistic concept and that the complexity of language required for the concept's expression in a particular language established the ceiling for acquisition expectancy.

Cromer's (1979) position has been supported through research aimed at teaching animals a language system akin to man's. These studies attempted to teach animals ranging from chimpanzees (Gardner & Gardner, 1969) to dolphins (Herman, Richards, & Wolz, 1984) syntactic language, and failed. Though many of the animals exhibited the ability to learn language typical of children in Piaget's sensorimotor stage of intelligence (intentional use of referential words), none has exhibited the ability to order words into various sentence structures that carry contrasting meanings. To Cromer this suggests that more than cognition is involved in learning to express complex and decontextualized meanings through acquiring understanding and application of the regularities of morphosyntactic language components (Highnam, 1994).

Summary

Within this section we have presented various forms of cognition theories, proposing that language results from cognitive growth and including the strong cognition hypothesis of Piaget (1955), the local homologies theory of Bates and colleagues (1979), and the weak cognition hypothesis of Cromer (1979). We have also reviewed research findings, which, while supporting a correlation between cognition and language, suggest that the relationship changes across time and skills. Bates' local homology theory, that language and nonlanguage behaviors that are related in structure and initial appearance probably result from the emergence of deep cognitive abilities, appears to be best supported by presently known research. Also, though necessary for language acquisition to some degree, cognition does not appear to be sufficient to explain various aspects of what Marion Blank and her colleagues (1978) call the "perceptual-language match" or to clarify organizational language matters like acquiring sentence-making strategies. Some theorists believe these latter concerns are best explained by more language-specific theories (Chomsky, 1981; Fodor, 1983.)

LANGUAGE AND THOUGHT

Despite strong evidence supporting the position of cognitive control on language development, one finds it hard to reflect on the language-thought relationship without sensing, conversely, that *language may influence thought*. Several relevant positions will be reviewed here to examine the possible degree of influence our language exerts on our thoughts.

Whorf—Cultural Influences

Benjamin Whorf (1941, 1956) developed a theory of the language-thought relationship that, though challenged and unproven, has been recurrently influential in a variety of professional arenas. As a result of his 1920 to 1930 investigations of native American "talk" and thinking styles, Whorf came to believe that speakers of a common language share a common world view. His position (called the Whorfian hypothesis) actually has two elements. The first, linguistic determinism, consists of the belief that all *higher* thinking is dependent on language. The second, referred to as linguistic relativism, is the notion that classification systems (primarily in the lexicon and syntax) of various languages are frequently so different that their speakers' thought systems (cognitive representation of the world—"reality") are also very diverse.

Whorf (1941) was interested in learning if such higher *concepts* as time, space, and matter developed out of universal experiences or out of the way they are expressed through the structures of a particular language. In studying the language and culture of the Hopi Indians of the American Southwest, he found striking differences between traditional Western cultures (including English and standard European languages) and the Hopi concerning concepts of time. Western cultures view time concepts as objectified and sequential units, measurable like space concepts. Such objectification affects both the lexicon (semantics—meaning) and syntax in a language, as well as cultural dealings with time and its effect on lives. Westerners express time concepts as proper and common nouns (1997, Spring, March, day, hour, minute, noon, etc.) through which one can progress forward or remember backwards (resulting in past, present, and future verb tense), in varying manners and degrees (re-

sulting in a prolific vocabulary of adjectives and adverbs: long, slow, many, few, old, young, etc.). The Hopi, on the other hand, express "temporal" concepts, similar to but different from our "time," as a distinctive part of speech, somewhat akin to English adverbs. Rather than verb tenses, Hopi utilize temporal measurement such as: *validity* (whether the temporal event was related to the speaker or witnessed by him), *aspect* (similar to duration, as "while morning phase is occurring"), and *mode* (which indicates "same time" or "later time" between experiences). Whorf believed that temporal expressions of the Hopi suggest their belief that days occur in a recurring cycle rather than new days in an endless chain (as viewed by most Western cultures), and that they can make "preparations" (perform elaborate ceremonies) that will influence future events.

Whorf (1941) also described differences in views of "matter" between the Hopi and Western cultures. To Westerners, thought about real world objects is simply a labeled picture held in the brain that represents the real object and can be stored as memory or consciously focused on. Such thought or mental imagery can have no physical effect on the real object. Hopi, on the other hand, believe that "thought" pervades the universe and that one's thoughts can "engage with" and affect objects directly.

Whorf (1941, 1956) was not much interested in child language development, focusing instead on the influence of a language on the thought or cognitive content of the culture that speaks it. He felt that cultures can change quickly through world events and innovations, but that the character of a language changes very slowly—and can confine flexibility of thought.

Vygotsky: Inner Speech and Verbal Mediation

While Whorf (1941, 1956) discussed the relationship of language to higher thinking, Soviet psychologist Lev Vygotsky (1962) was interested in the development of "inner speech." Vygotsky believed "inner speech" is the private process of thinking in words that allows the management and direction of one's behavior through mental comments, reactions, imaginings, organizing/hypothesizing, and planning. Expressions of inner speech are always "new information," as there is no need to restate old information for one's self, unlike outer speech directed to a listener. Therefore, inner speech, if spoken aloud, would sound telegraphic or fragmentary: "Now put this here. OK. Got it. Pretty good!"

Vygotsky (1962) became interested in structural similarities between adult inner speech and the "egocentric speech" heard in preschoolers who seem to verbally direct themselves as they play. Piaget's (1955) view of egocentric speech was that it was an expression of preschool egocentric thought (view of the world that permitted only the child's immature preoperational perspective), with preschoolers assuming their speech was understood by others. Because decentered thought (viewing the world through a variety of perspectives) develops during early elementary years (part of concrete operational thinking) and, in most normal children, egocentric speech disappears during the same period, Piaget felt supported in his correlation of the two. Vygotsky, however, had a suspicion that there was developmental continuity between egocentric speech and inner speech and set out to prove it.

Vygotsky's (1962) hypothesis was that preschool self-directed speech was not a reflection of Piagetian egocentric thought but a functional self-communicative and directive verbal mechanism or "tool" that later "goes underground" to become inner speech. In other words, Vygotsky believed that egocentric speech grows out of the basic social functions of early-stage speech, which gradually takes two directions: a continued social, communicative, and interactive function and a new nonsocial, private, and "managerial" function. This latter egocentric speech gradually comes to be internalized as mental talk/thinking, or inner speech, according to Vygotsky.

With his student Luria, Vygotsky (1956) set out to prove their view of the self-managerial purposes of preschool egocentric speech as opposed to Piaget's theory of expressed egocentered thought with quasi-social functions. Under conditions not conducive to social communication (background with loud noise and communication partners that were difficult to communicate with, such as speakers of other languages), egocentered speech decreased in preschoolers. Under conditions requiring simple problem solving, egocentric speech increased. Such findings appeared to support Vygotsky's perception of egocentered speech as self-directing and an outward means of planning and problem solving and to disprove the Piagetian view of such private speech as semisocial. Vygotsky went on to demonstrate changes in the form and length of egocentric speech that supported its movement from a socialized origin to the underground-thought usage; he demonstrated a greater length and social-like form at age 3 that decreased to one- to two-word utterances before it disappeared from overt use around age 6 (Dale, 1972).

Vygotsky's (1962) ideas about language development in infants and young children have been supported through the 1960 to 1980 studies (Nelson, 1973; Snow, 1986) revealing the importance of social interaction and parental roles in the language-learning process—and concepts from his work have been expanded for intervention processes (Norris & Hoffman, 1990). Interest in metacognition as a verbally recruited skill or tool for improving academic ability has additionally grown out of Vygotsky's work (Forrest-Pressley & Waller, 1984). Within social interactionist theory, Vygotskian concepts have been integrated in a variety of dynamic and practical clinical and educational applications (Palincsar, Brown, & Campione, 1994).

Other Evidence Regarding the Language-Thought Relationship

An interesting finding about language's facilitation of thought development was made by Premack (1971) in his comparative study of language-trained and non-language-trained chimpanzees. Premack found that language-trained chimpanzees could problem solve in ways that other animals could not: they could match proportions of unlike substances, do causal analyses, attribute intentions, and solve analogies (Highnam, 1994). Because none of the monkeys ever possessed syntactic ability, Premack felt it was possession of the abstract symbol system—or lexicon—(and not a syntactic-rule system) that resulted in such improved problem solving, and that developing language increased the animal's reasoning capacity.

Marion Blank and colleagues (1964, 1974, 1978) posit that the language-cognition relationship is largely constrained by decontextualization and abstraction ability. Younger and less able students, she noted, require highly concrete visual/spatial support to focus and learn—or talk coherently—during interactions, suggesting that cognition is a primary factor at this level of complete contextualization. In learning about concepts that are not visually apparent but realized through abstract ideas, Blank proposes that language plays the leading role. Studies with preschoolers by Blank and colleagues (1964) supported her thesis that early problem solving is easiest with concrete cues or materials to manipulate. Her Perceptual-Language Match Hierarchy (or Scale of Abstraction for Discourse—see Westby chapter on School-Age Language) provides structure for providing appropriate contextualization so that children can obtain the most benefit during an adult's teaching, reading to/with, or conversing with a child.

Summary

While Whorf's (1941, 1956) hypothesis views language as confining flexibility to learn/understand new concepts or different cultural perspectives, Vygotsky (1962) and others (including Premack, 1971) viewed language as having more positive effects on cognition, enabling self-control, planning, reasoning, and abstract thinking. Blank and colleagues' (1978) theory, that of contextualization

requirements for learning resulting in a seesaw effect in primacy between cognition and language, is more and more recognized for its importance in clinical and academic circles (Norris & Hoffman, 1993; Westby, 1994).

INTERACTIONISM: BRINGING IT ALL TOGETHER

Two extreme points of view regarding the development of language and thought are represented in the theories just covered: Piaget's cognitive determinism and Whorf's linguistic determinism, with related but milder versions of these also being discussed. In the last two decades, interactionist theory has proposed a more reconciliative view of the cognition-language relationship: that language and thought emerge in the same relative time frame, each facilitating the development of the other (Highnam, 1994). Interactionist as a term is also used to indicate that element of language-acquisition theory that focuses on the value of early, guiding, social interchanges between caretakers and children for developing important component skills and thus enabling language. However, from the cognitive-language perspective, the interactionist hypothesis proposes that a nonlanguage (cognitive) concept may emerge and that language eventually comes to code this; this is, of course, consistent with cognitive first thinking. But—within interactionist theory—a language expression may emerge first (without the coding concept purpose)—and its use result in contexts that cause the forming of new cognitive concepts. Such learning is aided by exposure to an adult-guided language environment; the impact of the social environment is an important element in interactionist theories.

Recall that within interactionist theory most of the information in the system is accessible to any part of the system at any time. In the course of processing information, attention, perception, cognition, memory, and language are all interdependent and interactant. Schema theory illustrates cognitive interactionism, with its flexibility for top-down (recognition of familiar input) and bottom-up (decoding of unfamiliar input) processing. Language and cognition interactions have a similar flexibility with this theory, with information from either domain influencing development and function in the other (Highnam, 1994).

Highnam (1994) sets the stage for illustrating interactionist theory by defining the terms *category, concept,* and *meaning.* He defines *category* as a nonlinguistic grouping of objects, events, actions, and relationships that, while not identical, elicit the same response. Categorically similar are a rocking chair and kitchen chair as they both elicit sitting. *Concept* refers to the mental representation that underlies the grouping principle for a category; in our examples, the concept is one of *furniture* for *seating one person. Meaning* is used to suggest the semantic referents or the concepts supposedly represented by words in the language. Meaning is *not* always mapped perfectly onto concepts. For example, "chair" appropriately references our examples, but would not reference a stool, swing, or desk even though they would all be included within the category and satisfy the grouping concept of seating.

Within early language acquisition, schema theory supports an interactionist framework. During repeated caregiving routines with orchestrated social engagements, infants develop cognitive information structures or "schemas." These schemas are made up of organized basic *concepts* tightly contextualized (confined) to the objects and events in the routine of occurrence. These concepts are *organizing principles* for eventual *categories* of objects, actions, and events, but initially the category members may have as few as *one* member and be recognizable as a concept only in the routine of occurrence. Also, the concepts are the basis for development of words (semantic referents) that *mean* or indicate them. The words become "mapped" on concepts, developing meaning for the child, as he participates repeatedly in the routine, hearing adults pairing words onto routine elements.

Highnam (1994) provides an example of thought (cognition) preceding language in his description of his son's mapping of the word "up" onto the event of being lifted from his crib during a repeated "awakening" routine provided by his parents. Highnam's son, during the latter half of his first year, would be approached as he awoke, greeted, and presented a signal (reaching out of arms) and word "Up?" as an offer for being removed from the crib confinement. The boy responded first by raising his arms (matching the concept), later paired this gesture with an approximation of "up" (mapping verbal meaning onto the concept) and later used both the nonlanguage recognitory concept (raising of arms) and language (word "up") in all contexts (morning, naptimes) of awakening (formed a category of "upness" within similar routines). Highnam proposes that his son's behavior well illustrates Slobin's (1973) example of new forms (new word—up) expressing an old concept or function (being lifted from confinement), as well as being an example of thought preceding language.

Examples of language preceding thought, conversely, can be provided through observations of toddlers during the period when vocabulary growth begins to increase in leaps and bounds. At a certain point, children seem to "catch on" to the adult strategy of referencing them to novel objects through the excited exclamation of "what's THAT?", pointing, and other various paralinguistic strategies that elicit interest. Soon enough, toddlers deduce this joint referencing usually leads to their being presented with a "word" to attach to the novel object. At this time they seize the language strategy for their own and go on a veritable "word-learning extravaganza" through the interminable asking of "wassat?, wasSAT?" of caretakers soon weary of repeatedly naming environmental objects for them. This is a classic example of using language to increase and extend thought. Another example can be provided through young children's attempts to clarify their concepts and categories by pointing to similar objects and expressing, in questioning intonation, the one word they have to label the concept they understand only in a single context. For example, my first son pointed to all real-life and toy wheeled vehicles and asked "cah?" until he had a firm concept and category for cars from the adult responses he gleaned: "no, not car—truck!" or "Yes—car." My 18-month-old daughter, whose toys were frequently "borrowed" by her older brother, usually responded with loud crying and distress. One day, she apparently made special note of my recovering a possession from her with "sorry, that's *mine.*" The next day she spent bringing her possessions to me and asking "mine?" repeatedly. Then, having firmly established this semantic relationship of possession, her responses to her brother's attempted appropriations of her toys resulted in her tightly gripping them and proclaiming loudly: "MINE!" Interactionally, language and thought had merged in a meaningful and functional relationship and strategy for her.

Bowerman (1989) adds another element to interactionist theory in her discussion of how different languages may provide various or restricted options for mapping meaning onto language. She illustrates by demonstrating that spatial terms in different languages do not represent space in ways that are easily compared. In English, for example, the concept of containment differentiates the relationship inherent in the concepts *in* and *on*. Spanish, however, makes no such distinction, and their word *en* would be used to describe both *in* and *on* in English. German has more discriminating semantic distinctions for English *on*, expressing *auf*, *an*, and *um* for *on* the table, the wall, or the finger—expressing orientation to either a horizontal or vertical surface and to encirclement.

The contrast in semantic meaning across language as discussed by Bowerman (1989) demonstrates that each language illustrates a different dimension and quality of perceptual reality. This suggests that the mapping of semantic meaning onto con-

cepts as well as attaching conceptual principles to words, is also dissimilar from language to language. Too, the extent of language and word use facilitation or organization of such concepts as space may be semantically influenced by specific language conventions. Bowerman illustrates that English children derive the meaning of the prefix *un* (*un*tie, *un*lock) from observing adult use of it within certain contexts and then inferring the categorization principle of negation + verb for these spatially oriented relationships. Korean children, she notes, are unable to "overextend" spatial meaning because their spatial reference system is so unlike that of English. Bowerman's work, to some degree, supports aspects of Whorf's (1941) linguistic relativism, but at a much lower language level.

Three researchers have already been presented who have commented on the changes in the language-cognition relationship from one of cognitive primacy to one where language has the greater role in thought; these include Blank (1974), Slobin (1973), and Vygotsky (1962). Within schema theory, Nelson (1985) provides a developmental stage system that also supports this movement. Her earliest stage, *Prelinguistic*, is a period when the child moves from episodic thoughts of routine events to develop and express contextualized labels that represent the whole event. During the middle stage (*Conceptual*), Nelson depicts the child as gradually parsing out individual parts of the whole event and determining the relationships between objects, actions, and events, while also decontextualizing and extending words (semantic mappings of meaning) for concepts. In the final stage (*Semantic*), the child's concepts are well organized into hierarchical categories, enabling the transition in thought referred to as the *syntagmatic-paradigmatic* shift. Younger children give more *noncategorical*, actionlike (syntagmatic) answers to word-association tasks such as dog—bite; banana—peel; while older school-age children respond more *categorically* (paradigmatically), for example, chair—table; books—school. Nelson and others believe that categories of synonymy (similarity), antonymy (opposition), inclusiveness (hierarchically higher or lower), or reciprocity (as in buy-sell) are developed during the Semantic period to aid in semantically based storage (Blewitt, 1983; Shipley, Kuhn, & Madden, 1983).

Summary

Within the interactionist hypothesis is the belief that language and cognition influence the development of each other in various ways. First, word meanings may be matched to preexisting, nonlinguistic ideas, as suggested by the cognitive hypothesis. Also, the pairing of verbiage and concepts during repeated, systematic, routine contexts results in development of contextualized word use that is mapped on the simultaneously developed concept. Children may also monitor word, word-class use, and even word-stem changes for regularities and may form corresponding concepts for which they, somewhat later, express the new word or morphologic change. Evidence also suggests a merging relationship of language and thought as children mature, a process that is most active during increased exposure to literacy and increased semantic categorization ability during early school years.

FROM THEORY TO APPLICATION: THERAPEUTIC IMPLICATIONS

How applicable are these theories to treatment goals, methods, and procedures in facilitating appropriate communication development or remediating linguistic weaknesses? One must have a firm grip of theoretic reasons for a management approach in therapy. An examination of possible theoretic applications of the theories presented follows.

Innatist Theory and Therapy

Within theories that propose a faculty or system "hard-wired" for processing language, most would view a youngster with language disability as having an underdeveloped, damaged, or dysfunctional faculty. Such a view could result in a rather pessimistic outlook for therapy benefits, but we will look at each researcher for possible elaboration. Remember, that within this theory, language and cognition develop independently, and language is viewed more as a "processor" that readies sensory information for linguistic use.

Chomsky's (1981, 1986) government-binding theory makes little effort to address language disabilities, but there does exist within the literature (Leonard & Loeb, 1988) some interpretive applications of his work. Leonard and Loeb, in their 1988 tutorial on government binding (GB) and its universal grammar (UG), review a couple of considerations. Within the linguistic rule economy of UG is the concept of a multilevel linguistic mechanism. A language-disordered child could, conceivably, exhibit a pattern of errors that could be accounted for within a single level of the UG, such as with phonetic forms (*PF* level) or semantic-syntactic interactions (*D-structures*) Highnam (1994). Within parameter setting, a youngster's errors of comprehension or production could be accounted for by his either failing to "set" a certain parameter such as adding -ed to past tense verbs—or by setting a parameter but then failing to develop the parameter exceptions required by his language, as actually changing the stem of the verb rather than inflecting the ending for irregular past tense (wake, woke).

While Chomsky's (1981, 1986) theories may offer explanations of error patterns and suggest a framework for approaching them clinically, the actual therapy for improving phonologic processes, linguistic rules, or verbal performance is likely to resemble existing procedures (Highnam, 1994).

Pinker's (1984) work does, however, offer a therapeutic hint worth considering. If children do indeed "bootstrap" or deduce syntactic usage and structure from semantic analysis of parental language models, then perhaps therapy should address word meaning while attempting to clarify grammatic violations within therapy (Pye, 1989). Meaning-based therapeutic approaches have grown in number since the early 1970s when Lois Bloom sparked the "semantic revolution" and are easily found in the literature.

While Pinker (1989) believes grammatic rules linking structures such as subject and verb are innately specified (universally given) and not learned, the semantic information necessary for the children to *understand* this relationship *is* learned and can be addressed in therapy. Pinker's conclusions are somewhat supported by Bates and colleagues (1988) who found semantics and syntax to be dissociable in normal children, providing more encouragement for addressing the two language systems as one therapeutically (Highnam, 1994).

Fodor (1983), within his modularity hypothesis, also offers little discussion about language disabilities, but again there are implications that can be made from his work. For example, researchers for decades have speculated that children with language disorders may have particular problems with the *perception of speech* (Eisenson, 1968; Mykelbust, 1954). More recent studies have made more specific claims. Tallal and colleagues (Tallal, 1978; Tallal & Stark, 1981; Tallal, Stark, & Mellits, 1985) have proposed the theory that children with language impairment have a deficient ability to process auditory information at an appropriate rate. Leonard (1989) has expressed a presently less precise theory that children with difficulty learning grammatical morphemes may be inefficient at perceiving auditory features with low phonetic substance. If such deficits are the results of damaged input systems (such as a vertical module of Fodor's), one might have doubts about the success of treatment. Recall, however, that while Fodor does emphasize limited central access and information encapsulation resulting in most of the module processing as bottom-up, he does allow some restricted top-down effect. Highnam (1994) suggests that linguistic information *can* be fed back down in a compensatory role, though the overall process would be notably slower, lacking the rapid rate of speed that charac-

terizes an intact module. Slowed interactions and the use of language cuing systems other than auditory could possibly benefit clients with damaged (Fodorian modular) systems in terms of comprehending language.

In general, innatist theories have perhaps the least to offer in terms of therapeutic approaches to communication disorders, but such theory is not without its implications and need not suggest limited treatment benefit (Highnam, 1994).

Clinical Implications of Cognitive Theories

The cognitive hypothesis has had a strong effect on the work of speech-language pathologists, as many states use it as a guiding factor in determining who qualifies for SLP services. Many states require that a child exhibit language abilities a year or more below their overall cognitive functioning in order that they meet criteria as language-impaired. As an overly general rule, this method of service determination has often proven somewhat problematic. For example, a child 3 years of age whose language is more than a year behind his cognitive functioning is significantly more impaired than a child 12 years of age with a similar delay. One would hope to provide facilitative developmental services to 3 year olds *before* their communication abilities are as much as a year behind and probably beginning to impact on social and conceptual development.

Highnam (1994) points out that research has indicated that children with language impairments frequently also have "substantial" impairment in cognitive areas (Johnston, 1988) such as Piagetian-type tasks (Snyder, 1978) and play development (Kennedy, et al., 1991). Nelson, Kamhi, and Apel (1987) reviewed such studies and included the following among cognitive weaknesses: less capacity and efficiency in processing verbal, as well as nonverbal, information; and perceptual, attentional, and/or representational disabilities. However, no conclusions have been made regarding which area (language or cognition) is a leading factor (Terrell, et al., 1984), and more, well-controlled studies focusing on contrasting populations of youngsters with language delays and disorders are indicated. Such studies should focus not just on the language-cognition relationship but on particular language characteristics and learning patterns seen in both high-incidence disabilities, such as Down Syndrome and Specific Language Impairment, and low-incidence populations, such as sensory impairment (both vision and hearing) and cerebral palsy.

Most obviously, SLPs and educators need to have an awareness of a student's cognitive level to provide services at a beneficial level. Assessment of such knowledge can be tricky, and standard IQ tests rarely give the kind of information needed. Essentially, one needs to assess both world knowledge the child may possess, strategies he or she has for the acquisition of new information, and strategies that are present for communicating in less conventional ways. Observation in natural environments, structured by tests of developmental norms such as the cognitive subtest of the *Early Intervention Developmental Profile* (Rogers, et al., 1981) and Westby's (1980) *Play Scale*, can reveal contrasts between language abilities, play schemas, and sensorimotor and early preoperational reasoning for young children. Wetherby and Prizant (1990) have developed a series of "communicative temptations" using naturalistic tasks for determining a variety of verbal and nonverbal symbolic behaviors in young children; their procedures are incorporated in a package called *Communication and Symbolic Behavior*. Other tools for comparing language and cognition in very young children include Dunst' (1980) adaptation of the Uzgiris-Hunt Scale (1975) and Olswang and colleagues' (1987) *Assessing Linguistic Behaviors*. For children at the preoperational and operational levels, various nonverbal cognitive tests are available for use such as the *Test of Nonverbal Behavior* (Brown, Sherbenou, & Dollay, 1982), which is designed for use with children of ages 5 and up. Korsten and colleagues (1995) provide a utilitarian assess-ment-to-intervention program for attempting to move prelingual children with severe disabilities to a level of conventionally recognized and intentional behaviors.

Once cognitive and language levels are established, the speech-language pathologist must determine what to emphasize in training: language, cognition, or both simultaneously. At this time, knowledge of the literature on gains in language subsequent to cognitive training can be beneficial. For example, some Piagetian concept training (means-end and schemes for relating to objects) has been found to benefit language development (Kahn, 1984). Research is ongoing in determining cognitive "readiness" for actual clinical training, but many interventionists are comfortable with new collaborative models that enable professionals, especially SLPs, to work together in supporting advancements across the developmental spectrum, and specifically cognition and language for children under the age of 3 years. Such collaboration involves parents and teachers, supported and enabled by speech-language pathologists in extending social-communicative and cognitive ability through repeated, facilatory, interactive routines.

Clinical Implications for Language Hypotheses

During the 1920s and 1930s, when Whorf's research was being accomplished, so-called linguistic study primarily focused on the vocabulary and syntax of a language. Since that time "language" has become a much more inclusive term, and linguistic anthropologists are much more interested in the ways words are used in everyday use—and within specific ethnocultural communities (Moerman, 1988). For some time Whorf's hypothesis of the controlling impact of language on cultural world views was accepted in a modified version in which conventions of a given language influence codability, or how easily or specifically ideas can be expressed (Highnam, 1994). Whorf's theories have more recently enjoyed a resurgence of interest, partially as a result of the growth in linguistic and cultural diversity in our country and others and partially because of growing interest in ethnographic discourse analysis in the field of communication disorders, linguistics, and anthropology. Particularly of interest to educators today is how influential language is on thought and learning; the Oakland (California) controversy regarding "Ebonics" (a current term for Black English Vernacular) is an illustration. Research goes forward in examining such issues as types of language use by specific cultural groups during social, vocational, and educational contexts and effects of dialectic differences and narrative experiences in regional and socioeconomically disadvantaged cultures (Heath, 1982; Labov, 1972; Michaels, 1991; Scollon & Scollon, 1981).

Vygotsky's theories about language's enabling and directive effects on thinking have also been reexamined and, in fact, are incorporated into many educational and communicative interventions today for both early intervention and services for school-aged, language-impaired children. Vygotsky's concept of inner speech as being an outgrowth of social supportive dialogue that becomes internalized as directive thought, along with his concept of a "zone of proximal development" (distance between independent functioning and functioning with adult support and scaffolding), are the underlying tenets of reciprocal teaching. This latter language and educational model is organized around "dialogues" in which teacher and student share the responsibility for discussing and exploring text (Palincsar, et al., 1994). Research into Vygotskian theoretic concepts has included the following: how language may serve to augment self-control in behavior (Karoly, 1977) and in problem solving (Hall, 1980); the effect of personal factors, task requirements, and strategy use on the upper limits of children's ability while using self-talk (Carlson & Wiedl, 1988); and the facility with which students learn from others and their flexibility of application of learning (Campione, et al., 1984). Nip-

pold's (1988) review of studies of later language development found evidence that linguistic knowledge may be important to the advancement of syllogistic reasoning (deductive reasoning, where conclusions are based on two premises) in particular. Though the *degree* of benefit of Vygotskian linguistic theory on communicative and academic functioning in particular populations of children with language weaknesses is not yet known, his procedures are recognized as worthwhile tools in our field.

Marion Blank's ideas about language's impact on the development of ideas have also been widely adapted in educational and therapeutic arenas. Blank and colleagues (1978) have developed an assessment tool (*Preschool Language Assessment Instrument*) and accompanying text (*The Language of Learning: The Preschool Years*) that have been found to be helpful tools in predicting and intervening with kindergarten children believed likely to have language and learning difficulty in elementary school. A number of intervention packets have been structured around or utilize ideas from the language-abstraction model of Blank and colleagues (Blank & Marquis, 1987; Zachman, et al., 1982; Norris & Hoffman, 1994; and Witt, 1988, 1992).

Clinical Implications of Interactionist Theory

From an interactionist standpoint, several variables may need to be considered in management of communication disorders. First, approaches that "connect" more linguistic knowledge (phonology, syntax, and morphology) with work on more conceptual language components (thematic, pragmatic, and world knowledge) are likely to result in both language and cognitive growth, a belief that largely underlies the set of philosophies we have come to call "whole" language. Next, Piaget (1955) and Blank (1974) have shown us that children's language development is benefitted through paying attention to their cognitive level and providing the types of concrete activities that are appropriate for them.

Later, abstract cognitive knowledge may be more assisted and dependent on language ability. Monitoring cognitive *and* language growth and gaps between should always be an important SLP function.

Interactionist therapies and interventions recognize that social aspects and repeated, natural routines are critical for ensuring both cognitive and language growth, and thus a family orientation is mandated by our current special-education service law. A variety of interactionist intervention processes have been organized around the construct of creating social contexts in which concepts and word meanings are systematically paired (play routines and the routines of daily living). These include the following: Snyder-McLean and colleagues' (1984) "joint action routines," Constable's (1986) "script play," and Hunt and Goetz's (1988) "interrupted behavior chains."

Narrative assessment and intervention have become an important focus of interactionist therapy for school-age children. Work organized around stories (and now extending into expository or teaching texts), enables a variety of benefits: repeated exposure to the permanency of print, with the supporting modifiability of oral language; extension activities from meaningful "themes" drawn from stories, which result in connections between print and real-life and expansion of concepts and categories; and the opportunity to write in Vygotskian-supported contexts about experiences repeatedly explored. Attention to text structure (such as the story grammars of Stein & Glenn, 1979) is believed to enhance information storage and retrieval. An example of this type of narrative-based approach includes the story-centered lesson plans and themes of Norris & Hoffman (1994). For older children and adolescents, interactionist language applications that appear to aid in improving academic and memory performance include such metacognitive strategies as "semantic organizers" (Pehrsson & Denner, 1988), "think aloud program" (Chabon & Prelock, 1989), and "cognitive behavior modification" (Marshall, 1985). Interactionist therapies are commonly accepted today and recognized for their efficiency in permitting goals for both linguistic and conceptual development.

CONCLUDING REMARKS

Four positions on the relationship between language and cognition have been discussed. The language faculty position proposes significant independence between structures of language and cognition. The cognitive hypothesis proposes that language is largely controlled by cognition, and the language hypothesis has the opposite notion—that language exerts control on cognition. Within the interactionist position is a view of a strong, beneficial interaction between the two. Each theory offers some benefit in terms of therapy considerations. While it is certainly helpful to examine all of these theories, it *is not* necessary to adopt one position as a unitary approach to management of communication disorders. Instead, as is recommended by Highnam (1994), choosing a therapy and the theory behind it to serve a particular individual should always be based on the individual's level of functioning, type of language problem, and particular disability. Moreover, monitoring of the changing findings in research on these matters, particularly as we learn more about specific populations and their learning and language characteristics, will be important in maintaining an appropriate level of competence in our field.

REFERENCES

Bates E, Benigni L, Bretherton I, et al. From gesture to the first word: on cognitive and social prerequisites. In: Lewis M, Rosenblum L, eds. Interaction, conversation, and the development of language. New York: Wiley, 1977.

Bates E, Bretherton I, Snyder L, et al. The emergence of symbols: communication and cognition in infancy. New York: Academic Press, 1979.

Bates E, Camaioni L, Volterra V. The acquisition of performatives prior to speech. Merrill-Palmer Q 1975;21:205–216.

Bates E, Bretherton I, Snyder L. From first words to grammar. Cambridge, England: Cambridge University Press, 1988.

Bates E, Snyder L. The cognitive hypothesis in language development. In: Uzgiris I, Hunt J, eds. Infant performance and experience: new findings with the ordinal scales. Urbana, IL: University of Illinois Press, 1987.

Beilin H. Studies in the cognitive basis of language development. New York: Academic Press, 1975.

Bickerton D. The language bioprogram hypothesis. Behav Brain Sci 1984;7:173–221.

Blank M. Cognitive functions of language in the preschool years. Dev Psychol 1974;10:229–245.

Blank M, Bridger W. Cross-modal transfer in nursery school children. J Comp Physiol Psychol 1964;58:277–282.

Blank M, Marquis AM. Directing discourse. Tucson, AZ: Communication Skill Builders, 1987.

Blank M, Rose S, Berlin L. The language of learning: the preschool years. New York: Grune & Stratton, 1978a.

Blank M, Rose S, Berlin L. The preschool language assessment instrument. New York: Grune & Stratton, 1978b.

Blewitt P. What determines the order of acquisition of object categories? Paper presented at the meeting of the Society for Research in Child Development, Detroit, April 1983.

Bloom L. One word at a time: the use of single-word utterances before syntax. The Hague, Netherlands: Mouton, 1973.

Bowerman M. Learning a semantic system: what role do cognitive predispositions play? In: Rice M, Schiefelbusch R, eds. The teachability of language. Baltimore: Brookes, 1989.

Brown R. A first language: the early stages. Cambridge, MA: Harvard University Press, 1973.

Brown R, Hanlon C. Derivational complexity and the order of acquisition in child speech. In: Hayes J, ed. Cognition and the development of language. New York: John Wiley, 1970.

Brown L, Sherbenou R J, Dollay SJ. Test of Nonverbal Intelligence. Austin, TX: PRO-Ed, 1982.

Bruner J. Early social interaction and language acquisition. In: Schaffer H, ed. Studies in mother-child interaction. New York: Academic Press, 1977.

Campione JC, Brown AL, Ferrara RA, Bryant NR. The zone of proximal development: implications for individual differences and learning. In: Rogoff B, Wertsch J, eds. New directions for cognitive development: the zone of proximal development. San Francisco: Jossey-Bass, 1984.

Carlson JS, Wiedl KH. The dynamic assessment of intelligence. In: Haywood HC, Tzurill D, eds. Interactive assessment. Hillsdale, NJ: Lawrence Erlbaum, 1988.

Chabon S, Prelock P. Strategies of a different stripe: our response to a zebra question about language and its relevance to the curriculum. Semin Speech Hear 1989;10:241–250.

Chomsky N. Aspects of a theory of syntax. Cambridge, MA: MIT Press, 1965.

Chomsky N. Cartesian linguistics. New York: Harper & Row, 1966.

Chomsky N. Language and mind. New York: Harcourt Brace Jovanovich, 1972.

Chomsky N. Rules and representatives. New York: Columbia University Press, 1980.

Chomsky N. Lectures on government and binding. Dordrecht, Holland: Foris, 1981.

Chomsky N. Knowledge of language: Its nature, origin and use. New York: Praeger, 1986.

Clark EV. Meaning and concepts. In: Musser P, ed. Handbook of child psychology. Vol. 3. New York: Wiley, 1983.

Constable C. The application of scripts in the organization of language intervention contexts. In: Nelson K, ed. Event knowledge: structure and function in development. Hillsdale, NJ: L. Erlbaum, 1986.

Corrigan R. Language development as related to stage 6 object permanence development. J Child Lang 1978;5:173–189.

Cromer R. Strengths of the weak form of the cognition hypothesis for language acquisition. In: Lea V, ed. Language development. New York: John Wiley, 1979.

Cromer RF. The cognition hypothesis revisited. In: Kessel F, ed. The development of language and language researchers. Hillsdale, NJ: Erlbaum, 1988.

Dale PS. Language development: structure and function. Hinsdale, IL: Dryden Press, 1972.

Dunst C. A clinical and educational manual for use with the Uzgiris and Hunt Scales of Infant Psychological development. Baltimore: University Park Press, 1980.

Eisenson J. Developmental aphasia: a speculative view with therapeutic implications. J Speech Hear Disord 1968;33:3–13.

Farrar M, Goodman G. Developmental differences in the relationship between scripts and episodic memory: do they exist? In: Fivush R, Hudson J, eds. What young children remember and why. New York: Cambridge University Press, 1991.

Ferreiro E, Sinclair H. Temporal relationships in language. Int J Psychol 1971;6:39–47.

Fodor J. Modularity of mind: an essay on faculty psychology. Cambridge, MA: MIT Press, 1983.

Forrest-Pressley DL, Waller TG. Cognition, metacognition, and reading. New York: Springer-Verlag, 1984.

Friel-Patti S. Auditory linguistics processing and language learning. In: Wallach GP, Butler KG, eds. Language learning disabilities in school-age children and adolescents. New York: Macmillan, 1994.

Frost SE. Basic teaching of the great philosophers. New York: Doubleday, 1962.

Gardner H. Frames of mind. New York: Basic Books, 1983.

Gardner H. "Multiple intelligences" as a catalyst. English J 1995;84(8):16–18.

Gardner R, Gardner B. Teaching sign language to a chimpanzee. Science 1969;165:664–672.

Ginsburg H, Opper S, eds. Piaget's theory of intellectual development. Englewood Cliffs, NJ: Prentice-Hall, 1979.

Gopnik A, Meltzoff A. Relations between semantic and cognitive development in the one word stage: the specificity hypothesis. Child Dev 1986;57: 1040–1053.

Gross T. Cognitive development. New York: Brooks/Cole, 1985.

Hall R. Cognitive behavior modification and information processing skills of exceptional children. Exceptional Education Q 1980;1:–15.

Harding C, Golinkoff R. The origins of intentional vocalizations in prelinguistic infants. Child Dev 1978;50:33–40.

Heath S. The dismantling of narrative. In: McCabe A, Peterson C, eds. Developing narrative structure. Hillsdale, NJ: Lawrence Erlbaum, 1991.

Herman L, Richards D, Wolz J. Comprehension of sentences by bottle-necked dolphins. Cognition 1984;16:128–219.

Highnam CL. Cognition. In: Haynes WO, Shulman BB, eds. Communication development: foundations, processes and clinical applications. Englewood Cliffs, NJ: Prentice-Hall, 1994.

Hoffman L, Paris S, Hall E, Schall, R. Developmental psychology today. 5th ed. New York: Random House, 1988.

Hunt P, Goetz L. Teaching spontaneous communication in natural settings through interrupted behavior chains. Top Lang Disord 1988;9:58—71.

Johnston J. On location: thinking and talking about space. Top Lang Disord 1981;2:17—31.

Johnston J. Speech language disorders in the child. In: Lass N, McReynolds L, Yoder D, eds. Handbook of speech pathology and audiology. Philadelphia: B.C. Decker, 1988.

Kahn J. Cognitive training and the initial use of referential speech. Top Lang Disord 1984;5:14–23.

Karoly P. Behavior self-management in children: concepts, methods, issues and directions. In: Herson M, Eisler R, Miller P, eds. Progress in behavior modification. New York: Academic Press, 1977.

Kennedy M, Sheridan M, Radlinski S, Burghly M. Play-language relationships in young children with developmental delays: implications for assessment. J Speech Hear Res 1991;34:112–122.

Korsten JE, Dunn DK, Foss TV, Francke MK. Every move counts. San Antonio, TX: Psychological Corporation, 1995.

Labov W. Language in the inner city: Studies in the black English vernacular. Philadelphia: University of Pennsylvania Press, 1972.

Labov W. Sociolinguistic patterns. Philadelphia: University of Pennsylvania Press, 1973.

Leonard L. Language learnability and specific language impairment in children. Appl Psycholinguist 1989;10:179–202.

Leonard L, Loeb D. Government binding theory and some of its applications: a tutorial. J Speech Hear Res 1988;31:515–524.

Liberman AM, Cooper S, Shankweiler DP, Studdart-Kennedy M. Perception of the speech code. Psychol Rev 1967;74:431–461.

Lowery L. Learning about learning: conservation abilities. University of California, Berkeley, ERA Program, 1977a.

Lowery L. Learning about learning: propositional abilities. University of California, Berkeley, ERA Program, 1977b.

Lowry R. The evolution of psychological theory. 2nd ed. New York: Aldine, 1982.

Mandler J. Stories, scripts, and scenes: aspects of a schema theory. Hillsdale, NJ: Erlbaum, 1984.

Mandler J, Johnson N. Some of the thousand words a picture is worth. J Exp Psychol [Hum Learn Mem] 1976;2:529–540.

Maratsos M. Decrease in the understanding of the word "big" in preschool children. Child Dev 1973;44:747–752.

Marshall K. Cognitive behavior modification in the classroom: theoretical and practical perspectives. In: Simon C, ed. Communication skills and classroom success. San Diego: College-Hill, 1985.

Michaels S. The dismantling of narrative. In: McCabe A, Peterson C, eds. Developing narrative structure. Hillsdale, NJ: Erlbaum, 1991.

Miller G. Spontaneous apprentices: children and language. New York: Seabury, 1977.

Miller J, Chapman R, Branston M, Reichly J. Language comprehension in sensorimotor stages 5 and 6. J Speech Hear Res 1980;4:1–12.

Miller L. The roles of language and learning in the development of literacy. Top Lang Disord 1990;10:1–24.

Miller PH. Theories of developmental psychology. San Francisco: W.H. Freeman, 1983.

Moerman M. Talking culture: ethnography and conversation analysis. Philadelphia: University of Pennsylvania Press, 1988.

Mykelbust H. Auditory disorders in children: a manual for differential diagnosis. New York: Grune & Stratton, 1954.

Nelson K. Making sense: the development of meaning in early childhood. New York: Academic Press, 1985.

Nelson K. Event knowledge. Hillsdale, NJ: Erlbaum, 1986.

Nelson LK, Kamhi AG, Apel K. Cognitive strengths and weaknesses in language-impaired children: one more look. J Speech Hear Disord 1987;52:36–43.

Nicolosi L, Harryman E, Kresheck J. Terminology of communication disorders: speech-language-hearing. 3rd ed. Baltimore: Williams & Wilkins, 1989.

Nippold M. Later language development: ages nine through nineteen. Boston: College Hill Press, 1988.

Norris JA, Hoffman PR. Whole language in school-age children. San Diego: Singular Press, 1993.

Norris JA, Hoffman PR. Storybook Centered Themes and Storybook Centered Lesson Plans. San Antonio, TX: Psychological Corporation, 1994.

Olswang L, Stoel-Gammon C, Coggins T, Carpenter R. Assessing linguistic behaviors. Seattle: University of Washington Press, 1987.

Owens RE. Language development: an introduction. 4th ed. Boston: Allyn & Bacon, 1966.

Palincsar AS, Brown AL, Campione JC. Models and practices of dynamic assessment. In: Wallach GP, Butler KG, eds. Language learning disabilities in school-age children and adolescents. New York: Macmillan, 1994.

Pehrsson R, Denner P. Semantic organizers: implications for reading and writing. Top Lang Disord 1988;8:24–37.

Penfield W, Robert L. Speech and brain mechanisms. New York: Atheneum, 1966.

Piaget J. The language and thought of the child. New York: Meridian Books, 1955.

Piaget J, Inhelder B. The child's conception of space. London: Routledge & Kegan Paul, 1956.

Pinker S. Language learnability and language development. Cambridge, MA: Harvard University Press, 1984.

Pinker S. The bootstrapping problem in language acquisition. In: McWhinney B, ed. Mechanisms of language acquisition. Hillsdale, NJ: Lawrence Erlbaum, 1987.

Pinker S. Learnability and cognition. Cambridge, MA: MIT Press, 1989.

Premack D. Language in chimpanzee? Science 1971;172:808–822.

Premack D. Gavagai! On the future of the animal language controversy. Cambridge, MA: MIT Press, 1986.

Pulaski MA. Understanding Piaget: an introduction to children's cognitive development. New York: Harper & Row, 1980.

Pye C. Synthesis/commentary: the nature of language. In: Schiefelbusch R, ed. The teachability of language. Baltimore: Brookes, 1989.

Ramsay D. Object word spurt, handedness, and object permanence in the infant. Unpublished doctoral dissertation, University of Denver, 1977.

Rogers SJ, Donovan CM, D'Eugenio DB, et al. Early intervention developmental profile. Ann Arbor, MI: University of Michigan Press, 1981.

Rosch E, Mervin C. Children's sorting: a reinterpretation based on the nature of abstraction in natural categories. In: Smart R, Smart M, eds. Readings in child development and relationship. 2nd ed. New York: Macmillan, 1977.

Rumelhart D. Toward an interactive model of reading. In: Dornic S, ed. Attention and performance. Vol. 6. Hillsdale, NJ: Erlbaum, 1977.

Rumelhart D. Schemata: the building blocks of cognition. In. Spiro R, Bruce B, Brewer W, eds. Theoretical issues in reading comprehension. Hillsdale, NJ: Erlbaum, 1980.

Schank R, Abelson R. Scripts, plans, goals, and understanding. Hillsdale, NJ: Erlbaum, 1977.

Scollon R, Scollon S. Narrative, literacy, and face in interethnic communication. Norwood, NJ: Ablex, 1981.

Shipley E, Kuhn I, Madden E. Mothers' use of superordinant category items. J Child Lang 1983; 10:571–588.

Shore C. Combinational play, conceptual development and early multi-word speech. Dev Psychol 1986;22:184–190.

Sinclair-DeZwart H. Language acquisition and cognitive development. In: Moore TE, ed. Cognitive development and the acquisition of language. New York: Academic Press, 1973.

Slobin D. Cognitive prerequisites for the development of grammar. In: Ferguson C, Slobin D, eds. Studies of child language development. New York: Holt, Rinehart & Winston, 1973.

Slobin D. Cognitive prerequisites for the development of grammar. In: Bloom L, Lahey M, eds. Readings in language development. New York: John Wiley, 1978.

Smolak L, Levine M. The effects of differential criteria on the assessment of cognitive-linguistic relationships. Child Dev 1984;55:973–980.

Snyder L. Communicative and cognitive abilities and disabilities in the sensorimotor period. Merrill-Palmer Q 1978;24:161–180.

Snyder-McLean L, Solomonson B, McLean J, Sack S. Structuring joint action routines. A strategy for facilitating communications and language development in the classroom. Semin Speech Lang 1984;5:213–228.

Steckol K, Leonard L. Sensorimotor development and the use of prelinguistic performatives. J Speech Hear Res 1981;24:262–268.

Stein J, ed. The Random House college dictionary. Revised edition. Toronto: Random House, 1980.

Stein N, Glenn C. An analysis of story comprehension in elementary school children. In: Freedle R, ed. New directions in discourse processing. Vol. 2. Norwood, NJ: Ablex, 1979.

Stevenson R. Models of language development. Philadelphia: Open University Press, 1988.

Tallal P. Relation between speech perception, language comprehension, and speech production in children with speech language delay. Allied Health Behav Sci 1978;1(2):220–236.

Tallal P, Stark RE. Speech acoustic cue discrimination abilities of normally developing and language-impaired children. J Acoust Soc Am 1981;69(2):568–574.

Tallal P, Stark RE, Mellits ED. Identification of language-impaired children on the basis of rapid perception and production skills. Brain Lang 1985;25:314–322.

Terrance H, Pettito L, Saunders R, Bever J. Can an ape create a sentence? Science 1979;206:891–902.

Terrell B, Schwartz R, Prelock P, Messick C. Symbolic play in normal and language-impaired children. J Speech Hear Res 1984;27:424–429.

Thal D. Language and cognition in normal and late-talking toddlers. Top Lang Disord 1991;11:33–42.

Tremaine R. Syntax and Piagetian operational thought. Washington, DC: University Park Press, 1975.

Uzgiris I, Hunt J. Assessment in infancy: ordinal scales of psychological development. Champaign-Urbana, IL: University of Illinois Press, 1975.

Vygotsky L. Izbrannyye psikologicheskiye issiedovaniya. Moscow: Izd-vo APN RSFSR, 1956.

Vygotsky L. Thought and word. In: Vygotsky LS, ed. Thought and language. Cambridge, MA: MIT Press, 1962.

Watson R. The great psychologists from Aristotle to Freud. New York: Lippincott, 1968.

Westby C. Assessment of cognitive and language abilities through play. Lang Speech Hear Serv Schools 1980;11(3):154–168.

Westby CE. Communication refinement in school age and adolescence. In: Haynes WO, Shulman BB, eds. Communication development: foundations, processes and clinical applications. Englewood Cliffs, NJ: Prentice-Hall, 1994.

Whorf B. The relation of habitual thought and behavior to language. In: Spier L, ed. Language, culture, and personality: essays in honor of Edward Sapir. Salt Lake City: University of Utah Press, 1941.

Whorf BL. Language, thought, and reality: Selected Writings of Benjamin Lee Whorf. Cambridge, MA: Technology Press of MIT and John Wiley, 1956.

Witt B. ENABLE: developing instructional language skills. Tucson, AZ: Communication Skill Builders, 1988.

Witt B, Morgan J. TOTAL-Revised. San Antonio, TX: Psychological Corporation, 1992.

Zachman L, Huisingh R, Barrett M, et al. Manual of exercises for expressive reasoning (MEER). Moline, IL: Linguisystems, 1982.

CHAPTER 7

The Development of Play

Janet L. Patterson and Carol E. Westby

Play is a universal human activity that blends cognitive, social, emotional, linguistic, and motor components. When children play, they enact and use their knowledge and skills as they vary and create activities. Observing children playing provides information about children's knowledge and views of the world. We can also observe how children communicate as they play. Play is also an effective context for teaching children. During play, children can learn new skills as part of whole, meaningful activities.

Knowledge about the development of play is needed to observe and interpret play effectively and to use play for teaching. Information about the development of play is presented in this chapter. First, the characteristics that differentiate "play" and "non-play" activities are presented, and the role of play in development is discussed. The following examples contrast play and non-play activities based on current definitions of play.

Roger, age 3, asks his mother for a cookie for his snack. He is disappointed when his mother says there aren't any cookies and offers him yogurt or raisins.

Later in the day, Roger plays with kitchen toys with his mother. She offers him a "cookie," a round plastic poker chip, which he happily accepts and pretends to eat.

Theresa, age 2½, watches her mother watering the garden using a spray nozzle on the garden hose. When her mother lays the hose down to answer the phone, Theresa walks over to the hose, picks up the end, and looks at the nozzle carefully. She pulls the trigger that operates the nozzle and, frowning with concentration, tries to spray the garden.

After spraying the garden for a few seconds, Theresa starts and stops the water flow several times and giggles while she points the nozzle in the air.

Jimmy, age 4, looks at all the moving parts of a toy helicopter. He twirls the helicopter blades by pushing them with his finger. Then he discovers a trigger under the body of the helicopter. He pushes and pokes at the trigger and finally pulls it, which makes the blades rotate. He rotates the blade twice more, using the trigger, and then starts to look at the working parts of a toy fire engine.

PLAY: THEORIES AND DEFINITIONS

Characteristics of Play

Although researchers differ on exactly how they define play, most would agree that in the preceding descriptions of children's activities, some involve play and some do not. As illustrated in the examples above, play and nonplay activities cannot be distinguished on the basis of the specific materials or actions involved (Garvey, 1977). Furthermore, the same knowledge structures or *schemas* are involved in play and nonplay activities (Piaget, 1962).

What distinguishes play from nonplay is the child's orientation and attitude toward the activity (Garvey, 1977; Rubin, Fein, & Vandenberg, 1983). Some characteristics of play include the following:

1. *Intrinsic motivation.* Children (and adults) play because they want to. Play activities are done for their own sake, not to achieve goals outside the play activity (Garvey, 1977; Johnson, Christie, & Yawkey, 1987; Rubin, et al., 1983).

2. *Process over product.* The individual is more focused on the ongoing activity than a goal. In other words, the focus is on the means rather than the ends of an activity, in contrast with nonplay activities (Piaget, 1962). The child playing with the garden hose switched from a focus on the product/end/goal (watering the garden) to a focus on the activity of manipulating the nozzle. As a result of focusing on the process rather than working for a particular product or goal, children's play activities often may appear more varied and flexible than their other activities (Johnson, et al., 1987; Rubin, et al., 1983).

3. *Child structured.* Children's purposes structure the activity, rather than properties and conventional uses of the materials they play with. During play, children rely "on internal tendencies and motives and not on incentives supplied by external things" (Vygotsky, 1978, p. 96). In contrast with exploration of objects, where the activity seems to involve questions of what the object is and what its functions are, play with objects is focused on what the child can use the object for (Rubin, et al., 1983). From the examples in this chapter, Jimmy's exploration of the helicopter was object-focused. In contrast, Fred started with an object focus, but then used the helicopter in a play activity. Children generally play with objects only after they have become familiar with the objects by exploring the properties and conventional uses of new objects (Johnson, et al., 1987), as in the example above.

4. *Active engagement.* This characteristic is used to differentiate play activities in children from quiet observation without direct participation in other's play, from simply lounging, and from daydreaming (Garvey, 1977). Although this distinction seems useful for children in the sensorimotor and preoperational stages, daydreaming may be viewed as a form of play in older children and adults (Johnson, et al., 1987; Rubin, et al., 1983; Vygotsky, 1978).

5. *Intrinsic rules and structure.* Freedom from externally imposed rules and direction is frequently mentioned as a characteristic of play (Rubin, et al., 1983). There are "rules" or structure in play, but the rules are internal to the play activity (Garvey, 1977; Vygotsky, 1978). The rules and structure of play activities are created by the child, or are negotiated and/or agreed on when two or more children play together. The contrast between internally and externally imposed rules and structure can be helpful in distinguishing some instances of play and nonplay. For example, a child who is told to build a high tower with blocks by an adult may not be playing, in contrast with a child who does so independently. Similarly, participating in a school play is generally highly structured by externally imposed rules, scripts, and directions, while the same children may also engage in elaborate pretend play on their own, negotiating rules, structures, and actions among themselves. Children who play games with rules, such as board games or tag, agree to a set of rules that apply to the play situation, but do not apply to the real world (Vygotsky, 1978). For example, the rules of chess do not apply to situations outside the game itself.

6. *Free choice.* This characteristic is closely related to the intrinsically motivated nature of play and the characteristic of intrinsic rules and structure. Young children in particular may not regard activities that are assigned by adults as play (Johnson, et al., 1987; King, 1986).

7. *Positive affect.* Children value play activities and often show positive affect during play (Garvey, 1977; Johnson, et al., 1987). Piaget's (1962) descriptions of his daughter's play contain many references to verbal and nonverbal expressions of pleasure, joy, happiness, and enjoyment.

8. *Nonliteral activity.* Play activities are treated differently than "real" activities. They are released from the rules, routines, and consequences of daily activity. Rough-and-tumble play and pretending to cook are examples of activities where a play orientation or "frame" allows different behaviors than the literal or real activity. The nonliteral aspect of play is particularly highlighted in pretend play, where an "as if" or nonliteral attitude is clear to observers (Garvey, 1977; Johnson, et al., 1987). See the example above in which Roger pretends to eat a poker chip *as if* it were a cookie.

Children frame an activity as nonliteral or playful and convey the message that an activity is play by gesture, facial expressions, body movements, and/or through language. The communication that an activity is play is a type of *metacommunication* (Bateson, 1971; Garvey, 1977; Sawyer, 1997). Smiles and acceptance of events without expected outcomes (e.g., "drinking" from an empty cup without distress) are forms of metacommunication that are used and understood by very young children. In addition to these forms of metacommunication, children begin to use language to identify activities as pretend (e.g., "Let's pretend we're making cookies") at about 3 years of age (Goncu, 1993).

The Roles of Play in Development

Definitions of play and views of the functions, attributes, and worth of play differ across cultures and historic contexts (Schwartzman, 1984; Sutton-Smith, 1986). In recent years play has been viewed positively in many Western cultures by those interested in the development and education of children, although not all types of play are equally valued. For example, teachers and parents are not likely to encourage aggressive play or play with explicit sexual themes. In contrast, constructive play, pretend play, and games with rules with "acceptable" content are often viewed positively and may be actively fostered by many parents and teachers.

Many studies have demonstrated relationships between *symbolic play* (pretend play) and various cognitive and social skills (Fein, 1981; Johnson, et al., 1987; Rubin, et al., 1983). Although play might simply reflect skills learned in other contexts, it appears that at least some cognitive and social skills develop in the context of play.

An important aspect of cognitive development that develops in symbolic play is the ability to *decontextualize* or to separate actions and objects from their usual contexts (Bates, Benigni, Camioni, et al., 1979). Children who can use actions in play and words in communication as *symbols* for objects, actions, and ideas are no longer bound to the immediate context in their thoughts, actions, or speech. In symbolic play, actions and objects are not "for real," but are used to represent events, objects, and people.

The importance of the separation of the child's motives and ideas from objects, particularly in symbolic play, is emphasized by Vygotsky (1978):

> In play thought is separated from objects and action arises from ideas rather than from things: a piece of wood begins to be a doll and a stick becomes a horse . . . This is such a reversal of the child's relation to the real, immediate, concrete situation that it is hard to underestimate its full significance. (p.97)

When children begin to represent hypothetical or "as if" situations through pretend play, it is an initial step toward understanding the attitudes and mental representations of others (Astington, 1994). Young children understand pretense as a special type of action, one in which the usual consequences do not hold, and they recognize when someone else is engaging in pretend versus real actions (Harris & Kavanaugh, 1993). Because understanding of pretend involves inferring someone else's attitude toward an activity, pretend play is seen as an important landmark in the development of a *theory of mind*, or knowledge about the mental experiences and mental representations of others (Leslie, 1993).

The course of development toward a theory of mind is summarized as follows by Astington (1994). Some time after pretend play begins, children start using terms to describe the emotions and internal states of themselves and others, between 2 and 3 years of age. Young children refer to these types of experience in real-world and pretend contexts (e.g., saying "my baby hungry" or "baby's sad"). Between 3 and 4 years of age, children make references to cognitive states and operations, using mental state verbs such as *know, remember, and forget*. At about 4 years of age, children recognize that different people can have different knowledge and perspectives. This is typically tested through tasks involving "false beliefs." For example, a child is shown a boy putting chocolate in a drawer. His mother moves it to a cupboard when he is playing outside. Before 4 years of age children say that the boy will look in the cupboard for the chocolate from the drawer when he comes in, indicating they do not mentally represent the boy's knowledge separately from their own. When children base their answers on information about others' mental states, rather than on their own information, at about 4 years of age, most researchers credit the child with having a theory of mind.

There is disagreement to date on whether young preschool children realize that pretend actions reflect a special type of mental representation. Just as children have feelings and knowledge before they talk about these types of mental experiences, it appears that children can pretend and recognize pretending before they identify the special mental processes involved in pretense. Lillard (1993) found that, at least until age 4 years, children base their judgements of whether someone is pretending on the actions they see the person carry out, rather than on what they are told about the actor's mental state. For example, if they are shown a man hopping and are told that the man has never seen a rabbit before and that he doesn't know that rabbits hop, young children still claim that the man is pretending to be a rabbit. Nonetheless, an understanding that there are situations in which people act "as if" rather than for real is an important step toward being able to understand the existence and importance of mental states (Astington, 1994). Because knowledge about the mental states of others provides us with a basis for understanding and predicting the actions of others, the development of theory of mind is an important component in social development.

In addition to its role in the sequence of development of theory of mind, pretend play with others (social pretend) is a context in which children practice and develop social skills. In social pretend play, children practice and refine communication of their "as if" meanings and intentions to one another. Howes (1992) suggests that once children have developed the ability to communicate meanings to one another in social pretend, usually by about 3 years of age, play then becomes a context for practicing negotiation and compromise in the coordination of more complex pretend activities, a focus of social pretend play during the preschool years.

Play is also an important context for the expression of affect, emotional states, and emotional themes (Fein, 1985; Greenspan & Greenspan, 1985; Howes, 1992; Motti, Cicchetti, & Sroufe, 1983; Paley, 1988). Use of symbolic play in therapy to address emotional issues is a common method used by various psychiatrists, psychologists, and counselors when working with children (for reviews see Guerney, 1984; Schaefer & O'Connor, 1983).

Pretend play is closely related to language development (McCune-Nicolich, 1981; Westby, 1980, 1988, 1991). There is a consistent co-occurrence of first words with early pretend play (Bates, Bretherton, Snyder, et al., 1980; Kelly & Dale, 1989), and word combinations and symbolic play scheme combinations also co-occur consistently (McCune-Nicolich & Bruskin, 1982; Shore, O'Connell, & Bates, 1984; Spencer, 1996). There is a general consensus that research should focus on relationships between specific dimensions of play and language, because general levels of sensorimotor and play development have not shown consistent relationships to general stages of language development (Bates, et al., 1979; McCune-Nicolich, 1981; Rice, 1983).

Among preschool children, relationships between language and symbolic play are at the level of texts, rather than at the level of words and word combinations within utterances. Sawyer (1997) draws parallels between the improvisational skills used in adult conversations and children's social pretend play. Preschool children practice linking and negotiating their individual ideas and roles in emerging performances in pretend play, just as adults improvise as they engage in conversations. Between 3 and 5 years of age, children's verbal contributions during social pretend play become more consistently linked to one another (Goncu, 1993).

Sawyer also points out similarities between children's social pretend and adults' improvisational performances in theater and jazz. In conversations and improvisational theater and jazz, individuals' contributions are woven into the group's performance moment-by-moment. Social pretend play provides a context for practicing improvisational skills needed in all of these endeavors (Sawyer, 1997). By 5 to 6 years of age, children participate in lengthy sociodramatic enactments. They use language to construct complex play episodes, to negotiate and argue, to refer to events

and issues outside the pretend frame, and to reestablish pretend play episodes when play is interrupted (Kane & Furth, 1993).

Parallels between fictional narratives and pretend play are also striking. Pretend play may function as a first context for entry into the world of fiction and drama (Harris & Kavanaugh, 1993). In pretend play and fictional narratives, an "as if" attitude is involved. In addition, there are two aspects or landscapes in fictional narratives (Bruner, 1986). One aspect of narratives is the events that occur in the story. The other is the subjective experiences of the characters; their feelings, motivations, perspectives, and knowledge. Understanding a story requires an understanding of how the actions in the story relate to the subjective experiences of the characters (Hewitt, 1994). These types of understandings are also seen in the development of pretend play.

Children draw on their real-world knowledge to make inferences and predictions about the physical aspects of actions in narratives told by others and to predict the pretend consequences of actions during pretend play (Harris & Kavanaugh, 1993). For example, if a child sees an adult overturn an empty cup that they have stated contains "tea," children will pretend to wipe up spilled "tea" in the area where it would have fallen in the real world. Thus, although there is an "as if" attitude in pretend play, real-world knowledge is used to make predictions and inferences about relationships among pretend events, just as real-world knowledge is used to make inferences in comprehension of narratives. Preschool children also make reference to the subjective experience of individuals in their pretend play. They relate the intentions and feelings of characters to the actions in pretend episodes. For example, a child might pretend to become angry after tea is spilled in a pretend scenario.

The ability to use both landscape of action and landscape of consciousness in play and narratives involves the use of *multiple voices*. To use multiple voices, children must be able to take multiple perspectives and to code each perspective linguistically

(Wolf & Hicks, 1989). Children as young as 3 years begin to distinguish voices in their play. For example, Jessica, a 4-year-old girl, received the book *Madeline's Christmas* and a Madeline doll. She then proceeded to act out the story with the Madeline doll and other dolls. In one voice Jessica described the action in the play, in a second voice she gave dialogue to the characters, and in a third voice she commented on the play activity itself:

Play Activity Recreation

Scenario ▶ *Jessica has her Madeline doll and 4 other dolls on the floor*

Narrative	Dialogue	Stage-Managing
Madeline came down to breakfast with all her friends.		
(J positions all the dolls around some dishes on the floor, then has the dolls talk.)		
	I don't feel very good. I don't worry either. Don't worry, I'll take care of you (said by Madeline)	They need to go to bed. Where's the bed?
(The clinician brings a doll bed out of a closet.)		
All the little girls went to bed. So Madeline took them soup. Madeline had to do all the cooking and cleaning.	This is hard. I wish I had someone to help me. I'm so tired.	I need a magician. You got a boy doll?
(Clinician gives Jessica a clown doll.)		
Then a magician knocked on the door. Madeline ran and opened the door.	Hi, I'm here to help you. What can I do?	

The voices have distinctive linguistic structures. The narrative voice is recounted in past tense with some temporal markers (so, then); the dialogue voice is recounted in present tense without temporal markers. In the narrative voice Jessica tended to make greater use of event verbs (came, took) and process verbs (knocked, ran), whereas in the dialogue she made greater use of state verbs (is, am, feel).

In summary, the development of pretend play is closely related to other areas of development, including social, cognitive, emotional, and language development. In the context of play, children practice abstract thought, creativity, and flexibility. They communicate at multiple levels of meaning, they assume and convey different roles, and they negotiate and construct interactions. They express affect, explore emotional issues, and enact subjective, as well as objective, experience in pretend play (Ellis, 1973; Howe, 1992; Vandenberg, 1986).

DEVELOPMENT OF PLAY

Types of Play

New types of play emerge over the course of development. This section provides an overview of the types of play seen in the sensorimotor, preoperational, and concrete operational periods.

Sensorimotor Period

Practice play, or *functional play*, which emerges in the sensorimotor period, consists of repetitive actions and movements carried out with or without objects (Rubin, et al., 1983). For example, Piaget's son began throwing his head back and looking at things from a new perspective at about 3 months of age. Two days later he began to throw his head back repeatedly, laughing and not seeming to focus on the new visual perspective. Piaget (1962) interpreted the repeated head movement as a form of early practice play since the focus seemed to be on the action and not on the result of the action. Examples of practice play involving objects include rolling a toy vehicle back and forth repeatedly and squeezing modeling clay without attempting to construct with it (Rubin, et al., 1983).

Although Piaget did not focus on social forms of play in the sensorimotor period, playful interactions between adults and infants have been an area of increasing interest and research in recent years (see Westby, Chapter 8). In mainstream United States culture, social play moves from face-to-face interactions between adults and infants in the first 4 months of life to ritualized games such as "pat-a-cake," to play with an object with another person in simple, repetitive activities (e.g., rolling a ball back and forth or taking turns operating a simple, mechanical toy).

During the sensorimotor period children play with sounds as a form of practice play and in the context of social play (Garvey, 1977). Babies repeat sounds over and over and vary sounds as a type of play, just as they repeat other actions during the sensorimotor period. They also produce sounds as part of social play with adults (see Westby, Chapter 8).

Preoperational Period

During the preoperational period, the growth of representational and symbolic abilities is reflected in children's play. *Symbolic play*, which begins to develop at the end of the sensorimotor period, continues to develop in the preoperational period. In symbolic play (1) activities are carried out without the usual materials,

contexts, or outcomes; (2) inanimate objects are treated as animate; (3) an object or gesture may be substituted for the real object or action; or (4) the child carries out an action usually done by someone else (Fein, 1981, p. 1096).

Children's play with language in the preoperational period includes practice play with words and sentences. Children play with language by repeating and varying words, phrases, and sentences while alone (Weir, 1962) and while playing with other children (Garvey, 1977). For example, one very talkative 4-year-old girl started rhyming words after her mother commented that a dog was barking, saying "barking, parking, tarking, sarking." Children also use sounds and language as part of pretend play. They make conventionalized sounds for objects (e.g., sirens, telephones ringing, running water), and they use language to establish a play frame with other children (Garvey, 1977). During the preschool years increasingly complex uses of language are seen in the development of play, including language used for dialogue and for setting the scene in pretend play, for directing other participants' play, and for planning and narrating play events (Westby, 1988, 1991).

During the preoperational period, *constructive play* with various materials, including blocks and modeling clay, develops. For example, children build bridges, roads, fences, and houses with blocks. Children's play with blocks and other construction type materials consists of practice play during the sensorimotor period. For example, sensorimotor play with blocks includes banging blocks together; lining up, stacking, and knocking over blocks; and putting blocks in containers.

Concrete Operations

Play involving *games with rules* develops toward the end of the preoperational period and continues in the school-age years. Prior to this, children have difficulty understanding and consistently following the rules of the game, and they require constant adult supervision and support to play most games. Games with rules include board games, card games, party games such as "Pin the Tail on the Donkey," playground games such as "Red Rover," various sports, and games with rules that children make up, negotiate, and adhere to. Although children who play together do not always agree on what rules to follow and disputes are common, there is a recognition that rules should be consistent, unlike earlier periods of development. More abstract approaches to games may occur in later years, with players developing systematic strategies and hypotheses about opponents' plans and actions.

Pattern of Development

When new types of play develop, "older" types of play do not disappear, although they decrease in frequency. For example, there is a progressive decrease in proportion of practice play during the preoperational period and an increase in symbolic and constructive play, but 5, 6, and 7 year olds still engage in occasional practice play (Monighan-Nourot, 1987; Rubin, et al., 1983).

Social Structure of Play

Social aspects of children's play with peers show changes over the course of development. Although children engage in solitary play at all ages, children's abilities to play with peers increase over time (Johnson, et al., 1983). As with the development of other aspects of play, the emergence of new forms of social play does not result in dropping out of all "old" forms of social play. Although research indicates there may be variation among individual children on the exact sequence of stages of social play (Rubin, et al., 1983), a developmental sequence of emergence of types of social play based on the works of Parten (1932) and Howes (1980) and on a review by Johnson et al. (1987) is presented.

Parallel Play

In parallel play, children play independently, but play near one another with similar toys or activities. They may engage in parallel play with mutual regard, showing some awareness of each other through eye contact.

Simple Social Play

Children engage in simple social bids, either by communicating through smiles, vocalization, or touching, or by simple object interactions such as giving or taking toys.

Group Play

In group play there is both active social engagement and shared use of materials. In the first type of group play, *associative play*, children engage in some reciprocal or complementary actions with others, using the same materials and activities. For example, children may roll a ball back and forth, or may exchange materials while pretending to cook, with one child mixing a cake and the other child stirring food in a pan on the stove. Associative play with peers occurs by about 3 years of age (Westby, 1980), but may appear by 2 years of age in mixed age groups if older children are involved in directing play activities (Dunn & Dale, 1984).

The more advanced form of group play is *cooperative play*, which appears by about 5 years of age (Westby, 1980). In this type of play, children collaborate in organizing their play activities, with complementary roles and activities contributing to the overall structure of the play. For example, roles and events in pretend play are coordinated—one child is the mother and one the father; they come home from work at the same time and agree to go get a pizza for dinner. In constructive collaborative play, children might plan to build a town with each child building a different structure.

Solitary Play

In group settings children also engage in some solitary play, unoccupied activities (e.g., wandering around the room), and onlooker activity (watching other children play). These nonsocial types of activities are not of concern unless they occur more frequently than in peers' behavior. For example, Rubin (1982) found that higher frequencies of unoccupied behavior, solitary practice play, and solitary pretend play were associated with lower cognitive and social skills in 4 year olds.

Parallel play seems to serve as a transition between solitary and group types of play. Monighan-Nourot (1987) reported that in her preschool classroom frequency of parallel play peaked at 4 years of age and decreased by 5 years of age when children engaged in more group play. Frequency of parallel constructive play was associated with higher cognitive and social skills in 4 year olds in a study by Rubin (1982), even though children at this age are beginning to engage in group play. Simple social play may also serve as another form of transition to group play, but its relationship to other forms of play has not been studied.

SYMBOLIC PLAY DEVELOPMENT

Sensorimotor Foundations

Children's exploration and play with objects moves from undifferentiated actions on single objects to specific functional uses of objects and combining of objects in play during the first year of life (Belsky & Most, 1981; Fenson, 1985; O'-Connell & Bretherton, 1984). Early inspection and action schemes include looking, touching, mouthing, banging, shaking, and dropping objects. By approximately 8 to 12 months of age more specific manipulation of parts of objects emerges such as flipping switches and pressing buttons (Fenson, 1985; Westby, 1980, 1991). Functional uses of objects such as rolling a toy car, holding a telephone receiver to the ear, and throwing a ball are seen at about 1 year of age (Bayley, 1969; Fenson, 1985; Nicolich, 1977). At about this same time, children combine two objects in play, for example, putting a lid on a box or placing a peg in a hole (Bayley, 1969; Belsky & Most, 1981; Fenson, 1985). Once schemes for appropriate object uses and object combinations appear, early representational play emerges, including constructive and symbolic play (Fenson, 1985).

Another precursor to symbolic play is the participation of infants in social games and routines such as "peek-a-boo" and "I'm gonna get you" chasing games. These games involve actions that are not "for real," but are clearly understood as play-hiding and play-chasing games by young children. This is an early version of the "as if" or nonliteral aspect of play (Ross & Kay, 1980).

Dimensions of Pretend Play

The development of symbolic play involves several dimensions, each of which has been the focus of various studies and theoretic questions (Bretherton, 1984; Fein, 1981). A multidimensional approach to pretend play is also useful in speech-language pathology and education. Research has shown some qualitative differences between the play of handicapped and nonhandicapped children (Hill & McCune-Nicolich, 1981), and clinical observations have indicated that children with developmental delays frequently show variability of development across dimensions of play (Westby, 1991). Four dimensions of symbolic play are addressed in the description of symbolic play development. In addition, developmental changes in language use during pretend play are described.

The dimension of *role* development involves the recipients and agents of pretend actions. The child's increasing ability to include other people and dolls in pretend play, as well as the child's ability to portray others' behaviors and characteristics, reflects changes in the ability to decenter and to represent others' perspectives (Bretherton, 1984; Fein, 1981; Fenson, 1984; Westby, 1988, 1991).

Another dimension that has been the focus of many studies is the nature of *props*. Children's early play involves realistic-appearing toys, but later they can use less realistic toys or substitute objects, or they use pantomime and language to "set the scene." This increasing ability to engage in symbolic play that is not bound to concrete contexts provided by realistic props is a form of decontextualization, which is an important process in cognitive and language development (Donaldson, 1978; Vygotsky, 1978; Westby, 1988, 1991). The development of increasing decontextualization in pretend play appears in two ways over time: (1) Children can use objects that are increasingly dissimilar to the things they represent, and (2) they can use pantomime and language to represent events with less and less support from other objects or props.

Organization of symbolic play is another important dimension that involves the elaboration and sequencing of children's pretend play activities. Pretend play progresses from early isolated pretend actions to complex sequences of detailed activities during the preschool years (Fenson, 1984; Westby, 1988, 1991).

The topics or *themes* of play also change over time. Early pretend play in toddlers involves common daily experiences in the child's life. Preschool children's play topics also include themes they have not directly experienced such as occupational roles (e.g., fireman) and fantasy play. (Some authors use the term "theme" to refer to a more abstract level than "topic." For example, an "averting threat" theme could include firefighters, police, or monster topics.)

As language and symbolic play develop, *language use* becomes more frequent during pretend activities (Bretherton, et al., 1984; Fenson, 1984; Sachs, Goldman, & Chaille, 1985). The ways language is used during pretend play also change over time, with increasing use of language for dialogue; for identifying substitute and imaginary props; and for negotiating, organizing, and narrating pretend settings, roles, and events (Westby, 1988, 1991).

Sequence of Pretend Play Development

A summary of developmental information on play is presented in Table 7.1. This table lists when new play behaviors in each dimension are seen in the child's spontaneous pretend play. Most normally developing, middle-class children incorporate the activities described by the age listed in the chart. For example, most children engage in autosymbolic play by 18 months.

The earliest pretend play consists of simple, isolated pretend actions involving

the child's own body (Belsky & Most, 1981; Nicolich, 1977). The child uses realistic toys or real objects to carry out these "autosymbolic" actions that represent activities the child experiences daily. For example, a child may pretend to drink by putting an empty cup to her lips and making smacking sounds. Piaget (1962) described his daughter pretending to sleep by placing her head on a cloth that resembled her pillow, smiling, and blinking her eyes several times. Many children engage in autosymbolic play toward the beginning of the second year (Nicolich, 1977), and by 18 months most children have begun autosymbolic play (Westby, 1980, 1988, 1991). Children in some studies (e.g., Bates, et al., 1980) have imitated autosymbolic actions at 10 to 12 months of age, following modeling and prompting by adults.

After autosymbolic play emerges, children's ability to pretend extends to involving others as recipients of pretend actions (Belsky & Most, 1981; Nicolich, 1977; Westby, 1980, 1988, 1991). For example, children will pretend to give a drink to a doll or to their mother, as well as to themselves. This was regarded by Piaget (1962) as the first instance of true symbolic play since pretend actions are no longer bound to the child's body and can be represented in other contexts. Children also begin to represent actions of others that they see regularly, such as reading a newspaper or mopping the floor (Nicolich, 1977). Soon after these single symbolic schemes emerge, children begin to use the same scheme on more than one recipient (Nicolich, 1977; Westby, 1980, 1988, 1991). For example, a child may pretend to comb a doll's hair and then the mother's hair. Children also use combinations of props at about the same time, such as picking up food with a spoon from a plate, rather than simply using a spoon in a pretend feeding activity. These types of play are seen in most children's spontaneous play by 19 to 22 months (Fenson, 1984; Westby, 1980, 1988, 1991), but are imitated by younger children (Fenson & Ramsay, 1981).

By 24 months of age most children engage in "multischeme combinations" in

Table 7.1	Summary of Symbolic Play Development				
Age	Props	Themes	Organization	Roles	Language Use in Play
By 18 months	Uses one realistic object at a time	Familiar everyday activities in which child is active participant (e.g., eating, sleeping)	Short, isolated pretend actions	Autosymbolic pretend (e.g., child feeds self pretend food)	Language used to get and maintain toys and seek assistance operating toys (e.g., "baby," "mine," "help")
By 22 months	Uses two realistic objects at a time	Familiar everyday activities that caregivers do (e.g., cooking, reading)	Combines two related toys or performs actions on two people (e.g., uses spoon to eat from plate; feeds mother, then doll)	Child acts on dolls and others (e.g., feeds doll or caregiver)	Occasional comment on toy or action
By 24 months	Uses several realistic objects		Multischeme combinations of steps (e.g., put doll in tub, apply soap, take doll out and dry)		Talks to doll briefly; describes some of the doll's actions (e.g., "baby sleeping")
By 30 months		Common but less frequently experienced or especially traumatic experiences (e.g., shopping, doctor)		Emerging limited doll actions (e.g., doll cries)	Talk to doll and commenting on doll's actions increase in frequency
By 3 years			Sequences of multischeme events (e.g., prepare food, set table, eat food, clear table, wash dishes)	Child talks to doll in response to doll's actions (e.g., "don't cry now," "I'll get you a cookie.")	Children may comment on what they have just completed or what they will do next (e.g., "Dolly ate the cake," "I'm gonna wash dishes.")

Table 7.1 *Summary of Symbolic Play Development (continued)*

Age	Props	Themes	Organization	Roles	Language Use in Play
By 3 1/2 years	Miniature props, small figures, and object substitutions	Observed, but not personally experienced activities (e.g., police, firefighter)		Brief complementary role play with peers (e.g., mother and child; doctor and patient) Attributes emotions and desires to dolls; reciprocal role taking with dolls (child treats doll as partner—talks for doll and as caregiver)	Children use dialogue for dolls and metalinguistic markers (e.g., "he said"); refer to emotions
By 4 years	Imaginary props (language and gestures help set the scene)	Familiar fantasy themes (e.g., Batman, Wonder Women, Cinderella, etc.)	Planned play events (e.g., child decides to play a birthday party and gathers necessary props and assigns roles)	Child or doll has multiple roles (mother, wife, doctor; firefighter, husband, father) Child can handle two or more dolls in complementary rolls (dolls are doctor and patient) Attributes thoughts and plans to doll	Uses language to plan and narrate the story line
By 6 years	Language and gestures can carry the play without props	Creates novel fantasy characters and plots	Multiple planned sequences (plans for self and other players)	More than one role per doll (doll is mother, wife, doctor)	Elaboration of planning and narrative story line

spontaneous play (Miller & Garvey, 1984; Nicolich, 1977; Westby, 1980, 1988, 1991) and in imitation of adult models (O'Connell & Gerard, 1985). The organization of pretend play includes details of common activities, usually performed in a sequence based on events the child has observed or experienced before. For example, a child may pretend to stir cake batter in a pan, place the pan in the oven, and then take the cake out and place it on the counter. Or a child may place a doll in a bathtub, rub it with soap, and then take the doll out of the tub and dry it off. Themes continue to involve familiar daily events.

Children show some evidence of purposefully looking for props at about 24 months (Nicolich, 1977; Westby, 1980, 1988, 1991). Although most props children use in spontaneous play are realistic toys and objects (Westby, 1980, 1988, 1991), some studies have found children using some substitute objects similar in form such as a screwdriver for a toothbrush in free play (Belsky & Most, 1981; Nicolich, 1977). By this time most children can imitate pretend actions involving a substitute object with similar form, or one with a dissimilar form. For example, children can substitute a clamshell or a block for a cup, but they seldom imitate actions involving two substitute objects at once (Fein, 1975; Jackowitz & Watson, 1980).

By 24 to 30 months of age, children also begin to give dolls a limited active role in play. This may be done verbally or by physically manipulating the doll. For example, they may say the doll is crying or is hungry, or they make the doll "walk" rather than simply placing the doll in new locations (Bretherton, O'Connell, Shore, & Bates, 1984; Fenson, 1984; Watson & Fischer, 1980; Wolf & Grollman, 1982). The doll is the recipient of many of the child's actions, but also begins to be treated as an agent.

At about 30 months children begin to include new themes in their play. In addition to daily household events, children begin to represent less frequently experienced events such as a visit to the doctor or shopping in multischeme combinations (Westby, 1980, 1988, 1991). For ex-

ample, a child may gather food from a grocery store shelf, take it to a toy cash register, and put the food in bags. Use of substitute objects similar in form (e.g., a cylindrical block for a baby bottle) appears in many children's spontaneous play (Fenson, 1984), in addition to the use of realistic toys.

By 3 years of age the most common themes are still household play and events the child has directly experienced and observed, but some episodes contain sequences of two or more multischeme events (Miller & Garvey, 1984; Westby, 1980, 1988, 1991; Wolf & Grollman, 1982). For example, a child might pretend to stir and bake a cake, then eat the cake at the table, feeding herself and a doll, and then wash the dishes. Children can also modify familiar schemes in play such as pretending to buy a toy the child's parents did not buy for him (Fein, 1985; Westby, 1980, 1988, 1991).

After modeling, children can also make one doll carry out several actions in free play (Watson & Fischer, 1980). For example, a "doctor doll" may check a doll with a stethoscope, give the patient a Band-Aid, and then call for an ambulance. Although children at this age do not yet act out scenes with dolls playing complementary or reciprocal roles, they do begin to engage in some complementary role play with their peers (Howes, Unger, & Seidner, 1989), often explicitly assuming roles such as "mother" and "child" (Miller & Garvey, 1984). Shared role play such as both children examining a doll in doctor play is still common among 3 year olds, however (Forys & McCune-Nicolich, 1984).

By 3 to 3½ years of age children use a doll or a puppet as a partner in reciprocal role play. They attribute emotions and desires to dolls (Wolf, Rygh, & Altshuler, 1984), and talk for the doll, alternating between dialogue for themselves and the doll (Miller & Garvey, 1984; Westby, 1980, 1988, 1991). A doll is typically treated as a baby, while the child takes the role of mother. Children vary their speech with different roles by 3½ to 4 years (Westby, 1980, 1988, 1991). For example, 3½- to 5-

year-old African-American girls from lower and middle socioeconomic groups used some longer utterances and more imperatives in their role play as mothers and older sisters than when they played "younger sister," and they used much shorter utterances and baby vocalizations (cooing, babbling) when playing a baby role (McLoyd, Ray, & Etter-Lewis, 1985). Features of "child directed speech" or "motherese" such as repetitions of simple utterances to baby dolls have been observed in many young preschool children's speech (e.g., Miller & Garvey, 1984).

Children engage in play involving events and themes they have not directly experienced by 3½ to 4 years, although household play themes are still frequent. Play themes include occupational roles such as police, firefighter, as well as familiar fantasy characters such as Batman, Wonder Woman, and Cinderella (Garvey, 1977; Paley, 1988; Westby, 1980, 1988, 1991). They can also use small, less realistically detailed replica toys in pretend play, such as Fischer-Price and Playmobile sets of abstract people figures, vehicles, and props for a village, fire truck, airport, and hospital (Westby, 1980, 1988, 1991).

By 3½ to 4 years, children's spontaneous play includes the use of substitute objects, as well as language and pantomime to designate props (Westby, 1980, 1988, 1991; Wolf & Grollman, 1982). For example, one girl we observed pretended to go to a drive-in movie. She sat on a stair step, pantomimed turning an imaginary key in the ignition, steering, and braking, and then announced she was watching a movie about a kitty as she indicated a stuffed dog a few feet away. Although most children can use substitute objects, gestures, and language for props by 4 years of age, individual children vary on how many substitute and imaginary objects they include in their play (Wolf & Grollman, 1982).

By 4 years children can act out scenes using dolls and puppets only, rather than participating in the play as a partner. For example, one doll can be the mother and the other her baby, rather than the child assuming the mother role to the baby doll. The child can also act out more than one aspect to a role in her own role play, or in roles taken by dolls (Westby, 1980, 1988, 1991). For example, a child might play mother to a baby, speak as a wife to her husband, and go to work. Many 4-year-old children develop an imaginary friend as a companion (Monighan-Nourot, 1987; Fein, 1981).

During group pretend play (sociodramatic play) in the preschool years, children's language use becomes an increasingly integral part of pretend activities. Language is used to plan and negotiate play, as well as to narrate some events rather than physically acting them out (Garvey, 1977; Westby, 1980, 1988, 1991; Giffin, 1984). Children can also use metalinguistic markers such as "He said. . . ." for narrating pretend dialogue in group or solitary pretend play (Bretherton, 1984; Westby, 1980, 1988, 1991). Preschool children use language to explicitly assign and assume roles ("I'm the mommy, and you're the baby"), and to plan play events ("Let's say baby's sick and she has to go to the hospital"). Children also set the scene by describing pretend past events (Giffin, 1984). For example, we observed a 6-year-old girl asking her 4-year-old brother if the cookies he was baking were ready. He replied, "Yes, and I ate them all up," momentarily deflecting his sister's persistent directions and questions about his play activities. Children also use language within role play to direct the events and actions of their peers. For example, a child said, "It's time for lunch. Here, eat it," as she offered an empty plate to an observer, simultaneously using language for dialogue in her role and steering her partner's action (Giffin, 1984). Language is also used for initiating pretend play (Scales, 1987) and for establishing a pretend frame (Bretherton, 1984; Garvey, 1977). For example, two boys were playing monsters, and one boy became increasingly boisterous. His partner asked "Be you like you?" to ask whether he had been pushed "for real" or as a play action (Fein, 1984). These and many other types of language used for metacommunication are described by Bretherton (1984), Garvey (1977), and Giffin (1984).

By 5 years of age children can engage in very complex solitary or group pretend play. They can plan and organize several roles and complex sequences of actions that may involve fantasy themes. Pretend activities can be carried out through language only, with language used to set the scenes, establish the roles, and narrate the events (Westby, 1980, 1988, 1991).

Multiple Media in Pretend Play

Preschool and kindergarten children include many types of representational and symbolic elements in their pretend play. After a period of stacking and lining up blocks, followed by simple bridging (using a horizontal block to roof two upright blocks), children begin to build simple enclosures (Hirsch, 1984), which are incorporated in children's pretend play as fences and simple houses at about 3 to 31/2 years (Westby, 1980, 1988, 1991). The next stage of block play is constructing three-dimensional structures, especially buildings (Hirsch, 1984), which are included in children's pretend play scenes by 4 years of age (Westby, 1980, 1988, 1991). Other construction materials that children use in pretend play include mud, sand, and modeling clay. Children also make drawings about their pretend play and narrate pretend scenarios about their drawings (Gardner, 1982).

Preschool and kindergarten children also include writing in their pretend activities. Jacob (1984) observed Puerto Rican kindergarten children making "shopping lists" and writing "prescriptions" in their play. Many children request or make their own signs to label block structures (Cuffaro, 1984).

Interaction of Dimensions in Pretend Play

There is some evidence of trade-offs among the dimensions of pretend play. Bretherton et al. (1984) found that when 20- and 28-month-old children imitated pretend actions using substitute objects, they used fewer different schemas, fewer sequenced schemas, and talked less than when they used realistic objects. Children play longer with peers and have longer conversations without interruptions of content during pretend household play than during play involving less familiar themes (Nelson & Seidman, 1984). Bretherton (1984) speculates that new developmental achievements in one dimension may occur in the context of less complexity in other dimensions. For example, sequenced multischeme events (*organization*) might initially occur in the context of familiar *themes* and realistic *props*.

Emotional Aspects of Pretend Play

Another aspect of pretend play is the affective or emotional component. Fein (1985) suggests there are two components in the development of play. One is the ability to store and represent events and actions in new contexts—the content of play. The other is the ability to store and represent emotions in new contexts. Thus a child who resents the arrival of a new sibling may represent the resentment, jealousy, and aggression in a variety of different pretend play activities, from the transparent (the baby is hurt in an accident) to apparently unrelated fantasy themes involving averting threats from monsters. Fein warns against literal interpretations of children's pretend play as representations of actual events they have experienced or as strictly reflecting knowledge about the world. Children's play reflects not only "real-world" knowledge but also emotions and creativity represented in a fluid, changing mixture.

VARIATION IN PLAY DEVELOPMENT

Although children go through similar sequences in play development, children's play is influenced by many factors, and individual children's preferences and styles of play vary. In this section differences among individual children, male-female differences, situational influences on play, and sociocultural differences in play are described.

Individual Differences

Differences in children's approaches to play activities were found in a longitudinal study of nine children. Some children, called *patterners*, consistently focused on the properties of objects, while *dramatists* were more focused on social aspects of situations (Wolf & Gardner, 1979). For example, two children slightly over 1 year old were presented with a toy tea set and several small dolls. One child engaged in several autosymbolic feeding and drinking actions, and then repeatedly fed her mother and the observer. She also "showed off" by walking around the room with a spoon in her mouth and making faces at the adults and by balancing a cup on her nose while looking at her mother. The other child gathered one doll, one cup, and one spoon, and briefly offered a spoon to the observer and her mother, but mostly spent her time grouping, stacking, and unstacking the plates, spoons, and cups (Wolf & Grollman, 1982). Preschool dramatists frequently included imaginary objects and actions, indicated by gestures and language in their play. The patterners did so much less frequently, showing a preference for using objects in their pretend play, even when they were capable of using imaginary objects (Wolf & Grollman, 1982). Parallel patterns of object or social focus were observed in the vocabularies, use of art and construction materials, and problem-solving strategies of patterners and dramatists (Wolf & Gardner, 1979). In play with blocks, for example, a preschool patterner would tend to make elaborate structures, while a dramatist might act out a pretend scene with two blocks (Gardner & Wolf, 1987). Johnson et al. (1987) suggest that the degree of focus on an object or social properties be viewed as a continuum rather than as two separate styles, as all children focus to some extent on each dimension.

Sex Differences

Studies of sex differences in play activities and play development have compared groups of girls and boys. Thus the information we have is on group trends, rather than on individuals. The results of the studies on group tendencies will probably not surprise anyone familiar with sex roles in our society. It is important to keep in mind that the studies discussed below do not address individual variation, even though we all know adults and children who do not mirror group trends.

Many studies of children's play activities and toy preferences have consistently shown that boys engage more often than girls in functional and rough-and-tumble play, while girls consistently engage in sedentary arts and crafts activities (e.g., playing with modeling clay) more often than boys. Boys and girls also differ on toy preferences and use in expected ways (e.g., boys prefer and play more often with vehicles, while girls prefer and play more often with dolls than boys do). Girls show a broader range of toy preferences and use than boys, however, including many "boy toys" in their preferences, while boys have a narrower range of toy use and preferences, which are restricted to "boy toys." This trend has been increasingly seen in studies done in the 1970s and 1980s as compared with earlier studies. Studies also indicate that boys' play is less boisterous than found in studies in the 1920s and 1930s, so the degree of some differences between boys' and girls' play activities may be decreasing (Johnson, et al., 1987; Rubin, et al., 1983).

Girls and boys of the same age generally do not differ in level of pretend play development, although some differences do show up when specific dimensions of pretend play are examined. Most studies have not shown differences in level of organization (Fiese, 1990; Johnson, et al., 1987; Rubin, et al., 1983), although one study involving a small number of children indicated that a higher level of play was seen in girls at 3½ and 5 years (Sachs, et al., 1985), and 20- to 31-month-old girls consistently use more multischeme combinations than boys (Fenson, 1984). If there are differences in organization of pretend play, it is possible that these may not emerge until approximately 2 years of age.

Differences between girls and boys have been found on other dimensions of pretend play. Girls' pretend play involves family/household themes more often than boys' pretend play, especially if dolls are used. Boys' pretend play involves other themes such as cowboys and superheroes more often than girls'. Girls use substitute objects and imaginary objects earlier than boys, and they have imaginary playmates more often than boys (Johnson, et al., 1987). Boys and girls prefer to play same sex roles, so the identity of roles played differs (Johnson, et al., 1987). Boys talk more frequently about the actions of characters than girls at the same level of play, who talk more frequently about internal states of characters such as emotions, desires, thoughts, and plans (Wolf, et al., 1984).

No differences between girls and boys in level of social play have been found. Children do show a preference for playing with same-sex peers by about 2½ years of age, and they continue to play more frequently with same-sex peers in preschool and school settings (Johnson, et al., 1987). Boys and girls often play in different areas in preschools due to their engagement in different types of activities. Changing the room layout to increase access between different areas such as blocks and the play house set has increased play with opposite-sex peers (Johnson, et al., 1987; Scales, 1987).

A number of studies have explored the differences in environmental and social influences on boys and girls. Mothers and fathers engage in different types of play with their children. For example, fathers do more physical play than mothers, so children's same-sex models differ. A number of studies have shown than mothers, fathers, preschool teachers, and peers encourage play associated with the child's sex and often discourage play associated with the opposite sex (Etaugh, 1983; Johnson, et al., 1987; Rubin, et al., 1983). In a study of 20 two-year-olds, mothers and older siblings initiated far more doll nurturing and household play with girls than with boys. They initiated play with vehicles with boys, but none with girls (Dunn & Dale, 1984). Studies inventory-ing children's toys show that sex-stereotyped toys predominate for both sexes, even before children are old enough to express preferences verbally (Johnson, et al., 1987; Rubin, et al., 1983).

Although these studies show strong social influences on types of play and play themes, they do not directly address the degree to which differences between boys and girls result from these influences, as we do not know what the child's contribution to the interactions are. In one study of 18 to 23 month olds, children played more actively with same-sex toys, regardless of parental level of involvement in their play. There was a higher frequency of negative comments by parents when cross-sex toys were presented, however, so parental influences were not eliminated (Caldera, Huston, & O'Brien, 1989). Parents may be partly responding to the likes and dislikes of their children, as well as contributing their own influences to their children's activities and preferences. Anecdotes abound of boys who prefer superheroes and girls who are fascinated with Cinderella, in spite of their parents' attempts to provide a wide range of toys and play experiences for their children. Nonetheless, many parents, other adults, siblings, peers, and the media provide a set of strong influences favoring sex-stereotyped play activities for boys and girls. In turn, the toys and activities children play with may have long-term influences on their further development. For example, frequent participation in quiet, craft play and household play for girls, and physical play and occupational and superhero pretend play themes for boys, may channel and support different learning and behavioral styles for boys and girls (Etaugh, 1983).

Environmental and Social Influences on Play Development

The influences of toys and of how they are presented to children are immense, as Rubin and Howe (1985) point out in a review of the literature. Studies exploring the influence of toys and of adult interactions with children on their play have shown complex and mixed results. This may be due to differential effects of social and environmental influences at different points in development.

Many studies show a positive influences of availability of toys in the home on social and cognitive skills in toddlers, although the correlations may appear at different ages for girls and boys of different racial backgrounds (Bradley, 1985). Studies of preschool children found that availability of fewer toys in the preschool classroom resulted in more social interaction, while social interactions of toddlers with peers most often occur in the context of examining toys and objects. The size of the room also influences types of play, with somewhat smaller classrooms decreasing rough-and-tumble play and increasing social pretend play and onlooker activity (Rubin & Howe, 1985).

Other studies have examined the effects of adults modeling pretend actions on children's subsequent pretend activity, either in free play or in response to prompting to imitate the adult. Although children typically engage in higher level play more frequently after modeling, the specific effects of modeling differ with the age of the child. For example, 12 month olds showed an increase in the use of components from adult models of sequences of simple pretend actions, but only 15 and 19 month olds showed an increase in sequencing the components (Fenson & Ramsay, 1981).

Young children's play when their mothers play with them is typically at higher developmental level than during solitary play, but specific effects vary with the age of the child. In a longitudinal study of children at 20 and 28 months, children's solitary play at home with a set of toys was compared with their play when their mothers were asked to play with them and show them how to use the same set of toys in a laboratory setting. The 20 month olds showed an increase in diversity of exploratory and combinatorial play with objects when their mothers played with them, while at 28 months the same children's diversity of symbolic play increased during play with their mother. Mothers gave more combinatorial than symbolic play suggestions and less exploratory play suggestions at both

ages, so the difference in effects was due to the children's selective responses to their mother's suggestions (O'Connell & Bretherton, 1984). In another study of 15 to 24 month olds, children's level of play increased in play with their mother compared with solitary play, and the mother's style of interaction with the child influenced subsequent play. When the mother asked questions or intruded on the child's play, switching his or her focus of attention, the child tended to engage more in exploratory play and was less likely to engage in symbolic play. When the child and mother engaged in turn-taking exchanges, symbolic play was more likely to occur (Fiese, 1990). (The effects of order of play conditions were not controlled for in this study, since the children first played alone and then with their mothers. Since children tend to engage in exploratory activities first with toys, followed by other play activities, including pretend play, the increase in developmental levels of play with the mother may have been at least partly due to the order of the play conditions.)

Not all aspects of play are maximally enhanced by adult interactions. Dunn and Dale (1984) found that 2-year-old children participated more in simple complementary role play with their older siblings than with their mothers. Methods of initiating and content of play also differed between play with mothers and play with siblings.

Socioeconomic and Cultural Differences

Studies of children from many different cultures have shown that children begin pretend play at about the same age (Fein, 1981). Studies examining level of play in children up to 2 years of age have shown no differences between children from lower- and middle-socioeconomic-status (SES) groups (Fein, 1981; Fiese, 1990). Many studies of preschool and early school-age children, however, have documented that children from lower-SES groups engage in less pretend play, especially sociodramatic play, than has been observed in the play of middle-class children (Shefataya, 1990). Fewer object substitutions and less incorporation of imaginary elements have also been observed. Some studies also document less constructive play and more solitary and parallel functional play in lower-SES children's play (see reviews by Fein, 1981; Johnson, et al., 1987; Rubin, et al., 1983). Studies of children in some other cultures have also reported little imaginative play (see a review by Schwartzman, 1984).

These studies, however, have been criticized on several grounds. First, the play of children from lower-SES groups typically has been observed in preschool and school classroom settings, which may differ from the school settings in which the middle-SES children were observed. Further, even if the school settings were equivalent, the contexts may have very different effects on lower- and middle-SES children. If lower-SES children have had less exposure to the play materials than the middle-class children, more solitary and parallel exploration and functional play would be expected for children who are less familiar with the toys. Similarly, the play of lower-SES children may have been inhibited by the presence of adult observers if they were accustomed to playing in other contexts. Furthermore, if observers lack knowledge about the cultural practices of the children studied, they may not recognize role-appropriate behavior.

In a study of the pretend play of 5-year-old lower-SES African-American girls, potential effects of the children's unfamiliarity with the setting and observers' unfamiliarity with the children's experiences were taken into account. Two pairs of acquainted girls were videotaped in a playroom. The girls had been allowed to explore the toys and the room in a previous session, and the researchers left them to play on their own with no adults present. In this setting, the girls engaged in extensive pretend play, with reciprocal roles, use of substitute and imaginary objects, and use of language to negotiate and plan play activities. They used language for dialogue appropriate to each of the family roles they took, with appropriate

speech style differences reflecting likely patterns of speech by their own family members (McLoyd, et al., 1985). These findings illustrate the importance of context in studying children's pretend play.

Schwartzman (1984) criticizes studies of children's play in other cultures as having an ethnocentric bias as to the materials, spaces, times, and types of play recognized. Thus the imaginative play that children engaged in may have been overlooked by many anthropologists as it did not closely resemble the contexts and materials expected in Western developed countries. Rich descriptions of some children's play can be found, however. Schwartzman cites work by Ammar (1954) describing girls' play that included making small dolls out of straw, clothing them, and enacting a variety of events and rituals such as cooking, marriage, circumcision, and social meetings. In the United States a landmark study by Labov (1972) documented the complex verbal games and rituals played by many urban African-American children. Previously, children from similar backgrounds were typically viewed as having linguistic deficits based on their verbal behavior in classrooms and on formal testing with unfamiliar adults.

In summary, the play of children from different cultures and socioeconomic backgrounds differs in some respects, especially after the age of 2 years. Relatively little is known about play in children from lower socioeconomic backgrounds and children from diverse cultures, however. There is a need for research that explores the development of play in children from different backgrounds using culturally appropriate definitions of play and observations of children in appropriate contexts.

Play Development in Children With Developmental Delays

In spite of numerous problems researchers must deal with in studying the development of play in various groups of children who have developmental delays, a few general findings have emerged from studies in the past 20 to 25 years. Plenty of unanswered questions remain, however, because of research design problems and there being relatively few studies on this topic (for a review of findings and problems in research in this area, see Quinn & Rubin, 1984).

Children with developmental delays go through the same general sequence of play development and show similar relationships of play to cognitive level as normally developing children. This has been found in studies of mentally retarded children (Casby & Ruder, 1983; Hill & McCune-Nicolich, 1981; Motti, et al., 1983; Whitaker, 1980; Wing, Gould, Yeates, & Brierly, 1977) and of a heterogeneous group of children with language delays and general developmental delays (Kennedy, Sheridan, Radlinski, & Beeghly, 1991). There are two areas of exception to this pattern. First, less combinatorial play has been observed in some mentally retarded children than would be expected based on their other abilities (Hill & McCune-Nicolich, 1981; Quinn & Rubin, 1984). Second, autosymbolic or self-directed pretend play appeared later than symbolic play actions on dolls and others in one study of children with Down syndrome (Hill & Mc-Cune-Nicolich, 1981). In general, however, the sequence of play development with Down syndrome is similar to that of normally developing children, and their development of pretend play is at a level expected based on their other cognitive skills and level of language development (Cicchetti, Beeghly, & Weiss-Perry, 1994).

A strikingly different pattern of development is found among autistic children. In a study of mentally retarded, nonautistic children and autistic children, the autistic subjects' onset of symbolic play was consistently delayed compared with other cognitive abilities, while mentally retarded children consistently showed pretend play by the time their other nonverbal cognitive abilities were at a 20-month level (Wing, et al., 1977). Autistic children who do engage in pretend play show qualitative differences such as less frequent, self-directed, pretend (McCune, 1986) and stereotyped, unvarying play routines (Wing, et al., 1977). In ad-

dition to impairments in symbolic play development, abnormal development of social relationships, affect, and communication are the distinguishing characteristics of autism. Ability to understand the mental states of other people is an important common element among these areas of difficulty (Leslie, 1987). The extreme difficulty autistic individuals have in all these areas has been termed "mind blindness" (Baron-Cohen, 1995). Deficiencies in symbolic play are seen as one manifestation of the difficulty autistic individuals have with understanding and representing subjective aspects of experience. Another manifestation is the difficulty that higher functioning, autistic individuals have with theory of mind tasks compared with their other cognitive abilities.

The focus of another group of studies is symbolic play development in children who have specific language delays but otherwise normal development. The question is whether these children have more generalized difficulty in the development of symbolic abilities, including pretend play, or if their difficulty is more specific to language acquisition. The symbolic play of 2- through 4-year-old children with language delays is behind that of children the same age with normal language development (Rescorla & Goossens, 1992; Terrell, Schwartz, Prelock, & Messick, 1984; Thal & Bates, 1988). When children with language delays are compared with younger children with similar levels of language development (language matches), the findings are mixed. The level of symbolic play of 2- through 4-year-olds with language delays is equal to or exceeds that of younger, language-matched children (Terrell, et al., 1984; Thal & Bates, 1988). In contrast, 5- to 7-year-olds with language impairments had lower levels of symbolic play than language matches (Roth & Clark, 1987).

In summary, children with language delays also show delays in another area of symbolic representation, symbolic play, when compared with peers. The relationship between delays in language and symbolic play is complex, however. The symbolic play of children with language impairments is not consistently at the same level as would be expected based on their level of language development. It also appears that specific dimensions of pretend play may be affected differently among children with language impairments. Thal & Bates (1988) found that the 2-year-olds who were using very few words ("late talkers") engaged in fewer different pretend actions than language matches, but they engaged in more sequenced actions following adult models than younger, language-matched children. Westby (1988, 1991) has also noted that various dimensions of play seem to be differentially affected among children with a variety of developmental disabilities, including language impairments.

The pretend play of deaf children is closely related to their language development, as is true of hearing children. In general, among deaf children, slower language development is associated with slower symbolic play. This is true regardless of whether the children are acquiring spoken or sign language (Blum, Fields, Scharfman, & Silber, 1994; Spencer, 1996). The relationship between language and play is not the same for every deaf child, however. In the study by Blum et al. one child, who used almost no spoken or sign language, acted out sequences of pretend play. In addition, the symbolic play of several deaf children varied a great deal in its complexity from one observation to the next, particularly among children with slower language and symbolic play development. In several cases it appeared that the waxing and waning of the children's pretend play was related to affective difficulties in relationships with the parents. These authors suggest that providing support for symbolic play development is an important part of early intervention programs for deaf children. This suggestion is appropriate for deaf children of hearing parents and deaf children of deaf parents who are enrolled in early intervention programs to support oral language acquisition. It does not appear relevant to deaf children of deaf parents, in general, because Spencer (1996) found that deaf children of deaf parents who used sign language with their children were as likely to have advanced play and language development as hearing children of hearing parents. In contrast, deaf children of hearing parents tended to be functioning at somewhat lower levels of language and symbolic play development in her study.

Social levels of play have received limited attention in research on children with developmental delays. Developmentally delayed children engage in less play actions directed toward teachers and peers than normal children of the same age (Field, Roseman, DeStefano, & Koewler, 1982), and mildly delayed preschool children engage in less group pretend play than normal peers (Johnson & Ershler, 1985).

There are some indications that children with developmental delays also show differences in level and quality of social play compared with younger normally developing children. Compared with normally developing children at similar developmental levels, developmentally delayed children with a variety of etiologies, including Down syndrome, did less initiating of interactions with their mothers in a room equipped with toys (Brooks-Gunn & Lewis, 1982). In a study of language-delayed, 5- to 7-year-old children, the language-delayed children engaged in more nonplay activities and less parallel play with peers than language-matched pairs of children 2½ to 3 years of age (Roth & Clark, 1987). The language-delayed and younger, normal children did not differ, however, on amount of simple social play. Both groups engaged in almost no cooperative play, which was a normal developmental finding for the 2½ to 3 year olds, but which constitutes a delay in social play skills for chronologic age in the older, language-delayed children. In summary, children with language delays and children with general developmental delays show lags in the development of social play abilities compared with peers, and there are some differences in frequency of various types of social play compared with children of similar developmental abilities.

PLAY ASSESSMENT

Play-based assessment is an invaluable approach to evaluating young children's development because play activities incorporate and integrate social, cognitive, motoric, communicative, and affective components. Play-based assessment is a naturalistic, functional method of evaluation for children up to 6 years of age (Linder, 1993a). Information about a child's communication, and social and cognitive abilities related to communication, can be obtained through observing children's play in the following ways. Observation of an infant's playful interactions with caregivers and participation in simple games and routines are an important component of a communication evaluation, especially for children functioning below 1 year of age. Observation of infant's play with toys can yield information on the child's sensorimotor cognitive development. Tool use and symbolic play are two important cognitive correlates with language in normally developing children (Bates, et al., 1979). Tool use, symbolic play, and language all rely on similar cognitive underpinnings that allow for mediated activity (Vygotsky, 1978). Tool use or symbolic play do not cause language development and do not function as perquisites for language development; however, because tool use, symbolic play, and language all depend on the ability to engage in mediated activity, in typically developing children they tend to emerge together. Hence, if you observe tool use in a child, you might also expect to see play and language; or if you observe communicative language, you would also expect to see tool use and pretend play. In some children with disabilities, however, this typical pattern is not observed. An autistic child may exhibit tool use skills but not pretend play and language because he experiences specific difficulty with symbolization essential for play and language. A child with specific language impairment may exhibit tool use and pretend play but lack language because he or she experiences a specific difficulty with linguistic coding.

For children who have begun to engage in pretend play, observation of pretend play can yield information about children's knowledge of social roles and event structures. If a child is observed with siblings or peers, information about social skills when interacting with children can also be gained. Play activities also provide an appropriate context for observation of communicative actions and recording speech samples for young children. Play assessments yield information about how the child uses skills in naturalistic and meaningful activities, rather than sampling isolated skills in a formal testing situation.

The contexts in which play assessments are conducted must be carefully considered because play activities are affected by many factors, including types of toys, spatial arrangements, and who the child is playing with. In addition, different contexts may be optimal for observing play depending on the child's age and cultural background. For example, Farver and Howes (1993) found that Mexican children frequently engage in pretend play with siblings, but their mothers seldom participate in pretend play with them. In this situation, play with an older sibling may be the best context for observation.

Play is by nature varied and flexible, so the focus of play evaluations is on characteristics of play rather than specific tasks. For example, if one child uses a block for a cup, and another child uses the block as a wallet, both would be described as being able to use substitute objects in play. Play observers must take a nonliteral approach to interpreting play activities, because children may improvise and create events in their play that they have never experienced (Fein, 1985). Thus the observer looks at children's ability to include different themes, organize play events, use props, and take roles, rather than seeing pretend play as directly reflecting children's knowledge of specific objects, events, and characters.

A variety of play assessment procedures have been developed in recent years with many different developmental and emotional focuses. A volume containing many play assessment procedures (Schaefer, Gitlin, & Sandgrund, 1991) includes procedures designed to assess children's attention and activity levels, social skills, parent-child interaction patterns, and infant temperament characteristics in the context of play activities. The types of diagnoses and problems these procedures are designed to address include physical and sexual abuse, thought disorders, attention deficit hyperactivity disorder, autism, and many family problems. In addition, there are many scales used to assess developmental levels of play. One such scale is the Westby Symbolic Play Scale, which was first published in 1980 and which was subsequently revised to detail the developmental progression of symbolic play across four dimensions of symbolic play (Westby, 1988) and to include presymbolic levels of play (Westby, 1991). This scale was developed to cover ages 8 months to 5 years, but can be used as a guide to describing the play of older children with language learning impairments and developmental delays. In addition, observers may make qualitative descriptions, including the amount of variety in a child's play, whether the child initiates or primarily responds to others, and whether the child clearly signals an "as if" or playful attitude (Westby, 1991). Restricted quality in these areas may indicate that a child has learned play behaviors, but is not playing, or that the child's communication and social aspects of play may need to be an area of focus to facilitate active participation with peers.

PLAY AND INTERVENTION

There are many reasons to include play in an intervention program for children with developmental delays. Although play is defined and regarded differently across different cultures and historical contexts, play is a universal aspect of human life (Sutton-Smith, 1980). In play, social, cognitive, communicative, emotional, and motor skills are integrated in enjoyable activities.

Sociodramatic and fantasy play training studies have shown increases on measures of creativity, flexible problem-solving, IQ scores, performance on language tasks, impulse control, perspective-taking, and social skills and social problem-solving, in addition to increases in the frequency and complexity of pretend play (Saltz & Saltz, 1986; Rubin, et al., 1983; Rubin, 1980). Although the children in these studies were normally developing children from lower and middle socioeconomic groups, it seems reasonable to predict that pretend play training would also be helpful with developmentally delayed children.

There are many resources and guides for supporting play development and for using play-based intervention methods to support development in multiple areas. Many parent guides and curriculum guides for early childhood and preschool programs for typically developing children have excellent ideas that can be used with children with special needs (e.g., Hagstrom, 1982; Hereford & Schall, 1991). Guides specifically designed for using play activities to facilitate various aspects of motor, cognitive, language, and social skills in children with developmental delays are also available (e.g., Linder, 1993b). In the following section we focus on the use of symbolic play in approaches to language intervention.

Play-Based Language Intervention

Play activities are widely used as a context for language therapy with young children (Fey, 1986; Hubbell, 1981; Owens, 1991; Snyder-McLean, Solomonson, MacLean, & Sack, 1984). Children are motivated to learn language forms, functions, and meanings and to use them in the naturalistic contexts of play, particularly pretend play (Culatta, 1994; Sonnenmeier, 1994). Pretend play is also a context that lends itself to inclusion of children with and without developmental difficulties, particularly among preschool children and children in primary grades.

Virtually any aspect of language can be taught within a play context (Culatta, 1994). Examples include using forms of the verb "to be" in questions and answers while playing grocery store (Culatta & Horn, 1982) and increasing the use of various types of words and different speech acts during play activities (Norris & Hoffman, 1990).

Pretend play also provides a context for facilitating children's cognitive and social development in ways that support the ability to use language successfully in response to the demands of school and in negotiating social relationships. Westby (1991) outlines five areas in which adults can foster such development in children's pretend play:

1. Encourage use of decontextualized symbols. In pretend play this includes the use of substitute objects and the use of language and gestures to stand for objects and actions.

2. Help children focus on the temporal, cause-effect, and social relationships that exist in situations in the world (home, doctor's office, restaurant, stores, etc.).

3. Promote children's ability to organize and monitor their own behavior so they can become independent, self-motivated learners.

4. Nurture children's ability to interpret the needs, desires, and roles of others and to recognize how to relate appropriately to these needs, desires, and roles so that they can play and work effectively with others.

5. Stimulate language used for reasoning, planning, and creating.

Examples of a few methods that can be used to foster development in some of these five areas follow. Adults can make suggestions such as "Let's pretend this is bread" (referring to a block) to model use of language for metacommunication and to support the use of decontextualized symbols in play (Westby & Rouse, 1985). To foster children's understanding of temporal relationships, adults can model and prompt sequences of related actions in pretend play. This is appropriate for children whose pretend play and stories consist of a series of isolated, unrelated actions and statements. Through pretend play, related actions can be enacted and temporal terms can be modeled simultaneously in a meaningful context (Culatta, 1994). Use of language for planning and solving problems can be prompted by providing obstacles in play

such as a ladder on a fire engine that is too short to reach the second story of the dollhouse (Culatta, 1994) and by planning the props and sequence of events before engaging in some pretend play sessions (Westby & Rouse, 1985).

Because pretend play and narratives share many characteristics (Christie, 1991; Westby, 1985), several intervention approaches combine play and story-telling activities. In one approach used in a preschool classroom that includes three children with special needs, each child dictates a story to the teacher, which all the children will enact later in the day. Because the children want to have their stories acted out by their peers, they are motivated to relate stories in a manner that is comprehensible (Paley, 1994). Culatta (1994) uses children's literature in her approach. She reads stories aloud to children, which they later act out in pretend play. Another method is to have children engage in pretend play and then to retell the pretend activity as a narrative at a later date.

It is important to provide children with materials and activities that are appropriate for their current level of development. Children whose play is at presymbolic levels will need a variety of manipulable exploratory toys. Children in the early stages of pretend play will respond well to realistic toys and daily-living themes. Children whose pretend activities are beginning to include some sequencing of multischeme episodes and an expanding variety of themes will benefit from the inclusion of some toys involving occupational roles (doctor, firefighter, etc.) and fantasy themes. They will also benefit from including some objects and materials that are not replica toys to enhance the use of substitute objects and the use of language and gestures to represent objects in play (McLoyd, 1986).

Toys can also be made or adapted for children with motor impairments and sensory impairments (Langley, 1982; Musselwhite, 1986). In addition, individual children will respond to and prefer different toys, so variety is also necessary, even for children functioning at approximately similar developmental levels (Wachs, 1982).

Methods for adults to facilitate pretend play with children's peers are reviewed in many resources (Johnson, et al., 1987; Rivkin, 1986; Rogers & Sawyers, 1988). The least intrusive method for using with children who are participating in some group play is to observe the children's play and provide new props or arrangements of materials to stimulate play. More intrusive methods may be needed, at least initially, however, as simply providing toys and playtime increases dramatic play only for children who are already accomplished players (Saltz & Saltz, 1986). Adults may pair children who are not participating in play with peers who are active participants in pretend play (Fein & Kinney, 1994). Another option is to suggest new themes, actions, or roles when a child or children seem "stuck." Some children may require even more directive intervention at first, with the adult participating in their play, modeling and prompting pretend actions at a level appropriate to the child's abilities (Rivkin, 1986; Westby & Rouse, 1985).

When symbolic play is used as a context for direct language intervention, clinician planning, modeling, and prompting of scripted play activities are appropriate. Themes, materials, script components, roles, and strategies for adults to use to guide the children's participation in pretend play are discussed by Culatta (1994) and Sonnenmeier (1994).

Although many play activities that are structured and encouraged by adults are helpful and fun for young children, every child should also have the opportunity to play alone and to play near or with other children with minimal adult involvement. Some of the benefits of group pretend play may stem from children's negotiations, explanations, and arguments when conflicts arise during play (Rubin, 1980; Howes, 1992).

Another reason for leaving children to play alone or together independently is that adults often use playtime as teaching time and encourage reality-based enactments during pretend play (Dunn & Dale, 1984). Although these are valuable activities, they should not replace the free, child-structured, imaginative, sometimes silly, sometimes aggressive play activities that come from children's own creativity, experiences, perspectives, and emotions.

CONCLUSION

Play is an important part of life and development. It is not something to do only when there is nothing else to do. Play is a reflection of learning and a way to learn.

> One of the most profound means available to children for constructing and reconstructing, formulating and reformulating knowledge is through play. It is a means for synthesis and integration in that it brings together the child's concept of reality with the inner world of fantasies and feelings. Play may be seen as the child's substitute for adult musing, contemplation, hypothesizing, meandering among ideas, and experiences. Play is the visible language of childhood wherein we see and hear the total child functioning, revealing individual concerns, conflicts, information and misinformation, ambivalences, wishes, hopes, pleasures, and questions (Cuffaro, 1984, p. 121).

REFERENCES

Ammar H. Growing up in an Egyptian village. London: Routledge & Kegan Paul, 1954.

Astington JW. Children's developing notions of others' minds. In: Duchan JF, Hewitt LE, Sonnenmeier RM, eds. Pragmatics: from theory to practice. Englewood Cliffs, NJ: Prentice-Hall, 1994; pp. 72–87.

Baron-Cohen S. Mindblindness. Cambridge: MIT Press, 1995.

Bates E, Benigni L, Camaioni L, et al. The emergence of symbols. New York: Academic Press, 1979.

Bates E, Bretherton I, Snyder L, et al. Gestural and vocal symbols at 13 months. Merrill-Palmer Q 1980;26:407–423.

Bateson G. The message "This is play." In: Herron R, Sutton-Smith B, eds. Child's play. New York: John Wiley, 1971.

Bayley N. Bayley scales of infant development. New York: Psychological Corp, 1969.

Belsky J, Most R. From exploration to play: a cross-sectional study of infant free play behavior. Dev Psychol 1981;17:630–639.

Blum EJ, Fields BC, Scharfman H, Silber DM. Development of symbolic play of deaf children, aged 1 to 3. In: Slade A, Wolf DP, eds. Children at play. New York: Oxford University Press, 1994; pp. 238–260.

Bradley R. Social-cognitive development and toys. Top Early Child Spec Educ 1985;5(3):11–30.

Bretherton I. Representing the social world in symbolic play: reality and fantasy. In: Bretherton I, ed. Symbolic play: the development of social understanding. Orlando, FL: Academic Press, 1984.

Bretherton I, O'Connell B, Shore C, Bates E. The effect of contextual variation on symbolic play: development from 20 to 28 months. In: Bretherton I, ed. Symbolic play: the development of social understanding. New York: Academic Press, 1984.

Brooks-Gunn J, Lewis M. Play behavior in handicapped and normal infants. Top Early Child Spec Educ 1982;2(3):14–27.

Bruner J. Actual minds, possible worlds. Cambridge, MA: Harvard University Press, 1986.

Caldera Y, Huston A, O'Brien M. Social interactions and play patterns of parents and toddlers with feminine, masculine, and neutral toys. Child Dev 1989;60:70–76.

Casby M, Ruder K. Symbolic play and early language development in normal and mentally handicapped children. J Speech Hear Res 1983;26:404–411.

Christie JF, ed. Play and early literacy development. Albany: State University of New York Press, 1991.

Cicchetti D, Beeghly M, Weiss-Perry B. Symbolic development in children with Down syndrome and in children with autism. In: Slade A, Wolf DP, eds. Children at play. New York: Oxford University Press, 1994; pp. 206–237.

Cuffaro H. Dramatic play—the experience of block building. In: Hirsch E, ed. The block book. Revised edition. Washington, DC: National Association for the Education of Young Children, 1984.

Culatta B. Representational play and story enactments: formats for language intervention. In: Duchan JF, Hewitt LE, Sonnenmeier RM, eds. Pragmatics: from theory to practice. Englewood Cliffs, NJ: Prentice-Hall, 1994; pp. 105–119.

Culatta B, Horn D. A program for achieving generalization of grammatical rules to spontaneous discourse. J Speech Hear Disord 1982;47:174–180.

Donaldson M. Children's minds. New York: W. W. Norton, 1978.

Dunn J, Dale N. I a daddy: 2-year-olds' collaboration in joint pretend with sibling and mother. In: Bretherton I, ed. Symbolic play: the development of social understanding. Orlando, FL: Academic Press, 1984.

Ellis M. Why people play. Englewood Cliffs, NJ: Prentice-Hall, 1973.

Etaugh C. Introduction: the influences of environment on sex differences in children's play. In: Liss M, ed. Social and cognitive skills: sex roles and children's play. New York: Academic Press, 1983.

Farver JM, Howes C. Cultural differences in American and Mexican mother-child pretend play. Merrill-Palmer Q 1993;39:344–358.

Fein G. A transformational analysis of pretending. Dev Psychol 1975;11:291–296.

Fein G. Pretend play in childhood: an integrative view. Child Dev 1981;52:1095–1118.

Fein G. The self-building potential of pretend play or "I got a fish, all by myself." In: Yawkey T, Pellegrini A, eds. Child's play: developmental and applied. Hillsdale, NJ: Lawrence Erlbaum, 1984.

Fein G. The affective psychology of play. In: Brown C, Gottfried A, eds. Play interactions: the role of toys and parental involvement in children's development. Skillman, NJ: Johnson & Johnson, 1985.

Fein G, Kinney P. He's a nice alligator: observations on the affective organization of pretense. In: Slade A, Wolf DP, eds. Children at play. New York: Oxford University Press, 1994; pp. 188–205.

Fenson L. Developmental trends for action and speech in pretend play. In: Bretherton I, ed. Symbolic play: the development of social understanding. New York: Academic Press, 1984.

Fenson L. The developmental progression of exploration and play. In: Brown C, Gottfried A, eds. Play interactions: the role of toys and parental involvement in children's development. Skillman NJ: Johnson & Johnson, 1985.

Fenson L, Ramsay DS. Effects of modeling action sequences on the play of twelve-, fifteen-, and nineteen- month-old children. Child Dev 1981; 52:1028–1036.

Fey M. Language intervention with young children. Boston: College-Hill, 1986.

Field T, Roseman S, DeStefano L, Koewler J. The play of handicapped preschool children with handicapped and non-handicapped peers in integrated and non-integrated situations. Top Early Child Spec Educ 1982;2(3):28–38.

Fiese B. Playful relationships: a contextual analysis of mother-toddler interaction and symbolic play. Child Dev 1990;61:1648–1656.

Forys S, McCune-Nicolich L. Shared pretend: sociodramatic play at 3 years of age. In: Bretherton I, ed. Symbolic play: the development of social understanding. New York: Academic Press, 1984.

Gardner H. Art, mind and society. New York: Basic Books, 1982.

Gardner H, Wolf D. The symbolic products of early childhood. In: Gorlitz D, Wohlwill J, eds. Curiosity, imagination, and play. Hillsdale, NJ: Lawrence Erlbaum, 1987.

Garvey C. Play. Cambridge, MA: Harvard University Press, 1977.

Giffin H. The coordination of meaning in the creation of a shared make-believe reality. In: Bretherton I, ed. Symbolic play: the development of social understanding. Orlando, FL: Academic Press, 1984.

Goncu A. Development of intersubjectivity in social pretend play. Hum Dev 1993;36:185–198.

Greenspan S, Greenspan N. First feelings. New York: Penguin Books, 1985.

Guerney L. Play therapy in counselling settings. In: Yawkey T, Pellegrini A, eds. Child's play: developmental and applied. Hillsdale, NJ: Lawrence Erlbaum, 1984.

Hagstrom J. Let's pretend: games of fantasy for babies and young children. New York: A & W Visual Library, 1982.

Harris PL, Kavanaugh RD. Young children's understanding of pretense. Monogr Soc Res Child Dev 1993;58(1):1–92.

Hereford NJ, Schall J. Learning through play: dramatic play. New York: Scholastic, 1991.

Hewitt LE. Facilitating narrative comprehension: the importance of subjectivity. In: Duchan JF, Hewitt LE, Sonnenmeier RM, eds. Pragmatics: from theory to practice. Englewood Cliffs, NJ: Prentice-Hall, 1994; pp. 88–104.

Hill P, McCune-Nicolich L. Pretend play and patterns of cognition in Down's syndrome children. Child Dev 1981;52:611–617.

Hirsch E, ed. The block book. Revised edition. Washington, DC: National Association for the Education of Young Children, 1984.

Howes C. Peer play scale as an index of complexity of peer interaction. Dev Psychol 1980;16:371–372.

Howes C. The collaborative construction of pretend: social pretend play functions. Albany: State University of New York Press, 1992.

Howes C, Unger O, Seidner L. Social pretend play in toddlers: parallels with social play and solitary pretend. Child Dev 1989;60:77–84.

Hubbell R. Children's language disorders. Englewood Cliffs, NJ: Prentice-Hall, 1981.

Jackowitz E, Watson M. Development of object transformations in early pretend play. Dev Psychol 1980;16:543–549.

Jacob E. Learning literacy through play: Puerto Rican kindergarten children. In: Goelman H, Oberg A, Smith F, eds. Awakening to literacy. Portsmouth, NH: Heinemann, 1984.

Johnson J, Christie J, Yawkey T. Play and early childhood development. Glenville, IL: Scott, Foresman, 1987.

Johnson J, Ershler J. Social and cognitive play forms and toy use by nonhandicapped and handicapped preschoolers. Top Early Child Spec Educ 1985;5(3):69–82.

Kane SF, Furth HG. Children constructing social reality: a frame analysis of social pretend play. Hum Dev 1993;36:199–214.

Kelly C, Dale P. Cognitive skills associated with the onset of multiword utterances. J Speech Hear Res 1989;32:645–656.

Kennedy M, Sheridan M, Radlinski S, Beeghly M. Play-language relationships in young children with developmental delays: implications for assessment. J Speech Hear Res 1991;34:112–122.

King P. Play and the culture of childhood. In: Fein G, Rivkin M, eds. The young child at play. Washington, DC: National Association for the Education of Young Children, 1986.

Labov W. Language in the inner city: studies in the Black English vernacular. Philadelphia: University of Pennsylvania Press, 1972.

Langley M. Selecting, adapting, and applying toys as learning tools for handicapped children. Top Early Child Spec Educ 1982;5:3:101–118.

Leslie AM. Pretense and representation: the origins of "theory of mind." Psychol Rev 1987;94412–426.

Lillard AS. Young children's conceptualization of pretense: action or mental representational state? Child Dev 1993;64:372–386.

Linder T. Transdisciplinary play-based assessment. Revised edition. Baltimore: Paul Brookes, 1993a.

Linder T. Transdisciplinary play-based intervention. Baltimore: Paul Brookes, 1993b.

McCune L. Symbolic development in normal and atypical infants. In: Fein G, Rivkin M, eds. The young child at play. Washington, DC: National Association for the Education of Young Children, 1986.

McCune-Nicolich L. Toward symbolic functioning: structure of early pretend games and potential parallels with language. Child Dev 1981;52:785–797.

McCune-Nicolich L, Bruskin C. Combinatorial competency in symbolic play and language. In: Pepler DJ, Rubin KH, eds. The play of children: current theory and research. Basel, Switzerland: S. Karger, 1982.

McLoyd V. Scaffolds or shackles: the role of toys in preschool children's pretend play. In: Fein G, Rivkin M, eds. The young child at play. Washington, DC: National Association for the Education of Young Children, 1986.

McLoyd V, Ray S, Etter-Lewis G. Being and becoming: the interface of language and family role knowledge in the pretend play of young African-American girls. In: Galda L, Pellegrini A, eds. Play, language and stories. Norwood, NJ: Ablex, 1985.

Miller P, Garvey C. Mother-baby role play: its origins in social support. In: Bretherton I, ed. Symbolic play: the development of social understanding. New York: Academic Press, 1984.

Monighan-Nourot P. Conversations with the real and imagined. In: Monighan-Nourot P, Scales B, Van Hoorn J, Almy M, eds. Looking at children's play: a bridge between theory and practice. New York: Teachers College Press, 1987.

Motti F, Cicchetti D, Sroufe L. From infant affect and expression to symbolic play: the coherence of development in Down's syndrome children. Child Dev 1983;54:1168–1175.

Musselwhite C. Adaptive play for special needs children. San Diego: College-Hill, 1986.

Nelson K, Seidman S. Playing with scripts. In: Bretherton I, ed. Symbolic play: the development of social understanding. New York: Academic Press, 1984.

Nicolich LM. Beyond sensorimotor intelligence: assessment of symbolic maturity through analysis of pretend play. Merrill Palmer Q 1977;23:89–99.

Norris J, Hoffman P. Language intervention within naturalistic environments. Lang Speech Hear Serv Sch 1990;21:72–84.

O'Connell B, Bretherton I. Toddlers' play, alone and with mother: the role of maternal guidance. In: Bretheron I, ed. Symbolic play: the development of social understanding. New York: Academic Press, 1984.

O'Connell BG, Gerard AB. Scripts and scraps: the development of sequential understanding. Child Dev 1985;56:671–681.

Owens R. Language disorders: a functional approach to assessment and intervention. New York: Merrill, 1991.

Paley VG. Bad guys don't have birthdays: fantasy play at four. Chicago: University of Chicago Press, 1988.

Paley VG. Every child a storyteller. In: Duchan JF, Hewitt LE, Sonnenmeier RM, eds. Pragmatics: from theory to practice. Englewood Cliffs, NJ: Prentice-Hall, 1994; pp. 10–19.

Parten M. Social participation among preschool children. J Abnorm Soc Psychol 1932;27:243–269.

Piaget J. Play, dreams and imitation in childhood. (C. Gattegno C, Hodgson FM, Trans.) New York: W.W. Norton, 1962.

Quinn J, Rubin K. The play of handicapped children. In: Yawkey T, Pellegrini A, eds. Child's play: developmental and applied. Hillsdale, NJ: Lawrence Erlbaum, 1984.

Rescorla L Goossens M. Symbolic play development in toddlers with expressive specific language impairment. J Speech Hear Res 1992;35: 1290–1302.

Rice M. Contemporary accounts of the cognition/language relationship: implications for speech-language clinicians. J Speech Hear Disord 1983;48:347–359.

Rivkin M. The teacher's place in children's play. In: Fein G, Rivkin M, eds. The young child at play. Washington, DC: National Association for the Education of Young Children, 1986.

Rogers C, Sawyers J. Play in the lives of children. Washington, DC: National Association for the Education of Young Children, 1988.

Ross H, Kay D. The origins of social games. New Dir Child Dev 1980;9:17–31.

Roth F, Clark D. Symbolic play and social participation abilities of language-impaired and normally developing children. J Speech Hear Disord 1987;52:17–29.

Rubin K. Fantasy play: its role in the development of social skills and social cognition. New Dir Child Dev 1980;9:69–84.

Rubin K. Nonsocial play: necessarily evil? Child Dev 1982;53:651–657.

Rubin K, Fein G, Vandenberg B. Play. In: Hetherington E, ed. Handbook of child psychology. Vol. 4. Socialization, personality, and social development. New York: John Wiley, 1983.

Rubin K, Howe N. Toys and play behaviors: an overview. Top Early Child Spec Educ 1985;5: 3:1–10.

Sachs J, Goldman J, Chaille C. Narrative in preschoolers' sociodramatic play: the role of knowledge and communicative competence. In: Galda L, Pellegrini A, eds. Play, language and stories. Norwood, NJ: Ablex, 1985.

Saltz R, Saltz E. Pretend play training and its outcomes. In: Fein G, Rivkin M, eds. The young child at play. Washington, DC: National Association for the Education of Young Children, 1986.

Sawyer RK. Pretend play as improvisation. Mahwah, NJ: Lawrence Erlbaum, 1997.

Scales B. Play: the child's unseen curriculum. In: Monighan-Nourot P, Scales B, Van Hoorn J, Almy M, eds. Looking at children's play: a bridge between theory and practice. New York: Teachers College Press, 1987.

Schaefer C, Gitlin K, Sandgrund A, eds. Play diagnosis and assessment. New York: John Wiley, 1991.

Schaefer C, O'Connor K, eds. Handbook of play therapy. New York: John Wiley, 1983.

Schwartzman H. Imaginative play: deficit or difference? In: Yawkey T, Pellegrini A, eds. Child's play: developmental and applied. Hillsdale, NJ: Lawrence Erlbaum, 1984.

Shefataya L. Socioeconomic status and ethnic differences in sociodramatic play: theoretical and practical implications. In: Klugman E, Smilansky S, eds. Children's play and learning. New York: Teachers College, 1990; pp. 137–155.

Shore C, O'Connell B, Bates E. First sentences in language and symbolic play. Dev Psychol 1984;20:872–880.

Snyder-McLean LK, Solomonson MA, McLean JE, Sack S. Structuring joint action routines: a strategy for facilitating communication and language development in the classroom. Semin Speech Lang 1984;5:213–225.

Sonnenmeier RM. Script-based language intervention: learning to participate in life events. In: Duchan JF, Hewitt LE, Sonnenmeier RM, eds. Pragmatics: from theory to practice. Englewood Cliffs, NJ: Prentice-Hall, 1994; pp. 134–148.

Spencer PE. The association between language and symbolic play at two years: evidence from deaf toddlers. Child Dev 1996;67:867–876.

Sutton-Smith B. Children's play: some sources of play theorizing. New Dir Child Dev 1980;9:1–16.

Sutton-Smith B. The spirit of play. In: Fein G, Rivkin M, eds. The young child at play. Washington, DC: National Association for the Education of Young Children, 1986.

Terrell B, Schwartz R, Prelock P, Messick C. Symbolic play in normal and language-impaired children. J Speech Hear Res 1984;27:424–429.

Thal D, Bates E. Language and gesture in late talkers. J Speech Hear Res 1988;31:115–123.

Vandenberg B. Play theory. In: Fein G, Rivkin M, eds. The young child at play. Washington, DC: National Association for the Education of Young Children, 1986.

Vygotsky LS. Mind in society. Cole M, John-Steiner V, Scribner S, Souberman E, eds. Cambridge, MA: Harvard University Press, 1978.

Wachs T. Toys as an aspect of the physical environment: constraints and nature of relationship to development. Top Early Child Spec Educ 1982; 5: 3:31–46.

Watson M, Fischer K. Development of social roles in elicited and spontaneous behavior during the preschool years. Dev Psychol 1980;16:483–494.

Weir R. Language in the crib. The Hague: Mouton, 1962.

Westby CE. Assessment of cognitive and language abilities through play. Lang Speech Hear Serv Sch 1980;11(3):154–168.

Westby CE. Learning to talk—talking to learn: oral-literate language differences. In: Simon C, ed. Communication skills and classroom success: therapy methodologies for language-learning disabled students. San Diego: College Hill, 1985.

Westby CE. Children's play: reflections of social competence. Semin Speech Lang 1988;9:1–14.

Westby C. A scale for assessing children's pretend play. In: Schaefer C, Gitlin K, Sandgrund A, eds. Play diagnosis and assessment. New York: John Wiley, 1991.

Westby C, Rouse G. Culture in education and the instruction of language learning-disabled students. Top Lang Disord 1985;5:4:15–28.

Whitaker C. A note on developmental trends in the symbolic play of hospitalized profoundly retarded children. J Child Psychol Psychiatry 1980;21:253–261.

Wing L, Gould J, Yeates S, Brierly M. Symbolic play in severely mentally retarded children and in autistic children. J Child Psychol Psychiatry 1977;18:167–178.

Wolf D, Gardner H. Style and sequence in early symbolic play. In: Smith N, Franklin M, eds. Symbolic functioning in childhood. Hillsdale, NJ: Lawrence Erlbaum, 1979.

Wolf D, Grollman SH. Ways of playing: individual differences in imaginative style. In: Pepler DJ, Rubin KH, eds. The play of children: current theory and research. Basel, Switzerland: S. Karger, 1982.

Wolf D, Hicks D. The voices within narratives: the development of intertextuality in young children's stories. Discourse Processes 1989;12:329–351.

Wolf D, Rygh J, Altshuler J. Agency and experience: actions and states in play narratives. In: Bretherton I, ed. Symbolic play: the development of social understanding. New York: Academic Press, 1984.

Processes and Applications of Communication Development

Part II contains six chapters that consider a basic chronologic development of communication. We take the child from birth to adolescence showing how basic communications that are present before the first birthday persist and are progressively refined as the child matures. Prelinguistic children communicate through gestures and vocalizations. Chapter 8 discusses the nature and types of these communications and how they change with development. Youngsters pass through a period in which their only output is single-word responses. Chapter 9 reviews the transitions from prelinguistic communication to the single-word period and the transition from single to early multiword combinations. Chapter 10 considers the first types of word combinations children produce as their utterance length expands. After the basic building blocks of a sentence are constructed in early word combinations, the child begins to apply function words and word endings to utterances. These morphological acquisitions are examined in Chapter 11. Chapters 12 and 13 comprise a thorough examination of more complex language development from late preschool through adolescence.

When all of the chapters are viewed together, they provide a detailed chronology of communication development. Through each chapter, an effort is made to weave the multiple interactive areas of cognitive, social, and linguistic developments together. So it is not surprising that a discussion of single-word development includes cognitive and social impacts. Similarly, basic morphological development is covered in Chapter 11, but is revisited in Chapter 12 as morphemes become more complex and are applied in different contexts. There are many other examples of the same areas that are addressed in different ways by the chapters, and the student will even see concepts from Part I, Foundations of Communication, woven into these sections on development. This consistent reworking of the same concepts in different contexts in different ways provides the student with good examples of the integrative nature of communication development. Chapter 13 extends the discussion by presenting information pertaining to communication development in the school-age and adolescent populations.

The chapters that follow in Part II all contain clinical applications. Thus, after we see how a child develops particular facets of communication, we present examples of how these developments have been applied to clinical work. Remember, these are just *glimpses* of clinical relevance, not in-depth treatments of the applications. They do, however, provide enough of an example to show students that *there is clinical relevance to the study of communication development,* which is a basic premise of this text. Students who will be embarking on their first clinical work should note that the clinical applications in assessment and treatment flow directly from a rationale that is based on the literature of communication development and communication theory.

CHAPTER 8

Social-Emotional Bases of Communicative Development

Carol E. Westby

anguage acquisition involves three
components: (1) the learning of well-
formedness, that is, the rules of grammar (syntax); (2) the capacity to refer and to
mean (semantics); and (3) communicative
function or intent, that is, the ability to get
things done with words (pragmatics). Language is a social activity. A primary function
of language is to sustain and maintain emotional attachments that are common to human beings. To understand why and how
children speak, we must understand how
language is influenced by social-motiva-
tional factors based in children's emotional
needs and external pressures of their social
world. The need to be attached and affili-
ated with other humans may be one of the
primary motivators for language development (Gleason, Hay, Cain, 1989). Children's intentionality drives their acquisition of language. Children's intentional
states—beliefs, desires, and feelings—drive
the ways they relate to others in everyday
events (Bloom, 1993). Language learning is
intimately connected to children's emotional life because infants learn to talk about
the things their feelings are about—the
persons, objects, and events that are the
causes and circumstances of emotion. Children talk to maintain social contact for no

other reason than to share an experience,
feeling, or thought with another person
(Bates, Bretherton, & Beeghly-Smith,
1982). This motivation for sharing reflects
the need infants have to sustain "intersubjectivity" or an interfacing of mind with
other persons. Intentionality drives language acquisition and intersubjectivity drives intentionality. Initially, this subjectivity
reflects the child's experience of emotions.
Gradually, however, children come to recognize others' experiences of emotions. Increasingly, this appreciation of intersubjectivity, or what has been termed a *theory of
mind* or *landscape of consciousness* contributes
to children's ability to predict behaviors of
others and to participate in effective social
conversation (Bretherton, 1991; Bruner,
1986; Hewitt, 1994).

Language is not only a tool to engage
and attract the attention of others, it is also
the medium though which children come
to understand their social world and acquire their culture. It enables them to share
and understand emotions, goals, and expectations (Bloom, 1990, 1993; Bretherton
& Beeghly, 1982; Dunn, Bretherton, &
Munn, 1987; Vygotsky, 1986). Language
acquisition cannot be understood by looking at only the child's cognitive and lin-

guistic abilities. The child's emotional development, which drives communication, must also be considered. In addition, because language acquisition is the acquisition of a culture, it can only be understood by also looking at the social interactions or cultural settings in which language occurs (Bruner, 1983). Chomsky (1959, 1965) proposed a Language Acquisition Device (LAD) that predisposed a child to acquire syntax. The LAD cannot function, however, without assistance given by adults who interact with children. These interactions, which are initially under the control of the adult, provide a Language Acquisition Support System (LASS) that frames or structures the input to the child. "It is the interaction between LAD and LASS that makes it possible for the infant to enter the linguistic community—and, at the same time, the culture to which the language gives access" (Bruner, 1983, p.19). Infants enter the world of language and culture with a motivation to find or invent systematic ways of dealing with social requirements and linguistic forms. Bruner (1983) proposed that the infant is predisposed in several ways to acquire culture through language:

1. Much of cognitive processing in infancy supports goal-directed activities.

2. Much of the child's development during the first year and a half is social and communicative.

3. Early infant actions take place primarily in familiar situations and show a high degree of order and regularity.

To acquire language children must be sensitive to the sound pattern and grammatical constraints of the language, to referential requirements, and to communicative intentions. Such sensitivity grows in the process of fulfilling certain general nonlinguistic functions—predicting the environment, interacting transactionally, getting to goals with the aid of another, et cetera. Bruner suggested that such functions must first be fulfilled by prelinguistic communicative means and that these means must reach certain levels before any language acquisition device will generate linguistic hypotheses. Hence, language acquisition cannot be understood apart from social-emotional development.

This chapter will discuss (1) the affective and social bases of communication, (2) the development of communicative intent and social uses of language, (3) conditions affecting the social/emotional bases of communication, and (4) methods for assessing and facilitating the social/emotional bases of communication and communicative competence.

EMOTIONAL AND SOCIAL BASES OF INTENTIONALITY

Dore (1986) maintained that conversational competence comprises four interlocking systems of competence that interact with one another. "The basic elements are the *feelings* between participants that motivate the utterance *forms* used to effect various intentional and sequential *functions* relative to the contextual *frames* in which they occur" (Dore, 1986, p.7). Affect or feeling is the major organizing concept for the infant's earliest communication experiences (Bloom, 1990, 1993; Thoman, 1983). Infants experience objects and events mainly in terms of the feelings they evoke in them. They do not experience them as objects in and of themselves or for what they do or are called (Stern, 1990). Assuming that affective forms of communication precede, influence, and subsequently become integrated with linguistic communication, disruption of early social-affective relations may be a prelude to later emotional and language disorders. Because communication is dependent on affective interactions between infants and adults, we must understand what children and adults bring to the interactive episode and the way these interactions are organized (Greenspan, 1992).

What the Child Brings to Interactions

Infants are not passive recipients of what people do to them. From birth, infants are capable of influencing their caregivers (Bell, 1968). Infants come with perceptual and motor abilities that permit them to engage in social interactions. In the first year of life infants become experts in maintaining and modulating the flow of social exchange. They appreciate the causes of their emotional states. They acquire the signals to engage, avoid, or terminate a social encounter, and they can participate in a series of interactive exchanges (Stern, 1977). Greenspan (1997) has proposed a developmental hierarchy of emotional abilities that underlie social-communication skills. Table 8.1 displays the stages of emotional development, related social-communicative skills, indications of social-emotional disorders.

Infant Engagement Tools

During the prelinguistic period children are developing not only the emotional intentionality that underlies the desire to communicate, but also the social behaviors that enable them to engage others and interact with objects in their environment. Newborns have reflexes that enable them to fixate on and follow an object. Infants are designed to prefer looking at faces over other objects (Sherrod, 1981) and to prefer speech over other sounds (Gibson & Spelke, 1983). Infants' ability to gaze at people and objects of interest and to convey internal emotions through facial expressions provide the bases for the beginning of normally developing social interactions.

Baron-Cohen (1995) proposed three mechanism that underlie infants' engagement abilities and a fourth mechanism that underlies children's ability to form mental representations of the mental states of others. These mechanisms reflect four properties: volition, perception, shared attention, and epistemic states (i.e., knowledge of thoughts and feelings). The first mechanism, the *Intentionality Detector* (ID), interprets self-propelled motion stimuli in terms of volitional mental states of goals and desires. The child uses vision, touch, or audition to differentially respond to animate and inanimate objects.

The second mechanism, the *Eye Direction Detector* (EDD), has three functions: it detects the presence of eyes or eyelike stimuli; it determines whether the eyes are "looking at me" or are looking toward something else; and it infers that if the other organism's eyes are directed at something, then the organism sees that thing. This mechanism enables infants to recognize that they are seen by their mothers. The ID and EDD permit dyadic representations, that is, the relationship between an agent and object or the agent and oneself. They do not, however, permit the infant to recognize that both the infant and adult are attending to the same object or event. For this function, the *Shared Attention Mechanism* (SAM) is necessary. The SAM uses the dyadic representations to build triadic representations in which children recognize that they and someone else are both attending to the same object (Fig. 8.1). This shared attention is essential if the infant is to communicate about a shared reality. The last mechanism, the *Theory of Mind Mechanism* (ToMM) is a system for inferring the full range of mental states from behavior. The ToMM is a way of representing mental states (such as pretending, thinking, knowing, believing, guessing, deceiving) and tying these mental states into a coherent understanding of how mental states and actions are related.

From birth to 9 months, the infant has the ID and the basic functions of EDD that allow for dyadic representations. Around 9 months, SAM becomes active, and, consequently, the child is now able to build triadic representations that make joint reference possible. SAM also links EDD with ID, thus enabling eye direction to be read in terms of basic mental states. With the emergence of SAM, children are able to open and close circles of communication. A circle of communication has three components: the child shows an interest, the parent responds to that interest, and the child builds on the parent's communication. For example, the child reaches toward an object, the adult comments on the object, and the child picks it up and shows it to the adult (Greenspan, 1992). Finally, ToMM's arrival is heralded by the onset of pretend play. This represents a qualitative change

Table 8.1	*Emotional Development and Social-Communicative Skills*		
Age Range	Emotional Development	Social-Communicative Skills	Indications of Disorder
Birth to 3 months	Regulation and interest in the world: maintains a level of calm that permits child to make sense of sensations in the world; attends to auditory or visual stimulus for 3 or more seconds	Shows interest in caregiver by looking/listening; shows interest when caregiver makes joyful facial expressions and vocal tones	Shows no interest in anyone; always upset or crying; does not respond to interesting stimuli or is overly excited by stimuli
By 5 months	Forming relationships: evidences positive affect toward caregivers; looks/smiles spontaneously	Responds to social overtures with pleasure or other affects; localizes source of voice; vocalizes to caregiver's facial expressions and sounds	Disinterested in people or overly clingy to caregivers—cries if not held; withdraws; flat affect
By 9 months	Intentional 2-way communication: interacts in a purposeful (intentional, reciprocal, cause-effect) manner; uses multiple sensory modalities and range of emotions	Initiates and responds to social gestures—opens and closes a circle of communication (e.g., looks and reaches for toy [opening circle], caregiver points to toy and vocalizes [This one?"], child nods, makes sound, and reaches [closing circle])	May interact but not purposefully; oblivious to caregiver's signals or inconsistent response; tantrums or withdraws if caregiver does not respond quickly
By 13 months	Behavioral organization: develops complex sense of self by organizing complex emotions and behavior chains of interaction	Strings together 3 or more circles of communication around different intentions (e.g., love, protest, exploration)	Rarely initiates behaviors or emotions; behavior and affect appear random; shows few socially meaningful behaviors; no or limited focused curiosity
By 18 months	Behavioral elaboration: elaborates sequences of interaction that convey emotional themes such as closeness, pleasure/excitement, assertiveness/exploration, fear, anger	Opens and closes 10 or more circles of communication and imitates others as part of dealing with emotional patterns	Marked passivity or usually out of control; rarely initiates, usually only responding; may take initiative, but is demanding and stubborn; repeats rather than develops new behaviors
By 24 months	Representational capacity: creates mental images of intentions and/or feelings	Uses pretend play, words, and gestures to convey need, wish, and intention	No or limited symbolic behavior; no or little capacity for social-emotional

Table 8.1   *Emotional Development and Social-Communicative Skills (continued*

Age Range	Emotional Development	Social-Communicative Skills	Indications of Disorder
			thoughts (can label but not say "I like")
By 30 months	Representational elaboration: elaborates a number of intentions or feelings beyond basic needs	Uses pretend play and words to convey two or more emotional ideas	No or limited sense of intention in use of symbolic mode; relates in a chaotic manner; no impulse control; narrow range of emotions; vulnerable to slightest stress
By 36 months	Emotional thinking: creates logical bridges between different emotional ideas; understand that emotions can be caused by situations	Pretend play and words convey two or more logically connected, emotional ideas (e.g., doll gets hurt and mommy fixes; ugly monster scares doll; plays out eating cookie he could not get in reality)	Failure to elaborate play; manipulates toys but does not take on roles of others in play
By 42–48 months	Elaborated emotional thinking: creates logical bridges between three or more emotional ideas. Bridges informed by concepts of causality, time and space; understands that beliefs can affect emotion	Pretend play with 3 or more logically connected ideas dealing with intentions, wishes, feelings, deals with causality, e.g., "Why did you hit your brother?" —"He hit me and took my cookie"; uses time and space to deal with intentions, wishes, feelings, e.g., "Where should we look for the toy you can't find?"—"In my garden; I was playing out there."	No sequence in play events; does not give intentions to dolls; does not relate play behaviors to play behaviors of others

Based on information in Greenspan S. Infancy and early childhood: the practice of clinical assessment and intervention with emotional and developmental challenges. Madison, CT: International Universities Press, 1992; and Greenspan S. The growth of the mind: and the endangered origins of intelligence. Reading, MA: Addison-Wesley, 1997.

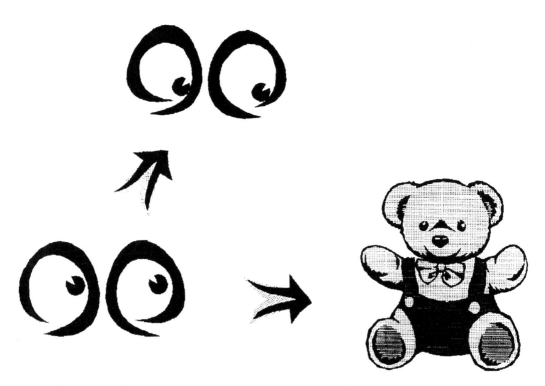

Figure 8.1.   Triadic representation: an example of the shared-attention mechanism.

in development because now children can begin to appreciate their own and other people's mental states, starting with pretending and progressing to "knowing" and "believing" over the next 2 years.

The development of these mechanisms can be witnessed in a variety of behaviors during infancy. At approximately 6 weeks, infants can visually fixate on their mothers' eyes, hold the fixation, and widen their own eyes. This fixation results in the mother feeling a greater sense of connection with the infant. With this eye fixation, social play between infant and adult begins in earnest. Infants cannot only seek out interaction, but can also terminate interaction. Infants can gaze directly into the adult's eyes, can turn their heads slightly so that they see the adult out of the corner of their eyes, or can lower their heads and turn far enough away to totally avoid visual contact. These engagement-disengagement behaviors enable infants to control the amount of stimulation they desire (Schaffer, 1984; Stern, 1977).

By the end of the third month infants' mature motor control of gaze direction gives them complete control over what they see. With this ability they can start or stop face-to-face interaction, because these interactions are built around mutual gaze. By looking at the mother, infants can start an encounter because the mother will look back. Children can continue the interaction by smiling or end it by averting their eyes or turning their heads away. Mutual gaze represents the turn taking that is later seen in verbal conversation. In these early months babies are learning the nonverbal basis of social interaction on which language is later built. They are able not only to fixate on an object, but also to pursue it. In the second half of the first year, infants become interested in objects as their increasing motor abilities enable them to reach, grasp, and manipulate the objects in their world. Once this occurs, the mother-infant interaction becomes a triadic affair between the mother, infant, and object.

Infants less than a week old can distinguish facial expressions such as happy, sad, and surprised, and they appear to imitate those expressions (Meltzoff &

Moore, 1977). Near the end of the first year they are able to engage in social referencing. They are able to perceive the link between a person's affect and the eliciting stimulus. Infants use this social referencing to make judgements about how to respond to a situation. They are particularly alert to a parent's indications of fear (Walden, 1993).

The infant's ability to convey emotional responses gives adults a topic for communication. The emotions of interest, joy, sadness, anger, surprise, disgust, and fear appear to be prewired into the system. In the first few weeks of life, the smile is reflexive, that is, internally triggered. By 6 weeks to 3 months, however, the smile becomes a social response elicited by external events. At this point the smile may take on an instrumental function; that is, the infant produces it to get a return smile from another person. The laugh is not present at birth. It first appears between 4 to 8 months in response to external stimuli. Initially the laugh is usually triggered by tactile stimulation such as tickling. From 7 to 9 months auditory events trigger the laugh, and from 10 to 12 months it is most readily triggered by visual events. The cry face is present from birth, and some observers believe that the cry may be used instrumentally as early as 3 weeks of age. By the third month, the infant has the major emotional expressions in place. These expressions and the sequence of behaviors associated with them help infants regulate interaction with their mothers.

These social-emotional characteristics lead infants to interact with adults in ways that are useful for language development. All normal babies exhibit these gaze and emotional expression behaviors. They do not, however, all respond in the same way to their social and physical environments.

Temperament

Babies come with their own personalities or temperaments. Temperament is defined as behavioral style or the how of behavior. Temperament significantly de-termines the pattern of interactions infants experience with their environments; it determines what infants respond to and how they respond. Variations in infant temperament involve differences in general mood, in activity level, and in adaptability to changes in routine. Large differences also exist between babies in the intensity of their responses, in their tendency to approach or withdraw from new experiences, in their persistence, and in their distractibility. Infants also vary in their regularity of sleeping and eating and in their sensitivity to stimulation.

Thomas and Chess (1977) described three temperamental patterns: *easy, slow-to-warm-up,* and *difficult.* Recently, more positive terms have been substituted: *flexible, fearful,* and *feisty.* Flexible babies have a regular overall pattern. They accept new experiences easily, exhibit mild reactions to discomfort, and make smooth adjustments to changes in routines. Fearful babies share some of the same style of easy babies, but tend to withdraw from new experiences. They will gradually adapt to new situations, but need to be handled sensitively in the process. Such babies generally cannot be pressured into new experiences. Feisty babies are easily distressed. They express their likes and, much more often, their dislikes in no uncertain terms. They react forcefully and negatively to new experiences and to even minor changes in routine, and they show little or no consistency in their schedule. It is hard for caregivers to predict their behaviors.

Infants' temperaments are a major factor in determining the nature of the interactions that infants experience with significant people in their environment. What is essential for the best development of children is that there be a "good fit" between infants and their caregivers. Flexible babies, who are so adaptable, can be reared by nearly anyone. Fearful and feisty infants take more sensitivity and insight on the part of caregivers. Goodness of fit results when the expectations and demands of the environment are in accord with the child's own capacities, motives, and behavioral style (Thomas & Chess, 1986). Poorness of fit occurs when there are dissonances between the two that may lead to incompatibility. An active, intense parent may be comfortable with an intense baby who cries vigorously with change. The parent may see the child as reflecting his/her own behavior patterns and have strategies to calm the child. A parent who expects the infant to have a regular time routine and be able to tolerate changes in caregivers may be unnerved by a feisty baby and have no idea of how to calm or interact with the child. Children with difficult temperaments can be perfectly normal children who can develop normal social behaviors, but their temperament does predispose them to developmental problems because their caregivers may not be able to establish effective communicative interactions with them. Infants who differ in temperament may experience identical stimulation much differently. Rough-and-tumble games may delight one child and overwhelm another. Lullabies may be ignored by one child, but provide great pleasure for another.

Mastery Motivation

Communicative competence is not merely a function of cognitive, linguistic, and social-emotional abilities, but also a function of motivation. (Scarr, 1981). *Mastery motivation* assumes that a child not only receives stimulation from the environment, but also initiates interactions that elicit stimulation from the physical and social environment. To engage in activities, children must feel comfortable and safe (Westby, Stevens-Dominguez, & Otter, 1996). The more children engage in mastery-motivation activities, the more exposures they have that will facilitate their social and intellectual competence. There are two aspects of mastery motivation: *mastery pleasure* and *persistence* (Brockman, Morgan, & Harmon, 1988; Yarrow, 1981). *Mastery pleasure* is defined as instances of positive affect during task-directed behavior or immediately following a solution. *Persistence* is defined as the amount of time a child works at or plays with toys in a task-directed man-

ner. Before 9 months of age, exploration and curiosity are identified as the best indicators of mastery motivation. Mastery motivation can be observed in a variety of situations from highly structured to free play, and from several sources, including direct observation of a child's behavior and parental, caregiver, or teacher ratings. Children who exhibit higher levels of mastery motivation increase the range and frequency of their experiences with the social and physical world and, as a consequence, provide themselves with more opportunities for communicative interactions.

What Caregivers Bring to Interactions

Children set the tone for interactions, but caregivers determine what children learn about interactions within the culture.

Mainstream Caregivers

The majority of information regarding socialization of communication comes from studies of white, middle-class families. Mainstream adults attend carefully to infants' smiles, noises, and movements as they play with them. In these interactions infants' excitement builds and then peaks. Infants may bring their hands to their mouths, suck on their tongues, or yawn in an effort to control their excitement as the play peaks. They begin to smile less and make fewer sounds and may even begin to grimace. Then they turn away slightly. They use the period of looking away to recover from their excitement. They then turn back to the parent, and the cycle begins again. When infants turn away, adults generally decrease their attention to the infants. When the infants turn back, adults begin to interact again, smiling and vocalizing (Schafer, 1977; Schaffer, 1984).

Most caregivers use a variety of behaviors to engage and maintain the interest of infants. When caregivers interact with infants, they often exaggerate their facial expressions in space and time. Caregivers may use an expression of mock surprise— opening their eyes wide, raising their eyebrows—and saying something like *oooooh* or *aaaaah* to signal a readiness to interact.

They may move their heads from side to side or toward the infant. The facial expressions are slow to form and are then held. Caregivers may play with the speed and rate of these behaviors, speeding up and then slowing down. As the interaction continues, they may smile to indicate that the interaction is going well, or they may use an exaggerated frown or pout when the interaction is running down or in trouble. The repertoire of facial exaggerations is limited, and a few patterns are repeated frequently. Stern (1977) suggested that these facial exaggerations facilitate infant's abilities to read facial expressions.

Mainstream caregivers also tend to engage in baby talk (Snow & Ferguson, 1977). They simplify syntax, use short utterances, use many nonsense sounds, transform words (e.g., pwitty wabbit for pretty rabbit), raise vocal pitch, and exaggerate loudness and intensity of vocalizations—ranging from a whisper to a loud "pretend scary" voice. Sometimes the speech is speeded up, and other times it is slowed down, elongating vowels on certain words, for example, *What a goooooooood little baby.* Pause times between utterances are also elongated, as though to allow time for the infant to respond. The caregiver appears to be shaping the infants turn-taking behavior to the form necessary when they become verbal. The mother also tends to repeat runs of interactions, *You're a pretty baby; you're such a pretty baby, you're the prettiest baby mommy has ever seen.* Many of these runs involve questions and answers, *Are you hungry? Are you? Huh? I think you are.* During each vocalization the mother brings her head closer to the infant. Between questions the mother moves away. Each question is accompanied by a distinct facial expression.

From the infant's birth, mainstream adults look for reasons for infants' behaviors and comment to the infants about possible intentions, for example, *You're so hungry. You don't like beets. You want mommy to pick you up.* When adults view infants as intentional, they attempt to find the object or event (referent) that is triggering the child's behavior (e.g., *You're looking at your teddy bear. You want your bot-*

tle.). In so doing, adults guide children into referencing (labeling) and requesting behaviors. As children develop the verbal ability to label and request, adults provide scaffolding questions to assist the children in producing more information. In mainstream homes, this scaffolding especially occurs during storybook reading as in the following example (Ninio & Bruner, 1978; Snow & Goldfield, 1981):

> **Mother**: Look!
> **Child**: (touches picture)
> **Mother:** What are those?
> **Child**: (vocalizes a babble string and smiles)
> **Mother:** Yes, they are rabbits
> **Child**: (vocalizes, smiles, and looks up at mother)
> **Mother** (laughs) Yes, rabbit
> **Child**: (vocalizes, smiles)
> **Mother:** Yes (Bruner, 1983, p. 78)

As children acquire the routine and begin to take over their pieces (e.g., labeling the picture), the adult ups the ante by asking a more complex question, for example, *What's the rabbit doing?* Once the child labels the object and what it is doing, the caregiver ups the ante again by asking, *Why is the rabbit is doing that?* or *How does he feel about what he is doing?* Through these social exchanges children come to understand how to take turns in conversations, maintain a topic, and provide information in their culture.

Cultural Variations in Caregiver-Child Interactions

Recently, anthropological studies have made it clear that cultures differ in their child-rearing practices. There are differences in views on infant capabilities, in who provides care for infants, the types of interactions between adults and children, and the role of the infant and young child in the family. Because of these variations, people of different cultures respond to and interact with infants and young children in different ways (Anderson & Battle, 1993; Blout, 1982; Briggs, 1984; Chisholm, 1983; Field, Sostek, Vietze, &

Leiderman, 1981; Greenfield & Cocking, 1994; Hale-Benson, 1986; Hanson & Lynch, 1992; Heath, 1983; Nugent, Lester, & Brazelton, 1989; Schieffelin & Eisenberg, 1984; Ward, 1971).

Some cultures do not view infants as capable of intentional behavior. Heath (1983) reported that Black working-class families in the Carolina Piedmont did not view infants as intentional and, hence, did not see them as conversational partners. Because infants were not seen as being able to communicate, their cries and vocalizations were not systematically attended to. When adults do not see infants as intentional, they are unlikely to talk with infants, provide labels, or ask questions. When they do not see toddlers and young children as information givers, they are less likely to support them in their attempts to produce lengthy topic-maintaining dialogues. (Heath, 1983; Whiting & Edwards, 1988). In such environments the major input to children from adults is likely to be directives. Expected responses from children is that they follow the directives, not that they talk.

In mainstream cultures early communicative functions are requesting and labeling. In cultures that do not view infants as intentional, one may find other early communicative functions. In the New Mexican Hispanic and Mexican American cultures studied by Briggs (1984) and Schieffelin and Eisenberg (1984) that did not perceive intentionality in infants, adults determined that the first words that should be used were polite and social words. Using the expression *dile* (say to him/her), adults gave children messages to repeat to someone else. What the adults told the children to say did not reflect the children's intentions, but instead, reflected the adults' beliefs concerning how different individuals should be addressed.

Some cultures that believe that infants are not intentional also believe that children learn to talk primarily by observing others, rather than by engaging in talk with adults. In these environments children are allowed to observe many adult interactions around them. They often begin talking by imitating words and phrases they hear. In these circumstances children's first words are likely to be those that attract their attention. Ochs (1982), reporting on child rearing practices in Western Samoa, reported that mothers frequently reported infants' first word as one that translated roughly as *shit* as the child's first word. Westby (1986), working in an inner city program, also found children whose first words represented words that might be considered profanity. Such words are usually spoken with increased loudness and intonation and in circumstances in which some important, emotionally laden event had occurred. All of this would focus the child's attention on such words. Heath (1983) observed that early language functions of Black children in the Carolina Piedmont included bossing, cussing, fussing, begging, and comforting—not the early communicative functions reported for mainstream children.

In much of the research literature it is assumed that the biological mother is the primary caregiver for the child and that the child must develop a particularly close attachment to this primary individual. Yet in many cultures infants may have multiple caregivers—grandparents, aunts, uncles, godparents, and older siblings also have major contributions to caregiving (Werner, 1984). Little information is available about the nature of communicative interactions in extended-family and sibling child-rearing cultures. When children interact primarily with other children, verbal exchanges may be structured differently than when children interact primarily with adults.

The remainder of this chapter will address the social-emotional bases of communication in mainstream children. Some principles are applicable to all children, but one must be alert to ways in which culture may affect the structure and functions of children's communications.

COMMUNICATING WITH OTHERS

Children's social-communicative abilities develop in two directions. *Vertical development* refers to increasing hierarchical development associated with increasing age and cognitive understanding. *Horizontal development* refers to the range of abilities or communicative functions within a particular developmental level.

Vertical Development

Intentionality

Using the theoretical framework of speech act theory (Austin, 1962), Bates (1976) described three stages in children's emergence of pragmatic or intentional communicative behaviors: *perlocutionary*, *illocutionary*, and *locutionary*. In the *perlocutionary* stage, from birth to approximately 9 months, infants have a systematic effect on adults without intending to. Adults interpret infant's smiles, cries, and coos as though they were intentional, although they are not. The infant does not intentionally cry or smile to seek a response from an adult, yet adults talk to the infants as though the infant is being intentional, *Oh, you want mommy to sing that again*, or *You don't want any more carrots. Mommy will take them away.* Perlocutionary behavior is sometimes referred to as functional communication. The infant's or child's behavior functions as a communication to adults, even though the child's behavior is not intentionally goal directed. Parents of older, handicapped children functioning in this perlocutionary stage may be quite adept at interpreting a child's behavior. Certain body movements may be correctly interpreted as the child needing to toilet or being thirsty or hungry.

Around 9 months, when infants are able to establish shared attention, they enter the *illocutionary* stage. Infants now use behaviors intentionally to gain the adult's attention. Many of these behaviors become conventionalized; that is, they are gestures that others would use (e.g., reaching, waving bye-bye). If a child wants a toy and his mother is not looking at it, he will point at the toy with his arm outstretched and index finger pointed, look toward the toy, and then shift his gaze to his mother's face, then look back and forth between the toy and his mother. A cry or vocalization is deliberately used to get another's attention. The child may whine, and then check to see if the adult is attending. If not, the child may escalate the whine to a cry, but again may stop to check if the adult is attending. During this stage one observes what Bates (1976) considered precursors to speech: the *protoimperative* and the *protodeclarative*. The *protoimperative* is defined as the child's use of a means to cause the adult to do something. It grows out of the child's attempts to do something themselves. Hence, the first protoimperatives involve instances of reaching and looking between the desired object and the event. Later the child may bring an object or toy to an adult seeking assistance with operating it. For example, the child recognizes a music box, but cannot wind it herself. She brings the box to an adult, hands it to the adult, and then waits expectantly for the adult to wind it.

A *protodeclarative* is defined as a preverbal effort to direct the adult's attention to some event or object in the world. Included here are showing objects or exhibiting oneself for the sole purposes of gaining attention. A child may bring a toy to an adult simply to capture the adult's interest and attention.

Between 13 to 18 months, children enter the *locutionary* stage. They begin to use conventionalized words to make things happen. The child who earlier pointed to the cookie now says, *cookie;* the child who simply handed mother a toy to wind now says, *help.*

Goal-Directedness

Development from perlocutionary, to illocutionary, to locutionary communication involves the development of goal-directed behaviors and the ability to share one's goals with others. Emotions that drive communication often arise from events related to goal achievement. Emotions rise and fall with success or failure to achieve one's goals. One generally experiences joy when a goal is achieved, anger when there is an obstruction to a goal, and sadness when a goal is lost or not achieved. Table 8.2, adapted from Wetherby and Prizant (1989) and Dunst and McWilliam

Table 8.2 *Goal-Directed Development and Interactive Competencies*

Level	Interaction Type	Goal	Description of Behaviors	Examples
I	Attentional interactions	No goal awareness	Attends to and discriminates between stimuli; diffuse fuss or movement to express emotion	Tracks objects moving in and out of field of vision; orients to sound; smiles at familiar face
II	Contingency interactions	Awareness of goal	Undifferentiated forms of behavior to initiate or continue a stimulus; manipulates physical properties of object or vocalizes toward person or object	Swipes at a mobile; reaches for object, picks it up, looks at it, and mouths it; vocalizes to get attention; anticipates events such as feeding when sees bottle or breast by showing excitement
III	Differentiated interactions	Simple plan designed to achieve a goal	Modifies and adjusts behavior to achieve goal; adapts to environmental demands and social expectations; uses motoric or vocal acts directed toward person	Raises arms to be picked up; shows and gives objects to others; pulls string to get toy; follows adult's visual line of regard to locate object; operates different buttons or knobs on busy box; anticipates social games, e.g., brings hand together for pat-a-cake; looks between adult and desired object
IV	Encoded interactions	Coordinated plan designed to achieve a goal	Uses conventionalized forms of behavior that are context bound and depend on concrete referents to evoke behaviors; uses combination of motoric and vocal acts or uses intermediary object to gain interaction	Points to desired objects; says words for objects he sees or wants in the environment; climbs on chair to get something out of reach; brings an object to caregiver as a way of getting attention

Table 8.2   Goal-Directed Development and Interactive Competencies (continued)

Level	Interaction Type	Goal	Description of Behaviors	Examples
V	Symbolic interactions	Alternative plans designed to achieve a goal	Uses conventionalized forms of behavior (language, pretend, sign, drawing) to refer to previous and future occurrences; modifies vocal signal or uses alternative strategy after unsuccessful attempt to achieve the goal	Uses words to label or request, e.g., "What's that?" "Gimme cookie"; pretends to drink from empty cup and eat from empty plate; repeats request louder if not attended to on first try
VI	Metapragmatic interactions	Mental awareness of plan to achieve goal	Plans out ahead of time strategies to use to achieve goal; reflects on success or lack of success	Child can verbalize plan: "Mom might give it to you if you ask real nice"; "I'll save my allowance till I have enough for the game"

Adapted from Dunst CJ, McWilliam RA. Cognitive assessment of multiply handicapped young children. In: Wachs TD, Sheehan R, eds. Assessment of young developmentally disabled children. New York: Plenum, 1988; and Wetherby AM, Prizant BM. The expression of communicative intent: assessment guidelines. Semin Speech Lang 1989;10:77–91.

(1988), presents a model of goal-directed development and interactive competencies that include both social and nonsocial aspects of development.

Attentional interactions refer to the child's capacity to attend to and discriminate between stimuli. These are behaviors that infants use to respond to and maintain stimulus inputs. Attentional behaviors can be manifested in a variety of ways, for example, looking at an object or person, orienting toward sound, smiling in response to a familiar person, laughing in response to an interesting event, tracking an object moving across the field of vision, and grasping an object placed in the child's hand. The interactions are triggered by environmental stimuli rather than initiated by the infant. The infant has no goal, or awareness of a goal. The infant uses a diffuse fuss or reaction to express emotion. When adults are aware that an infant is responsive to environmental events and is attempting to maintain these events, attentional interactive competencies enable adults to reinforce the child for gaining and maintaining control over stimuli.

Contingency interactions. Contingency interactive behavior is the infant's capacity to initiate and sustain interactions with the environment. At this stage infants begin to have awareness of a goal. They engage in repetitious behavior to maintain an event produced by their own actions. These behaviors are called undifferentiated because the child will attempt the same behaviors such as vocalizing, touching, or batting regardless of the stimuli. Contingency interactive behaviors may included batting at a mobile to produce a sound, touching an adult's mouth to get the person to repeat an interesting sound, or vocalizing to get attention. Contingency behaviors elicit an environmental stimulus, unlike attentional interactions that are elicited by environmental events. In this stage infants are capable of dealing with the world. Their hand-eye coordination and their hand-to-hand coordination permit them to reach and grasp and manipulate the world of inanimate objects.

Children in this stage are beginning to structure their social world. They are becoming aware that they are agents, that is, that they can make things happen, and that they are separate physical beings from their mothers. They are beginning to sense that they have feelings, like happiness or hunger. They are starting to construct in their minds a world of people, including themselves. There are distinct people in it—the infant, mother, father, those involved in the infant's everyday life. Greenspan and Greenspan (1985) suggest that this is the *falling in love stage*. The infant recognizes familiar people and rewards them with smiles. These behaviors lead to three important developmental competencies: *contingency awareness, predictability,* and *controllability. Contingency awareness* refers to infants' awareness of their own capabilities, that is, that they can produce interesting effects in the environment. *Predictability* refers to infants' awareness that certain behaviors can repeatedly produce the same effects in interactions with social and nonsocial environments (Lamb, 1981). *Controllability* refers to infants' capacity to understand that certain aspects of the environment can be affected as a function of their attempts to produce environmental consequences.

Differentiated interaction refers to the infant's ability to coordinate and regulate (e.g., modify and adjust) behavior to achieve goals. Children have a simple plan to achieve a goal. Children's interactions match or approximate social standards and expectations (e.g., raising arms to be picked up, rolling a toy car, drinking from a cup). Children are now in the illocutionary stage and have purposeful communicative intentions. They know when they want something, and they may have several strategies for getting what they want. They may crawl to it and pick it up; they may pull a cloth on which it is resting and draw the object toward them; or they may pull a string attached to the object. They may fuss and look between the desired object and an adult. They also know that another person can have the same intention. If the child's mother has a cookie, and the child wants it, she may reach toward the cookie, looking back and forth between her mother and the cookie. If that does not work, she may pull on her skirt and vocalize with increasing loudness. The behaviors children acquire are in part affected by the environmental demands placed on the them. In the previous stage the infant engaged in the same types of behaviors with all objects, for example, hitting, mouthing. Now children use different behaviors with different objects. Soft furry objects are patted, balls are thrown, cars are rolled. They also exhibit different interactional behaviors with different persons. They expect rough-and-tumble games with dad and quiet sit-down activities with mom.

Encoded interactions represent the beginning of the locutionary stage. The child coordinates a plan to achieve a goal using a variety of both motoric and verbal behaviors. Encoded interactions are preplanned rather than the result of trial and error. They use conventionalized forms of behavior, for example, verbal language, that are based on a set of rules that govern their construction. These interactions are tied to the immediate context and will not be used in unfamiliar contexts or when people or objects are not present (e.g., the child uses the word *dog* only to refer to his own dog or will ask for a cookie only when he sees a cookie). With encoded behaviors children can both initiate and sustain interactions and adapt and respond to requests and demands.

In *symbolic interactions* children can design alternative plans to achieve goals. If one plan is not successful, the child tries another. For example, if the child's verbal request was not responded to, the child may revise the request. They may repeat it louder, add *please*, or in later preschool rephrase the request. The behaviors are termed symbolic because the child uses words, images, or drawings as signifiers for objects, persons, and events. In contrast to encoded behaviors, which are tied to the immediate demands of the environment in which the child is currently functioning,

symbolic behaviors permit the recollection of previous events or evocations of future events. Symbolic interactions are rule-governed, conventionalized behaviors that are used to describe, request, and enact persons, objects, and events in the absence of reference-giving cues.

Once children have established symbolic behaviors, they can reflect on these behaviors, developing a *metapragmatic awareness* of a plan to achieve a goal. By the age of 3 years they can reflect on the means to achieve a goal and their success or failure in achieving it. They may comment on what may work or not work, for example, *She'll give it to you if you say, pretty please; or tell him you'll trade him four Matchbox cars for one turtle.*

At each level the child has the potential for *engaging* and *modulating* behavioral functions. The child uses *engaging* behaviors to initiate an interaction or to sustain or repeat an interactive episode. The *modulating* function refers to behavior a child uses to regulate or adapt to an interaction. Regulating behaviors are used to terminate input or to reinstate input. Adapting behaviors are used to respond to others' efforts to establish interactions or to get the child to respond to adult requests or comments. The nature of the interpersonal context will affect the engaging and modulating behaviors of infants (Lamb, 1979). Attachment behavior and stranger anxiety are more likely to be manifested indoors than outdoors (Blurton-Jones, 1972) and to be more intense in a laboratory setting than in a child's home (Lamb, 1979).

Referencing and Requesting

To engage in illocutionary and locutionary behavior, children must be able to reference. People use referencing to manage and direct each other's attention by linguistic means. Although emotions trigger early communication, children do not talk about the emotions. Instead, they talk about and draw attention to the people, objects, and events they have feelings about.

Referencing involves the superimposition of linguistic attention management on prelinguistic means; that is, the child names an object in addition to looking and pointing at it. Development of the ability to reference depends on the children's mastery of discourse and dialogue rules as much as on skills of linking percepts with sounds and with representations of the world in their head. Reference presupposes four things:

1. That individuals can signal to one another that they have a referential or indicating intent.

2. That reference can vary in precision, from a vague point to an explicit definition.

3. That reference is a form of social interaction having to do with the management of joint attention.

4. There is a goal structure in referring. One must not only have an intent to refer, but also a means for doing so if one is to be successful (Bruner, 1983).

Initially the management of joint referencing is under the control of the adult. The caregiver highlights objects by moving them into the infant's view. Once the infant's attention can reliably be gained by showing objects, the caregiver begins to prepare the child for the object by calling the child's name or saying, *Oh, look,* or *See what I have.* Between 8 to 12 months infants discover that the adult's speech signals that the adult is looking at something, and the infants begin to follow the adults' line of regard. By 12 months infants follow the adult's line of regard, search for an object, and if they find none, they look at the adult's face again and then again look outward. Shortly after this the child begins to point. Once pointing and consistent words appear, caregivers initiate *what* and *where* games (*What's this? Where did it go?*).

Once children can reference, they can request. Requesting provides a means of not only getting things done with words, but of operating in the culture. This entails not only coordinating one's language with the requirements of action in the real world, but of doing so in culturally prescribed ways. Bruner (1983) distinguished three types of early requests:

1. Request for an object

2. Invitation or request to an adult to share a role relationship in play or in a game

3. Request for supportive action in which the child tries to recruit an adult's skill or strength to help him achieve a desired goal

The caregiver's role is different in each of these requests. In the first, the caregiver must figure out what the child wants; in the second what the invitation is for; and in the third what kind of help the child needs. Requests for visible and near objects occur before a year of age. Requests for remote or absent objects and for supportive action or assistance explode around 18 months when children develop representational capacity. Once children are using words to request absent objects and supportive actions, caregivers begin to enforce the cultural expectations for requests. Children are expected to really need the object or the assistance and not request something they can get or do for themselves. Requests should not require unreasonable demands from caregivers (e.g., I can't go upstairs and find your book now, I'm fixing dinner), and the child must respect the voluntary nature of responses to requests (caregiver requires the child to say thank you after the request is fulfilled). Certain requests are related to time and can only be fulfilled within a particular time frame (e.g., You can't have cookies before dinner).

Verbal requests can be of three types:

Direct requests: Gimme that! More milk. Please pass the butter.

Indirect requests: Could you get that pencil? Why don't you close the door?

Hints or nonconventionalized requests: It's cold in here. I haven't gotten my allowance yet.

Successful requesting requires that children gain attention, that their requests are clear and persuasive, that they maintain the desired or expected social relationships, and that they have strategies for making repairs when their request is not understood (Ervin-Tripp & Gordon, 1986). In addition, children must produce requests that recognize the following:

1. The social status or the relative power of the speaker and the addressee. People with higher status should be addressed more politely.

2. The intrusiveness of the request. If a request is intrusive, one should be more polite. Requests can intrude on listeners in three ways: they interrupt an ongoing conversation, they may entail a disruption of plans or of an ongoing activity, and they may demand valuable goods or unusual services. Direct requests are normal in situations where speakers and listeners are engaged in a familiar routine or cooperative activity. Adults, however, provide justification and increased politeness when they perceive their requests to be intrusive.

3. Possession. One must be more polite when asking for property that belongs to others.

4. Rights and obligations. One need not be as polite in situations where the one has a right to expect service and the service provider has the obligation to provide the service. For example, parents and teachers are expected to perform certain services for children (Gordon & Ervin-Tripp, 1984).

In general, children are sensitive to roles, rights, and possessions by the age of 2 years. They have limited awareness of intrusiveness before school age. Lawson (as cited in Ervin-Tripp & Gordon, 1986) reported that a 2-year-old child used different forms of speech to her father, mother, and children at nursery school, depending on whether they were her own age or older. She used direct imperative requests to 2 year olds, and embedded requests or requests with tags such as please or OK. Ervin-Trip and Gordon (1986) reported that 60% of 2- and 3-year-old children's requests to outsiders used politeness markers, whereas only 1% of requests to mothers and 14 to 24 % of requests to other children were polite. These researchers suggested that children assume that mothers must be available for services, whereas older children and visitors do not have to be available. Requests for objects that belonged to others were usually polite even to mothers and siblings.

Children 2 and 3 years of age seldom provide justifications for their requests. A marked increase in justification of requests occurs around age 4 (e.g., *I need a red crayon cause mine is broke*). At this age children begin to challenge adults' refusals of requests. They later use information gained from adults' reasons for their refusals to persuade adults of their needs, desires, or intents (e.g., *I'll eat all my dinner if I can have a popsicle now*).

As children become sensitive to the social rules underlying requests, they produce more indirect and nonconventualized requests. Between ages 4 and 8, children not only use politeness modifications for issues of status and rights, but also become sensitive to how their requests might intrude on activities of others. Children understand direct and indirect requests during the preschool years, but they are around 8 years of age before they comprehend nonconventualized requests or hints. Conventionalized requests (directives and indirectives) can be learned as formulas. Caregivers can tell a child what to say in a particular situation. Nonconventionalized requests require greater cognitive and social knowledge.

Horizontal Development

Once children engage in illocutionary and locutionary behavior they communicate a variety of intentions. A number of taxonomies have been developed to code communicative intents. The categories vary depending on the age of the children studied, the philosophical orientation of the researcher, or the degree to which discourse and social context are considered (Chapman, 1981). Taxonomies may classify gestures or language at the following levels:

1. *The utterance level.* Each utterance is considered independent of the relationship of the utterance to other utterances and is coded based on what the speaker is doing at the moment. Are they labeling, requesting, warning, promising, or ordering?

2. *The discourse level.* In this taxonomy the utterance is categorized according to its relationship to other utterances. Does the utterance initiate a conversation, maintain the conversation, acknowledge another speaker, clarify an utterance, or terminate the conversation? Utterances coded at the utterance level can also be coded at the discourse level. An utterance may function as a label at the utterance level and as a topic initiator at the discourse level. At the discourse level, utterances may also be considered in terms of how they manage the conversation. Does the utterance function to get a turn, hold one's turn, or allow another person to take a turn?

3. *The social level.* The utterance can be placed in its social context. Language varies according to the setting and the roles of the participants in these settings. This is particularly true with politeness and argumentative behavior. How does the utterance function to soften or strengthen the communication?

Communication in the illocutionary and early locutionary phases involves efforts to regulate another's behavior for purposes of achieving a goal, to seek social interaction, or to establish joint attention for the purpose of sharing information (Bruner, 1981). Table 8.3 presents communicative intents, coded at the utterance level, that have been reported during the illocutionary and early locutionary stages (Coggins & Carpenter, 1981; Dore, 1975; Halliday, 1975; Wetherby & Prizant, 1989, 1991). Communicative intentions in this stage can be gestures or verbal utterances that serve to (1) regulate behavior, (2) engage in social interaction, and (3) establish joint reference.

Wetherby and her colleagues (Wetherby, Cain, Yonclas, & Walker, 1988) reported that the number of different communicative functions are comparable at the prelinguistic and one-word stage, but increase during the multiword stage. Even during the illocutionary stage, children are likely to use all three major functions. As they move into the multiword locutionary stage, requests for social routines and showing decrease, and calling, requesting permission, acknowledging, requesting information, and requesting clarifications increase. Rate increases substantially between the early illocutionary and multiword locutionary stages. Children displayed an average of about one act per minute during the prelinguistic stage, about two acts per minute in the one-word stage, and about five acts per minute by the multiword stage.

Halliday reported the following six communicative functions manifested gesturally or verbally between 10 and 18 months:

Instrumental: Seeks satisfaction of material needs, i.e., obtains objects

Regulatory: Controls others' behavior, i.e., requests actions

Interactional: Establishes interactions with others

Personal: Expresses feelings and attitudes

Heuristic: Questions, investigates the - environment

Imaginative: Creates a world through language

Around 24 months a seventh function emerges:

Informative: Shares information about nonpresent objects and events

Halliday's categories can be subsumed in the categories listed in Table 8.3. Instrumental and regulatory categories regulate others' behaviors. The heuristic and personal categories include intents for establishing joint attention, and the interactional category establishes social interaction. As children develop, these functions combine into other functions. Instrumental, regulatory, and interactional functions combine into a pragmatic function for the language of request used to act on one's environment. The mathetic function emerges out of the personal, heuristic, and informative functions. This function is used to learn about oneself and the environment. The mathetic function is critical for the types of learning demanded in schools.

During the preschool years, communicative functions become less tied to the concrete environment and more related to language referring to language. Table

Table 8.3   *Early Communicative Intents*

A. Behavioral regulation

    1. Request for specific object—demands an object

    2. Rejection of an object—refuses an object

    3. Request for action—commands someone to perform an action (e.g., raises arms to be picked up)

    4. Protest of action—refuses an activity by someone

B. Social interaction

    1. Greeting—gains attention, indicates notice of initiation or termination of activity (e.g., *hi, bye*)

    2. Request for social routine—initiates routines such as peek-a-boo or pat-a-cake

    3. Showing off—attracts attention

    4. Calling—gains attention of someone

    5. Acknowledging—indicates that the speaker's communication was received

    6. Requests permission—seeks approval to carry out an activity[a]

    7. Personal—expresses moods or feelings

C. Joint attention

    1. Transferring—places an object in another's possession

    2. Comment on an object—directs someone's attention to an object

    3. Comment on an action or event—directs someone's attention to an event

    4. Request for information—seeks information, explanations, or clarifications[a]

    5. Clarification—utterances used to clarify previous communication[a]

[a]Intention generally appears only in the locutionary period.

8.4 presents Dore's schema (1978) for coding communicative functions for preschool-aged children.

DISABILITIES AFFECTING SOCIAL/EMOTIONAL BASES OF COMMUNICATION

Social/emotional aspects of communication can be disrupted by factors within the environment or factors within the child.

Factors in the Environment

In some instances parents may be less able to read children's cues, may be less available to engage in interaction with children, or may misinterpret an infant's behavior (Field, 1987). Hinde (1976) sug-gested that "What a person thinks about a relationship may be more important than the interactions that actually occur" (p.4). Parents interpret an infant's behavior (which may be perfectly normal) according to their own values, intentions, repulsions, et cetera. Robson (1967) reported a case of a mother, who when she looked at her 3-week-old son's attempts to capture her gaze declared, "He looks daggers." With such an attitude, the mother avoided making eye contact with her infant.

Some parents may simply be poor matches with their infants. They may not be able to cope effectively with the temperamental style of their infants. They march to the beat of different drummers. The parents may overstimulate or under-

Table 8.4 *Communicative Functiion in Preschool Children*

Requests	For information	Where's Michael going?
	For action	Get me some more paste.
	For acknowledgement	You know what?
Responses to requests	Providing information	(Why isn't Karen here?) She's sick.
	Expressing acceptance, denial, or acknowledgement	Okay.
		You can't have it.
Descriptions of past and present facts	Labeling or describing objects and actions	I'm eating all my lunch. Anna spilled her milk.
	Describing properties and locations	My candle has lots of red paint on it. I put it in my cubbie.
Statements	Of facts or rules	It's not nice to grab.
		We have to share the wagon.
	Of explanations, reasons, causes	Sara can't go swimming cause she's got a cold
Acknowledgements	Recognizing responses	Okay, yes, right.
	Evaluating responses	That's not what teacher said.
Organization devices	Regulates contact and conversation	Hi, bye, my turn, sorry.
Performatives	Accomplish event by speaking (protests, jokes, claims, teases, warnings)	Stop. Don't touch it. Josh is a baby.

stimulate their infants. Adults who overstimulate tend to engage in overcontrolling intrusive behaviors with infants. Overstimulating adults may fail either to read or to respond to infants' efforts to control stimulation. What the baby does matters relatively little. In such interactions infants lose opportunities to discover that they can regulate the external environment, and as a byproduct, their internal state through emotional communication. In the face of consistent and marked overstimulation, the baby can go limp or develop a pattern of staring through the adult (Stern, 1977).

Depressed, emotionally disturbed, or intellectually limited parents may understimulate an infant. A depressed mother may go through daily caregiving activities, but not engage in a range of communicative intensity to attract and hold her infant's attention. She is likely to fail to use exaggerated expressions, vocal shifts, or repeated escalating vocal patterns to attract her infant's interest. Young or intellectually limited parents may have few ideas of how to interact with infants. Once they have gone through their repertoire, they may stop.

Children reared in abusive and/or emotionally neglectful circumstances may experience fewer instances of positive social interactions, and even when such an interaction is available, the children may be in such a constant state of fight or flight that they cannot attend to the communication (Perry, 1997). Such children may suffer long-lasting social-behavioral-communicative deficits. Perry (1997) suggests that lack of appropriate affective experiences in early life can result in neurologic differences and associated malorganization of attachment capabilities. During development, abused/neglected children spend so much time in a low-level state of fear that they are constantly focusing on nonverbal cues. Such children feel no emotional attachment to other humans, and they fail to develop appropriate social-interactive relationships and communication skills (Alessandri & Lewis, 1996).

Infants with understimulating or overstimulating caregivers have fewer opportunities to participate in satisfying social interactions and to discover ways they can affect their environments through communication. Infants and toddlers from welfare families hear fewer words and receive more discouragements and fewer encouragements for talking than children from professional and working-class families (Hart & Risley, 1995). As a consequence, one might also expect to find differences in social-communicative interactions.

Factors Within the Child

Children with cognitive, syntactic, or semantic deficits are also likely to show delays and differences in social or pragmatic aspects of communication. Children who were born prematurely, have significant medical problems, or are mentally retarded are less able to engage in the conversational dance during infancy, and hence, are at risk for pragmatic deficits beyond what would be expected based on their cognitive abilities alone. Some conditions particularly affect the social-emotional or pragmatic aspects of communication development. A number of factors may result in the child being less able to be involved in communicative interactions or for the adult to be less able to read the child's involvement.

Blindness

Early social interactions, gesturing, and the development of referencing are all dependent on vision. Blind children are generally delayed in acquisition of first words and may not use them for communication. They repeat words to themselves and fail to produce them to initiate interactions until well into their third year (Urwin, 1983). By 6 months of age the sighted infant has developed a large repertoire of social interactions. Blind children, however, have no way of watching their mothers' facial expressions or of engaging in joint attention to visual events with her. Also, because blind babies stop looking at their mothers after the end of the reflex period, mothers do not pick them up as often (Bovet, Parrat-Dayan, & Voneche, 1989). Consequently, infants miss opportunities for communicating.

Lack of vision particularly affects the development of joint attention, which is essential for establishing referencing that is necessary for communicating. The ability to reference requires the following:

1. Attracting attention to oneself

2. Assessing the listener's focus of attention

3. Directing attention to external referents (Mulford, 1983)

Blind children may have difficulty determining whether their intended listeners are attending to them, or even if the persons are present. Knowing that the person is present, however, is no guarantee that he/she is paying attention. Even if the person is present and has been listening, the child has no way of knowing if the person's attention has shifted to something else. The child must gain the listener's attention. The blind child does not have the option of establishing mutual gaze or gesturing. They must, instead, either touch the listener or vocalize. For normal-sighted children, vocalizing to gain attention and establishing joint referencing are initially superimposed on earlier gestural strategies. Without vision, blind children develop few gestural communications. The blind child also may not be certain if the referent exists in the environment or if the listener is attending to it.

Many of the blind child's early referents are names of people rather than names of objects. Use of language for requesting purposes appears in sighted children by the end of the first year, but closer to the end of the second year in blind children. Because blind children's nonverbal behavior so often fails to provide topics for comment, parents frequently adopt a questioning mode of interaction. Although questioning may facilitate an early form of turn taking between parent and child, because the initiative is always with the adult, the practice inhibits the child's development of awareness of his or her own agency, that is, awareness of the ability to make things happen in the environment (McGurk, 1983). Despite these early deficits, blind children, who have no other handicapping conditions and who have adults who are alert to the interaction of blindness and language, can develop normal communicative interaction patterns during the preschool years. Many, however, show patterns of delays and disorder in communicative interactions.

Autism

Autism is probably the condition most commonly thought of as affecting social/emotional communication. Early ideas about the cause of autism suggested it was due to poor parent-child interactions. Although the exact cause or causes of autism are still unknown, it is accepted that the deficiency lies within the neurological or biological functioning of the child (Anderson & Hoshino, 1987; Golden, 1987; Ornitz, 1987). Autistic children exhibit a fundamental failure in socialization. The social disfunction observed in autistic children is never observed in normal children of any age and cannot be accounted for on the basis of mental retardation alone. Autistic children show deficits in three areas related to social engagement: sociability and social communication, attachment, and understanding and expressing emotions (Cohen, Paul, & Volkman, 1987).

Deficits in socialization may be noted early. Many of the social-communicative deficits exhibited by autistic children reflect deficits in SAM and ToMM (Baron-Cohen, 1995). Many autistic children exhibit deviant patterns of gaze from early infancy. Young autistic children may avoid eye gaze, while some older children may stare fixedly and inappropriately (Rutter, 1978; Wing, 1976). Deficits in joint attention and referential pointing, which depend on SAM, readily discriminate autistic from nonautistic toddlers (Lord, 1993). Without a functioning SAM, ToMM cannot be triggered. Without ToMM, autistic children have difficulty recognizing the goals and beliefs of others; and without ToMM much of the social world would appear unpredictable.

Many autistic children fail to show differential attachment to familiar people and may show less distress with strangers and separation from family members than normal children. Autistic children tend to show a greater interest in objects than in people, unlike normal children who show a greater interest in people than objects. Autistic children exhibit deficits in gestural forms of communication, as well as in verbal communication. Some autistic children never acquire oral language. Of those that do acquire oral language, primary deficits are in use of language, not in the form of language (Bartolucci, Perce, & Streiner, 1980; Boucher, 1976; Trager-Flusberg, 1981). Autistic children exhibit a sparsity of intentional communicative behaviors. Even when they possess good syntactic language skills, they do not use language well for communication and interaction. Autistic children use fewer communicative acts during interactions. Many of the communicative intentions they do use are not conventionalized. For example, some autistic children use echolalia (repetitions of words and phases they have heard spoken) to request something, for example, saying *Do you want a drink?* instead of *I want water*. They use a high degree of nonreciprocal speech, fail to listen, make irrelevant comments, fail to leave a topic of obsessive interest, and fail to look for cues in the listener as to his or her interest or desire to take a turn

(Dewey & Everard, 1974). They tend to be poor at initiating conversation, although they may not be unresponsive if another person initiates it (Loveland, Landry, Hughes, Hall, & McEvoy, 1988). When they do bring up a topic, it is often related to their own preoccupations, and their remarks or questions are usually uttered without varied inflection (Rutter & Garmezy, 1983). They are likely to interrupt and respond inappropriately in conversations (Paccia-Cooper, Curcio, & Sacharko, 1981). Some engage in persistent and perseverative questioning that does not serve the purpose of requesting information (Hurtig, Ensrud, & Tomblin, 1980). Although some basic intention to communicate exists, autistic children have little skill in participating in communicative activities involving joint reference of shared topics, and particularly in supplying new information relevant to the listener's purposes (Paul, 1987).

Autistic children lack a normal affective range. They do not show normal transitions from calm to aroused states. Some are too calm and undemanding, never showing any needs. Others are exceedingly irritable and inconsolable. In addition to the difficulties in showing their own feelings, they fail to understand the feelings of others. Harris (1989) suggested that deficits in understanding and expressing emotions may account for many of the communicative and pretend-play deficits that are observed in autistic children. In studies by Hobson (1993) autistic children could match a drawing of a facial expression to a facial expression they had seen in a film. They could not, however, match a gesture, a vocalization, or an emotional context with a facial expression. They did much worse than normal and retarded children matched for mental age. The autistic children had difficulty recognizing that different emotional signals—a gesture, a facial expression, a tone of voice, or an emotionally charge situation—can all signify the same emotional state.

But how would a deficit in reading other people's emotional expression result in a lack of play and poor communicative interactions? Harris (1989) argued that an understanding of emotion depends on an understanding of other mental states, particularly desires and beliefs. Without a ToMM, autistic children have less awareness of psychological states, particularly desires. When children were asked to tell a story about a sequence of pictures, the autistic children made many fewer references to mental states of the story characters, including desires, than did normal and retarded children matched for cognitive level. Although a normal child might begin a story by saying, "The boy is putting the sweet in the box so nobody won't find it," an autistic child would simply describe the action with no reference to the character's motive.

If autistic children do not understand other people's expressions of emotion, they will find it difficult to form normal relationships with them. They will find people unpredictable and perhaps even frightening. They may understand physical or mechanical forces in the world but not psychologic forces. Understanding of a person's mental state and pretense have important similarities. Numerous studies have reported that autistic children exhibit difficulty with symbolic pretend (Harris, 1993). Pretend requires awareness of a mental world apart from a physical world. Pretend involves a willingness to entertain temporarily a false proposition. Leslie (1987) suggested that autistic children unlike normal children cannot temporarily disengage from reality and entertain pretend or nontruths.

When language first emerges in normal children, it is used along with gestures. For example, children point to an object and look back and forth between the object and the person whose attention they are trying to direct while saying a word. The implication is that they realize that other people may not be following their gesture, and they look to see whether the gesture is being registered and responded to. The combination of pointing plus looking suggests that the children appreciate that other people can have visual experiences like their own, provided they look in the same direction and that their attention can be directed by gestures such as pointing. Compared with normal and retarded children, autistic children are less likely to check that the adult is paying attention to the same object or event as themselves. They point less often and show objects to adults less often, and when they hold an object or watch an interesting toy, they rarely look to the adult (Mundy, Sigman, Ungerer, & Sherman, 1986; Sigman, Mundy, Sherman, & Ungerer, 1986). Thus they establish joint attention less frequently than normal children. As discussed earlier, joint attention is an important precursor to early conversation. A child who could not engage in such joint attention, or who avoids it, would have difficulty in grasping early language functions.

Communication requires that one be able to conceive of another's sharing an interest about an object or topic. A key symptom of autism is the child's inability to enter into joint attention and affective contact with other people. Although the difficulties of autistic children have a cognitive basis, they also have a social/emotional basis.

Language and Social Impairments

A strong correlation exists between language skills and social-emotional behavior (Baker & Cantwell, 1987; Britton & Fujiki, 1993; Camarata, Hughes, & Ruhl, 1988; Giddan, 1991). Although there is agreement that, in most instances, language and social impairments are causally linked, there is less agreement about the nature and direction of this relationship. Based on the information presented in this chapter, it should be clear how early disruptions in social-emotional development can disrupt language learning. Some children, however, may exhibit early appropriate social-emotional interactions, but later experience difficulty in developing the linguistic code. Problems in word finding, constructing requests or comments, repairing communication breakdowns, or comprehending what is said may adversely affect social skills. Children with language impairments are less willing to engage in conversation, and they are more likely to be ignored or rejected when they do attempt to communicate (Fujiki, Brinton, & Todd, 1996; Rice, 1993).

The current, predominant view of the cause-effect relationship is that for many students with social and language impairments, the impairments interact and affect each other during development. There may be a biological or neurophysiological factor that underlies both the social-emotional and linguistic difficulties. Deficits in one area further deficits in the other area. In addition, deficits in social and language skills frequently result in reduced opportunities for social interaction (Rice, 1993). Because social interactions are so critical in driving language and social development, the child with social and language impairments experiences further delays in development.

ASSESSING SOCIAL/EMOTIONAL BASES FOR COMMUNICATION

Assessment of children's communicative functions and intentions should consider the number of different communicative intentions they use, the proportion of each function, the rate of communicative intentions, and the child's developing theory of mind. The rate of communication may be a particularly useful measure of communicative development in language-impaired children who are using few or no words (Wetherby, Cain, Yonclas, & Walker, 1988). A lack of developing communicative functions may be a warning sign of broad-based communicative impairment. The use of gestural communicative intents in advance of linguistic abilities may be suggestive of specific language impairment. Assessment of children's communicative intentions can include observation of caregiver-child/teacher-child interactions, interviewing of family members and teachers regarding the child's communicative behavior, observation of children's language use in naturalistic settings and in activities structured to trigger a variety of communicative intentions, and for older preschool and school-age children the use of standardized tests.

Caregiver-Child Interaction

Children's development of the social-emotional/intentional basis of communication is dependent on their interactions with those around them and with their own personality and abilities. Because communication in infancy is so related to caregiver-child interaction, when a young child is referred for communication evaluation, it may be desirable to observe the nature of the caregiver-child interaction. Children require different types of interaction with caregivers at various stages of development. Greenspan (1992) described behaviors that indicate disordered caregiver functioning that can affect child development. Table 8.5 presents behaviors that represent disordered caregiver functioning at various stages of the child's social-emotional development.

Klein and Briggs (1987) developed a brief 10-item observation form to use in observing mothers and infants. They list 10 caregiver behaviors to observe:

1. Provides appropriate tactile and kinesthetic stimulation (e.g., gently strokes, pats, caresses, cuddles, rocks baby)

2. Displays pleasure while interacting

3. Responds to child's distress (changes verbalization, changes infant's position, provides positive physical stimuli)

4. Positions self and infant so eye-to-eye contact is possible (attempts to make eye contact, reciprocates eye gaze)

5. Smiles contingently at infant

6. Varies prosodic features (uses higher pitch, talks more slowly, exaggerates intonation)

7. Encourages conversation (uses rising intonation questions, waits after saying something, imitates child's sounds, answers when infant vocalizes)

8. Responds contingently to infant's behavior (vocalizes after infant movement or vocalization)

9. Modifies interaction in response to negative cues from infant (changes activity, reduces intensity of interaction, terminates interaction)

10. Uses communication to teach language concepts (interprets infant's behaviors appropriately, e.g., *You're hungry, aren't you?*; comments on infant's attention to something in environment, matches infant's vocalization or word with slightly more elaborate language)

For each category, Klein and Briggs provide additional descriptions of components of behavior. The observer is to rate the interaction on a scale of *rare, sometimes, often,* or *optimally.* This scale reflects ideas from mainstream literature on caregiver-child interactions and assumes that the mother is the primary caregiver. When using it with nondominant cultural groups, one will want to observe the infants with others who may be their caregivers and will want to observe other families from a similar cultural or socioeconomic level before interpreting the results of the observations.

Naturalistic Observations

The majority of studies on children's intentional communication have relied on naturalistic social contexts, having children interact with familiar people and allowing children to converse about topics of their choosing (Coggins, Olswang, & Guthrie, 1987). It has been assumed that nonobstrusive observation provides the best opportunity to obtain a representative sample of children's language use. This technique may, however, provide an incomplete picture of a child's capabilities. A combination of both natural, unstructured activities and structured activities designed to elicit particular communicative functions may be the best way of sampling children's capabilities. Children reportedly have produced different intentions under these two conditions. Children are more likely to use requests in structured conditions and comments during free-play situations (Coggins, Olswang, & Guthrie, 1987). In low-structured activities toys are readily

Table 8.5   *Potentially Disordered Caregiver Behaviors*

Child's Age	Child Stage of Social-Emotional Development	Indications of Disordered Caregiver Functioning
Birth to 3 months	Functional approach to caregivers— Homeostasis	Unavailable to comfort infant (e.g., self-absorbed, depressed) or intermittently available (can comfort for brief periods when infant not too upset); hyperstimulating—undermines infant's own regulatory capacities;
2–4 months	Functional approach to caregivers— Attachment	Unavailable; lacks emotional warmth (disinterested; does not look at, smile, talk to or touch infant) or intermittent interest (some looking, cuddling, talking, but may be limited to one modality—look only or talk only); intrusive, hyper-manic quality; impervious to infant's moods; overly anxious and overprotective (always smiling, stroking)
3–9 months	Functional approach to caregivers— Purposeful communication	Fails to recognize or respond purposively to infant's signals or responds intermittently; mis-reads or overresponds to infant's signals; tends to confuse own feelings with infant's feelings
10–17 months	Functional approach to caregivers— Behavioral organization and initiative	Unavailable when child organizes complex behaviors (feels "the child doesn't need me any-more"); becomes confused and disorganized when child's behavior & affect becomes complex (e.g., adult can't switch with child from one game to another or switches too quickly; or can't tolerate intensity of emotions or becomes easily ashamed of themes such as sex or aggression); can interact when not under stress
17–30 months	Functional approach to caregivers— Representational capacity and elaboration	Lacks capacity to engage child symbolically or engages in a concrete manner (feeding and clean-liness but does not describe feelings or represent people activities with dolls); some symbolic interactive capacity, but limited to some themes e.g., dependency but no curiosity or assertiveness; or acts symbolically but only according to own agenda

Table 8.5	*Potentially Disordered Caregiver Behaviors (continued)*

Child's Age	Child Stage of Social-Emotional Development	Indications of Disordered Caregiver Functioning
26–36 months	Functional approach to caregivers— Representational differentiation and consolidation	Unable to use symbolic mode in causal manner (can't complete play sequences, e.g., if child shows a doll being "naughty, mother cannot show how doll is punished or learns lesson); disorganized play pattern; does not set limits in response to childs anger; doesn't use language to help child see consequences of actions

Based on information in Greenspan S. Infancy and early childhood: the practice of clinical assessment and intervention with emotional and developmental challenges. Madison, CT: International Universities Press, 1992.

accessible, and caregivers follow the child's leads; hence there is little need for children to request. In such situations the child is in control and desires to share the experience with the adult. Consequently, the child is more likely to use comments to gain adult attention in nonstructured settings and less likely to use requests. Elicitation tasks are adult controlled, and the adult manipulates the materials to direct the child's attention. The child does not need to gain the adult's attention, but to gain access to the materials the children has to request.

Young children will most readily communicate with familiar people in familiar settings. For infants and toddlers it is best to carry out naturalistic observations of the child during daily routines at home—eating, bathing, and playing. This is especially critical for children functioning below the symbolic level of interactions because their communications are context dependent. When this is not possible, one can arrange naturalistic activities in a center and have the child's significant others (parents, grandparents, and siblings) carry out activities like they might do at home. When a situation is unfamiliar, children are not likely to produce their usual language in the first observations. Consequently, at least two observations should be scheduled (Wetherby, et al., 1988). Ideally, the child's communicative intents and functions

should be coded as they emerge from the situation, rather than forcing data into predetermined categories. In practicality, most clinicians do use predetermined categories. Tables 8.3 and 8.4 in this chapter can be used as checklists. A notation should be made each time a communicative behavior occurs. When using predetermined checklists, however, one should not feel compelled to make the child's responses fit the predetermined categories. The clinician should add new categories as necessary to explain the data.

In a completely naturalistic evaluation, children may not show the full range of intentionality that they are capable of. For this reason, one might want to structure the environment and interactions to trigger particular communicative functions. The activity may be loosely structured in that the adult selects the materials and may make leading comments or openended comments that could lead the child into using a particular communicative function. Shulman (1986) suggested some guidelines evaluators should consider when obtaining a language sample for analysis of communicative behaviors:

1. Avoid using direct questions that interrupt a child's activities.

2. Interact at the child's play and language level during the experience—act as the child's playmate.

3. Use open-ended questions (e.g.,

What would happen if. . . .), directives, (*tell me about . . .*) and conversational place-holders (*uh-huh, oh, hmmm, I see*) to maintain the flow of the conversation.

4. Avoid games, puzzles, and picture books that tend to elicit a narrow or routine set of utterances.

5. Select materials that allow for a child to construct a variety of relationships and meanings (playsets such as farms, airports, hospital, et cetera, with animals and bendable people are particularly useful).

As adults play with the child, they may attempt to trigger requesting by not providing all the parts of a toy that are necessary, predicting by commenting, I wonder what the fireman will do, or projecting feelings by commenting, I wonder how the baby feels, et cetera.

The evaluator may want to use even greater structure and plan to present specific activities and interactions that might trigger specific communicative intentions. For young or impaired children Wetherby and Prutting (1984) suggested activities that might tempt the child to communicate. Some of their suggestions include the following:

1. Eating a desired food in front of a child without offering any.

2. Activating a toy, letting it wind down, and then handing it to the child.

3. Opening a jar of bubbles, blowing some, and then closing the jar tightly and giving it to the child.

4. Initiating a pleasurable social game that the child enjoys; when child is showing enjoyment, stopping the activity and waiting.

5. Placing the child's hands in a cold, wet, or sticky substance such as jello, pudding, or paste.

6. Engaging child in putting together a puzzle; after child has put in several pieces, offering one that does not fit.

7. Waving bye to an object when removing it from the play area. Repeating twice more with another toy and then doing nothing when removing a fourth toy.

Preschool and school-age children's communicative intentions can also be evaluated through the use of observational checklists. The scale in Table 8.6 developed by Erickson (1986) assesses both speech acts/communicative functions and discourse skills. Children in school should be observed in several contexts (reading class, math class, cafeteria, playground) and with both adults and peers.

The intent or function of a gesture or verbalization cannot be determined from the child's behavior alone. One must also take into account other aspects of the situation and the communicative context. Wetherby and Prizant (1989) proposed several factors to consider in determining communication intentions and functions while noting both the nonverbal, as well as the verbal, aspects of the interactions and the linguistic and nonlinguistic context of the communication. What occurred prior to or following the behavior? How does the act relate to what came before and after? Does it repeat a prior behavior, respond to it, provide further information, et cetera? Did the child give clues that he was attempting to communicate; for example, did he orient his body to another person, look toward another, or attempt to clarify a behavior? Following the child's behavior, did he wait as though expecting a response?

Interviews

A formal observational evaluation—whether it be nonstructured or structured—can be quite useful, but does not tell about the variety and consistency of a child's behaviors in familiar environments. Although it may be possible to conduct an evaluation in the child's home or in the classroom, it is not possible to follow children in every aspect of their daily lives. Interviewing of significant others in children's lives can provide one with information regarding how children actually use their language. Schuler, Peck, and Willard (1989) proposed an interview format for five communicative functions that appear early in children's repertoires: (1) requests for affection/interaction, (2) requests for adult actions, (3) requests for ob-

Table 8.6   *Observational Analysis of Communicative Competence*

Client _____   Clinician _____   Date(s)_____

Naturalistic Evaluation Circumstances: Interactors: _____

   Setting(s) _____

   Topic(s) _____

I. Discourse skills

   Starts a conversation

   Shows listening behavior

   Passes turns

   Receives turns/follows

   Responds with appropriate content

   Interrupts legitimately

   Stays on topic

   Changes topic appropriately

   Appropriately ends conversation

   Recognizes listener's viewpoint

   Demonstrates topic relevancy

   Uses appropriate response length

   Comments and examples of inappropriate conversational styles:

II. Speech Acts/Communicative Functions

   Labels things/actions

   Asks for things/actions

   Describes things/actions

   Asks for information

   Gives information

   Asks permission

   Promises

   Agrees

   Threatens

   Warns

   Apologizes

   Protests/argues/disagrees

   Shows humor/teases

   Gives greetings and leavings

   Pleads

   Commands/orders

   Comments and examples of inappropriate language usage:

jects, food, (4) protests, and (5) declaratives/comments. The range of possible communicative behaviors are described. Such intentional behaviors may include crying, pulling another's hand, touching/moving another's face, grabbing, walking away, vocalizing, pointing, facial expression, shaking head yes or no, echoing something someone else said, using a single word or single sign, and using phrase or sign combinations. Specific situations are presented and the adult is asked to describe what the child would do. Table 8.7 presents the cue questions and situations.

Standardized Tests

Standardized tests are useful when there is a need to compare an individual or group with some standard, as for example, screening students at risk for communication deficits. Formal, standardized tests may also be more time efficient than observational approaches. The use of standardized tests for evaluating pragmatics is, however, controversial. Adults have control in testlike situations, and, consequently, children may not produce the same types and range of communicative intentions they may produce in more natural situations. This is particularly true for children who are unfamiliar with testlike situations and unfamiliar with the examiner-examinee role in testing (Westby, 1994). A diagnosis of communicative impairment or a plan for an intervention program should not be based solely on a test score, but a poor test performance may suggest those students who are at risk for communicative difficulties in mainstream environments.

Standardized tests of pragmatics may use structured or scripted interactions or require judgements of what should be said in particular situations. The *Test of Pragmatic Skills* (Shulman, 1986) is designed for children 3 years to 8 years of age. The child participates in four guided play interactions through which pragmatic behaviors are assessed. The examiner introduces the child to puppets and engages the child in a conversation about a favorite TV show, requests that the child complete a drawing task, carries out a conversation with the child on two toy telephones, and interacts with the child during a block-building activity. The test provides the examiner with a script to follow that should engage the child and trigger communication for greeting, answering, informing, requesting, naming, calling, and rejecting (Table 8.8).

The *Communication and Symbolic Behavior Scales* (CSBS) (Wetherby & Prizant, 1990) combines the benefits of naturalistic observations with the advantages of a standardized test. It can be used with children functioning in the 8- to 24-month developmental range. It is designed to be used for identification of infants and toddlers who have, or are at-risk for developing, communication impairment; to establish a profile of communication, symbolic, and affective functioning; to provide directions for further assessment; to plan intervention; and to monitor changes in abilities over time (Prizant & Wetherby, 1990). The CSBS uses a standardized but flexible format that includes a parent interview; a direct, elicited sample of nonverbal and/or verbal communication (using communicative temptations as described by Wetherby and Prutting, 1984); and observation of relatively unstructured play activities. The assessment battery provides the examiner with information regarding the child's range of communicative functions, the systems the child uses to convey intention, repair strategies the child uses when efforts to express intentions are unsuccessful, and the child's signaling of social affect through gaze and positive and negative affect.

Emotional Awareness and Theory of Mind

The assessments discussed so far have focused on the nature of the parent-child interaction and the language functions (reasons for communicating) used by the child. Because intersubjectivity (the ability to appreciate the emotions, intentions, and beliefs of others) is so critical to the social basis of communication, it is useful to eval-

Table 8.7   *Cue Questions for Communicative Function*

1. Requests for affections/interaction: What if child wants:

   Adult to sit near?

   Peer to sit near?

   Nonhandicapped peer to sit near?

   Adult to look at him?

   Adult to tickle him?

   To cuddle/embrace?

   To sit on adult's lap?

   Other:

2. Requests for adult action: What if child wants:

   Help with dressing?

   To read a book?

   To play ball/a game?

   To go outside?

   Other:

3. Requests for object, food, or things: What if child wants:

   An object out of reach?

   A door/container opened

   A favorite food?

   Music/radio/TV?

   Keys/toys/book?

   Other:

4. Protest: What if

   Common routine is dropped?

   Favorite toy/food is taken away?

   Taken for ride with/without desire?

   Adult terminates interaction?

   Required to do something doesn't want to?

5. Declaration/Comment: What if child wants:

   To show you something?

   You to look at something?

   Other:

Table 8.8   *Script from Test of Pragmatic Skills Revised*

Examiner Probe	Sample Response	Observe For
(Clinician gives a toy telephone to the child).		
1. Let's talk on these telephones. Rrrring!	Hello	Greeting
2. Hi! How are you?	Fine	Answering/responding
	Okay	Answering/responding
3. Tell me about what you did today.	I played with my toys.	Informing
	I went to school.	Informing
	Play with the ball.	Informing
4. Guess what?	What?	Requesting information

uate children's abilities to recognize and interpret the emotions and beliefs of others. One should expect the majority of 4 year olds to be able to identify the expressions of happy, mad, sad, surprised, and afraid, and by ages 4 or 5 years they should be able to match expressions to situations that would cause the expressions (Michaelson & Lewis, 1985). One can ask children to identify emotions of characters in wordless picture books such *as One Frog Too Many* (Mayer & Mayer, 1975) or *A Boy, A Dog, and A Frog* (Mayer, 1967); videos such as *Max the Mouse* (1989); or interactive computer story programs such as *The Berenstein Bears Have a Fight*. Videos and interactive computer programs provide additional movement and sound cues that signal emotions. One can also ask the child why the characters feel as they do and what they might do next. By 8 years of age the majority of children should be able to explain the reasons for the feelings and to predict what the characters will do in response to the emotion.

A number of strategies have been used to assess children's theory of mind, that is, their awareness and understanding of mental states in themselves and others. Children must understand that one can know only if one has been provided with information, either directly by seeing, hearing, or touching or indirectly by being told information from someone else.

One can only remember or forget if one knew something originally. Understanding of these metacognitive terms such as knowing, remembering, forgetting, and guessing can be assessed with tasks such as the following (Wellman, 1985):

• Ernie (puppet) puts its coat in one of two closets. Ernie leaves and then comes back and correctly chooses the closet with the coat.

Ask the child: Did Ernie remember? Did Ernie forget? Did Ernie guess?

• Bert puts Ernie's coat in one of two closets when Ernie is not watching. Later when Ernie needed his coat, he went to the correct closet.

Ask: Did Ernie remember? Did Ernie forget? Did Ernie guess?

Understanding of these basic mental processes is essential if a child is to make predictions about what people will do in particular situations. The following tasks can be used to assess children's understanding of how persons' beliefs affect their behavior (Perner, Frith, Leslie, & Leekman, 1989):

Implicit False-Belief Task

The adult produces a Smarties box (candy) from her bag and asks the child, "What do you think is in here?" (Expected answer: Smarties). The adult opens the box, but the contents are not Smarties

(Adult: No, look, there are colored pencils).
She puts the pencils back in the box, closes
the box, and then asks two prompt ques-
tions (reality prompt—What's in here [pen-
cils]; and memory prompt—When I first
asked you, what did you say? [Smarties]

Then the child is asked about the next
child to come into the room (Who will come
after you?). The adult then follows with
she/he hasn't seen this box. When she/he
comes in, I"ll show her/him the box just like
this and ask what's in here? (Prediction
prompt—What will (name) say? [correct an-
swer: Smarties]; then a reality check—Is that
what's really in the box? [correct answer:
No]. What's really in the box? [correct an-
swer: pencils]; than a memory check—Do
you remember when I took the box out of my
bag and asked you what was in it, what did
you say? [correct answer: Smarties].

The child must understand that he or
she has information that is not known to
the next child. The next child's behavior
will be directed by a false belief. Typically developing 5 year olds from high-
print homes respond correctly to these
false-belief tasks. A large number of
children with autism, even at much older
ages, have difficulty with false-belief
tasks.

PHILOSOPHY OF INTERVENTION FOR SOCIAL-COMMUNICATIVE DEFICITS

Current intervention approaches for
social-communicative deficits use a
functional or naturalism/ecology-based
framework (Hayes, Ladzik, & Healy,
1982; Hunt & Goetz, 1988; MacDonald,
1989; Manolson, 1985; McLean & Snyder-McLean, 1978). Three aspects of the
social use of language are essential components of these language-intervention
programs: the social context in which intervention occurs, the embedding of communicative goals and objectives in daily
activities, and the inclusion of caregivers
(or children's significant others [SOs]—
parents, siblings, grandparents, and
teachers) in the intervention. Some programs such as the Ecological Communi-

cation Organization (ECO) Program
(McDonald, 1989) and the Hanen Early
Language Parent Program (Manolson,
1985) focus on intervention with family
members. Other approaches such as the
milieu approach and the activity-based
approach are two naturalistic intervention
strategies that have been widely used in
infant, toddler and preschool programs.
Milieu teaching uses everyday instances
of social-communicative exchanges as opportunities to teach elaborated language
and capitalizes on natural consequences as
reinforcers (Kaiser, Henderson & Alpert,
1991). Activity-based intervention is similar to milieu teaching, but is often directed to a group rather than an individual child and addresses all aspects of
development, not just communication
(Bricker & Cripe, 1992). Ecologically
based programs such as these have some
common assumptions:

1. SOs are facilitators, not trainers.
The significant others in the child's life
are language facilitators, not language
trainers. As a facilitator they do not teach
or control interactions with demands or
questions. Instead, they follow the child's
lead. For children who do not yet intentionally communicate, SOs imitate the infants' behavior. The facilitator looks for
behaviors in the child and responds appropriately to the content and intent of
the child's behavior. The child controls
and initiates the conversational topics.
The SO's job is to reinforce and maintain
the communication naturally by responding in semantically and pragmatically
contingent ways. Responses to children's
behavior should be natural consequences.
Thus a request for a cookie should be followed by giving the cookie and by words
such as *Ok*, or *just one*, or *what kind*, but
not by *good talking*.

2. Interactions should be contextualized and familiar. The learning context
should be meaningful to the child. Facili-
tory activities should occur in natural encounters throughout the day in the child's
usual environments with familiar people
and materials, not in contrived, therapeutic settings.

The goals for children with social-communicative deficits are as follows:

1. To establish interactional functions. Turn taking is essential for communication. SOs begin to establish turn-taking routines by attending to a child's behavior, responding to it, pausing and waiting for the behavior to recur, and then responding again. Turn taking can occur in games in which the SO nuzzles the infant; stops; watches for the infant to smile, vocalize, or laugh; and then nuzzles the infant again; or it can occur in play exchanges in which the SO and child roll a car back and forth, take turns stacking blocks, or take turns placing rings on a stand or dropping blocks in a bottle.

2. To establish a clear intentional signaling system. SOs treat an observed infant behavior as intentional (even when it is not) and respond accordingly. If the infant looks toward a toy, the SO may say, *You want your teddy. Here it is,* as she brings the toy to the infant. If the infant moves its arms, the SO may say, *You want up,* raise the infant's arms, and then pick the infant up. When adults respond consistently to children's behavior, children discover that they have an effect on their environment, and in time their gestures and sounds acquire meaning because they elicit a predictable response.

3. To develop socially appropriate and conventionalized signals. Once the child is indicating intentions through gaze, vocalizations, or reaching, the adult begins to shape the behaviors by modeling appropriate gestures and words.

4. To increase the variety and frequency of communicative intentions. As the child becomes successful in indicating intentionality, SOs provide communicative temptations that will encourage active participation of the child.

Highly routinized sequences of behavior have been shown to promote the development of intentional communication (Goetz, Gee, & Sailor, 1985). A strategy termed *interrupted behavior chain* can be used to trigger communicative behaviors. The SO participates with the child in a familiar activity such as eating cereal, washing hands, or putting a doll to bed. The SO interrupts the behavior chain by delaying presentation of an item necessary for completion of the routine, placing a needed item just out of the child's reach, or preventing the child from obtaining the desired object or person (by holding an object down, stepping back out of the child's reach, preventing the child from going outside by putting hand on child). For example, the child may begin the hand-washing activity by turning on the water, picking up the soap, and getting his hands wet and soapy. The adult may then turn off the water before the child rinses her hands. Because the routine is highly familiar, the child may comment that she has not rinsed her hands or that her hands are sticky or may request that the water be turned back on. Adults must be conscious of a wide range of communicative functions and model them contingently in response to the child's behavior.

CONCLUSION

Communication is basic in the sharing of affect. Children will not use semantics and syntax meaningfully if they do not develop goals to share their emotional responses. To facilitate development of the social-emotional bases of communication, adults must be alert to children's emotional cues and respond to them in such a way that children discover they can influence their environments. Linguistic skills are then superimposed on this social-cognitive understanding.

REFERENCES

Alessandri SM, Lewis M. Development of the self-conscious emotions in maltreated children. In: Lewis M, Sullivan MW, eds. Emotional development in atypical children. Mahwah, NJ: Erlbaum, 1996.

Anderson NB, Battle DE. Cultural diversity in development of language. In: Battle DE, ed. Communication disorders in multicultural populations. Boston: Andover, 1993.

Anderson GM, Hoshino Y. Neurochemical studies of autism. In: Cohen DJ, Donnellan AM, eds. Handbook of autism and pervasive developmental disorders. New York: Wiley, 1987.

Austin J. How to do things with words. Cambridge, MA: Harvard University Press, 1962.

Baker L, Cantwell DP. A prospective psychiatric follow-up of children with speech/language disorders. J Am Acad Child Adolesc Psychiatry 1987;26:546–553.

Baron-Cohen S. Mindblindness. Cambridge, MA: MIT Press, 1995.

Bartolucci G, Pierce SJ, Streiner D. Cross-sectional studies of grammatical morphemes in autistic and mentally retarded children. J Autism Dev Disord 1980;10:39–50.

Bates E. Language in context. New York: Academic Press, 1976.

Bates E, Bretherton I, Beeghly-Smith M, McNew S. Social bases of language development: a reassessment. In: Reese HW, Lipsett LP, eds. Advances in child development and behavior. Vol. 16. New York: Academic Press, 1982; pp. 7–75.

Bates JE. Temperament in infancy. In: Osofsky JD, ed. Handbook of infant development. 2nd ed. New York: Wiley, 1987.

Bell RQ. A reinterpretation of the direction of effects in studies of socialization. Psychol Rev 1968;75:81–95.

Bloom L. Developments in expression: affect and speech. In: Stein NL, Leventhal B, Trabasso T, eds. Psychological and biological approaches to emotion. Hillsdale, NJ: Erlbaum, 1990.

Bloom L. The transition from infancy to language: acquiring the power of expression. New York: Cambridge University Press, 1993.

Blout BG. Culture and language socialization: parent speech. In: Wagner DA, Stevenson HW, eds. Cultural perspectives on child development. San Francisco: Freeman, 1982.

Blurton-Jones NG. Nonverbal communication in children. In: Hinde R, eds. Nonverbal communication. Cambridge: Cambridge University Press, 1972.

Boucher J. Articulation in early childhood autism. J Autism Child Schizophr 1976;6:297–302.

Bretherton I. Intentional communication and the development of an understanding mind. In: Frye D, Moore C, eds. Children's theories of mind. Hillsdale, NJ: Erlbaum, 1991.

Bretherton I, Beeghly M. Talking about internal states: the acquisition of an explicit theory of mind. Dev Psychol 1982;18:906–921.

Bricker D, Cripe JJ. An activity-based approach to early intervention. Baltimore: Paul Brookes, 1992.

Briggs CL. Learning how to ask: native metacommunicative competence and the incompetence of fieldworkers. Lang Soc 1984;13:1–28.

Brinton B, Fujiki M. Language, social skills, and socioemotional behavior. Lang Speech Hear Serv Sch 1993;24:194–198.

Brockman LM, Morgan GA, Harmon RJ. Mastery motivation and developmental delay. In: Wachs TD, Sheehan R, eds. Assessment of young developmentally disabled children. New York: Plenum, 1988.

Bruner J. The social context of language acquisition. Lang Commun 1981;1:155–178.

Bruner J. Child's talk. New York: WW Norton, 1983.

Bruner J. Actual minds, possible worlds. Cambridge, MA: Harvard University Press, 1986.

Chapman R. Exploring children's communicative intents. In: Miller JF, ed. Assessing language production in children. Austin, TX: Pro-Ed, 1981.

Camarata SM, Hughes CA, Ruhl KL. Mild/moderate behaviorally disordered students: a population at risk for language disorders. Lang Speech Hear Serv Sch 1988;19,:191–200.

Chess S, Thomas A. Temperament in clinical practice. New York: Guilford Press, 1986.

Chisholm JS. Navajo infancy: an ethnological study of child development. New York: Aldine, 1983.

Chomsky N. Review of *Verbal behavior* by B.F. Skinner. Language 1959;35:26–58.

Chomsky N. Aspects of a theory of syntax. Cambridge, MA: MIT Press, 1965.

Coggins TE, Carpenter RL. The communicative inventory: a system for observing and coding children's early intentional communication. Applied Psycolinguistics 1981;2:235–251.

Coggins TE, Oslwang LB, Guthrie J. Assessing communicative intents in young children: low structured observation or elicitation tasks? J Speech Hear Disord 1987;52:44–49.

Cohen DJ, Paul E, Volkman FR. Issues in the classification of pervasive developmental disorders and associated conditions. In: Cohen DJ, Donnellan AM, eds. Handbook of autism and pervasive developmental disorders. New York: Wiley, 1987.

Dewey M, Everard M. The near normal autistic adolescent. J Autism Child Schizophr 1974;4:348–356.

Dore J. Holophrases, speech acts and language universals. J Child Lang 1975;2:21–40.

Dore J. Requestive systems in nursery school conversations: analysis of talk in its social context. In: Campbell R, Smith P, eds. Recent advances in the psychology of language: language development and mother-child interaction. Plenum Press: New York, 1978.

Dore J. The development of conversational competence. In: Schiefelbusch R, ed. Language competence: assessment and intervention. San Diego: College-Hill, 1986.

Dunn J, Bretherton I, Munn P. Conversations about feeling states between mothers and their young children. Dev Psychol 1987;23:132–139.

Dunst CJ, McWilliam RA. Cognitive assessment of multiply handicapped young children. In: Wachs TD, Sheehan R, eds. Assessment of young developmentally disabled children. New York: Plenum, 1988.

Erickson JG. Analysis of communicative competence. In: Cole L, Deal V, eds. Communication disorders in multicultural populations. Washington, DC: American Speech-Language-Hearing Association, 1986.

Ervin-Tripp S, Gordon D. The development of

requests. In: Schiefelbusch RL, ed. Language competence: assessment and intervention. San Diego: College-Hill, 1986.

Field T. (1987). Affective and interactive disturbances in infants. In: Osofsky JD, ed. Handbook of infant development. New York: Wiley, 1987.

Field T, Sostek AM, Vietze P, Leiderman PH. Culture and early interactions. Hillsdale, NJ: Erlbaum, 1981.

Fujiki M, Brinton B, Todd CM. Social skills of children with specific language impairment. Lang Speech Hear Serv Sch 1996;27:195–202.

Gibson EJ, Spelke E. The development of perception. In: Flavell JH, Markman EM, eds. Handbook of child psychology. Vol. III. Cognitive development. New York: Wiley, 1983.

Giddan JJ. School children with emotional problems and communication deficits: implications for speech-language pathologists. Lang Speech Hear Serv Sch 1991;22:291–295.

Gleason JB, Hay D, Cain L. Social and affective determinants of language acquisition. In: Rice ML, Schiefelbusch RL, eds. The teachability of language. Baltimore: Paul Brookes, 1989.

Goetz L, Gee K, Sailor W. Using a behavior chain interruption strategy to teach communication skills to students with severe disabilities. J Assoc Pers Severe Handicaps 1985;10:21–30.

Golden GS. Neurological functioning. In: Cohen DJ, Donnellan AM, eds. Handbook of autism and pervasive developmental disorders. New York: Wiley, 1987.

Gordon D, Ervin-Tripp S. Structure of children's requests. In: Schiefelbusch RL, Pickar J, eds. The acquisition of communicative competence. Baltimore: University Park Press, 1984.

Greenfield PM, Cocking RR. Cross-cultural roots of minority child development. Hillsdale, NJ: Erlbaum, 1994.

Greenfield P, Smith J. The structure of communication in early language development. New York: Academic Press, 1976.

Greenspan S. Infancy and early childhood: the practice of clinical assessment and intervention with emotinoal and developmental challenges. Madison, CT: International Universities Press, 1992.

Greenspan S. The growth of the mind: and the endangered origins of intelligence. Reading, MA: Addison-Wesley, 1997.

Greenspan S, Greenspan ND. First feelings. New York: Penguin, 1985.

Hale-Benson J. Black children: their roots, culture and learning styles. Baltimore: Johns Hopkins University Press, 1986.

Halliday MAK. Learning how to mean: explorations in the development of language. London: Edward Arnold, 1975.

Harris PL. Children and emotion: the development of psychological understanding. New York: Basil Blackwell, 1989.

Harris P. Pretending and planning. In: Baron-Cohen S, Tager-Flusberg H, Cohen DJ, eds. Understanding other minds: perspectives from autism. New York: Oxford University Press, 1993.

Hart B, Risley TR. Meaningful differences in the everyday experiences of young children. Baltimore: Paul Brookes, 1985.

Hayes S, Ladzik K, Healy L. Conestoga language interaction program. Tucson: Communication Skill Builders, 1982.

Heath SB. Ways with words. Cambridge: Cambridge University Press, 1983.

Hewitt LE. Narrative comprehension: the importance of subjectivity. In: Duchan JF, Hewitt LE, Sonnenmeier RM, eds. Pragmatics: from theory to practice. Englewood Cliffs, NJ: Prentice-Hall, 1994.

Hinde R. On describing relationships. J Child Psychol Psychiatry 1976;17:1–19.

Hobson RP. Autism and the development of mind. Hillsdale, NJ: Erlbaum, 1990.

Hunt P, Goetz L. Teaching spontaneous communication in natural settings through interrupted behavior chains. Top Lang Disord 1988;9:58–71.

Hurtig R, Ensrud S, Tomblin JB. Question production in autistic children: a linguistic pragmatic perspective. Paper presented at the University of Wisconsin Symposium on Research in Child Language Disorders, Madison, WI, 1980.

Kaiser AP, Yoder PJ, Keetz A. Evaluating milieu teaching. In: Warren SF, Reichle J, eds. Causes and effects in communication and language intervention. Baltimore: Paul Brookes, 1992.

Klein MD, Briggs MH. Observation of communicative interaction. Los Angeles, CA: California State University, 1987.

Lamb M. The effects of social context on dyadic social interaction. In: Lamb M, Suomi S, Stephenson G, eds. Social interactions analysis. Madison: University of Wisconsin Press, 1979.

Lamb M. The development of social expectations in the first year of life. In: Lamb M, Sherrod L, eds. Infant social cognition. Hillsdale, NJ: Erlbaum, 1981.

Leslie AM. Pretense and representation: the origins of "theory of mind." Psychol Rev 1987;94:41.

Lord C. The complexity of social behavior in autism. In: Baron-Cohen S, Tager-Flusberg H, Cohen DJ, eds. Understanding other minds: perspectives from autism. New York: Oxford University Press, 1993.

Loveland KA, Landry SH, Hughes SO, et al. Speech acts and the pragmatic deficits of autism. J Speech Hear Res 1988;31:593–604.

Lynch EW, Hanson MJ. Developing cross-cultural competence. Baltimore: Paul Brookes, 1992.

Max in Motion/Adventuresome Max. Chicago, IL: SVE Videoplus 1989.

MacDonald JD. Becoming partners with children: from play to conversation. San Antonio: Special Press, 1989.

Manolson A. It takes two to talk: a Hanen early language parent guide book. Toronto: Hanen Early Language Resource Centre, 1985.

Mayer M. A boy, a dog and a frog. New York: Dial Press, 1967.

Mayer M, Mayer M. One frog too many. New York: Dial Press, 1975.

McGurk H. Effective motivation and the development of communicative competence in blind children. In: Mills AE, ed. Language acquisition in the blind child: normal and deficient. San Diego: College-Hill, 1983.

McLean JE, Snyder-McLean LK. A transactional approach to early language training. Columbus: Merrill, 1978.

Meltzoff A, Moore W. Imitation of facial and manual gestures by human neonates. Science 1977;198:75–78.

Miller PJ. Amy, Wendy, and Beth: learning language in Baltimore. Austin, TX: University of Texas Press, 1979.

Mulford R. Referential development in blind children. In: Mills AE, ed. Language acquisition in the child: normal and deficient. San Diego: College-Hill, 1983.

Mundy P, Sigman M, Ungerer J, Sherman T. Defining the social deficits of autism: the contribution of nonverbal communication measures. J Psychol Psychiatry 1986;27:657–669.

Ninio A, Bruner JS. The achievement and antecedents of labelling. J Child Lang 1978;5:1–15.

Nugent JK, Lester BM, Brazelton TB. The cultural context of infancy: biology, culture, and infant development. Norwood, NJ: Ablex, 1989.

Ochs E. Talking to children in Western Samoa. Lang Soc 1982;11:77–104.

Ornitz EM. Neurophysiologic studies of infantile autism. In: Cohen DJ, Donnellan AM, eds. Handbook of autism and pervasive developmental disorders. New York: Wiley, 1987.

Paccia-Cooper J, Curcio F, Sacharko G. A comparison of discourse features in normal and autistic language. Paper presented at the Boston University Child Language Conference, Boston, 1981.

Paul R. Communication. In: Cohen DJ, Donnellan AM, eds. Handbook of autism and pervasive developmental disorders. New York: Wiley, 1987.

Perner J, Frith U, Leslie A, Leekam S. Exploration of the autistic child's theory of mind: knowledge, belief, and communication. Child Dev 1989; 60:689–700.

Perry PD. Incubated in terror: neurodevelopmental factors in the "cycle of violence." In: Osofsky JD, ed. Children in a violent society. New York: Guilford, 1997.

Prizant BM, Wetherby AM. Assessing the communication of infants and toddlers: integrating a socioemotional perspective. Zero to Three: Bull Natl Center Clin Infant Prog 1990;11:1–12.

Robson KS. The role of eye-to-eye contact in maternal attachment behavior. J Child Psychol Psychiatry 1967;8:13–25.

Rutter M. Diagnosis and definition. In: Rutter M, Schopler E, eds. Autism: a reappraisal of concepts and treatment. New York: Plenum, 1978.

Rutter M, Garmezy N. Developmental psychopathology. In: Hetherington EJ, ed. Handbook of child psychology. Vol. IV. Socialization, personality, and social development. New York: Wiley, 1983.

Scarr S. Testing for children: assessment and the many determinants of intellectual competence. Psychol Rev 1981;66:297–323.

Schaffer HR. Mothering. London: Open Books, 1977.

Schaffer HR. The child's entry into a social world. New York: Academic Press, 1984.

Schieffelin BB, Eisenberg AR. Cultural variation in children's conversation. In: Schiefelbusch RL, Pickar J, eds. The acquisition of communicative competence. Baltimore: University Park Press, 1984.

Schuler AL, Peck CA, Willard C, Theimer K. Assessment of communicative means and functions through interview: assessing the communicative capabilities of individuals with limited language. Semin Speech Lang 1989;10:51–62.

Sherrod LR. Issues in cognitive-perceptual development: the special case of social stimuli. In: Lamb ME, Sherrod LR, eds. Infant social cognition: empirical and theoretical approaches. Hillsdale, NJ: Erlbaum, 1981; pp. 11–36.

Shulman B. Test of pragmatic skills—Revised. Tucson: Communication Skill Builders, 1986.

Sigman M, Mundy P, Sherman T, Ungerer JA. Social interaction of autistic, mentally retarded and normal children and their caregivers. J Child Psychol Psychiatry 1986;27:647–655.

Snow CE, Ferguson CA. Talking to children: language input and acquisition. Cambridge: Cambridge University Press, 1977.

Snow CE, Goldfield B. Building stories: the emergence of information structures from conversation. In: Tannen D, ed. Analyzing discourse: text and talk. Washington, DC: Georgetown University Press, 1981.

Stern D. The first relationship: infant and mother. Cambridge, MA: Harvard University Press, 1977.

Stern DN. Diary of a baby. New York: Basic Books, 1990.

Thoman EB. Affective communication as the prelude and context for language learning. In: Schiefelbusch RL, Bricker DD, eds. Early language: acquisition and intervention. Baltimore: University Park Press, 1983.

Thomas A, Chess S. Temperament and development. New York: Brunner/Mazel, 1977.

Trager-Flusberg H. On the nature of linguistic functioning in early infantile autism. J Autism Dev Disord 1981;11:45–56.

Urwin C. Dialogue and cognitive functioning in the early development of three blind children. In: Mills AE, ed. Language acquisition in the blind child: normal and deficient. San Diego: College-Hill, 1983.

Vygotsky L. Thought and language. Translated and edited by A. Kozulin. Cambridge, MA: MIT Press, 1986.

Ward MC. Them children: a study of language learning. New York: Holt, Rinehart & Winston, 1971.

Walden TA. Communicating the meaning of events through social referencing. In: Kaiser AP, Gray DB, eds. Enhancing children's communication: research foundations for intervention. Baltimore: Paul Brookes, 1993.

Werner EE. Child care: kith, kin and hired hands. Baltimore: University Park Press, 1984.

Westby CE. Cultural differences affecting communication development. In. Cole L, Deal V, eds. Communication disorders in multicultural populations. Washington, DC: American Speech-Language-Hearing Association, 1986.

Westby CE. Multicultural issues in speech and language assessment. In: Spriesterbach D, ed. Diagnostic methods in speech and language pathology. San Diego: Singular, 1994.

Westby CE, Stevens-Domingues M, Otter P. A performance/competence model of observational assessment. Lang Speech Hear Serv Sch 1996; 27:144–156.

Westby CE. There's more to passing than knowing the answers. Lang Speech Hear Serv Sch 1997;28:274–287.

Wetherby AM, Cain DH, Yonclas DG, Walker VG. Analysis of intentional communication in normal children from the prelinguistic to multiword stage. J Speech Hear Res 1988;31:242–252.

Wetherby AM, Prizant BM. The expression of communicative intent: assessment guidelines. Semin Speech Lang 1989;10:77–91.

Wetherby AM, Prizant BM. Communication and symbolic behaviors. San Antonio: Special Press, 1990.

Wetherby AM, Prutting C. Profiles of communicative and cognitive-social abilities in autistic children. J Speech Hear Res 1984;27:364–377.

Whiting BB, Edwards CP. Children of different worlds. Cambridge, MA: Harvard University Press, 1988.

Wiig E. Let's talk inventory for adolescents. Columbus: Merrill, 1982.

Wing L. Early childhood autism. New York: Pergamon, 1976.

Yarrow LJ. Beyond cognition: the development of mastery motivation. Zero to Three: Bull Natl Center Clin Infant Prog 1981;1(3):1–4.

CHAPTER 9

Single-Word Communication: A Period of Transitions

William O. Haynes

Bloom (1973) wrote a classic volume in language development entitled *One Word at a Time: The Use of Single Word Utterances Before Syntax.* In that text she was describing a particularly fascinating period of language development when a child speaks largely in one-word utterances. It is almost as if the child has an expressive processing channel that is open only wide enough to encompass a single linguistic unit and isolated words are all that can pass from the child's mind into the environment. Another reason why this period is fascinating is because it is the first time that a child actually uses words as communicative symbols. This stage of development is especially interesting to researchers because they wonder how and why a child moves from being unable to use conventional language to being able to communicate with words. What goes on cognitively, socially, and linguistically to permit this kind of ability to develop? Although the expression of language is limited to single words, a child in the single-word period often evidences the ability to understand some connected speech and to follow directions involving more than single linguistic units (Griffiths, 1986; Leopold, 1939).

The period in which children talk in single-word utterances appears to last until the child has accumulated an expressive vocabulary of about 50 words (Nelson, 1973), and then these utterances are expanded into early word combinations. Thus the period lasts in normally developing children from about 12 months of age until the child is nearly 2 years old. Children, of course, have not read the developmental literature indicating exactly when they should enter and leave the single-word stage, so there is considerable variability among youngsters in traversing the single-word period.

It is perhaps misleading to refer to this period of development as simply the single-word stage because there is so much more going on in communication development than merely the onset of single words. As the title to the chapter indicates, this is a period of transitions, and the single-word utterance stage is only a relatively brief plateau in the child's constantly changing communication system. In actuality we can see the single-word period as being sandwiched in between two important transitional stages. Thus the single-word period is not static, but dynamic. The single-word period and the transitional stages surrounding it can be superficially sketched as follows (Fig. 9.1):

Prelinguistic →	Transition 1 →	Single-word usage →		Transition 2 →	Early multiwords
Babbling	Vocalizations stabilized in specific situations	True-word approximations		True words combined with vocalizations	True-word combinations

Figure 9.1. A period of transition.

First, a child is unable to use words to communicate or even gestures to make needs known. The child is said to have no intentionality, which means there is no attempt to communicate to solve a problem or perform a particular function. Second, the child then begins to use gestures and sometimes couples these gestures with vocalizations while interacting with others; however, no words are used. Third, the child begins to use vocalizations more consistently in certain situations, and this marks the beginning of what we will call Transition 1, or the transition before the onset of single-word speech. Fourth, the child begins to use word approximations in communicative attempts and amasses a vocabulary or lexicon of words used to perform a variety of functions. This is what most authorities call the "single-word period." Fifth, The child begins to combine various phonemes, syllables, and even some words with items from the current lexicon under the same intonation pattern. These combinations of a word and another vocalization do not necessarily qualify as two-word utterances for a variety of reasons, which we will explore later. The point here is that the child has entered Transition 2, or the movement from single words into early multiwords. Finally, the early multiword period is characterized by productive two-word combinations used for a variety of communicative functions. Thus the reader can see that the single-word period is somewhat of a misnomer in terms of what actually occurs during this time. The term makes it seem that the period is a static one in which children only use single words, and this is not true. Soon after children are competently using single words for communication, they are already beginning to transition out of this mode of communicating.

The present chapter will begin by talking about "true words" and some of the current issues surrounding the single-word period and its associated transitions. A section will be devoted to Transition 1 developments that precede the use of single-word communication. Another section will focus just on single-word communication and some issues surrounding this period such as construction of the first lexicon, overextensions/underextensions, the vocabulary spurt, cognitive influences, phonological influences, and the functions of single-word communication.

The final part of normal development will consider Transition 2 and the ways children begin to expand their single-word utterances into primitive word combinations. The last section of the chapter will be devoted to a discussion of single-word utterances in language-impaired children, to the consideration of single-word utterances in assessment, and to how this period is dealt with in language intervention.

WHAT IS A TRUE WORD

Most speech-language pathologists wish they had a dime for every parent who reported that their child spoke its first word at the age of 6 months. Parents typically scan the output of their infants with great interest early on for evidence of the first word, because this marks the beginning of verbal communication. It was Charles Van Riper who used to say that "speech is man's most human characteristic." He was probably referring to the use of speech as seen in most adults, but this message also applies to children as well. A baby truly becomes a "person" when verbal communication begins. There is an important difference, however, between a 6 month old uttering "mama" in a variety of random situations, and an adult using many words in specific, consistent, and appropriate contexts. For instance, Kamhi (1988) has written about the first-word myth in which parents report the unusually early occurrence of their child's first word. Kamhi indicates that their criteria for the first word probably are phonological and not semantic in nature. So, if a word sounds like an adult word, the child is given credit for using it even though it may have been semantically or contextually inappropriate. Thus the notion of a true word should be separate from the mere uttering of a bisyllable by an infant. In babbling, infants often approximate an adult word (e.g., "DI"), and parents might say "Didn't he just say 'dish'?" when actually it was just a phonetic accident that the child could never duplicate. Owens (1996) has suggested some criteria for true words that help us to discriminate between lucky phonetic productions, routines, and imitations. According to Owens (p. 199), a true word has to have "a phonetic relationship to some adult word" and also the child must "use the word consistently to mark a particular situation or object." These criteria rule out babbling that is not similar to adult words, and it also specifies some criterion of consistency, which indicates that the word must occur repeatedly to code a particular object or event. Thus, when we talk of the single-word period, we are referring to the point at which a child uses true words.

SOME ISSUES IN THE SINGLE-WORD PERIOD

Lest the reader believe that there are no unresolved problems in the single-word period, a little space must be devoted to dispelling this notion. The single-word period is controversial in many respects. For instance, some of the following questions plague researchers and theorists (Barrett, 1985): What is the specific relationship between babbling and words? That is, does the amount of babbling a child does, or the way it is done, relate to the types of words, syllable shapes, phonetic components of first words, or transition-1 behaviors? What is the method by which a child acquires first words, and what is the nature of their meaning? What is the relationship between cognitive attainments and the onset of first words and early word combinations? Are there certain communication functions for which first words are used and how do these relate to prelinguistic gestures? For the present, we must say that the above relationships are not known for certain; however, researchers around the world are currently exploring many interesting connections, which we will mention in the remainder of the present chapter.

PRELINGUISTIC COMMUNICATION AND TRANSITION TO SINGLE WORDS

Babbling

Although there is much that we do not know about the relationship between babbling and first words (Locke, 1987), a number of studies have shown that babbling does appear to have some connection to later speech development (Oller, 1980; Stark, 1980; Stoel-Gammon & Cooper, 1984; Boysson-Bardies, de Sagart, & Durand, 1984; Vihman, Macken, Miller, et al., 1985; Vihman, 1996; Boysson-Bardes & Vihman, 1991). Locke (1987, p. 8) indicates the following:

> There is now a fair amount of evidence that babbling and early speech often are phonetically identical (Locke, 1983, 1986, 1987; Vihman, 1986). There also is some evidence that children's early lexical targets correspond to patterns of phonetic bias detectable in the preceding stages of (late) babbling (Messick, 1984).

Some researchers divide the babbling period into prelinguistic babbling, which is prior to the onset of the first words, and postlinguistic babbling, which refers to babbling produced in the first-word period (Elbers & Ton, 1985). As mentioned above, Locke and others have suggested ties between prelinguistic babbling and early words. Several studies have examined this relationship in an unusual way by examining language development in children who have been tracheostomized prior to the onset of speech and lacked the capability of babbling, since they were breathing through a tracheal tube (Ross, 1982; Lenneberg, 1967; Simon, Fowler, & Handler, 1983; Locke, 1987). All of these studies suggested that language development was delayed in the tracheostomized children. In the Locke (1987) study the child was intubated from birth until 18 months of age and developed normally in all respects but language. When the tube was removed, the child began vocalizing in a manner similar to a child about a year younger than her chronological age. A comparable finding was reported by Lenneberg (1967). This suggests that prelinguistic babbling may involve the child practicing the use of the consonants and syllabic shapes available in its repertoire for forming first words and that the lack of this practice slows first-word acquisition. Locke (1986, p. 148) talks about more general aspects of the relationship between babbling and first words:

> What I am attempting to say is that babbling and speaking may be similar processes not merely because they share certain psychological substrates which emerge, for example, in turn-taking, but because the motives for babbling and speaking are not altogether different. Children frequently use words playfully, as in babbling, or fabricate new words with the contents of their babbling repertoire, or utter unintelligibly their best rendering of a 'standard' word . . . My contention is that babbling becomes developmentally significant when its similarity to speech is noticed by the infants themselves and by their caretakers. It is at this point, I believe, that both parties begin to do things a bit differently.

In the postlinguistic babbling period, Elbers and Ton (1985) report a reciprocal relationship between babbling and word production in that babbling does not disappear after the onset of first words.

Both babbling and word production coexist for a period that Elbers and Ton call concurrent babbling. In fact, Vihman (1986) indicates that babbling accounts for about two-thirds of vocalizations in children who have a vocabulary of over 30 words. Elbers and Ton studied a Dutch child in the concurrent period and concluded the following (1985, p. 562):

> The data and interpretations presented in the previous sections suggest that there is an interplay between both systems: words acquired by the talking system may influence and shift the course of babbling, whereas babbling in its turn may predispose the talking system towards selecting words of a certain form (i.e., towards developing "phonological preferences").

As mentioned at the beginning of this section, the research is incomplete on the exact relationship between babbling and first words; however, many studies support the notion of a continuity between these two periods, and we await more information on the issue.

Communicative Gestures

One of the most important principles that has been emphasized in the literature is the notion that function precedes form in the development of language. Most current authorities agree that children communicate via gestures and vocalizations prior to using words to fulfill these same functions (McLean & Snyder-McLean, 1978; Muma, 1986; Caselli, 1990; Morford & Goldin-Meadow, 1992). The idea that a child communicates for a particular reason is based on the assumption that the child has an intent to communicate. This notion of intentionality has been studied extensively in cognitive and pragmatic development. Bates (1976) defines the sequence of development of early communicative functions as consisting of three phases. First is the perlocutionary stage, which can be present from approximately birth to near the end of the first year. In this stage the infant primarily behaves in a particular manner, and the adult infers a communicative intent. For instance, a child looks at a toy, and the adult infers that the child wants it. Thus communication has taken place, but the child has not necessarily intended a specific message to the adult.

The second stage is the illocutionary period. In this period the child displays intentionality in communication primarily through gestures, pointing, showing objects to others, and giving objects to others. Two major reasons that children attempt to communicate are (1) to regulate joint attention and (2) to regulate joint action (Bruner, 1975). In other words, a child will repeatedly show an object to an adult to gain attention. Similarly, a child will repeat an activity (banging) and will alternate his or her gaze between the adult and the activity to gain attention. It is clear that the child's goal is to gain attention, and objects and gestures are used to accomplish this end. Bates (1976) calls this operation the protodeclarative because it is a primitive form of trying to influence the attention and attitude of an adult. The second major category of communicative function is the regulation of adult action. An example of this would be when a child wants to be picked up or have a wind-up toy activated. This type of regulation is typically seen as physical manipulation by the child (moving the adult's hand to the toy). This has been called the *protoimperative* by Bates (1976). A major difference in this stage (illocutionary) from the prior one (perlocutionary) is that the child has clear intention to communicate, and it is not merely an adult inferring a communicative intent. The illocutionary stage is typically characterized by the child using gestural communication or using gestures accompanied by vocalizations that are not necessarily correct word approximations.

Finally, there is the locutionary stage in which words replace the gestures, and the child uses oral language to manipulate adult attention and action. This would be exemplified by a child saying "up" and extending the arms toward the adult in an attempt to be picked up. Another example would be a child who points at a dog entering the back yard and says "doggie" in an attempt to regulate adult attention to the oncoming canine.

Zinober and Martlew (1985) reviewed literature and studied the development of communicative gestures in children. They found that gestures tended to revolve around four basic functions. *Expressive gestures* indicated positive and negative emotional states and were manifested in the form of arm flapping, hand clapping, foot stomping, and whole body movements such as the child propelling backward. *Instrumental gestures* were used to control the behavior of an adult and included extending arms toward an adult, alternating gaze with changing facial expression, and opening and closing the fist while reaching. *Enactive gestures* were those that symbolically represented actions of people and objects such as pretending to sleep and eat. These were initially associated with the child's own body and later with dolls and other people. Finally, *deictic gestures* were noted, which were largely the showing of objects to other people or pointing at an object. The first types of gestures to emerge developmentally were expressive and instrumental. Eventually, all of these gesture types are coordinated with vocalizations, and, finally, words supersede the gesture system or at least accompany these movements. Zinober and Martlew (1985) noted that the children they studied combined vocalizations with gestures in all categories except deictic starting at the age of 10 months. Deictic pointing at age 9 months was typically not accompanied by vocalization, but by 14 months there was coordination. Pointing has perhaps been the gestural type that has been linked most closely with the onset of language, and communicative pointing has been viewed by some as a strong predictor of the onset of single-word usage (Bates, et al., 1980; Zinober & Martlew, 1985). Masur (1980, 1983) suggests that single-word usage may not occur until the child has coordinated two nonverbal behaviors. An example might be to point at an object while alternating gaze between parent and the object of interest.

The basic progression that occurs in normally developing children therefore, is that the flow of intentional communication begins around 8 months of age with gestures being the predominant response mode. The gestures then become paired with vocalizations, and, finally, the vocalizations and some gestures are replaced by or occur concomitantly with early single words. In a chapter on single words it might seem strange to speak first of gestural communication, but much research supports a basic continuity between these earlier modes and the use of single words (Bates, et al., 1975, 1980; Lock, 1978).

Prelexical Transition Utterances

As we mentioned in the introduction, children progress from a period of babbling to a point at which they begin to stabilize certain vocalizations around specific situations, events, and objects. These vocalizations have been called various names by researchers, including the following: "protowords" (Halliday, 1975), "prelexical forms" (Bates, 1976), "phonetically consistent forms" (Dore, Franklin, Miller, & Ramer, 1976), "vocables" (Creaghead, 1989), and "sensorimotor morphemes" (Carter, 1979). These vocalizations do not meet the criteria for classification as true words because they may not resemble adult productions. Prelexical transition utterances are more associated with a situation than a particular referent. They are regarded by many as simply a part of an activity rather than language that is referential in nature.

Some examples of prelexical utterances are provided by Dore et al. (1976) in which these vocalizations are called "phonetically consistent forms" (PCF). Dore et al. indicate that these forms have the following characteristics: (1) they are isolatable units bounded by pauses, (2) they occur repeatedly, (3) they are correlated with recurring conditions, and (4) they are phonetically more stable than babbling but not as stable as word productions. One example of a PCF is an "affect expression" in which a child stabilizes a vocalization around an emotional reaction such as anger, frustration, joy, protest, or some other affective situation. It is important to note that these PCFs are not necessarily to be construed as attempts at word approximation, and they

are highly individual to specific children. A child might say "na na na" every time he protests. Another child may say a different vocalization for protest, but the point is that the vocalization will be similar for each protest situation. A second PCF is an "instrumental expression" in which a child vocalizes a consistent pattern whenever he is attempting to regulate adult behavior to obtain goods or joint activity. An example would be a child who vocalizes "uh" whenever he or she is attempting to regulate an adult. Again, a child who says "uh" to be lifted up is not necessarily saying "up" because the same vocalization is produced when the adult is enlisted to open a jar or wind a toy. A final example of a PCF is an "indicating expression." The indicating expression is produced in concert with pointing where the goal is the direction of adult attention and not necessarily the regulation of action. The child may say "ba" every time he points to an object to direct adult attention. These PCFs stabilize around situations and are viewed as *part of* the situation they occur in (e.g., saying "ba" is part of the act of pointing and regulating adult attention).

Gillis and DeSchutter (1986) studied a single child during the period of using PCFs. They noted that initial acquisition of a PCF occurred in the following manner (p. 132):

> . . . someone pushes the car around and utters the PCF, then the child tries to imitate the action with the object and the PCF. So, he experiences them together in the adult model he imitates . . . so, we assume that the child at first associates a PCF with a holistic structure, called a script and the utterance of the PCF is part of the execution of the script. The execution of the script is determined by the presence in the situation of one (or more) elements of the script . . .

Gillis and DeSchutter go on to make the point that PCFs are initially part of a specific context involving both an object and an action. Later in development the child begins to generalize the PCF to similar contexts with objects and actions that bear a perceptual and functional resemblance to the original components. Also, even though the "script" for a PCF begins as a wholistic entity, the child starts to separate the function and object parts of the context as development occurs so that generalization can occur to either functionally or perceptually similar items.

Several other types of prelexical vocalizations have been reported in the literature. Peters (1977) reports "gestalts," which are multiword utterances that are stabilized around situations such as "uh-oh" and "open the door." Peters also discusses words said in the context of joint book-reading activities between parents and children; however, these responses are contextually tied to the book-reading activity and not used in other situations. Nelson and Lucariello (1985, pp. 62–63) state the following:

> We classify this kind of labeling as a third type of prelexical usage because, like the first two, its use is primarily procedural, not referential . . . There is no evidence in these exchanges that the child attaches any meaning to these labels beyond their association with the familiar routine . . . The mental representation of a lexicon requires that words be established as symbols that stand for meaning independent of the specific conditions of their use. There is little evidence that the prelexical kinds of word use described here, which occur primarily in the first half of the second year, are symbolic in this way.

Dore et al. (1976) suggest that these types of phonetically consistent forms aid the child in moving toward true language use. They provide the child with the advantage of stabilizing a vocal production around a specific situation or object, which in a basic sense is a "prerequisite" for the use of words. When we use words, we use them either in the presence of certain objects and events or to refer to these referents. When we use words, we learn that certain words can only be appropriately used with a specific range of situations. This is grossly analogous to the child's using the same vocalization for a variety of types of regulation of adult action and attention. The child has the luxury of producing these consistent vocalizations without the

complexity of applying semantic, syntactic, or phonological rules. Thus prelexical vocalizations as "procedural" rather than "referential" allow the child to inject consistent vocal behaviors into daily routines. When examined in this light, this transition appears to be part of a logical progression that a child follows on the way to becoming a verbal communicator.

SINGLE-WORD COMMUNICATION

The period of single-word communication refers to the time that children are speaking primarily "one word at a time." We can consider several aspects of this period. First, the structure of the early lexicon can be described as to the types of words present and what linguistic catagories they represent. Second, a cross-cultural perspective will be presented that compares lexicons of children from around the world. This will give some insight into any consistent commonalities in development of the first lexicon and also bear on various theories about why children initially develop the types of words they do. Third, the functions of these single-word communications can be analyzed in terms of the communicative intents children use early word forms to fulfill. Fourth, the phenomenon of the "vocabulary spurt" will be reexamined. Fifth, the nature of children's overextensions and underextensions will be discussed. Finally, phonological influences on the first lexicon will be addressed. Much data exist on each topic. For instance, an entire chapter of the present textbook could be devoted just to the literature on overextensions and the theories proposed to account for them.

Structure of the First Lexicon

Two classical studies have longitudinally examined the development of children's first vocabularies, and these investigations are mentioned in virtually every complete account of this period. Nelson (1973) followed 18 subjects from approximately the age of 1 until they were 2 years old. Part of Nelson's study focused on the point at which each child had attained a 50-word vocabulary. The mean age for acquisition of this 50-word lexicon was 19.75 months (range = 15 to 24 months). Nelson noted that the children exhibited significant variability in the length of time it took them to progress from their first word to attainment of the fiftieth vocabulary word (4 to 13 months). Thus some children accumulate lexical items rapidly, while others take more time. Benedict (1979) studied eight children from the age of 9 months until they had an MLU of 1.10 or reached the age of 2 years, whichever came first. The Nelson and Benedict studies both used similar classification schemes for the types of words used in the children's first lexicons. A third study (McGonagle, Haynes, & Haynes, 1989) also used the Nelson classification system to analyze the first 50-word lexicons of 17 children in the single-word period. The catagories (Nelson, 1973) were as follows:

1. *Specific nominals:* Refer to a specific exemplar of a category whether or not it is a proper name (e.g., mommy, daddy, pet's name, etc.).

2. *General nominals:* Refer to all members of a category and include classes such as objects, substances, animals, people, letters, numbers, pronouns, and abstractions.

3. *Action words:* Used to describe or demand an action.

4. *Modifiers:* Refer to properties or qualities of things or events such as attributes, states, locations, or possessives.

5. *Personal-social words:* Express affective states and social relationships such as assertions (e.g., no, yes, want) and social expressive words (e.g., please, ouch).

6. *Function words:* Refer to items that serve a grammatical function in relating to other words (e.g., what, is, for, to).

In examining the data from these three studies it is striking that the percentages of the children's first lexicons are remarkably similar. Table 9.1 compares the percentages of the first 50 words in each investigation that represent the categories described above.

Thus there seems to be some correspondence in the composition of the structure of early vocabularies according to these three studies. It is important to remember that these percentages refer only to the proportions of the lexicon and may not represent the actual *use* of the word types. That is, although a child's lexicon only has 9% action words, this does not mean that action words are used only 9% of the time. The small number of action words could actually be used more than words from a category that comprises a much larger percentage of the child's total vocabulary. Gopnik (1981, p. 94) studied nine children between the ages of 15 and 21 months and found the following:

> All nine children used non-nominal expressions in their earliest recorded speech. In fact, some children used non-nominals before they used names. Furthermore, non-nominal expressions were used more frequently than names in the early recordings.

There are several additional points to emphasize about the onset of single-word communication. Benedict (1979) provides a table of raw data on eight children that clearly illustrates these concepts (Table 9.2). In the table the number of

Category	Nelson (1973)	Benedict (1979)	McGonagle, Haynes, & Haynes (1989)
General nominals	51	50	50
Specific nominals	14	11	12
Action words	14	19	23
Modifiers	9	10	7
Personal-social	9	10	6
Function words	4	0	1

Table 9.1   *Structure of the First Lexicon in Three Studies (in Percent)*

Table 9.2   Data From Benedict (1979) on Single-Word Development

Number of Words	Craig		Elizabeth		Amy		Michael		Diana		William		David		Karen		Mean Age at Acquisition	
	C	P	C	P	C	P	C	P	C	P	C	P	C	P	C	P	C	P
0	0;9.0[a]	0;10.26	0;10.8	1;3.9	0;10.15	1;2.11	0;9.28	0;11.11	0;10.21	1;0.28	0;10.24	1;2.13	0;10.10	0;11.24	1;0.8	1;6.16	0;10.14	1;1.21
20	0;9.21	0;11.30	0;11.10	1;3.29	0;11.13	1;4.13	0;10.14	1;1.0	0;11.13	1;3.11	1;0.7	1;3.17	0;11.5	1;1.5	1;2.3	1;8.2	0;11.15	1;3.6
30	0;10.1	1;1.15	0;11.26	1;4.12	0;11.28	1;5.13	0;11.11	1;1.28	0;11.26	1;4.29	1;0.16	1;5.22	1;0.1	1;2.15	1;3.11	1;9.5	1;0.3	1;4.14
40	0;10.14	1;3.21	1;0.16	1;5.0	1;0.5	1;6.3	1;0.8	1;2.17	1;0.14	1;6.2	1;0.26	1;7.19	1;0.23	1;3.11	1;3.15	1;9.19	1;0.19	1;5.16
50	0;10.20	1;5.2	1;0.17[a]	1;6.0	1;0.21	1;6.29	1;0.23	1;3.0	1;1.7	1;7.1	1;1.18	1;8.20	1;1.19	1;5.5	1;4.5[b]	1;10.0	1;1.5	1;6.15
60	0;11.2	—	1;0.20	—	1;0.26	—	1;0.25[c]	—	1;2.5	—	1;2.13	—	1;3.0	d	d	—	—	—
80	1;0	—	1;1.5	—	1;0.26[c]	—	1;0.26	—	1;2.19	—	1;2.30	—	1;3.11	—	—	—	—	—
100	1;0.17	—	1;2.11	—	1;0.26	—	1;2.17	—	1;3.5	—	1;3.19	—	d	—	—	—	—	—
150	1;1.15	—	1;2.29	—	1;2.13	—	d	—	d	—	d	—	—	—	—	—	—	—
200	1;3.24	—	d	—	1;3.16	—	—	—	—	—	—	—	—	—	—	—	—	—
Words added per month	28.06	6.43	29.85	14.76	37.70	8.71	19.35	10.96	20.09	6.53	19.60	6.42	13.94	7.42	10.26	11.49	22.23	9.09

Reprinted with permission from Benedict H. Early lexical development: comprehension and production.
[a] 10 words understood prior to start of study, age is estimate based on mother's report.
[b] Karen did not reach 50 words understood by the end of the study. However, her mother continued to keep a record to 50 words understood.
[c] The introduction of the word checklist at 0;12.5 caused rapid inflation in total corpus for several of the children (notably Amy, Elizabeth, and Michael).
[d] The child did not reach this vocabulary level during the first phase of the study.

words acquired in either comprehension or production is arrayed in the left margin. Then each child's age (year, month, day) is provided for attainment of comprehension or production. For instance, Craig comprehended 50 words according to the parental diaries provided at age 10 months, 20 days. He did not produce 50 words until he was age 1 year, 5 months, and 2 days. Several things are important to notice about Benedict's data. First, there is considerable variability shown in the attainment of a productive lexicon of 50 words. Karen could produce 50 words at 22 months, while Michael could do it at 15 months. Variability is one of the striking things noted throughout the table. A second clear finding is that comprehension precedes production in single-word acquisition; also, comprehension development appears to be more rapid than production. Clearly, children are adding significantly more words to their receptive vocabularies than they are to their productive repertoires between the ages of 9 and 18 months. Early in development, comprehension appears to lead production by an approximate ratio of about 4:1 in word acquisition. The final thing to notice from the table is the difference in overall rates of development. Some children are faster than others in both comprehension and production of single words.

A Cross-Cultural Perspective

The picture that emerges from the information provided above is that children develop first lexicons that are largely composed of nouns (Bates, Marchman, Thal, et al., 1994). Gentner (1982) reported the proportions of grammatical classes in the early vocabularies of children speaking Mandarin Chinese, Japanese, Kaluli, German, English, and Turkish. In all cases the percentage of the first lexicon represented by nominals in these languages was significantly higher than other word classes (e.g., action words, modifiers, etc.). This is similar to the results of first lexicon studies in English.

There must be some reason for the preponderance of nominals in children's first lexicons cross-culturally. The fact that the high percentage of nouns is not language specific suggests that there may be some other reason to account for this observation. Gentner explored several possible language-based explanations. For instance, frequency of occurrence cannot explain why more nouns are learned. Adults use more nouns, but since there is a larger variety, they are used less frequently than the smaller group of verbs in a language (Goldfield, 1993). Thus the pattern should be reversed (more verbs than nouns) because they hear the smaller number of verbs more often than the larger number of nouns. Word order also cannot account for the high percentage of nouns. In English, nouns occupy the most salient positions in sentences (S-V-O). Cross-linguistic studies have shown that some languages such as German, Kaluli and Turkish have verb-final sentence arrangements (S-O-V; O-S-V). Yet, children learning these languages have lexicons that are predominantly made up of nominals. Another explanation is "morphological transparency," which has to do with the number of inflections that can be attached to a root word. In English there are many more word endings that can be attached to verbs as compared with nouns. Unfortunately, this argument does not hold up in accounting for the preponderance of nouns in early vocabularies because languages vary in their morphological transparency and there is still no difference in the domination of early nominals. A final explanation might lie in the way parents teach language to their children. However, in Kaluli, parents are not particularly interested in teaching object names to their children. This is in sharp contrast to English parents who emphasize object names in interactions with their children. Yet, there is little difference in the early lexicons of children from these two disparate cultures. Gentner (1982) proposes "the natural partitions hypothesis," which states among other things that there are cognitive-perceptual distinctions between nominals and verbs. Nouns represent more perceptually stable entities, and verbs represent more dynamic events. Nouns are more concrete and verbs actually presuppose nouns when we are talking about an action. The reverse may not be true. We do not know why children tend to acquire more nouns than verbs; however, the fact that most children have a preponderance of nominals in their early vocabularies has been fairly well accepted in the literature.

Functions of Single-Word Communication

The previous section concentrated on the structural components of the child's early vocabulary. This portion considers the reasons children use the lexical items that they are capable of producing. We know that children are good communicators even when they have no words at all. They exhibit a variety of communicative functions that are served at first by gestures, then by gesture plus vocalization, and, finally, by word approximations. Chapter 9 of the present volume reviews much work on the development of communicative function/intent. Basically, children use early word productions to regulate adult attention and regulate adult action. These functions of communication were previously coded using gestures such as pointing, showing, giving, or pulling. Thus it can be seen that the first lexicon is largely used to continue serving the functions of communication that have been well established during the prelinguistic period.

Overextension and Underextension

Parents and researchers have noted for years that children in the single-word period often "misuse" the words in their vocabularies. The term "misuse" is only appropriate if one subscribes to the assumption that children are attempting to use adult meanings and that their vocabularies are similar to the adult lexicon. Actually, children possess very limited vocabularies, and their meanings are not necessarily similar to those of adults. The single-word child's lexicon is in an almost continual state of flux. Thus, when a child calls a cow "doggie," he is exhibiting the limitations of his vocabulary and applying the most applicable item he has available to this new referent. It is important to also consider that a child's conceptual system is reflected in semantic organization, and if a word is "misused," it could be due to an incomplete concept of the referent just as easily as an incomplete semantic system. Thus a child may not know that cows and dogs are different animals and may make a conceptual error when calling a cow "doggie" rather than a semantic error. When a child uses a word too broadly to refer to referents that may be similar in structure or function, it is called an *overextension.* Some examples might be calling the moon a ball, or calling a strange man "daddy." On the other hand, some meanings are too narrow, and these are called *underextensions.* An example is the use of the word "car" only for a particular vehicle but not for other automobiles encountered during the day. Clark (1993) estimates that overextensions/underextensions occur frequently and can represent up to one-third of a child's early vocabulary between the ages of 1 and 2 years. As mentioned previously, the child may overextend or underextend lexical items for a variety of reasons, some of which are not semantic. For instance, Hoek, Ingram, and Gibson (1986, p. 492) studied overextensions and report six possible factors that may lead to overextensions:

> (1) the use of a known word for an unknown word; (2) the use of a known (older) word for a more recently acquired word; (3) the incomplete knowledge of the defining features of two or more similar meaning words; (4) the overextensions of a preferred word; (5) the use of a phonologically simple word (in production) for one that is more difficult; (6) the use of a word for a more natural class than the one in its adult meaning.

Although some authorities feel that overextensions are only present in the production of words and not comprehension (Fremgen & Fay, 1980; Owens, 1996), some researchers clearly report overextension in both comprehension and production (Hoek, Ingram, & Gibson (1986).

Dore (1985, p.30) discusses the stages in developing "meaningfulness" in single-word children. He indicates that, in development, the baby acquires a "series of insights" about meaning:

> (1) That his early cries, squeals, babbles, etc., are attended to and responded to in routine ways; (2) that he can produce vocal forms intentionally to indicate aspects of an activity; (3) that specific combinations of vocal forms denote classes of items in contrast to other classes; and (4) that one form class can be used to comment about another which is presumed to be shared with others.

Dore calls the first "insight" or phase mentioned above *protocommunicative signals*, which refers to vocalizations used in particular situations. These may simply be a part of a routine as opposed to manifestations of communicative intent. Table 9.3 gives some examples from Dore (1985). The second phase involves use of *indexical signs*, which were "wordlike" forms that appeared to be unstable in terms of the context in which they were used. Dore also says that indexical signs are organized into "protosemantic" domains. The indexical signs are not completely clear semantic categories as seen in Table 9.3 ("k k " is used for a variety of things ranging from a cookie to pantry doors opening or closing). The third phase is called *denotative symbols* in which words are more semantically contrastive, and the words are more "tightly organized into perceptually and functionally related sets (p. 36)." In essence, the child appears to use particular words to refer to more specific categories. This stage is associated with the vocabulary spurt, which obviously is related to the development of more linguistic diversity. The final stage involves the child using words as *predictive syntagmas*. This suggests that the child may have several appropriate words for a given occasion and chooses only one to use from this available group. For instance, a child may be able to say "doggie"

for the family pet, but elects to say "spot" (the dog's name) instead.

Several theories have been put forward that have used overextensions to support their explanations of semantic organization in single-word children. One theory is the *Semantic Feature Hypothesis* (Clark, 1973, 1975), which basically states that children classify and organize referents in terms of perceptual features such as size, shape, animateness, texture, etc. This could explain some overextensions in which a child generalizes a word based on perceptual similarity (e.g., ball—moon), but would have difficulty accounting for overextensions based on function. The other major theory involving overextensions is the *Functional Core Hypothesis* (Nelson, 1974, 1977) in which words are overextended because of the actions or functions performed on objects rather than the perceptual features of the referents. Thus a child may say the word "rake" when a person is sweeping since the actions are similar.

It is important to note that no single theory of semantic organization has been universally supported by research or descriptions of early lexicons. Criticisms of the existing theories are numerous, but each theory appears to be able to account for at least some overextensions and underextensions in early language. It is possible that a combination of existing theories may come closest to explaining early word use and organization since human behaviors, especially mental abilities, are seldom simple and unidimensional. Specific examples of overextensions and underextensions tend to support some theories and act as negative evidence for others. No one really knows what goes on in the heads of single-word children, how they mentally organize the world, or how their semantic systems really work, but these theories provide interesting insights into potential explanations.

Phonological Influences on Single-Word Usage

When children are in the single-word period they utter words that are not phonologically complete. These approxi-

Table 9.3   *Stages of Development of Meaning*

Examples of Phase 1 "protocommunicative signals" produced by a child between 11 and 15 months:

Behaviors/Tones	Interpreted Functions
Usually abrupt contour	Apparent desire or need for something
While grasping for objects	As if to point out something
Invariably successive occurrences	

Examples of "indexical signs" produced by a child between 15 and 20 months for food-related items only:

Form	Application
/ku/ /kʌkə/	Cookies, crackers, or candies; bags of other sweets or dried fruits; jars; when pantry doors are opened or closed
/baba/	Bottles and jars of liquid; glasses, cups, containers

Examples of "denotative symbols" produced by a child from 20 to 23 months:

Form	Extension
/ku/	Cookies, crackers, and potato chips
/baba/	His bottle only
tea	Cups
beer	Anything father drinks
/ænə/	Bananas; zucchini

Adapted from Dore, J. Holophrases revisited: Their "logical" development from dialog. In: M. Barrett (Ed.) *Children's single word speech.* New York: John Wiley & Sons, 1985.

mations of adult productions typically have a CV, VC, or CVCV syllable shape. The single-word child seems to have a constraint on the number of syllables that can be chained together in meaningful words that results in limited syllable shapes, typically under three syllables. The child at this stage of development has incomplete vowel and consonant systems, so words must be produced with the phones that are in the child's repertoire. The consonants and vowels typically seen in children during the single-word period (14 to 22 months) are as follows: k, g, t, d, p, b, m, n, w, h, and sometimes f and s. The vowels are /I/, /a/, and /u/ (Stoel-Gammon, 1985; Ingram, 1976; Ingram, 1981; Irwin & Wong, 1983). There is great interchild variability in the phonemes produced and the word posi-

tions in which they occur. Thus incomplete phonetic inventories account for some word approximations.

There is an extensive literature on the occurrence of phonological processes or patterns of simplification in early child language (Bernthal & Bankson, 1993; Ingram, 1976; Grunwell, 1982). It is clear that children reduce the complexity of adult productions in characteristic ways. This tendency to simplify is especially seen in early word productions and then diminishes as the child develops language (Kahn & Lewis, 1986). Some authorities and researchers have even suggested that children tend to avoid words containing phonemes that they do not have in their phonemic inventories (Reich, 1986; Ferguson & Farwell, 1975; Leonard, et al., 1982; Schwartz &

Leonard, 1982; Hoek, Ingram, & Gibson, 1986).

Thus it can be seen that children's early word productions in the single-word period will be simplified versions of the adult model. These simplifications are for the most part predictable, and the words produced are influenced by the child's particular phonetic inventory, simplification tendencies, and constraints on the developing processing systems (motoric, linguistic, memory, etc.).

Cognitive Development and First Words

Just as there appears to be a particular level of cognitive development for the onset of early gestural communication, some researchers have suggested that specific cognitive attainments may relate to the onset of single-word communication. The studies of this relationship can be categorized in a variety of ways. For instance, Bloom, Lifter, and Broughton (1985) discuss "correspondence studies" in which correspondences between language and sensorimotor behaviors are described. An example might be that the onset of single-word utterances corresponds to the successful performance of certain sensorimotor stage-V or stage-VI tasks involving object permanence, space, imitation, and causality. The other type of research on the cognition-language relationship discussed by Bloom et al. (1985) was "correlational studies." In these investigations data are gathered on children in longitudinal studies on both cognitive and linguistic development, and statistical procedures are performed to determine relationships among variables (e.g., Bates, et al., 1980).

Gopnik and Meltzoff (1986) examined the research in a slightly different manner compared with Bloom et al. (1985). These researchers discuss the cognition-language research in terms of three basic thrusts. First, there are studies in which general communicative development relates to some particular area of cognitive development. They cite as an example the Bates et al. (1980) finding that the emergence of prelinguistic communicative gestures re-

lates to the attainment of stage-V means-ends skills. A second research thrust is that general cognitive development relates to some particular linguistic development. They cite the Corrigan (1978) finding that attainment of a stage-6 sensorimotor cognitive level may be prerequisite to specific types of linguistic acquisitions (e.g., the naming explosion). A final point of view is called the "specificity hypothesis" and is promoted by Gopnik and Meltzoff (1986). This hypothesis suggests that there are certain cognitive attainments that are linked quite specifically to linguistic developments. For instance, they feel that specific object permanence acquisitions on a cognitive level are linked to the use of disappearance words such as "all gone" or "gone."

In this section we are particularly interested in the research on the cognition-language relationship that has focused on the single-word period. It seems that two major linguistic variables have received the most attention in the single-word period. These variables are (1) the onset of "first words" and (2) the occurrence of the "vocabulary spurt." These variables will be dealt with separately in the following sections.

Cognition and Onset of First Words

Piaget (1962) has indicated that children produce their first single words during stage V of the sensorimotor period. More recent investigations have also shown that single words begin to emerge when children attain stage V (Ingram, 1977; Bates, et al., 1975). Bloom et al. (1985) found first words to emerge in stage V for two of the three children studied. In the third child, first words did not develop until late stage VI. This suggests that cognitive development to the stage V level does not *ensure* that single words will be acquired and that there are both cognitive, as well as linguistic, skills to be learned by a child. In essence, stage V cognitive development may be "necessary, but not sufficient" for the development of single-word usage. Bloom et al. (1985, p. 161) indicate the following:

Ingram (1978) concluded from his review that stage 5 in general is critical for the occurrence of first words, and Harding and Golinkoff (1979) specified stage 5 causality as a prerequisite for development of the intention to communicate. Most recently, Lifter (1982) reported that two of the children she studied began to say their first words at the same time that they were performing those tasks on the Uzgiris and Hunt object permanence scale that are comparable to Piaget's late stage 5 behaviors. Different investigators, then, have observed that different kinds of elicited stage 5 behaviors (means-ends, object permanence, causality) are coextensive with the beginning of communication that is both intentional and conventional. However, we do not have, as yet, an explanatory model of what it means for stage 5 developments in sensorimotor thought to coincide with first words.

Many authors continue to report specific behaviors that appear to herald the beginning of single-word use in children. For instance, Bloom et al. (1985) noted that their three subjects engaged in "constructing" activities such as assembling nesting cups just prior to the onset of first words. As mentioned previously, Bates et al. (1980) found that the use of communicative gestures was strongly associated with the onset of first words.

The present author is unaware of any research reports of children in stage IV using words. There are many variables in the cognitive, social, temperamental, gestural, and play areas that are currently being explored by researchers. It is only through more longitudinal and cross-sectional research that specific relationships between cognitive and linguistic attainments can be more clearly delineated.

Cognition and the Vocabulary Spurt

After a child says the "first word," there is a period in which vocabulary growth is rather slow and a small lexicon of items is used repeatedly. Most children will then exhibit what has been variously referred to by researchers as a "vocabulary spurt," a "naming insight," a "nominal insight," or a "naming explosion." All of these terms refer to a discernable rapid increase in the number of words a child is using and a rise in a child's "interest" in learning words.

Researchers have defined the vocabulary spurt in slightly different ways. For instance, Bloom and Capatides (1987) indicated a vocabulary spurt had occurred when a child had an increase in at least 12 new words in a particular monthly sampling session. Gopnik and Meltzoff (1987) used a criterion of 10 new names acquired in a sampling session to indicate the presence of a naming explosion. Thus there seems to be at least some agreement not only that there is a vocabulary spurt, but that it is indicated by an increase of from 10 to 15 words between monthly sampling sessions.

Bloom and Capatides (1987) found that their 12 subjects had a mean age at first words of 13.6 months with a range of 305 to 510 days. The mean age of the onset of the vocabulary spurt was 19.6 months with a range of from 392 to 755 days. In the Gopnik and Meltzoff study of 12 children, the mean age for the naming explosion was 18.33 months with a range from 472 to 652 days. The Bloom et al. (1985) study of three children found the vocabulary spurt to occur somewhere between 16 and 20 months. McGonagle, Haynes, and Haynes (1989) studied 17 children longitudinally and found the vocabulary spurt to occur at a mean age of 16.79 months (range = 14 to 20 months). The younger ages in this study may have been due to the use of a parent questionnaire to determine use of words, while some other studies used live language sampling.

It appears therefore that the naming explosion occurs within 6 months of the first words for the average experimental subjects and that, for most children, it is likely to occur between 14 and 20 months of age. There is, of course, much variability in these developments between children. Further research can more closely pinpoint central tendency and variability data that can be applied to large groups of children for normative purposes.

Some studies have reported significant relationships between attainment of certain sensorimotor stages in object permanence/means end and the vocabulary spurt. For instance, Gopnik and Meltzhoff (1987) found a significant correlation between stage VI object-permanence ability and the age of vocabulary spurt. McGonagle et al. (1989) found significant relationships between the vocabulary spurt and both stage VI means-end and object-permanence abilities. The subjects in the Bloom et al. (1985) study all had attained stage VI object permanence prior to the onset of the vocabulary spurt.

Some researchers have noted the correspondence between specific cognitive and play acquisitions and the onset of the naming explosion. For instance, Bloom et al. (1985) found the following:

> Of all the language behaviors observed, the vocabulary spurt was most consistently related to developments in object play. For all three children, a precipitous increase in vocabulary occurred after the shift from separating activities to a balance between separating and constructing activities. The vocabulary spurt was after or coextensive with (1) the shift from predominantly given to predominantly imposed relations, (2) the transformation in the content of imposed constructing activities from general to specific relationships, and (3) an increased ability to locate objects for their constructing activities that were out of view and independent of prior action schemes.

Separating and constructing activities involved taking things apart and putting objects together (e.g., putting nesting boxes together and separating them). The researchers noted that separating activities occurred first, then constructing activities, and, finally, a balance between the two. They also noted that when children shifted from given to imposed relations, the vocabulary spurt soon followed. Given relations are the experimenter's original demonstrations of object manipulations (e.g., placing pegs in a board) and imposed relations are those that the child invents or generalizes (e.g., loading pegs into a truck). Finally, imposed activities could be general (e.g., putting a bead in a box) or specific (e.g., putting a bead on a string) in which the qualities of the two

objects are specifically related in the activity. Similar results regarding constructing activities and specific constructions were found with a larger sample of 14 children by Lifter and Bloom (1989) and with a sample of 17 children by McGonagle, Haynes, and Haynes (1989).

Another view of the vocabulary spurt is given by Gopnik and Meltzoff (1987) in which they found a relationship between active categorization and the naming explosion. Active categorization involves the child's ability to "sort objects into two spatially distinct groups, placing all the balls in one pile and all the boxes in another pile.(p. 1524)." Gopnik and Meltzoff (1987, p. 1529) conclude the following:

> There was evidence of a specific relation between the development of the highest level of categorization (level 3, two category grouping) and the development of the naming explosion. First, none of the children achieved a naming explosion before they displayed level 3 categorization. Second, children frequently developed a naming explosion very shortly after they first produced level 3 categorization. In fact, five of the 12 children first produced level 3 categorization in the very same session in which a naming explosion was first recorded. The mean gap between these two developments was only 33.17 days, suggesting that the two developments occur fairly closely together. Third, there was a large and significant correlation between the age of the naming explosion and the age of development of level 3 categorization ($r = 0.78$, $p<.005$).

McGonagle, Haynes, and Haynes (1989) also examined categorization abilities in 17 children as they related to the vocabulary spurt, using essentially the same procedure as Gopnik and Meltzoff (1987), but found no significant relationships between the two developments. While all of the subjects in the former study achieved the vocabulary spurt, less than half achieved the categorization skill reported by Gopnik and Meltzoff (1987).

Another related research area that is emerging is the study of temperament and its relation to language acquisition. For instance, Bloom and Capatides (1987) studied expression of affect and its relationship to the onset of first words and the vocabulary explosion. They found that the more frequently the children expressed emotion during language development, the longer it took them to achieve language milestones. The children who spent more time in "neutral affect" talked earlier. The researchers indicate that perhaps the expression of positive and negative emotions detracts from the "reflective stance" that enhances a child's ability to recall and to recognize words. The research on temperament and language development has only just begun, and this may be a fruitful avenue of exploration.

The kind of research we have been discussing is only in its beginning stages; however, some relationships have started to emerge that show connections among cognitive and linguistic acquisitions. Some inconsistencies in research may be due to small sample sizes and some methodological variations. These researchers are not necessarily attempting to establish "causal" connections between cognitive and linguistic skills. Certainly, these skills can emerge simultaneously, and one may not be prerequisite to the other. The more we know about these correspondences of the various domains of child development, the clearer the picture will become. It is almost certain that the relationships will be multivariate and include cognitive, social, temperamental, biologic, and environmental components.

THE TRANSITION FROM SINGLE WORDS TO EARLY MULTIWORD UTTERANCES

Dore et al. (1976) noted that children do not simply move from saying single words to uttering multiword combinations. They noted a transitional period between single and multiword use in which children produce single words combined with "nonwords." We have called this "Transition #2." To appreciate this transitional period, we must reflect on what a "syntactic" utterance is composed of. First, a syntactic utterance is two or more "true" words that are combined under a single intonation contour. That is, there is no pause between the words, and they are clearly meant as a word combination. Another criterion of a syntactic utterance is that the two words form a relation between each other that is beyond their individual meanings. For instance, a child that says "daddy chair" to refer to his father's recliner has combined two words that have individual meanings, and there is an additional "third meaning." In essence, the specific combination of the words creates a meaning (possession) that is larger than the meanings of the words considered individually. There are probably other criteria for defining a syntactic utterance, but Dore et al. (1976) focus on these two. Any utterance that does not meet these criteria should not be considered a syntactic utterance.

Dore and his colleagues found several specific types of "transitional phenomena" produced by children just after the single-word period. On the surface these utterances may have appeared to be multiword combinations, but they did not meet the criteria for a syntactic utterance. We will mention these below:

1. *Dummy Element Productions:* These are productions that extend an utterance phonetically, but do not have relational meaning. In other words, it is a combination of a real word with a nonword, and this does not meet the criteria of being a syntactic utterance. Some examples are the combining of a vowel production with a real word, such as [I cat] or [ae ball]. It is important to note here that the child is not necessarily attempting to say "a ball," as in the use of the indefinite article "a." The child is simply combining a vowel with a real word in some consistent pattern. This only serves to put two elements under an intonation pattern, but they have no relational meaning.

2. *Dummy Form Productions:* These are similar to dummy element productions; however, instead of just placing a vowel before a real word, a consonant-vowel combination is placed there. For instance, a child might say [di ball] or [bae doggie].

The child is not trying to say "this ball" or "bad doggie." The phonetic combinations that precede the word could just as easily have been [wuh] or [mae]. The point is that only one real word was included in the utterance along with a vocalization.

3. *Reduplication Productions:* These are single words produced repetitively two or three times under the same intonation contour. For instance, a child might say [doggie doggie] under the same intonation pattern. This meets one of the syntactic criteria, but not the other having to do with relational meaning.

4. *Empty Form Productions:* These are stable productions that "lack identifiable reference and appear in a wide range of contexts" (Dore, et al., 1976). In other words, these productions appear to be "meaningless" in terms of connecting them with a particular referent or action. An example is reported by Bloom (1973) where her daughter repeatedly combined [widə] with other words, and it was never clear what [widə] meant. Leonard (1975) reports a child who used [gɔkin] in combination with other words. These empty forms serve to combine two elements under the same intonation pattern; however, there is no perceivable relational meaning.

5. *Rote Productions:* These are combinations of two or more real words, but the words never occur in combination with other words (Hickey, 1993; Perez-Pereira, 1994; Plunkett, 1993). For instance, a child who says [no way] and never combines "no" with another word, or "way" with another word has a rote production. Rote productions are highly practiced word combinations that appear to be routines or formulas rather than generative language. Therefore, they may meet the two criteria for a syntactic utterance, but they do not meet another criteria some people feel is important called "productivity" (Leonard, Steckol, & Panther, 1983). Word combinations are productive when each word in the combination can be generatively paired with other words to make novel constructions.

6. *Vertical Constructions:* Scollon (1976) published a book entitled "Conversations with the One Year Old" in which he provided detailed documentation of the single and early multiword period of a child named Brenda. Scollon described four types of "transitional" utterances that he called vertical constructions. Essentially, these are utterances that are leading to early multiword combinations. The first two types of vertical constructions are initiated and produced by the child alone, while the second two types rely on discourse with an adult. Type A vertical constructions involve two real words said individually and separated in time by a pause (e.g., "car. . . . . . go"). Although the words were not included under the same intonation pattern, they certainly would have been syntactically related if the child shortened the pause time. The type B vertical construction involves repetition instead of a pause (e.g., "car car car go go go"). The type C vertical construction is a product of conversation with another person. In this construction an interaction might go like this:

Child: "doggie"
Mother: "yeah, that's a doggie"
Child: "run"

This type of construction is transitional because the adult takes a child-initiated word and responds in such a way to allow the child to produce a second utterance that could logically be combined with the initial word into a semantic relation. The type D construction is a combination of types B and C in which a child uses repetition and also may benefit from conversational cues:

Child: "milk"
          "milk"
Mother: "yeah, milk"
Child: "cold"

These conversational constructions and the utterances built up by the child alone are transitional because they begin to relate words in time and conversational proximity just prior to the ability to combine elements under the same intonation pattern. Other researchers have noted similar patterns in single-word children (Greenfield, Reilly, Leaper, & Baker, 1985; Greenfield & Smith, 1976; Branigan, 1976). Greenfield et al. (1985) suggest that some children get into "constructive" patterns in which they use these buildups as a transitional mechanism. Other children do more "breaking down" of elements and then recombine them with other words.

Garman (1979) has characterized these approaches as "synthetic and analytic" transitional processes. It would be interesting indeed to discover the sources of children's individual variability in using the different types of transitional phenomena in language acquisition. What is it that makes one child analytic and another synthetic and others a combination of the two approaches? Does it have to do with environmental influences or the neuropsychologic organization of the child? Only further research will illuminate these issues.

We have seen how a child learns to gradually develop the ability to use words for communication. It begins with nonverbal communicative gestures and then progresses to incorporate vocalizations, then a few words, a vocabulary spurt, and, finally, the beginnings of two-word combinations. The process involves the coordination of cognitive development, pragmatic rules, semantic rules, social skills, phonological development, and caretaker-child interaction. The process does not always unfold without difficulty. In the next section we will discuss how information on single-word development is applied to children with language impairment.

APPLICATIONS: SINGLE WORDS AND THE CHILD WITH LANGUAGE IMPAIRMENT

Children with language impairment pass through a single-word period that is quite similar to that experienced by normal-language youngsters. In fact, one way

to characterize children with language impairment is to determine at which level they are operating in terms of utterance length (McLean & Snyder-McLean, 1978; Haynes & Pindzola, 1998). For instance, children with language impairment can fall into four basic groups (nonverbal, single-word users, early multiword users, and syntax users). It is important to note that when a child with a language impairment is in the single-word period, he or she is typically going through this stage at an older chronological age than normal-language children. A normally developing child usually is in the single-word period, as mentioned above, somewhere between the ages of 9 and 21 months. This, of course, includes the transitions in and out of the actual period of single-word usage. Children with language impairment, on the other hand, may be passing through this stage when they are 2 to 3 years old. Some severe cases may still be in the single-word stage when they are 4 or 5 years old. Whenever the child with language impairment traverses the single-word period, many of the same phenomena can be observed in terms of transitions and of the progressions from babbling to single words and from single words to early multiwords. The structure of the lexicon also may be similar in children with language impairment in that their vocabularies are basically constructed of similar types of words (e.g., nominals, action words, etc.). Also, the child with language impairment typically develops language faster in comprehension than production just as seen in normal language development. Most of the evidence appears to suggest that children with language impairment are delayed, rather than deviant in their acquisition of language (Leonard, 1979), and this means that they can be expected to exhibit similar patterns of linguistic development to normal-language youngsters. At any rate, children with language impairment definitely pass through a single-word period, and the data gathered on normal-language children is useful in predicting what types of words, functions of lexical items, cognitive/social influences, and transitions will be seen in this population.

APPLICATION OF THE SINGLE-WORD PERIOD TO ASSESSMENT

There are some extremely important applications from normal development to the clinical assessment of a child with language impairment who is talking in single-word utterances. First, since we can usually expect that these children will be exhibiting language that is similar to that used by normally developing children at an earlier age, we can use some of the same measurements that researchers have taken in studying the single-word period. There presently are no standardized tests that provide complete information on the single-word period. There are also vocabulary tests, but these largely focus on vocabulary comprehension and not production. Because they use drawings as stimuli, many of these tests could not be used on normal-language children at age 1½ and thus may not be appropriate for an older, language-impaired child who is chronologically 3 years old, but functioning communicatively at age 1½. As a result, we are left primarily with informal measures, spontaneous language sampling, and detailed parent interview data as the mainstays of single-word assessment.

One major goal in assessing language-impaired children at the single-word level is to determine the size of the lexicon. This is difficult to do in a clinical sampling session because a child will obviously not have occasion to use every word he has in his vocabulary during a 2-hour period. Most clinicians rely on parent reporting to help in determining the size of a child's vocabulary and the types of words represented in the lexicon. A popular method is to use large checklists of words on which parents only need to circle or somehow mark the words their child has said in the home environment (Fenson, Dale, Reznick, et al., 1993; Rescorla, 1989). These checklists are made up largely from the data on normally developing children during the single-word period, and, generally, there is a good correspondence in the types of utterances between language delayed and normal-language children during the single-word period.

The reader will also recall that in normally developing children the lexicon may reach about 50 words and then the child begins to transition into early multiword utterances. A similar criterion can be examined in children with language impairment. If their lexicon is only 10 words as determined by parental reports and language sampling, we may not consider training early multiword combinations. Perhaps a more logical goal would be to add to the child's lexicon before emphasizing word combinations. On the other hand, if the child's vocabulary is 75 words, then we might consider targeting some multiword utterances in treatment.

From the checklist of words used by a child, a clinician can also determine the types of lexical items in the vocabulary. Many clinicians use the categories of Nelson (1973) and Benedict (1979) to categorize individual words. This is important because a child with language impairment needs to have enough words of different kinds to code many aspects of the environment (possession, location, action, labels, greetings, etc.). A variety of words is typically present in the early lexicon of normally developing children, and we can only assume that it is equally important in those with language impairment as well.

We can also assume that the articulatory productions of single words by a child with language impairment will be similar to those of normal-language children at an earlier age. The same phonological processes have been shown to exist in language-impaired children as are seen in normally developing youngsters (Leonard, 1979).

Some aspects of the single-word period have not been adequately studied in children with language impairment. For example, we suspect that similar cognitive variables influence the development and use of single words in children with language problems; however, more research needs to be done to determine specific effects. It seems prudent to suggest that attainment of at least late stage IV or early stage V in sensorimotor intelligence is a requisite to single-word use, since we can find no reports of such utterances in normal children or subjects with language impairment prior to their attaining these levels of cognitive development.

Also, some phenomena such as the vocabulary spurt that is seen in normally developing children are masked by language intervention, which is typically begun with language-disordered children at an early age. Although overextensions and underextensions have been frequently reported in children with language impairment, more research must be done to fully illuminate this area and how the data relate to the various theories of lexical development.

Another aspect of single-word assessment might be to determine not only the types of words used, but also the uses the words normally have. For instance, we would want to know if a child uses his single words to regulate attention, to regulate action, to question, to greet, or to practice or for the other functions as reported by Dore (1976) and Halliday (1975). Some clinicians do a "form-function analysis" in which the single-word utterances are arranged next to the function they served in a spontaneous language sample. The clinician can thus determine not only the *types* of words used by the child, but also the reasons *why* they were used:

Form	Function
"up" (arms extended)	regulating behavior
"bye" (waving)	greeting
"tape" (after daddy)	imitation
"horsie" (pointing)	regulating attention

Another important aspect of the single-word period is to note the presence of transitional phenomena in the child with language impairment. These may indicate a move into a more sophisticated level of language development. There are no standardized tests for transitional phenomena, so the clinician is again in the position of having to rely on knowledge of normal language development to determine the status of a child with language impairment at the single-word level.

APPLICATIONS: TREATMENT OF THE CHILD WITH LANGUAGE IMPAIRMENT

In dealing with a child who is nonverbal, one of the initial considerations of the speech-language pathologist is the construction of a first lexicon or "core vocabulary." Most clinicians combine two sources of information to construct the training vocabulary for use with a language-impaired child. First, the clinician considers the research done on the single-word period in normally developing children. The work of Nelson (1984) and others is studied to determine the types of words used by single-word speakers. Many child language researchers have reported actual transcripts of language used by children in the single-word period, and these are a rich source of potential words to include in a first lexicon for a handicapped child. The second source of information a clinician considers is a study of the child's environment and daily routine to determine which words will be especially functional for the child. If we know anything about the development of language it is that the symbol system is acquired because it is useful and the child learns to manipulate the environment efficiently with it. Obviously, we would not want to teach a word like "cow" as one of the first lexical items to a child living in an urban area. Holland (1975) and Lahey and Bloom (1977) report specific suggestions for a first lexicon to be used in language training, and they draw their suggestions primarily from the single-word period. They also recommend that the vocabulary words be functional to the child.

Once the vocabulary items are decided

on, there are various ways in which clinicians have utilized them therapeutically. Certainly, most therapy methods recommend that the child's caretakers use and model the core vocabulary often to stimulate the development of these specific forms in the child. Other approaches use play therapy and in addition to stimulating the single-word vocabulary words, they set up situations in which the child can use them. For instance, a vocabulary word might be "ball." The clinician might withhold the ball from the child in a reciprocal ball-rolling activity until the child "requests" the ball by making an approximation of the word. Still other treatments are even more structured and require the child to imitate the lexical items in more drill-oriented activities. Whatever the approach, data from the single-word period are used to construct the first lexicon and determine play situations in which it will be used.

CONCLUDING REMARKS

The single-word period is an exciting phase of development for both parents and researchers. A child moves from nonverbal communication to developing speech—one of our most human characteristics. It is a highly complex time of transitions and complex acqusitions in which there are general patterns of development common to all children, yet different pathways taken by subgroups of youngsters. Multiple influences from cognitive, affective, interactive, motoric, and linguistic domains interact to account for the compexity in this interesting period. As research continues on the single-word period, the applications of this knowledge will have impacts on theory as well as clinical practice.

REFERENCES

Barrett M. Children's single word speech. Chichester: John Wiley, 1985.

Bates E. Language in context: the acquisition of pragmatics. New York: Academic Press, 1976.

Bates E, Camaioni I, Volterra V. The acquisition of performatives prior to speech. Merrill-Palmer Q 1975;21:206–226.

Bates E, Bretherton I, Snyder L, et al. Vocal and ges-

tural symbols at 13 months. Merrill-Palmer Q 1980;26:407–423.

Bates E, Marchman V, Thal D, et al. Developmental and stylistic variation in the composition of early vocabulary. J Child Lang 1994;21:85–123.

Benedict H. Early lexical development: comprehension and production. J Child Lang 1979;6:183–200.

Bernthal J, Bankson N. Articulation disorders. Englewood Cliffs, NJ: Prentice-Hall, 1993.

Bloom L. One word at a time. The Hague: Mouton, 1973.

Bloom L, Lifter K, Broughton J. The convergence of early cognition and language in the second year of life: problems in conceptualization and measurement. In: Barrett M, ed. Children's single word speech. Chichester: John Wiley, 1985.

Bloom L, Capatides B. Expression of affect and the emergence of language. Child Dev 1987; 58:1513–1522.

Boysson-Bardies B de, Sagart L, Duranc C. Discernable differences in the babbling of infants according to target language. J Child Lang 1984;11:1–15.

Boysson-Bardies B de, Vihman M. Adaptation to language: evidence from babbling and first words in four languages. Language 1991;67:297–319.

Branigan G. Sequences of single words as structured units. Papers Reports Child Lang Dev 1976; 12:60–70.

Bruner J. The ontogenesis of speech acts. J Child Lang 1975;2:1–19.

Carter A. Prespeech meaning relations: an outline of one infant's sensorimotor morpheme development. In: Fletcher P, Garman M, eds. Language acquisition. New York: Academic Press, 1979.

Caselli M. Communicative gestures and first words. In: Volterra V, Erting C, eds. From gesture to sign in hearing and deaf children. New York: Springer-Verlag, 1990.

Clark E. What's in a word? On the child's acquisition of semantics in his first language. In: Moore T, ed. Cognitive development and the acquisition of language. New York: Academic Press, 1973.

Clark E. Knowledge, context and strategy in the acquisition of meaning. In: Dato D, ed. Developmental psycholinguistics: theory and application. Washington, DC: Georgetown University Press, 1975.

Clark E. The lexicon in acquisition. Cambridge: Cambridge University Press, 1993.

Corrigan R. Language development as related to stage 6 object permanence development. J Child Lang 1978;5:173–189.

Creaghead N. Development of phonology, articulation and speech perception. In: Creaghead N, Newman P, Secord W, eds. Assessment and remediation of articulatory and phonological disorders. Columbus, OH: Merrill, 1989.

Dore J. Holophrases, speech acts and linguistic universals. J Child Lang 1975;2:21–40.

Dore J, Franklin M, Miller R, Ramer A. Transitional phenomena in early language acquisition. J Child Lang 1976;3:13–28.

Elbers L, Ton J. Playpen monologues: the interplay

of words and babbles in the first words period. J Child Lang 1985;12:551–565.

Fenson L, Dale P, Reznick J, et al. The MacArthur communicative development inventories: users guide and technical manual. San Diego: Singular Publishing Group, 1993.

Ferguson C, Farwell C. Words and sounds in early language acquisition: English initial consonants in the first fifty words. Language 1975;51:419–439.

Fremgen A, Fay D. Overextensions in production and comprehension: a methodological clarification. J Child Lang 1980;7:203–211.

Garman M. Early grammatical development. In: Fletcher P, Garman M, eds. Language development. Cambridge: Cambridge University Press, 1979.

Gentner D. Why nouns are learned before verbs: linguistic relativity versus natural partitioning. In: Kuczaj S, ed. Language development: Vol. 2. Language, thought and culture. Hillsdale, NJ: Lawrence Erlbaum, 1982.

Goldfield B. Noun bias in maternal speech to one year olds. J Child Lang 1993;20:85–89.

Gopnik A. Development of non-nominal expressions in 1–2 year olds; why the first words aren't about things. In: Dale P, Ingram D, eds. Child language: an international perspective. Baltimore: University Park Press, 1981.

Gopnik A, Meltzoff A. Relations between semantic and cognitive development in the one word stage; the specificity hypothesis. Child Dev 1986; 57:1040–1053.

Gopnik A, Meltzoff A. The development of categorization in the second year and its relation to other cognitive and linguistic developments. Child Dev 1987;58:1523–1531.

Greenfield P, Reilly J, Leaper C, Baker N. The relationship between single word speech and multiword speech. In: Barrett M, ed. Children's single word speech. Chichester: John Wiley, 1985.

Greenfield P, Smith J. The structure of communication in early language development. New York: Academic Press, 1976.

Grunwell P. Clinical phonology. London: Aspen, 1982.

Halliday M. Learning how to mean. New York: Elsevier, 1975.

Haynes W, Pindzola R. Diagnosis and evaluation in speech pathology. Boston: Allyn and Bacon, 1998.

Hickey T. Identifying formulas in first language acquisition. J Child Lang 1993;20:27–41.

Hoek D, Ingram D, Gibson D. Some possible causes of children's early word overextensions. J Child Lang 1986;13:477–494.

Holland A. Language therapy for children: some thoughts on context and content. J Speech Hear Disord 1975;40:514–523.

Ingram D. Phonological disorders in children. New York: Elsevier, 1976.

Ingram D. Sensorimotor intelligence and language development. In: Lock A, ed. Action, gesture and symbol: the emergence of language. New York: Academic Press, 1977.

Ingram D. Procedures for the phonological analysis of children's language. Baltimore, MD: University Park Press, 1981.

Kahn L, Lewis N. Kahn-Lewis phonological analysis. American Guidance Service, 1986.

Kamhi A. Three popular myths about language development. Child Lang Teach Ther 1988;4(1):1–12.

Lahey M, Bloom L. Planning a first lexicon: which words to teach first. J Speech Hear Disord 1977;42:340–350.

Lenneberg E. Biological foundations of language. New York: John Wiley, 1967.

Leonard L. On differentiating syntactic and semantic features in emerging grammars: evidence from empty form usage. J Psycholinguist Res 1975; 4:357–364.

Leonard L. Language impairment in children. Merrill Palmer Q 1979;25:205–232.

Leonard L, Schwartz K, Chapman L, et al. Early lexical acquisition in children with specific language impairment. J Speech Hear Res 1982;25:554–564.

Leonard L, Steckol K, Panther K. Returning meaning to semantic relations: some clinical applications. J Speech Hear Disord 1983;48:25–35.

Lifter K, Bloom L. Object knowledge and the emergence of language, infant behavior and development. 1989;12:395–423.

Lock A. Action, gesture and symbol: the emergence of language. London: Academic Press, 1978.

Locke J. The linguistic significance of babbling. In: Lindblom B, Zetterstrom R, eds. Precursors of early speech. New York: Stockton, 1986.

Locke J. Linguistic significance of babbling: evidence from tracheostomized infants. Paper presented to the convention of the American Speech Language Hearing Association, New Orleans, 1987.

Masur E. The development of communicative gestures in mother-infant interactions. Papers Reports Child Lang Dev 1980;19:121–128.

Masur E. Mother's responses to infants' object-related gestures: influences on lexical development. J Child Lang 1982;9:23–30.

McClean J, Snyder-McClean L. A transactional approach to early language training. Columbus, OH: Merrill, 1978.

Morford M, Goldin-Meadow S. Comprehension and production of gesture in combination with speech in one word speakers. J Child Lang 1992;19:559–580.

Muma J. Language acquisition: a functionalistic perspective. Austin, TX: Pro-Ed, 1986.

Nelson K. Structure and strategy in learning to talk. Monogr Soc Res Child Dev 1973;38 (Serial No. 149).

Nelson K. Concept, word, and sentence: interrelations in acquisition and development. Psychol Rev 1974;81:267–285.

Nelson K. The conceptual basis of naming. In: Mac-Namara J, ed. Language learning and thought. New York: Academic Press, 1977.

Nelson K, Lucariello J. The development of meaning in first words. In: Barrett M, ed. Children's single word speech. Chichester: John Wiley, 1985.

Oller D. The emergence of the sounds of speech in infancy. In: Yeni-Komshian G, Kavanagh J, Ferguson C, eds. Child phonology. Vol. 1: Production. New York, Academic Press, 1980.

Owens R. Language development: an introduction. Boston: Allyn and Bacon, 1996.

Perez-Pereira M. Imitations, repetitions, routines, and the child's analysis of language: insights from the blind. J Child Lang 1994;21:317–337.

Peters A. Language learning strategies: does the whole equal the sum of the parts? Language 1977;53:560–573.

Piaget J. Play, dreams and imitation. New York: Norton, 1962.

Plunkett K. Lexical segmentation and vocabulary growth in early language acquisition. J Child Lang 1993;20:43–60.

Reich P. Language development. Englewood-Cliffs, NJ: Prentice-Hall, 1986.

Rescorla L. The language development survey: a screening tool for delayed language in toddlers. J Speech Hear Disord 1989;54:587–599.

Ross G. Language functioning and speech development of six children receiving tracheostomy in infancy. J Commun Disord 1983;15:95–111.

Schwartz R, Leonard L. Do children pick and choose? An examination of phonological selection and avoidance in early lexical acquisition. J Child Lang 1982;9:319–336.

Scollon R. Conversations with a one year old: a case study of the developmental foundations of syntax. Honolulu: University of Hawaii Press, 1976.

Simon B, Fowler S, Handler S. Communication development in young children with long-term tracheostomies: preliminary report. Int J Pediatr Otorhinolaryngol 1983;6:37–50.

Stark R. Stages of speech development in the first year of life. In: Yeni-Komshian G, Kavanagh J, Ferguson C, eds. Child phonology. Vol. 1: Production. New York, Academic Press, 1980.

Stoel-Gammon C, Cooper J. Patterns of early lexical and phonological development. J Child Lang 1984;11:247–271.

Stoel-Gammon C. Phonetic inventories, 15–24 months: a longitudinal study. J Speech Hear Res 1985;28:505–512.

Vihman M. Individual differences in babbling and early speech. In: Lindblom B, Zetterstrom R, eds. Precursors of early speech. New York: Stockton, 1986.

Vihman M. Phonological development: the origins of language in the child. Oxford: Basil Blackwell, 1996.

Vihman M, Macken M, Miller R, et al. From babbling to speech: a reassessment of the continuity issue. Language 1985;61:397–445.

Zinober B, Martlew M. The development of communicative gestures. In: Barret M, ed. Children's single word speech. Chichester: John Wiley, 1985.

CHAPTER 10

Development of Early Multiword Utterances

William O. Haynes

Thus far, we have seen how a child progresses in communication development from nonverbal signals to the consistent use of a variety of single-word utterances. The child has also passed through a transitional period in which single words are combined with nonword elements as a prelude to producing legitimate, generative multiword combinations. This chapter deals with the very complex period in which the child first begins to link individual words together forming primitive sentences. There are several reasons why we say this period is complex. First, there has been controversy surrounding even the basic issue of *how* to describe these early multiword utterances. In the past 2 decades, many systems have been suggested for use in linguistic notation when classifying these word combinations. Second, the early multiword period is controversial because it represents a child's first use of syntax, or rules for combining words. Researchers are interested in what strategies children use in these primitive constructions and what role cognitive and/or social mechanisms play in developing word combinations. Finally, theorists have debated the nature of the underlying mechanisms that govern initial primitive word combinations and how these processes change over time to ultimately drive adultlike syntactic organization. We will briefly discuss these and other issues, as well as the clinical applications of the literature concerning the early multiword period.

THE ISSUE OF METRIC

The method used to describe early multiword utterances has been a continuing source of controversy in the developmental literature for the past 3 decades, and there has been a progressive evolution of metrics or measuring systems advocated by authorities in language development. One method would attain a degree of popularity in the literature for a brief time and then would be relinquished by authorities as more discriminating methods were developed or as the field of language development began a new theoretical trend. Some methods were rejected because they proved to be incomplete or inaccurate. For instance, a particular method purported to be a grammatical account of utterances in the early multiword period, and early data from the language acquisition literature supported it. Later, exceptions were noted in research data, and the method was found to be inadequate or inaccurate. Some of the methods used to deal with early multiword utterances were descriptive in nature. That is, they were designed merely to describe early child multiword utterances. Other methods were designed as grammars that were alleged to map the underlying system that generated the early word combinations.

In the 1950s most early multiword utterances were accounted for descriptively, but provided little detailed information about these word combinations. For example, one could describe early utterances simply by referring to their length (e.g., most early multiword utterances are two to four words in length). While noting a child's utterance length would undoubtedly be accurate, it does not provide a great deal of information to students or clinicians. What types of words are in the utterances? What order are they in? Why were they said? Thus a length metric may be descriptive, but not very informative.

Another example of a way to describe early multiword utterances is *telegraphic speech* (Brown & Bellugi, 1964). This type of metric is based on the assumption that the production of early multiword utterances is under a length constraint, just as a person sending a telegram is under a money constraint. The more words you send in a telegram, the more money you have to pay, so you eliminate those words that are unnecessary. Similarly, the child at the two- to three-word stage is under a length constraint in that the processing channel can only deal with utterances of a certain maximum length. Thus the child must eliminate words that are not really necessary for communication. The proponents of telegraphic speech noted that in both telegrams and early multiword utterances the content words (nouns, verbs, adjectives, etc.) are retained and the function words (prepositions, word endings, articles, etc.) are eliminated. So, a general description of early multiword communications using telegraphic speech might be

that the child retains content words and eliminates function words. This is certainly more descriptive than the length measure mentioned above, but still not very informative.

A major problem emerges when systems are designed not only to try to describe the types of utterances seen in early combinations, but also to divine the system that the child uses to generate these utterances. In the 1960s there were several popular methods proposed to describe and account for early multiword utterances. For instance, Braine (1963) attempted to account for early multiword utterances in children cross-culturally using a positional strategy called *pivot grammar*. Early researchers initially found pivot grammar to be useful in describing early multiword combinations (McNeil, 1966; Miller & Ervin, 1964). We must consider that when we refer to a grammar, we are suggesting a systematic way to account for the majority of child utterances and a way to even predict future word combinations. For instance, English grammar indicates the sentences that are acceptable in the language, and knowledge of the grammar could be used to basically predict all acceptable utterances in the language. If sentences are generated that the grammar would not predict or are in violation of the grammar, then one must question the validity of the grammatical system. Regarding pivot grammar, Braine postulated that certain words were "pivot words," which occurred exclusively in either the first or second position in a two-word utterance. For example, the word "go" might be a pivot word in the second position (P2) in the utterances "mommy go," "doggie go," and "daddy go." Similarly, the word "more" might be a pivot word in the first position (P1) in the utterances "more milk," "more juice," and "more play." The integrity of pivot grammar depends on the child's utterances conforming to the particular system (grammar) and on certain words only being used in specific positions. Unfortunately, many researchers found exceptions to pivot grammar in that violations to the grammar occurred and it did not account for many utterances found in language samples from children cross-culturally. Ultimately, many authorities forcefully rejected the notion of pivot grammar (Brown, 1973; Slobin, 1971) as a reasonable or accurate method for describing early multiword utterances. We only bring it up here to provide an historical perspective.

It was also controversial when authorities attempted to impute adult grammatical categories from Chomsky's (1965) transformational grammar to children's utterances during the early multiword period. Bowerman (1973, p. 199) outlined many reasons why adult transformational grammars have difficulty accounting for early multiword utterances. One of the most potent reasons was that the adult grammatical categories were too abstract; that is, "subjects of English sentences play such diverse semantic roles as agent (as in *John* opened the door), object involved (the *door* opened), instrument (the *key* opened the door), person affected (*John* wants milk) and location (*Chicago* is windy)." As Peters (1986, p. 309) puts it, "The argument against using adult grammatical constructs (e.g., noun phrase, subject of sentence) as a descriptive framework is basically that much grammatical machinery is not needed, and is in fact, much too powerful at the early stages and that semantic relations or case categories fit the data much better." If a child said "mommy sock" as her mother is putting on a sock, "umbrella boot" while pointing to an umbrella sitting inside a boot, and "daddy coat" as she picks up her father's jacket, these utterances would all be described as "noun + noun." If we were to analyze the contexts of these utterances one by one, it would be clear that the child is referring to a different meaning relationship with each utterance. In the first utterance the child is referring to the relationship between an actor (mommy) and an object (sock). In the second utterance the child is referring to a particular entity (umbrella) and its relationship to a location (boot). In the final utterance, the

child refers to the relationship between a possessor or owner (daddy) and a possession (coat). Thus calling all of these utterances "noun + noun" describes the grammatical category of the words, but does not provide a description of what the child means in the utterance. This means that a grammatical notation such as noun + noun may be descriptive, but does not really provide a rich interpretation (Brown, 1973) of a child's early utterances and give credit for the variety of meanings that can be expressed.

In the 1970s the semantic revolution pervaded the language acquisition literature. It became popular to describe early multiword utterances using variants of adult, semantically based grammars (Fillmore, 1968; Chafe, 1970). Most authorities in the current literature on language development and assessment still use some variant of these semantically based grammars to describe two- and three-word utterances of children. These grammars take into account the meaning relationship the child is trying to communicate with early two-word combinations. To use semantically based grammars, one has to take into account two aspects: (1) the utterance and (2) the context in which the utterance was spoken. Earlier in this chapter we provided some examples of two-word utterances that were described as "noun + noun," but differed significantly in their meaning relationship. While the use of variants of semantically based grammars still enjoys popularity into the 1990s, this metric has not been immune from criticism (Duchan & Lund, 1979; Howe, 1976, 1981; Rodgon, 1977). Generally, the critics are concerned with whether the semantic relations used to analyze children's speech really reflect the legitimate operational meanings in their utterances. Most authorities suggest that before we ascribe adult semantic categories to a child's speech, we need to acquire evidence from multiple samples in a variety of contexts that the categories are operative (Bloom, Capatides, & Tackeff, 1981; Leonard, 1984; Braine, 1976; Ingram, 1981). Essentially, some evidence of productivity would be the clear generative use of many different words to produce a particular semantic relation (e.g., agent + action using "mommy run," "Johnny eat," "doggie jump," etc.) and use of novel, generative utterances the child could not have heard from adult speakers (e.g. "open banana," "open shoe"). We must be very careful, however, because child categories may be more specific or general than adult categories. For example, Leonard (1984, p.13) cites a rule found by Braine (1976): ". . . . Braine has reported evidence for a word-combining rule that might be characterized as Act-of-Oral-Consumption + Object-Consumed (e.g., "Eat banana," "Bite banana," "Eat cookie," "Bite cookie." This is to say that positional consistency obtained only in word combinations related to the acts of eating and drinking."

The issue of which metric is the most accurate or appropriate to use in describing and accounting for early multiword utterances may never be totally resolved. It is always difficult to prove what is actually going on inside a child's head as an utterance is generated. There are many books, chapters, monographs, and articles dealing with the theoretical aspects of what kind of metric to use in describing early multiword utterances. To date, however, many authorities have voiced their uncertainty regarding the exact nature of what two-word utterances actually represent:

> Two word utterances may represent (1) memorization of a number of combinations into which particular words may enter; (2) productive rules applied only to specific words; (3) productive rules conveying meanings that cross lexical boundaries, but narrower than traditional semantic relation categories, as well as (4) semantic relation rules of a traditional type (Leonard, 1984, p. 13).

Reich (1986, p. 82) also reflects this point of view:

> The categories used by the child to generate sentences may differ from adult categories in the same way that child meanings may differ from adult meanings. Relative to adult categories, the child's category may theoretically be identical,

more specific, more general, overlapping, entirely nonoverlapping, nonexistent, or totally unrelated to any adult class.

For professionals who are going to be dealing with language-impaired youngsters, the theories underlying the various metrics may not yet be clinically applicable, and we will not spend time reviewing them in detail here. For those who are interested in the more sophisticated aspects of linguistic theory as it relates to the early multiword period, we have cited many references that provide this information.

TYPES OF EARLY WORD COMBINATIONS FOUND BY RESEARCHERS

We have indicated above that the metric currently used to refer to early word combinations is some variation of a semantically based grammar. It is interesting that children from many cultures have been studied during the early multiword period and that there are significant similarities in their types of early word combinations (Brown, 1973; Braine, 1976). Children speaking American English, Finnish, Swedish, Samoan, Spanish, French, German, Hebrew, Japanese, Korean, Luo, Russian, and Mandarin have been investigated, and generally their early multiword combinations are similar. This lends strong support to the notion that there are certain "universals" operating at the onset of language development. Depending on which theorist one reads, these universals can be innate linguistic capacities, behavioral principles, modes of caretaker-child interaction, the nature of cognitive development, or the structure of language itself. In the present chapter, however, it is enough to note that children from various parts of the world begin to combine words in a basically similar fashion and that there are a limited number of early multiword utterance types. Table 10.1 provides some definitions and examples of semantic cases typically mentioned in the two-word utterances of children. These cases can be combined with one another to make two-word utterances such as "mommy run" (agent +

Table 10.1   *Semantic Categories*

Action A perceivable movement or activity engaged in by an agent (animate or inanimate).

Entity (One-term utterances only) Any labeling of the present person or object regardless of the occurrence or nature or action being performed on or by it.

Entity (Multiterm utterances only) The use of an appropriate label for a person or object in the absence of any action on it (with the exception of showing, pointing, touching, or grasping); or someone or something which caused or was the stimulus to the internal state specified by a state verb or any object or person which was modified by a possessive form. (Entity was used to code a possession if it met either of the preceding criteria.)

Locative The place where an object or action was located or toward which it moved.

Negation The impression of any of the following meanings with regard to someone or something, or an action or state: nonexistence, rejection, cessation, denial, disappearance.

Agent The performer (animate or inanimate) of an action. Body parts and vehicles, when used in conjunction with action verbs, were coded **Agent.**

Object A person or thing (marked by the use of a noun or pronoun) that received the force of an action.

Demonstrative The use of demonstrative pronouns of adjectives, *this, that, these, those,* and the words *there, right there, here, see,* when stated for the purpose of pointing out a particular referent.

Recurrence A request for or comment on an additional instance or amount; the resumption of an event; or the reappearance of a person or object.

Attribute An adjectival description of the size, shape, or quality of an object or person; also, noun adjuncts which modified nouns for a similar purpose (e.g., *gingerbread* man).

Possessor A person or thing (marked by the use of a proper noun or pronoun) that an object was associated with or to which it belonged, at least temporarily.

Adverbial Included in this category were the two subcategories of action/attribute and state/attribute.

Action/Attribute A modifier of an action indicating time, manner, duration, distance, or frequency. (Direction or place of action was separately coded as **Locative, Repetition** and **Recurrence.**)

State/Attribute A modifier indicating time, manner, quality, or intensity of a state.

Quantifier A modifier which indicated amount or number of a person or object. Prearticles and indefinite pronouns such as *a piece of, lots of, any, every,* and *each* were included.

State A passive condition experienced by a person or object. This category implies involuntary behavior on the part of the **Experiencer,** in contrast to voluntary action performed by an **Agent.**

Experiencer Someone or something that underwent a given experience or mental state. Body parts, when used in conjunction with state verbs, were coded **Experiencer.**

Recipient One who received or was named as the recipient of an *object* (person or thing) from another.

Beneficiary One who benefited from or was named as the beneficiary of a specified action.

Name The labeling or request for naming of a person or thing using the utterance forms: *my, (his, your,* etc.) *name is* _____ or *what's* _____ *name?*

Created Object Something created by a specific activity, for example, a *song* by singing, a *house* by building, a *picture* by drawing.

Comitative One who accompanied or participated with an agent in carrying out a specified activity.

Instrument Something which an **Agent** used to carry out or complete a specified action.

Reprinted with permission from Miller J. *Assessing language production in children.* Baltimore: University Park Press, 1981; p. 44.

action) and "hit ball" (action + object). Table 10.2 shows some of the frequently cited studies of the early multiword period and the two-word utterances they have reported in children cross-culturally. These researchers refer similarly to some utterances, and on other word combinations there are terminological differences.

Various authorities have divided the early semantic categories into two subsets. Brown (1973) defined *nomination, recurrence, and nonexistence* as basic operations of reference, while other semantic categories such as *agent, action, object, state, locative, possessive, dative, locative*, etc. were viewed as semantic relations. Similarly, Bloom (1973) called nomination, recurrence, and nonexistence "functional relations," and the other

cases cited above by Brown as semantic relations were called "grammatical relations" by Bloom. Schlesinger (1971) also called nomination, recurrence, and nonexistence "operations" and the other cases "relations." Interestingly, as pointed out by Muma (1986, p. 167), ". . . it is precisely these basic grammatical relations that comprise a semantic base; or as Bloom . . . said, 'semantic primitives' that together constitute a subjective-verb-object (SVO) grammatical core for the emergence of syntax. This semantic base is agent-action-object."

As we will mention in a later section, the basic operations of reference are typically among the first types of word combinations to appear in development, and the semantic relations seem to appear later. Some re-

Table 10.2   *Early Two-Word Combinations Seen in Brown's Stage 1*

Basic Operations of Reference[a]	Examples
Nomination + X	That ball; A ball
Recurrence + X	More eat; Nother bite
Nonexistence + X	No kitty (when kitty missing)
Rejection + X	No wash (when Mom is washing)
Denial + X	No rain (when Mom said it was)

Semantic Relations[a]	
Agent + Action	Mommy run
Action + Object	Hit ball
Agent + Object	Timmy ball (while kicking)
Entity + Attribute	Big doggie
Possessor + Possession	Daddy shirt
Entity + Locative	Chair outside
Action + Locative	Run kitchen
X + Dative	Give Mommy
Experiencer + State	Me hungry
Instrument + Action	Broom sweep
Action + Commitive	Go Mommy (going with Mommy)
Conjunction	Mary Mommy

[a]These operations and relations were derived from a variety of sources (Brown, 1973; Bloom, 1970, 1973; Schlesinger, 1971; Braine, 1976; Leonard, 1976). Some of these relations and operations were addressed using slightly different terms by the researchers listed above (e.g., Brown refers to "Big doggie" as attribute + entity, while Schlesinger refers to this as modifier + head).

search has suggested that the basic operations of reference serve a cognitive, as opposed to a grammatical, function (Gopnik, 1981; McCune-Nicolich, 1981). Gopnik (1981) noted that nonnominal expressions did not appear to be used to serve social or instrumental functions, but rather had an egocentric quality as if they were being used to note or mark objects and relationships. Anisfeld (1984) notes that, in the Bloom et al. (1975) data, of the 87 utterances in the demonstrative + naming category "none of these utterances involved an instrumental purpose. They were uttered in the context of the child's pointing to something, holding it, or picking it up, not in the context of trying to get something or asking for it (p.133)." Werner and Kaplan (1963) also noted that children had a preponderance of naming in their early utterances, and this may actually be part of developing categorization skills, as opposed to a communicative effort. Similarly, Anisfeld (1984, p.139) reports on another basic operation of reference, recurrence:

Of all the semantic relations, recurrence would seem most naturally suited for the expression of instrumental goals . . . What I found was that even in the recurrence category, the cognitive function predominates. For the four children studied by Bloom et al. (1975, pp. 41–74), the ratios of comments (i.e., a cognitive function) to requests (i.e., an instrumental function) were: 27:1, 32:6, 25:5 and 32:2. That is, the children used recurrence sentences much more often to give expression to their observations than to ask for goods and services.

Muma (1986, p. 176) draws an interesting parallel concerning the categories of functional and grammatical relations:

. . . assume, for the moment, that such early grammatical relations yield a structural core or base for learning grammatical systems for "point making" and that functional relations provide a means of problem solving. Under these assumptions, it appears that Bloom's distinction between grammatical relations and functional relations are vestiges of what Halliday (1975) regarded as the *pragmatic* and *mathetic* functions of language respectively.

You will recall from prior chapters that the functions studied by Halliday and others are present at the single-word, and even at the nonverbal, levels of communication development. It is interesting how patterns of reorganization can be uncovered throughout the language acquisition process.

UTTERANCES LONGER THAN TWO WORDS

According to Muma (1986, p.169), the SVO construction "seems to be a core underlying structure that is realized only as two units early on because of a fixed programming capacity." Additionally, the child has a limited processing capacity to produce longer utterances. Peters (1986) indicates that the child must overcome such processing constraints as memory limitations, limited articulatory control, and primitive lexical/semantic knowledge. Progressively more of the SVO base is verbally realized as the child develops a larger processing capacity. As Muma (1986) and Greenfield and Smith (1976, p.64) have suggested, the process of grammatical development is an "accretion process whereby progressively more of the base structure is given verbal realization." It is important to note that children in stage I of language development have more tools at their disposal than simply to add length to their word combinations. For instance, we have known for years that children tend to heavily depend on the physical context of communication in both comprehension and production processes (Bloom, 1974; Greenfield & Smith, 1976). Children make use of pointing to or glancing at objects, stress patterns, intonation contours, and other mechanisms that make three-word utterances unnecessary. An example might be when a child holding a banana looks at mother, extending the fruit, and says "mommy eat." In this utterance, the banana is implied by the context and it is not necessary to lexicalize it. Greenfield and Smith (1976) and other researchers have shown that children tend to encode the aspects of the communication that provide the most information to the listener. They can presuppose certain elements that are physically present or redundant in the interaction and only lexicalize the most informative aspects of the message. One can see that the SVO construction can easily be reduced to SV, VO, or SO if the child can presuppose knowledge on the listener's part of the missing element. Weisenberger (1976) has shown that selecting the most informative element is a process that is present even at the single-word level of communication, and it is evident that the process is reorganized at the two- and three-word levels as well. The notion of new information has also been explored in the context of stress patterns in early multiword utterances. Weiman (1976) studied stress patterns in two-word utterances and found that most utterances had stress differences depending on the composition of the utterance. Wieman found a hierarchy of stress assignment that goes from most likely to least likely to receive stress: new information, locative, possessive, objective, attributive, verbal, and agentive. So, given this hierarchy, locative would be most likely stressed in an utterance such as "Fire truck *street*." On the other hand, if someone asked a child "What's in the street?", the child may not stress the locative, but the new information as in "*Fire truck* street." Thus children appear to be sensitive to the context and the needs of the listener and some of this ability allows them to verbally encode only certain portions of the SVO grammatical base.

Roger Brown (1973) indicated the types of three-word combinations typically seen after the two-word period. As a child's length of utterance expands, the two-word utterances are broadened into three units. Two of the most commonly seen three-word combinations are *agent + action + object* and *agent + action + locative*. It is Brown's contention that these three-word combinations are not totally new knowledge. They represent the adding of some of the two-word combinations the child has already learned. For instance, *agent + action + object* may be

the "summing" or recombining of *agent + action* and *action + object*, which were learned in the two-word period. Owens (1988, p.222) finds parallels in other expansions:

> In contrast, other semantic relations expand from within to express attribution, possession, or recurrence. The noun term is expanded. For example, within the recurrent "more cookie," the noun portion could be expanded to "big cookie," resulting in "more big cookie."

Ramer (1977) wanted to determine if there was a universal sequence of emergence of grammatical relations leading to SVO. Ramer noted five groups of utterances in development, and they are directly quoted in the following:

> Group 1: One grammatical relation expanded
> SS (expanded subject) "rocking chair"
> VV (expanded verb) "want go"
> CC (expanded complement) "down stairs"
> Group 2: Two grammatical relations
> SV "mommy come"
> SC "daddy hospital"
> VC "play sand"
> Group 3: Two grammatical relations: one expanded
> SSV "her foot stuck"
> SSC "the money inside"
> VVC "want see that"
> SVV "baby go sleep"
> SCC "dolly this carriage"
> VCC "see boat outside"
> Group 4: Two grammatical relations: both expanded
> SSVV "my mommy want see"
> SSCC "that hat on Ernie"
> VVCC "want see the car"
> Group 5: Three grammatical relations
> SVC "mommy hit ball"

Ramer found that the order of emergence of the various groups mentioned above was 1, 2, 3, 5, and 4. She indicated that the inversion of groups 4 and 5 in development may relate to utterance length since group 4 utterances are longer than group 5.

Brown indicates that the three-word

combinations may be further expanded by inserting a possessor, attribute, or recurrence element in the three-word utterance. For instance, this fourth element would be inserted in an *agent + action + object* utterance between the action and the object. So, an utterance like "mommy hit ball" could be expanded to "mommy hit daddy ball" (possessive), "mommy hit big ball" (attribute), or "mommy hit more ball" (recurrence).

Brown refers to the acquisitions in his stage I as being the basic building blocks of adult sentences. While they are telegraphic in nature, they can communicate most meanings that a person requires for meeting basic needs. The rest of the acquisitions in the later stages of development serve to expand on this basic sentence form by applying word endings, function words, rearranging words, and increasing utterance length.

DEVELOPMENTAL ORDER OF EARLY MULTIWORD UTTERANCES

Almost all authorities in the area of language acquisition acknowledge that children proceed through the stages of development in grossly similar, yet different manners. By this statement we mean that while the general order of development is consistent among children, individual youngsters employ individual strategies within these general progressions. For instance, all children go through Brown's stage I in which they use the types of early multiword utterances (semantic relations) described in the prior section. However, there are some individual differences that have been reported as well. For example, we know that a large percentage of children, perhaps as many as half, use significantly more pronouns in constructing their early multiword utterances (Bloom, Lightbrown, & Hood, 1975). These pronominal children may say "me go" instead of "Johnny go," or "hit it" instead of "hit ball." Thus they are constructing semantic relations, but they are doing it in a slightly different way as compared with children who use more nominals. We can

even find some general correspondence among children in stage I in terms of order of development of certain semantic relations. For instance, many authorities indicate that what Brown calls basic operations of reference (nomination + X; nonexistence + X; recurrence + X) tend to be acquired before some of the two-term semantic relations involving action, attribution, possession, and location. Thus we can see that there is a general correspondence among children in developing basic operations of reference first and then some other two-term relations. There is, however, considerable individual variability in the developmental order *within* the category of two-term semantic relations and even in the basic operations of reference. So, the developmental order can be said to be similar, yet different in some respects.

Specifically, Bloom and Lahey (1978, p. 162) report the following:

> The reflexive object relations existence, nonexistence, and recurrence preceded development of verb relations and the encoding of interobject relations. Within verb relations, action events (action and locative action) preceded state events (locative state, state and notice), and action preceded locative action for 2 of the children. The categories of possession and attribution were variable among the children and appeared to be later developments . . .

Reich (1986, p. 83) reports that the developmental order is roughly (1) expressions of reference (that car); (2) expressions of events (Eva read); (3) expressions of attributions, location, and possession (big water; stick car; Andrew book); and (4) expressions of experiencing and instrument (Kimmy see; eat fork).

Similar orders were reported by other researchers (Bloom, et al., 1975; Braine, 1976; Leonard, 1976).

THE COGNITIVE-SEMANTIC CONNECTION

One of the attractions of the semantic metric for describing early multiword utterances is that some of the semantic categories grossly resemble concepts developed during the sensorimotor period of cognitive development. Muma (1986, p.166) indicates "Armed with cognitive categories via knowledge of the world (Bruner, 1981), which provides the bases of semantic knowledge or semantic categories, the child is on the threshold of grammatical knowledge." This idea that basic semantic categories depend on underlying cognitive bases has been advocated by many authorities in language development (Bloom, 1973; Bowerman, 1978; Brown, 1973). It has been suggested that the rather primitive, yet critical, meanings developed in the sensorimotor period are more reasonably described by a semantically based system rather than a syntactically based system that is far more abstract. For instance, children in early cognitive development clearly acquire concepts of someone who does something (agent), actions (action), location (locative), and attribute (attribute). They understand the physical experience of possessing something and learn which members of the family have ownership of specific items. As we stated in a prior section, a syntactic system using terms such as noun or subject is cognitively more distant from the conceptual framework of the child leaving the sensorimotor period. One can think of the subject of a sentence as being an umbrella that could incorporate many nouns; however, noun is also a broad umbrella that could include many individual semantic cases such as possessor, entity, agent, instrument, and experiencer, as well as some others. One advantage of the semantic grammars, then, is that they appear to be more concrete and, on a very general level, more related to the basic concepts acquired in the sensorimotor period. It is logical that children would develop language systems that move from concrete to abstract, and semantically based grammars appear to be more concrete at a descriptive level. In discussing the semantic notions developed in the single-word period, Leonard (1976, p.123) found some relationship between cognitive development and order of emergence of these word classes:

> The sequence in which the semantic notions emerged in the speech of the eight children studied in this volume appeared generally consistent with the course followed by cognitive development. Notions such as nomination and notice represent general non-core relations showing some parallel to attainments during the third stage of sensorimotor intelligence. Notions such as agent and action may be viewed as specific non-core relations resembling attainments of the fifth stage of sensorimotor intelligence. Semantic notions such as attribution and possession might be taken to represent the child's ability to view relationships independently of relevant action. Experience and experiencer would be expected to emerge later because they do not deal with overt activity, the source of information for the child during the period of sensorimotor intelligence.

Certainly, much more research needs to address the relationship between cognitive development and early multiword communication.

WORD ORDER IN EARLY UTTERANCES

Early in stage I, children begin to produce two-word combinations, and these multiword utterances soon become stabilized in a consistent word order. Interestingly, the word order that becomes stabilized is similar to that which is dominant in the adult language. In fact, violations of adult word order are the exception and not the rule in early multiword utterances of English, as well as other languages (Brown, 1973). Even in languages that allow variable word order (Finnish, Hebrew, Russian), children typically produce the dominant word order in the language.

Braine (1976) studied the acquisition of word order and provided some insight into how it develops. Initially, according to Braine, children may produce word combinations in variable orders. He called this a *groping pattern* in which no specific word order has been learned. A child may say "mommy run" one day and "run mommy" the next day. Specifically, Braine (1976, p. 90) says the following:

> A groping pattern is a set of combinations — usually not a large set — in which

the child is attempting to express a particular kind of meaning before he has acquired a rule that specifies the positions of the words. The word order is variable in the set because no order has yet been learned. A groping pattern is an early and temporary phenomenon and is always followed by a positional productive pattern expressing the same meaning, once the child has acquired a formula that determines the order of constituents.

Another pattern noted by Braine is a *positional associative pattern* in which the child has noted the "frequent occurrence of the constant term in a particular position in phrases in adult speech and learned a fair-sized batch of phrases of the type, but without acquiring a formula for coining new phrases (p. 90)." These are similar to rote productions and not analogous to the rule learning typically associated with stage I language. A child may say "no way" or "stop it," but have no mechanism to generate more utterances of these types since no productive rule exists.

The pattern that characterizes most stage I utterances that are truly generative language are *positional productive patterns.* Braine says the following (p.90):

> Each productive pattern results from the child acquiring a rule, here called a "limited-scope formula," that maps meaning into form by specifying where in the surface structure the words . . . should be placed. Some of these formulae are of the constant plus variable type, as in the "pivot construction" of earlier literature; in other common formulae both components are variable (e.g., actor + action, possessor + possessed). A high proportion of the combinations of most early corpora fall into positional productive patterns.

There is some evidence that a lexical influence is operative in stabilizing the positional productive pattern in that words learned earlier are used in the positional productive patterns. This probably occurs because the child has had more time to discern their meaning and is more comfortable with using them (Brown & Leonard, 1986).

THE CONTINUITY PROBLEM

One difficulty shared by many linguists is the problem of how to account for a child's transition from a semantically based system to a syntactic grammar (Bowerman, 1982; Gleitman & Wanner, 1982. If, as we said earlier, a child's early utterances are best described from a semantic grammar perspective because it is concrete and more related to a child's cognitive organization, then when does the child move to a syntactic grammar and how is this done? While the change from semantic to syntactic organization appears to be discontinuous and difficult to explain, some authorities have suggested that the child may be going through a series of reorganizations that, when viewed together, make the transition to syntax less of a mystery. For instance, we have evidence that reorganization is common in cognitive development (Piaget, 1952), phonology (Ferguson, 1978; Moskowitz, 1973), and morphology (Cazden, 1968; deVilliers & deVilliers, 1978). In these cases prior knowledge is reorganized in light of new experiences. Gleitman and Wanner (1982, p. 31) indicate "it could be that there are a succession of learners, each of whom organizes the linguistic data as befits his mental state. This is a kind of metamorphosis, or tadpole-to-frog, hypothesis." Muma (1986, p. 159) discusses this point as it relates to semantic categories:

> Moreover, there is other evidence (besides verbal) that prior learning becomes reorganized. Piaget's theory of stages of cognition is a prime example . . . It appears that the central nervous system is "hard wired" such that a *repertoire* of certain capacities comprises a key to unlock subsequent capacities (Schlesinger, 1977). In the instance of semantic capacities, it may not be a padlock but a combination lock. That is, it is only after children attain a variety of semantic categories and *combinations* of them that they become ready to learn the formal mechanisms of language.

For some authorities, the notion of reorganization goes a long way toward solving the problem of discontinuity between semantic and syntactic organization in early utterances. For instance, Peters (1986, p. 310) suggests ". . . if the child indeed periodically reorganizes the grammatical system she is building, and if there are enough small reorganizations, no sharp organizational shift could take place." Peters believes that the child will integrate the limited scope formulae into a smaller and more manageable set of patterns. That is, the specific patterns typically referred to in semantic grammar will be grouped into more general patterns that incorporate the specific ones. Peters (p. 321) cites some concepts referred to by Ewing (1982) as being clearly relevant to the reorganization processes postulated in the early multiword period:

> Ewing (1982) calls these processes *vertical* and *horizontal integration.* Vertical integration is accomplished by noticing that two limited patterns such as big/little + X and hot + X can be combined into a single pattern involving the same number of elements, but where the fixed term is generalized to a limited *class*, e.g., PROPERTY + X. This sort of integration is already possible at the two-unit stage. Horizontal integration involves the realization that one pattern can be added to another to create a longer pattern, e.g., big/little + X and see + X can be combined into see + big/little + X, or actor + action and action + object can be combined into actor + action + object.

Ewing has studied children's early utterances using a model involving vertical and horizontal integration and has been able to make some impressive predictions about early multiword combinations using this paradigm.

CLINICAL APPLICATIONS: THE LANGUAGE-DISORDERED CHILD

When children are language-impaired, they tend to exhibit delays in the onset of early multiword combinations. Indeed, staying too long in the single-word period may be a primary symptom that prompts parents or physicians to make a referral to a speech-language pathologist. Leonard (1979) has shown that most language-im-

paired children tend to be delayed in language development as opposed to traveling a deviant course of linguistic acquisition. This means that a 3 year old with a language impairment who is talking in two-word utterances should be exhibiting a similar early multiword system to a normal child who may be chronologically 1 year younger. Most research comparing language-disordered and normal children has balanced groups of these children on mean length of utterance (MLU) and then examined samples of their communication to determine similarities and differences. For instance, a group of language-impaired children may be 3 years old and have an average MLU of 1.95. This group might be compared with a group of normally developing children with an MLU of 1.95, but who are 2 years old. The researchers would then take language samples from each group and determine which semantic relations are present in the normally developing and language-impaired populations. If the samples are generally similar, it might be said that the language-impaired children exhibit a delay in language development because they are similar to normally developing children of a younger chronological age who are speaking at an identical MLU. If the samples show strikingly different patterns, the language-impaired children are thought to be deviant in their course of language development because they do not appear to simply be arrested in the normal developmental progression. Leonard (1979), after reviewing much research on this issue, concluded that most studies show language-impaired children to be delayed in their language development as opposed to deviant.

Several investigations have concentrated specifically on the early multiword period of language development. For instance, Leonard, Bolders, and Miller (1976) compared semantic relations in samples from normally developing and language-impaired children balanced for MLU and found that there were no significant differences between the groups in the types of semantic relations present. Freedman and Carpenter (1976) also examined semantic relations in language-impaired and normally developing children and found that there were no major differences in the use of semantic relations between the groups. They indicated that since there were no major differences in the types of semantic relations, and since semantic relations are based on a child's underlying conceptual organization, there probably were also no major differences in their concepts underlying language. Leonard, Steckol, and Schwartz (1978) studied semantic relations in groups of language-impaired and normally developing children. Although they found similarities in the semantic relations used in the two groups, there were also some differences. For example, the language-impaired group tended to use earlier developing relations (agent + action; action + object) more frequently than the normals, while the normals exhibited more frequent use of some of the later developing relations (e.g., experiencer + state). This suggests a less-mature system of semantic relations, but also affirms that the language-impaired children do use many of the same semantic relations seen in chronologically younger normals.

Thus it can be seen that the speech-language pathologist will be working with language-impaired children who need some help in developing early multiword utterances, since there have been many reports of delay in acquisition of these word combinations. When language-impaired children do develop early word combinations, however, they tend to learn types that are similar to those acquired by normally developing children. The clinician, therefore, needs to be familiar with the normal developmental data reviewed in this chapter to perform effective assessment and treatment on this population.

CLINICAL APPLICATIONS: ASSESSMENT

In many areas of language assessment there are formal tests that may be used to gain insight into a child's linguistic abili-

ties. The area of early multiword utterances, however, has no test available that has been widely accepted by clinicians. There are several reasons for this. First, children at the age of 2 to 3 years are not noted for their ability to cooperate in formal testing procedures. Second, since semantic relations are a product of a *context* of real communication, it is very difficult to contrive situations in which a child would express all the different types of relations he or she knows. Third, we want to get an idea of not only the types of semantic relations the child uses, but *why* they are used (communicative functions). Does the child use agent + action only in imitation, to regulate others, to answer questions, or to label activities? The three concerns addressed above are not dealt with on any formal test in speech-language pathology. Thus to gain insight into a child's early multiword system, the clinician should plan to obtain language samples over several sessions for later analysis. Most of the time the samples are taken in play activities, sometimes involving the parent as a play partner and sometimes during interaction with the clinician. At certain points in the play the clinician may produce specific prompts calculated to elicit certain semantic relations (e.g., "where's the ball?" to elicit entity + locative). These interactions are typically videotaped, since semantic relations can only be identified when the utterance plus the context is considered. For instance, if a child said "mommy box," we would not know if the child meant possessor + possession, entity + locative, or agent + object unless we were familiar with the context in which the utterance occurred. A major goal of the assessment of an early multiword child would be to get an inventory of the types of word combinations the child produces. Obviously, if the child can generate many different types of semantic relations seen in the early speech of normally developing children, it is a favorable prognostic sign. On the other hand, if the child can only produce some of the basic operations of reference and no two-term semantic relations, then the clinician can see that there is work to be done on the child's early multiword system. Targets such as common, early developing, semantic relations can be selected for stimulation or more direct work in treatment. When doing an early multiword analysis we must always remember that one instance of a particular semantic relation is not sufficient to credit this construction to the child's system. Many authorities suggest that we must obtain some evidence of *productivity* of these relations where they are produced with a variety of different words or some novel utterances that cannot be attributed to rote productions (Braine, 1976; Ingram 1979; Leonard, Steckol, & Panther, 1983).

At the conclusion of assessment, the clinician should have a reasonable idea about the child's inventory of two-, three-, and four-word combinations in terms of the semantic relation types produced. The clinician should also know the types of speech acts or communicative functions in which the relations are produced. A list of semantic relations that are missing can be used in designing specific probes for later sessions to determine if certain relations are not present simply due to sampling error. Those relations that are not produced can be targeted in treatment through language stimulation and provision of cues.

CLINICAL APPLICATIONS: TREATMENT

Since normally developing children acquire a variety of semantic relations prior to their transition into more syntactically regulated utterances, we assume that this is also important for language-impaired youngsters. As mentioned earlier, the elements of SVO are gradually realized verbally through the use of different semantic cases, and these different semantic relations are eventually subsumed under the more abstract and broad umbrellas of syntax. Thus it is probably good practice to try and establish as many different types of normally occurring se-

mantic relations as possible in language-impaired children so they can generate utterances about many facets of their environment. We have also indicated that many three- and four-word utterances are thought to be recombinations of early two-word operations and relations, so establishment of these combinations may be a good investment for later increases in MLU.

Many programs and paradigms for language treatment can be found in the extant literature. These programs tend to follow the theoreticalmphases that were popular at the time they were written. For instance, there are many programs from the 1960s that have a syntactic orientation in which they trained children to produce N + N and N + V combinations with no mention of the semantic relations that compose these grammatical combinations. Programs can also be found that stressed pivot grammar. Most current approaches to language therapy tend to emphasize assessing and training of the semantic relations discussed throughout the present chapter (Bloom & Lahey, 1978; MacDonald & Nickols, 1974; McLean & Snyder-McLean, 1978; Miller, 1981; Leonard, Steckol, & Panther, 1983).

The actual training of semantic relations can be done in a variety of ways ranging from highly structured treatment to more child-directed approaches (Fey, 1986). In the less-structured approaches the clinician selects specific semantic relation targets after a thorough assessment and then focuses stimulation on these during naturally occurring activities in the home or classroom. After the child has had the opportunity to hear the various relations used in their appropriate contexts, he or she often will begin to use them spontaneously during similar activities. If the child does not spontaneously produce the semantic relations being emphasized in the stimulation, the clinician can begin to provide some cues or prompts that are calculated to elicit the particular relation targeted. Sometimes a child is even encouraged to imitate specific relations during natural activities early in treatment, and then the clinician's model is faded in the hope the child will later use the relation spontaneously. Activities are often set up to emphasize specific relations; for instance, if entity + locative is the target, the activity can focus on objects being located in different places and finding them. More structured approaches use a drill-work mode usually involving imitation to establish the semantic relations. Later treatment moves toward more natural activities to generalize the word combinations to everyday situations. Whatever the approach, one can easily see that information from normal development is critical in understanding the language-impaired child at the early multiword stage and thus to effectively conduct assessments and plan treatment.

REFERENCES

Anisfeld M. Language development from birth to three. Hillsdale, NJ: Lawrence Erlbaum, 1984.

Bloom L. Language development: form and function in emerging grammars. Cambridge, MA: MIT Press, 1970.

Bloom L. One word at a time: the use of single word utterances before syntax. New York: Humanities Press, 1973.

Bloom L. Talking, understanding and thinking. In: Schiefelbusch R, Lloyd L, eds. Language perspectives: acquisition, retardation and intervention. Baltimore, MD. University Park Press, 1974.

Bloom L, Lightbrown P, Hood L. Structure and variation in child language. Monogr Soc Res Child Dev 1975;40:Serial 160.

Bloom L, Capatides J, Tackeff J. Further remarks on interpretive analysis: in response to Christine Howe. J Child Lang 1981;8:403–412.

Bloom L, Lahey M. Language development and language disorders. New York: Wiley, 1978.

Bowerman M. Reorganizational processes in lexical and syntactic development. In: Wanner E, Gleitman L, eds. Language acquisition: the state of the art. New York: Cambridge University Press, 1982.

Bowerman M. Structural relationships in childrens' utterances: syntactic or semantic? In: Moore T, ed. Cognitive development and the acquisition of language. New York: Academic Press, 1973.

Bowerman M. Semantic and syntactic development: a review of what, when and how in language acquisition. In: Schiefelbusch R, ed. Bases of language intervention. Baltimore, MD: University Park Press, 1978.

Braine M. The ontogeny of English phrase structure: the first phase. Language 1963;39:1–14.

Braine M. Childrens first word combinations. Monogr Soc Res Child Dev 1976;41:Serial 164.

Brown R. A first language: the early stages. Cambridge, MA: Harvard University Press, 1973.

Brown R, Bellugi U. Three processes in the acquisition of syntax. Harvard Educ Rev 1964;34:133–151.

Brown R, Leonard L. Lexical influences on children's early positional patterns. J Child Lang 1986;13:219–229.

Bruner J. The social context of language acquisition. Lang Commun 1981;1:155–178.

Cazden C. The acquisition of noun and verb inflections. Child Dev 1968;39:433–448.

Chafe W. Meaning and the structure of language. Chicago: University of Chicago Press, 1970.

Chomsky N. Aspects of the theory of syntax. Cambridge, MA: MIT Press, 1965.

deVilliers J, deVilliers P. Language acquisition. Cambridge, MA: Harvard University Press, 1978.

Duchan J, Lund N. Why not semantic relations? J Child Lang 1979;6:243–251.

Ewing G. Word order invariance and variability in five children's three-word utterances: a limited-scope formula analysis. In: Johnson C, Thew C, eds. Proceedings of the Second International Congress for the Study of Child Language. Vol. 1. Washington, DC: University Press of America, 1982; p. 316.

Ferguson C. Learning to pronounce: the earliest stages of phonological development in the child. In: Minifie F, Lloyd L, eds. Communicative and cognitive abilities: early behavioral assessment. Baltimore, MD: University Park Press, 1978.

Fillmore C. The case for case. In: Bach E, Harms R, eds. Universals in linguistic theory. New York: Holt, Rinehart & Winston, 1968.

Freedman P, Carpenter R. Semantic relations used by normal and language-impaired children. J Speech Hear Res 1976;19(4):784–795.

Gleitman L, Wanner E. Language acquisition: the state of the art. In: Wanner E, Gleitman L, eds. Language acquisition: the state of the art. New York: Cambridge University Press, 1982.

Gopnik A. Development of non-nominal expressions in 1–2 year olds: why the first words aren't about things. In: Dale P, Ingram D, eds. Child language. Baltimore, MD: University Park Press, 1981.

Greenfield P, Smith J. The structure of communication in early language development. New York: Academic Press, 1976.

Halliday M. Learning how to mean. New York: Elsevier, 1975.

Howe C. The meanings of two-word utterances in the speech of young children. J Child Lang 1976; 3:29–48.

Howe C. Interpretive analysis and role semantics: a ten-year mesalliance? J Child Lang 1981; 8: 439–456.

Ingram D. Early patterns of grammatical development. In: Stark R (ed). Language behavior in infancy and early childhood. New York: Elsevier North-Hooland, 1981.

Leonard L. Normal language acquisition: some recent findings and clinical implications. In: Holland A, ed. Language disorders in children. San Diego, CA: College-Hill Press, 1984.

Leonard L. Meaning in child language: issues in the study of early semantic development. New York: Grune & Stratton, 1976.

Leonard L. Language impairment in children. Merrill Palmer Q 1979;25:205–232.

Leonard L, Bolders J, Miller J. An examination of the semantic relations reflected in the language usage of normal and language disordered children. J Speech Hear Res 1976;19:371–392.

Leonard L, Steckol K, Schwartz R. Semantic relations and utterance length in child language. In: Peng F, Von Raffler-Engel W, eds. Language acquisition and developmental kinesics. Tokyo: Bunka Hyoron, 1978.

Leonard L, Steckol K, Panther K. Returning meaning to semantic relations: some clinical applications. J Speech Hear Disord 1983;48:25–36.

MacDonald J, Nickols N. The environmental language inventory. Columbus, OH: Nisonger Center, Ohio State University, 1974.

McLean J, Snyder-McLean L. A transactional approach to early language training. Columbus, OH: Merrill, 1978.

McCune-Nicolich L. The cognitive bases of relational words in the single word period. J Child Lang 1981;8:15–34.

Miller J. Assessing language production in children. Baltimore: University Park Press, 1981.

Moskowitz A. The two-year-old stage in the acquisition of English phonology. In: Ferguson C, Slobin D, eds. Studies in child language development. New York: Holt, Rinehart & Winston, 1973.

Muma J. Language acquisition: a functionalistic perspective. Austin, TX: Pro-Ed, 1986.

Peters A. Early syntax. In: Fletcher P, Garman M, eds. Language acquisition: studies in first language development. Cambridge, MA: Cambridge University Press, 1986.

Piaget J. The origins of intelligence in children. New York: International Universities Press, 1952.

Ramer A. The development of syntactic complexity. J Psycholinguist Res 1977;6:145–161.

Reich P. Language development. Englewood-Cliffs, NJ: Prentice-Hall, 1986.

Rodgon M. Situation and meaning in one- and two-word utterances: observations on Howe's "The meanings of two-word utterances in the speech of young children." J Child Lang 1977;4:111–114.

Schlesinger I. The role of cognitive development and linguistic input in language acquisition. J Child Lang 1977;4:153–170.

Schlesinger I. Production of utterances and language acquisition. In: Slobin D, ed. The ontogenesis of grammar. New York: Academic Press, 1971.

Slobin D. Data for the symposium. In: Slobin D, ed. The ontogenesis of grammar. New York: Academic Press, 1971.

Wieman L. Stress patterns of early child language. J Child Lang 1976;3:283–286.

Weisenberger J. A choice of words: two-year-old speech from a situational point of view. J Child Lang 1976;3:275–281.

Werner H, Kaplan B. Symbol formation. New York: Wiley, 1963.

CHAPTER 11

Morphology

Brian B. Shulman

As discussed in previous chapters, communication is a complex process evolving from different theoretical orientations. Studying young children's communication development requires us to examine separate components of language behavior. Our understanding of these components permits us, in turn, to initially assess and, if indicated, design an appropriate intervention program that benefits the child who exhibits poor communication development.

Many researchers (Bloom & Lahey, 1978; Hopper & Naremore, 1978; Lahey, 1988; Owens, 1988) have described components of language behavior. Regardless of the specific model used, language behavior is typically comprised of three components: language *form*, language *content*, and language *use*. To review, language form can be described relative to how sounds are sequenced and ordered into meaningful words (phonology). Furthermore, language form also can be described according to how words are ordered in an utterance (syntax). Moreover, language form includes the study of morphemes, the units of meaning that are words or inflections. Language content refers to

semantics, a system of rules governing the meaning of words and word combinations. Language use or pragmatics involves a set of rules governing language used within the communicative context (Bates, 1976a, 1976b). Pragmatics, therefore, is based on the function or purpose of language rather than on its specific structure.

This chapter focuses on one aspect of language form, namely, morphology. Discussion focuses on how morphology develops in young children, why it is important to communication development, and how knowledge about morphology is used in the assessment and treatment processes.

DEFINITION

Compare the following two sets of utterances obtained from the same child at age 18 months old and, again, at age 3 years old.

18 Month Old	3 Year Old
Cookie.	I eat cookies.
Two coat!	I have two coats.
Jump!	She is jumping!

Answer the following three questions about these two sets of utterances:

1. What was different about the two sets of utterances?
2. At what age did the child's language appear to be more complex?
3. What information did you use to determine language complexity?

By definition, the study of morphology involves morphemes, the smallest units of meaning. Morphology deals with words and their parts. Moreover, it refers to the language rules for combining these words and their parts. As humans develop language competence, two types of words are typically used. Berko-Gleason (1989) referred to these words as *content* (or *open class*) words and *functor* (or *closed class*) words. Content words are composed primarily of nouns, verbs, and adjectives, while functor words include prepositions, articles, and pronouns, among others. There are two types of morphemes, *free* and *bound*. Free morphemes can stand alone and convey meaning. For example, the word "cup" is a free morpheme because it can stand alone and generate meaning. Bound morphemes, however, are morphemes that must be attached to free morphemes to be meaningful. Bound morphemes are *grammatical markers* that cannot function independently. Prefixes (e.g., un-, in-, pre-, trans-) and suffixes (e.g., -ly, -est, -er, -ness) are examples of *derivational* bound morphemes, while the "-s" and "-ing" endings on the words

"coats" and "jumping" are examples of *inflectional* bound morphemes. Derivational morphology can be used to change one word into another word resulting in the emergence of a different part of speech. For example, when the bound morpheme *-ness* is added to the adjective *happy* (a free morpheme), the word becomes *happiness*. Inflectional morphemes do not change the overall meaning of words but rather modify words that may be used, for example, as *plural* markers (e.g., "coat**s**") or as *tense* markers (e.g., "jump**ing**" or "jump**ed**"). Since the use of free and bound morphemes has a potential effect on changing the *grammaticality* of language, it can be further stated that the study of morphology may be viewed as an aspect of syntactic (or grammatical) development. Figure 11.1 illustrates morpheme classes and provides additional examples.

MORPHOLOGIC DEVELOPMENT

During the preschool years the child's communication development extends beyond the single-word stage into a simple, early multiword combinatory stage. It is at this stage in the developmental process where we can *begin* to observe the child comprehending and understanding morphologic rules. Let's explore just how children develop these rules.

Roger Brown (1973) conducted a longitudinal study based on three children and determined certain critical stages of syn-

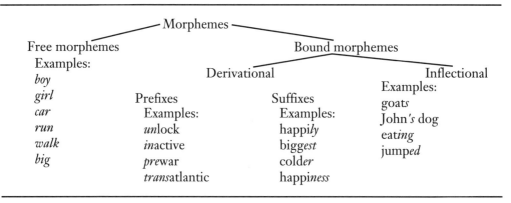

Figure 11.1. Morpheme Classes and Examples.(Adapted from Owens RE. Language development: An introduction. 2nd ed. Columbus, OH: Merrill, © 1988 All rights reserved.)

tactic development. These stages were characterized by changes in the child's utterance length and, in turn, syntactic complexity. Termed *Mean Length of Utterance* in morphemes (*MLU-M*), Brown denoted changes in MLU-M across each stage. MLU-M is a measure of utterance length based on the average number of free and bound morphemes contained in a designated set of spontaneously produced utterances. Length is determined by the number of *morphemes* rather than words. To calculate MLU-M, first determine the total number of free and bound morphemes in the language sample. Then divide the morpheme total by the number of utterances analyzed. The quotient obtained is the MLU-M. Brown provides a specific set of rules/guidelines to be used when calculating MLU-M (see the Clinical Applications section of this chapter for specifics).

Brown asserted the MLU-M measure was a reliable index for predicting a young child's grammatical development. In doing so, he determined a set of stages illustrated below in Table 11.1. Each of these stages is characteristic of certain changes in grammatical development.

In Stage I the child's language is primarily comprised of single-word utterances. Additionally, we can observe the child beginning to combine two words such that the two words are meaningfully related to one another. For example, in "Mommy eat," the child is ordering these two words to signify that Mommy is the person performing the act of eating. Thus the child is beginning to make word associations that convey meaningful information about the world around him. Brown and Fraser (1963) described these early two-word utterances as *telegraphic*. These utterances contain open-class words or content words (i.e., nouns, verbs, and adjectives) and lack closed-class or functor words making them resemble telegrams (e.g.,"no more"; "Daddy book"; "all wet"; "more cookie"; "no more"; "bye-bye Papa").

Early word combinations are extended in Stage II and further characterized by the appearance of grammatical morphemes that serve to add *syntactic specificity* to the child's language. In contrast to Stage I, the child in Stage II will typically produce utterances like "Mommy eat**ing**" or "**in** car" to mark the syntactic relations implied by the word order.

In a related study by de Villiers and de Villiers (1973), grammatical morpheme acquisition was investigated in a sample of 21 children. More adultlike utterances were observed in young children's language with simple sentences emerging in Stage III along with the child's use of yes/no and wh-

Table 11.1 *MLU Stages*		
Stage	MLU	Approximate CA (in Months)
Early I	1.01–1.49	19–22
Late I/Early II	1.50–1.99	23–26
II	2.00–2.49	27–30
III	2.50–2.99	31–34
Early IV	3.00–3.49	35–38
Late IV/Early V	3.50–3.99	39–42
Late V	4.00–4.49	43–46
V+	4.50–4.99	47–50
V++	5.00–5.99	51–67

Adapted from Miller J. Assessing language production in children. Baltimore, MD: University Park Press, 1981. *MLU*, Mean length of utterance; *CA*, chronological age.

question forms, imperative statements, and negatives. Stage IV is characterized by refinements in sentence complexity. Namely, the child begins *clausal* and *phrasal embedding*. Here, for example, the child places a clause such as "who smiled" within another sentence to create a sentence such as "The boy, *who smiled*, spilled the milk." As the child enters Stage V, syntactic modifications are exhibited in the form of compound sentences (e.g., "Mom dusted and I swept."). Table 11.2 illustrates grammatical morpheme production as a function of Brown's (1973) stages.

Retherford (1987) provides additional data relative to production of negative

sentences, yes/no questions, wh-questions, noun/verb phrase elaboration, and the development of complex sentences across Brown's (1973) stages.

A set of 14 grammatical morphemes, based on the longitudinal research of Brown (1973) and Cazden (1968), has been described in the literature and is presented below in Table 11.3.

It is important to note here that young children develop additional morphemes within Brown's stages. However, such morphemes were not studied by Brown and were, consequently, not represented in the above list. In turn, less is known about their acquisition. Such morphemes

Table 11.2 *Description of Grammatical Morpheme Production Organized by Brown's Stages*

Stage	MLU-M	Age (in Months)	Grammatical Morphemes
Early I	1.01–1.49	19–22	Occasional use
Late I/Early II	1.50–1.99	23–26	Occasional use
II	2.00–2.49	27–30	1. Present-progressive tense of verb, **-ing**
			2. Regular plural, **-s**
			3. Preposition, **in**
III	2.50–2.99	31–34	4. Preposition, **on**
			5. Possessive, **'s**
Early IV	3.00–3.49	35–38	No others mastered
Late IV/Early V	3.50–3.99	39–42	No others mastered
Late V	4.00–4.49	43–46	6. Regular past tense of verb, **-ed**
			7. Irregular past tense of verb
			8. Regular third-person singular of present tense
			9. Definite and indefinite articles
			10. Contractible copula
V+	4.50–4.99	47–50	11. Contractible auxiliary
			12. Uncontractible copula
			13. Uncontractible auxiliary
			14. Irregular third-person singular
V++	5.00–5.99	51–67	No data

Adapted from Guide to analysis of language transcripts by Kristine Retherford. Eau Claire, WI: Thinking Publications, © 1993 by Thinking Publications. Reprinted with permission. *MLU-M*, Mean length of utterance in morphemes.

Table 11.3 *Brown's 14 Grammatical Morphemes: Order and Mastery of Acquisition*

Grammatical Morpheme	Sample Utterance	Age[a]	Mastery Age (in Months)
1. Present progressive	-ing	"I go**ing**"	19–28
2. Preposition	in	"**in** car"	27–30
3. Preposition	on	"**on** nose'	27–30
4. Regular plural	-s	"see boy**s**"	24–33
5. Irregular past tense	came	"Mommy **came**"	25–46
6. Possessive	's	"John**'s** car"	26–40
7. Uncontractible copula	is	"He **is** nice"	27–39
8. Articles	a, the	"**a** dog"/"**the** boy"	28–46
9. Regular past tense	-ed	"She push**ed**"	26–48
10. Third-person regular tense	-s	"He sit**s**"	26–46
11. Third-person irregular	has, does	"She **has** cookie"	28–50
12. Uncontractible auxiliary	is	"**Is** he eating?"	29–48
13. Contractible copula	's	"He**'s** nice"	29–49
14. Contractible auxiliary	's	"He**'s** eating."	30–50

Adapted from Bellugi & Brown (1964); Brown (1973); Miller (1981); and Owens (1988).
[a]Used correctly 90% of the time in obligatory contexts.

include (1) pronouns (e.g., "I," "it," "one," "some," "other," "him," "her"), (2) other auxiliary verbs (e.g., "have + -en," "will"/"can"/"may" + Verb), and (3) noun and adjective suffixes (e.g., the adjectival comparative and superlative "-er" and "-est", respectively, as in "cold**er**" and "cold**est**").

The process of acquiring these major grammatical morphemes is gradual and lengthy (Tager-Flusberg, 1989). While these morphemes are initially observed in the child's linguistic repertoire on reaching an MLU-M of 2.0, all are not *consistently* used until after the child enters school. As grammatical morphemes continue to develop into Stage III, the child also begins to develop different types of sentences in the form of negatives (e.g., "no eat cookie") and questions (e.g., "Where Mommy go?"). Chapter 12 provides an extensive discussion of sentence development from its most simple stages to more advanced complex stages.

In studying his three subjects, Brown noted remarkable similarities in the order in which these grammatical morphemes were acquired. Since Brown's initial landmark longitudinal study, other researchers have investigated MLU-M (Miller, 1978; Miller & Chapman, 1975, 1979, 1981; Klee & Fitzgerald, 1985; Klee, Schaffer, May, et al., 1981). Miller and Chapman (1981) found a positive correlation between chronologic age and MLU. In comparing the data obtained by Brown with their own data, Miller and Chapman (1981) observed some general differences in syntactic growth.

More specifically, in comparing Brown's subject Eve with Miller and Chapman's subjects Adam and Sarah (Fig. 11.2), it can be noted that Eve's MLU-M increased markedly, while Adam and Sarah's language developed more gradually.

While MLU-M has typically been used to describe young children's *morphosyntactic* abilities, it was not intended to be used to describe the development of

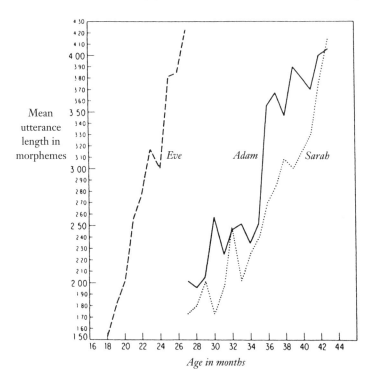

Figure 11.2. MLU Data: Eve, Adam, and Sarah. (Reprinted with permission from Brown R. *First language.* Cambridge, MA: Harvard University Press, 1973.)

complex syntactic structures used by older school-age children (see Chapter 12). Furthermore, while MLU has been criticized in the literature as a viable index of syntactic development (Crystal, 1974), it has proven to be an extremely useful measure in classifying young children's early syntactic competence.

A child's productive use of grammatical morphemes is evidence that he has acquired a set of rules and, in turn, the acquisition of these morphologic rules means that the child has acquired a rule-governed system. Berko (1958) studied preschool and first-grade children's productive control of English morphology using a set of "creatures" performing certain actions. Termed the *"Wug Test,"* a sentence completion task (or *structured elicited production task*) was employed to facilitate the child's use of invented (or nonsense) words containing grammatical morphemes in the form of plurals, possessives, the third-person present tense, past tense, and the present progressive tense.

Two sample items from the Wug Test are illustrated in Figure 11.3.

The children in the study performed well and led Berko (1958) to state that young children internalize knowledge about the English morphologic system such that they can add correct morphemes to novel words. In turn, this study further demonstrated that children do not simply learn grammatical morphemes through imitation, but rather they have acquired a rule-governed morphologic system.

CLINICAL APPLICATIONS

Since the study of morphology impacts the child's language comprehension and production abilities, a number of assessment instruments are available for evaluating a child's morphologic competence. Furthermore, for children who exhibit deficits in acquiring grammatical morphemes at age-appropriate levels, various intervention techniques are also available.

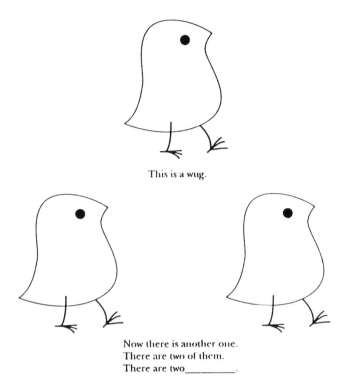

This is a wug.

Now there is another one.
There are two of them.
There are two_____.

Figure 11.3. The Wug Test: Sample Items. (Reprinted with permission from Berko J. The child's learning of English morphology. Word 1958;14:150–177.)

Instruments Available for the Assessment of Morphology

Many commercially available standardized instruments may be used to assess, in part, children's comprehension and/or use of grammatical morphemes.

By definition, a standardized or *norm-referenced* test is an instrument that evaluates a child's performance on specific tasks when compared with other children of the same chronologic age and/or grade level. Such tests are developed with specific standards for administration along with scoring guidelines and interpretation procedures that must be followed precisely to obtain optimum results. Details regarding test administration, scoring, and interpretation of results are described in the test's manual and must be followed so that the test may be used in the manner described by the developers of the instrument (Overton, 1992). For the purposes of this chapter, a brief description of six commercially available instruments that

evaluate English morphology are described below.

Test for Examining Expressive Morphology (TEEM)

The *TEEM* (Shipley, Stone, & Sue, 1983) is a 54 item norm-referenced instrument that examines a child's use of six major grammatical morphemes: (1) present progressive, (2) regular and irregular plurals, (3) possessives, (4) regular and irregular past tenses, (5) third-person singular verb forms, and (6) derived adjectives (e.g., -er, -est). The child is presented with individual picture cards corresponding to each item and is asked to complete a stimulus phrase with a response containing one of the above targeted morphemes. The child's performance is compared with data obtained on over 500 children between the ages of 3 and 8 years by the authors during the standardization process.

Miller-Yoder Language Comprehension Test (MY)

The *MY* (Miller & Yoder, 1984) formerly called the *Miller-Yoder Test of Grammatical Comprehension* (Miller & Yoder, 1972) provides the speech-language clinician with an awareness of how children, ranging in chronologic age from 4 through 8 years, understand short, simple sentences by using a variety of grammatical forms presented within a picture-choice paradigm. Furthermore, the *MY* can assist the clinician in determining a child's overall language comprehension performance. The *MY* contains 84 sentences presented as 42 sentence pairs, representing 10 basic grammatical forms some of which include such grammatical morphemes as prepositions, possessives, and noun plural forms.

Test for Auditory Comprehension of Language-Revised (TACL-R)

The *TACL-R* (Carrow-Woolfolk, 1985) is a standardized language assessment instrument that assesses a child's language comprehension across three different linguistic categories, each represented by a separate subtest (i.e., a part of a test that measures skills in a particular area/domain): word classes and relations, grammatical morphemes, and elaborated sentences. In the Grammatical Morphemes subtest, the child's comprehension of numerous grammatical morphemes presented within one of three picture choices is evaluated. Such morphemes include (1) auxiliary verbs, (2) plurals, (3) prepositions, and (4) derivational suffixes, among others. Normative data obtained from over 1000 children, between the ages of 3 and 12 years, are provided in the test manual. Figure 11.4 displays the portion of the *TACL-R* score sheet that emphasizes the Grammatical Morphemes subtest.

Patterned Elicitation Syntax Test (PEST)

The *PEST* (Young & Perachio, 1983) is a language assessment instrument standardized on children ranging in chronologic age from 3 years through 7 years and

6 months. While listening to three sentences or phrases produced by the clinician, the child is asked to look at three related pictures and is required to imitate the sentences with the aid of the pictures. A total of 44 syntactic structures are assessed with the *PEST*, including specific grammatical morphemes such as (1) present progressive verb forms, (2) plurals, (3) articles, (4) uncontractible copulas, (4) regular and irregular past-tense verbs, (5) possessives, and (6) third-person singular verb forms. Figure 11.5 illustrates a sample *PEST* score form containing a list of the grammatical morphemes (and related grammatical structure) and the corresponding test sentences.

Multilevel Informal Language Inventory (MILI)

The *MILI* (Goldsworthy, 1982) was designed to measure a child's ability to use syntactic (and semantic) rules. The *MILI* attempts to describe such skills in children between the ages of 4 and 12. In part, this instrument examines a child's use of the following grammatical morphemes: (1) present progressive, past regular/irregular, and third-person regular/irregular verb forms, (2) use of the copula and auxiliary, (3) regular/irregular plurals, (4) articles, and (5) prepositions. Other commercially available instruments that evaluate, in part, morphosyntactic abilities include the *Assessment of Children's Language Comprehension (ACLC)* (Foster, Giddan, & Stark, 1973); the *Bankson Language Test-2 (BLT-2)* (Bankson, 1990) [formerly the *Bankson Language Screening Test (BLST)* (Bankson, 1977)]; *Berko's Test of English Morphology* (Berko, 1971); the *Carrow Elicited Language Inventory (CELI)* (Carrow, 1974); the Grammatical Closure subtest of the *Illinois Test of Psycholinguistic Abilities (ITPA)* (Kirk, McCarthy, & Winifred, 1968); the *Northwestern Syntax Screening Test (NSST)* (Lee, 1971); the *Oral Language Sentence Imitation Screening Test (OLSIST)* (Zachman, Huisingh, Jorgensen, & Barrett, 1977); the *Oral Language Sentence Imitation Diagnostic Inventory (OLSIDI)* (Zachman, Huisingh, Jorgensen, & Barrett, 1978); the *Preschool*

BASAL AND CEILING RULES:
    BASAL: Four (4) consecutive correct at an age level.
    CEILING: Three (3) consecutive incorrect.

Section II. GRAMMATICAL MORPHEMES

	RESPONSE	STIMULUS
	NR ① 2 3	1. The cat is in the box.
3.0—3.11	NR 1 ② 3	2. The cap is on the toothpaste.
	NR 1 2 ③	3. The farmer is big.
	NR 1 ② 3	4. The girl is jumping.
	NR 1 ② 3	5. The boy is beside the car.
	NR ① 2 3	6. The dog is in front of the car.
4.0—4.11	NR 1 ② 3	7. The man sees the children play.
	NR 1 2 ③	8. The cat is between the chairs.
	NR 1 ② 3	9. The fish are eating.
	NR 1 ② 3	10. She feeds the birds.
	NR ① 2 3	11. The ball is under the book.
5.0—5.11	NR 1 ② 3	12. The rope is through the box.
	NR 1 ② 3	13. Father said, "I have these."
	NR 1 2 ③	14. She feeds her.
	NR ① 2 3	15. The circle is around the car.
	NR ① 2 3	16. Show me the shortest man.
6.0—6.11	NR 1 2 ③	17. She jumped rope.
	NR 1 ② 3	18. He rode the bicycle.
	NR ① 2 3	19. He feeds himself.
	NR 1 2 ③	20. His dog is big.
	NR 1 2 ③	21. She is pointing at the pencil.
7.0—7.11	NR 1 2 ③	22. The cat drank milk.
	NR 1 ② 3	23. The girl said, "We're eating popcorn."
	NR 1 2 ③	24. The lady said, "This shoe is mine."
	NR 1 ② 3	25. The boy said, "I want this."
	NR 1 2 ③	26. They swam.
8.0—8.11	NR 1 2 ③	27. Mother gave the ball to her.
	NR ① 2 3	28. There is the baby elephant.
	NR 1 2 ③	29. The man painted the house.
	NR ① 2 3	30. The men ran.
	NR 1 2 ③	31. She sewed the dress.
	NR 1 ② 3	32. The fish swim away.
	NR ① 2 3	33. There is the grandfather's clock.
	NR 1 ② 3	34. Here is the pianist.
9.0—9.11	NR ① 2 3	35. She is going to shop.
	NR 1 2 ③	36. The deer eats apples.
	NR ① 2 3	37. The deer is drinking.
	NR ① 2 3	38. She will hit the ball.
	NR 1 2 ③	39. The man has been cutting trees.
	NR ① 2 3	40. She would have jumped.

SUGGESTED STARTING POINT

TOTAL CORRECT [ ]

Section II. GRAMMATICAL MORPHEMES RAW SCORE

Figure 11.4. Test for Auditory Comprehension of Language-Revised (TACL-R): Grammatical Morphemes Subtest Score Form. (Reprinted with permission from DLM Teaching Resources Carrow-Woodfolk © 1985)

Patterned Elicitation Syntax Test
Response Sheet

Directions: For each item, read the three phrases or sentences while pointing to the pictures. Then ask the child to tell you about the pictures. Score each phrase or sentence with "+" or "0" to indicate whether the **bold italic** portion was correct. Only the third response is calculated in the raw score.

Demonstration Item   Tie a shoe   Write a letter   Kiss a baby

Structure	Test Sentences	Score	Structure	Test Sentences	Score
1. progressive verb	a baby *playing* / a boy *sitting* / a girl *combing*		13. subjective pronoun (plural)	*We* wear boots. / *We* eat ice cream. / *We* drink milk.	
2. auxiliary + negative	*Don't* scream. / *Don't* fall. / *Don't* drop.		14. auxiliary + progressive verb (plural)	They *are flying*. / They *are eating*. / They *are riding*.	
3. indefinite pronoun	You eat *it*. / You throw *it*. / You read *it*.		15. irregular past tense verb	The boy *caught* the ball. / The girl *saw* the bird. / The man *broke* the dishes.	
4. possessive pronoun	The cat is *hers*. / The balloon is *hers*. / The baby is *hers*.		16. possessive	a *boy's* jacket / a *dog's* collar / a *girl's* hair	
5. modal + verb	I can *talk*. / I can *read*. / I can *jump*.		17. subjective pronoun	*She* is sleeping. / *She* is washing. / *She* is eating.	
6. WH question: what	*What* is in the box? / *What* is in the basket? / *What* is in the bag?		18. infinitive	He wants *to ride*. / He wants *to blow*. / He wants *to swing*.	
7. progressive verb + object	girl *brushing teeth* / boy *eating banana* / man *reading paper*		19. copula + prepositional phrase	The ball *is on the table*. / The rabbit *is in the box*. / The dog *is under the chair*.	
8. plural	I have *rabbits*. / I have *socks*. / I have *dolls*.		20. copula + adjective (plural)	The balls *are round*. / The pigs *are fat*. / The babies *are little*.	
9. WH question: where	*Where* is the shoe? / *Where* is the cat? / *Where* is the apple?		21. progressive verb + noun phrase	He is *eating a sandwich*. / He is *beating a drum*. / He is *reading a paper*.	
10. copula + adjective	This *is round*. / This *is broken*. / This *is open*.		22. interrogative reversal	*Is* the boy playing? / *Is* the girl talking? / *Is* the boy watching?	
11. article	Take *a* bath. / Ring *a* bell. / Hit *a* ball		23. negative + progressive verb	The baby is *not walking*. / The dog is *not barking*. / The girl is *not swimming*.	
12. auxiliary + progressive verb	She *is reading*. / He *is climbing*. / She *is drinking*		24. indefinite pronoun + copula + negative	*It is not* big. / *It is not* good. / *It is not* open.	

Figure 11.5. Portion of Patterned Elicitation Syntax Test (PEST) Score Form. From the Patterned Elicitation Syntax Test. (Copyright © 1993 by Communication Skill Builders, a division of the Psychological Corporation. Reproduced by permission. All rights reserved.)

Language Test (PLT) (Hannah & Gardner, 1974); the *Preschool Language Scale-3 (PLS-3)* (Zimmerman, Steiner, & Pond, 1992); the *Sequenced Inventory of Communication Development (SICD)* (Hedrick, Prather, & Tobin, 1975); and the *Test of Syntactic Abilities* (Screening) and the *Test of Syntactic Abilities (TSA)* (both instruments by Quigley, Steinkamp, Power, & Jones, 1978).

Owens, Haney, Giesow, et al. (1983) described the content of test items across 14 commercially available language instruments and four language sampling procedures (Table 11.4).

It can be noted that all 14 of Brown's (1973) grammatical morphemes (among other grammatical components) are evaluated across all tests and language sampling procedures presented. This table is particularly important because it provides the speech-language pathologist with numerous instruments to use in assessing a child's morphosyntactic competence within the context of a comprehensive language test. Secondly, data obtained from the administration of these tests and language sampling procedures provide the speech-language pathologist with a vast amount of information regarding the child's morphosyntactic (and overall language) competence from which to design an appropriate language intervention program, if indicated.

An observable disadvantage to solely using standardized tests for morphosyntactic assessment is that there are often only a few bound morphemes being assessed in any given instrument. These instruments can, however, provide a general description of the child's morphologic development, but probably should not be the sole basis for determining whether he is a candidate for intervention.

Language Sampling and the Assessment of Morphology

A language sample is a systematic collection and analysis of an individual's utterances used as part of a regular diagnostic procedure (Nicolosi, Harryman, & Kresheck, 1989). More specifically, the language sample should be obtained in a variety of naturalistic settings to observe the child's range of language proficiency and difficulty (Lund & Duchan, 1988). In doing so, therefore, descriptions about the child's morphosyntactic, as well as semantic and pragmatic, language competence can be made. When collected appropriately, the language sample may provide the best picture of the child's language production abilities (Stickler, 1987). Numerous procedures are available for analyzing a child's morphosyntactic ability during spontaneous language sampling. These include *Developmental Sentence Scoring (DSS)* and *Developmental Sentence Types (DST)* (Lee, 1966; 1976); *Language Sampling, Analysis, and Training (LSAT)* (Tyack & Gottsleben, 1974); *Language Assessment, Remediation, and Screening Procedure (LARSP)* (Crystal, Fletcher, & Garman, 1976); and Miller's (1981) *Assigning Structural Stage* procedure.

As discussed at the beginning of this chapter, Roger Brown's (1973) work represented the foundation for studying and analyzing children's syntactic development. Brown's description of MLU was based on observable syntactic changes in children's productions on the basis of increases in utterance length. Rules for assigning morphemes to utterances have been described in the literature by Brown (1973) and are presented in Figure 11.6.

These rules are typically used by speech-language pathologists in determining the child's MLU in morphemes (MLU-M). As discussed previously, the MLU-M is a measure of the child's morphologic development based on Brown's (1973) work (see Table 11.1). Each intelligible utterance in the language sample is analyzed based on length and grammatical complexity. After analyzing approximately 100 utterances and calculating the MLU-M, the speech-language pathologist compares the obtained MLU-M with the data presented in Table 11.1 to determine if the child's morphosyntactic development is appropriate, inappropriate, or advanced for his chronologic age. For example, language samples from three children aged 3 years, 5 months old (i.e., 41

Table 11.4 *Morphosyntactic Assessment: Standardized Tests and Language Sampling Procedures*

Test/Tool	Nouns				Verbs																
	Possessives	Plural (reg.)	Plural (irreg.)	Derivational Suffix	Present	Present Participle	Present Progressive	Past (reg.)	Past (irreg.)	Future	Present Perfect	Past Perfect	Past Progressive	Present Perfect Prog.	Passive	Modals	Copula	Auxiliary Verbs	Third Per. Sing. (reg.)	Third Per. Sing. (irreg.)	Infinitives/gerunds
ACLC						X															
BLST		X	X		X	X	X				X	X							X	X	
Berko	X	X		X			X	X	X										X		
CELI		X	X		X		X	X	X	X	X	X		X	X	X	X	X	X	X	X
ITPA	X	X	X	X			X	X	X							X					
Miller-Yoder	X	X			X		X	X		X			X				X	X			
NSST	X	X	X		X		X	X		X	X				X		X	X			
OLSIDI	X	X			X		X	X	X	X				X		X	X	X	X	X	X
OLSIST	X	X			X		X	X	X	X				X		X	X	X	X	X	X
PLST					X											X	X	X			
SICD		X	X		X	X		X		X						X	X	X			
TACL		X		X	X	X	X	X	X	X				X	X		X	X	X		
TSA				X	X		X	X	X	X					X	X	X	X	X	X	X
TSA, Screening				X			X	X	X	X						X		X		X	
Sampling tools: ASS	X	X			X		X	X	X	X	X	X					X	X	X	X	
DSS					X	X	X	X	X	X	X	X	X	X	X	X	X	X	X	X	X
DST	X	X			X		X														
LSAT	X	X			X		X	X	X	X	X	X					X	X	X	X	X

Owens RE, Haney MJ, Giesow VE, et al. Language test content: a comparative study. Lang Speech Hear Serv Sch 1983;14(1):7–21.

Table 11.4 *Morphosyntactic Assessment: Standardized Tests and Language Sampling Procedures (continued)*

GRAMMATICAL · OTHER

Column groupings — **Pronouns:** Subject Pronouns, Object Pronouns, Possessive:Nom./Deter., Indefinite Pronouns, Reflexive Pronouns · **Adjectival:** Adjectives, Demonstratives, Articles, Comparatives, Superlatives · Adverbs, Prepositions · **Clausal:** Wh-Questions, Yes/No Questions, Embedding, Coordinated.Conjunction, Negatives, "Do" Insertions · **Other:** Response to Commands, Quantity, Body Parts, Common Nouns, Color, Categorization, Miscellaneous

Subject Pronouns	Object Pronouns	Possessive:Nom./Deter.	Indefinite Pronouns	Reflexive Pronouns	Adjectives	Demonstratives	Articles	Comparatives	Superlatives	Adverbs	Prepositions	Wh-Questions	Yes/No Questions	Embedding	Coordinated.Conjunction	Negatives	"Do" Insertions	Response to Commands	Quantity	Body Parts	Common Nouns	Color	Categorization	Miscellaneous
					X						X								X					
X	X	X			X			X	X	X					X			X	X	X	X	X	X	X
					X			X	X															X
X	X	X	X	X	X	X	X	X	X	X	X	X	X	X	X	X	X				X	X		
	X				X		X	X	X	X											X			
X	X						X			X					X				X			X		
X		X					X			X		X	X			X	X				X			
X	X	X				X				X		X	X	X	X	X	X							
X	X	X				X				X		X	X	X	X	X	X							
					X			X	X	X		X			X	X		X				X		X
X	X	X			X					X	X	X	X	X	X	X		X	X	X	X	X		
X	X	X			X		X	X	X	X	X	X			X		X		X		X	X		
X	X	X	X					X				X	X	X	X									
X	X	X	X					X				X	X	X	X	X								
X		X			X	X	X					X	X			X	X							
X	X	X	X	X	X	X						X	X	X	X	X	X							
X	X	X			X	X	X					X			X	X	X		X		X			
X		X			X	X	X			X	X	X	X	X	X	X					X			X

Rules for Calculating Mean Length of Utterance

1. Start with the second page of the transcription unless that page involves a recitation of some kind. In this latter case start with the first recitation-free stretch. Count the first 100 utterances satisfying the following rules.
2. Only fully transcribed utterances are used; none with blanks. Portions of utterances, entered in parentheses to indicate doubtful transcription, are used.
3. Include all exact utterance repetitions (marked with a plus sign in records). Stuttering is marked as repeated efforts at a single word; count the word once in the most complete form produced. In the few cases where a word is produced for emphasis or the like (*no, no, no*) count each occurrence.
4. Do not count such fillers as *mm* or *oh*, but do count *no, yeah,* and *hi.*
5. All compound words (two or more free morphemes), proper names, and ritualized reduplications count as single words. Examples: *birthday, rackety-boom, choo-choo, quack-quack, night-night, pocketbook, see-saw.* Justification is that no evidence that the constituent morphemes function as such for these children.
6. Count as one morpheme all irregular pasts of the verb (*got, did, went, saw*). Justification is that there is no evidence that the child relates these to present forms.
7. Count as one morpheme all diminutives (*doggie, mommie*) because these children at least do not seem to use the suffix productively. Diminutives are the standard forms used by the child.
8. Count as separate morphemes all auxiliaries (*is, have, will, can, must, would*). Also all catenatives: *gonna, wanna, hafta.* These latter counted as single morphemes rather than as *going to* or *want to* because evidence is that they function so for the children. Count as separate morphemes all inflections, for example, possessive {s}, plural {s}, third-person singular {s}, regular past {d}, progressive {in}.
9. The range count follows the above rules but is always calculated for the total transcription rather than for 100 utterances.

Figure 11.6. Rules For Calculating Mean Length of Utterance. (Used with permission from Brown R. First language. Cambridge, MA: Harvard University Press, 1973.)

months) were obtained and analyzed revealing the following MLU-Ms:

Child 1: 2.76
Child 2: 3.87
Child 3: 4.54

Using the MLU-M acquisition data presented in Table 11.1, answer the following questions relative to the child's chronologic age and corresponding MLU-M data:

1. Which child's MLU-M is age-appropriate?
2. Which child's MLU-M is advanced?
3. Which child's MLU-M is below age expectations?

The MLU-M for Child 2 is age-appropriate, while the MLU-M for Child 3 is advanced, and the corresponding MLU-M for Child 1 is below age expectations. MLU-M data along with formal data corresponding to a child's performance on standardized, norm-referenced tests described earlier are typically used by the speech-language pathologist to determine the need for language intervention.

Language Intervention for Morphosyntactic Deficits

After determining that a child's morphosyntactic development is impaired based on the administration of standardized tests and language sampling procedures, the speech-language pathologist typically designs an intervention program with the goal of bringing the child's morphosyntactic development up to an acceptable, age-appropriate level of functioning. Deficits that significantly affect the child's level of communicative functioning should be targeted first for intervention. To meet this objective, the speech-language pathologist may identify a variety of procedures based on commercially available language intervention programs and/or may design activities that emphasize grammatical morphemes and facilitate the child's comprehension and use of these morphemes within the context of spontaneous conversation.

Much of what takes place during lan-

Table 11.5   *Sample Morphosyntactic Intervention Techniques*

Directed tasks	1. Have the child retell stories that are chosen for the variety of morphologic forms. "Three Little Kittens," for example, is likely to elicit *plurals*, and "The Three Bears" has many possibilities for *possessive* forms.
	2. Create the unexpected. Ask the child to do something on the pretense that you are not aware he is doing it or it has been done. This can be effective in eliciting *copulas* and *auxiliary verbs*. ("Come and sit down." "I am sitting down." "Shut the door." "It is shut.")
Patterned practice	Create a pattern and have the child follow it.

I'll say:

(Past tense)

I see it today.	You say:	I saw it yesterday.
I know it today.	You say:	I knew it yesterday.

(Possessive)

That cat belongs to Tom.	You say:	That's Tom's cat.
That hat belongs to Ann.	You say:	That's Ann's hat.

Elicited imitation	Construct sets of sentences that present the question in several forms and contexts

For auxiliaries

(is)	The boy *is* throwing the ball.
(are)	The kids *are* riding on the bus.
(am)	The girl said "I *am* going home."
(were)	The dogs *were* swimming in the lake.
(was)	The baby *was* sleeping by the door.
(will)	The men *will* take away the trash.
(can)	We *can* sit on the steps.
(should)	The cook *should* wash his hands.
(has)	The lady *has* cut the grass.
(have)	We *have* eaten our breakfast.
(did)	We *did* like the new cereal.
(don't)	Cats *don't* like to get wet.
(doesn't)	He *doesn't* mind if we play here.

From Lund NJ, Duchan JF. Assessing children's language in naturalistic contexts © 1988 by Allyn and Bacon. Reprinted/adapted by permission.

guage intervention is based on the creativity with which the clinician can design materials and implement them to meet intervention objectives. For young children who exhibit morphosyntactic deficits, therapy should initially focus on facilitating the emergence of Brown's (1973) 14 grammatical morphemes. It is important to remember that children should typically be able to comprehend a particular linguistic structure (in this case, a specific grammatical morpheme) prior to being expected to express the structure. Consequently, language intervention should be approached from a *comprehension to production* paradigm. Brown (1973) asserted that the 14 grammatical morphemes were basically acquired in the order in which they are listed. Therefore, the speech-language pathologist should attempt to apply such a developmental progression when designing intervention tasks.

Teaching Morphology Developmentally (Shipley & Banis, 1981) is a commercially available program that approaches intervention for morphologic impairments from a developmental perspective. Specific grammatical morphemes emphasized in the program include (1) present progressive, (2) regular and irregular plurals, (3) possessives, (4) past tenses, (5) third-person singular tense, and (6) derivational morphemes. A total of 523 stimulus cards are provided to teach over 700 morphologic concepts.

Lund and Duchan (1988) describe three techniques to use in remediating morphologic deficits. These include the use of (1) directed tasks to elicit specific morphologic structures, (2) patterned practice, and (3) sentence imitation tasks. The specifics of each are presented in Table 11.5.

Owens (1991) also provides some general guidelines that can be used in intervention to improve the child's morphosyntactic abilities. Specific techniques are described relative to verb tensing, and pronoun/plural/article/prepositional usage. Additional suggestions are given to train word order and sentence types within the context of spontaneous conversation.

It is important to remember that the suc-cess of intervention varies with the particular linguistic structure trained, the manner and duration of the training, and the characteristics of the individual child (Leonard, 1981). As in assessment, it is also important for the speech-language pathologist to approach intervention from a developmental perspective. Development is a gradual process with much overlap between structures; it is not "domain-specific" (Kamhi & Nelson, 1988). Changes in one linguistic component can affect other areas.

Intervention should always be fun and challenging. Every attempt should be made to use dyadic conversational interaction within the framework of any intervention task. The child should always be exposed to how a particular linguistic structure is used in everyday conversation. Furthermore, to facilitate generalization and overall communicative competence, the child must be given the opportunity to experiment conversationally with the structure(s) taught. According to Lucas (1980), the child must be an active speaker who engages in communicative behavior that is effective at changing the attitude, beliefs, or behavior of the listener. Intervention that does not attempt to include such a "pragmatic" orientation is incomplete, to say the least.

REFERENCES

Bankson NW. Bankson Language Screening Test. Baltimore, MD: University Park Press, 1977.

Bankson NW. Bankson Language Test-2. Austin, TX: ProEd, 1990.

Bates E. Language and context: the acquisition of pragmatics. New York: Academic Press, 1976a.

Bates E. Pragmatics and sociolinguistics in child language. In: Morehead D, Morehead A, eds. Normal and deficient child language. Baltimore, MD: University Park Press, 1976b.

Berko J. The child's learning of English morphology. Word 1958;14:150–177.

Berko J. Berko's test of the child's learning of English morphology. In: Bar-Adon A, Leopold W, eds. Child language: a book of readings. Englewood Cliffs, NJ: Prentice-Hall, 1971; pp. 153–167.

Berko-Gleason J, ed. The development of language. Columbus, OH: Merrill, 1989.

Brown R. First language. Cambridge, MA: Harvard University Press, 1973.

Brown R, Fraser C. The acquisition of syntax. In: Cofer CN, Musgrave B, eds. Verbal behavior and learning: problems and processes. New York: Mc-Graw-Hill, 1963.

Carrow E. Carrow Elicited Language Inventory. Austin, TX: Learning Concepts, 1974.

Carrow-Woolfolk E. Test for Auditory Comprehension of Language—Revised. Allen, TX: DLM Teaching Resources, 1985.

Cazden C. The acquisition of noun and verb inflections. Child Dev 1968;39:433–438.

Crystal D. Review of R. Brown, "A first language." J Child Lang 1974;1:289–307.

Crystal D, Fletcher P, Garman P. The grammatical analysis of language disability. New York: Elsevier North-Holland, 1976.

de Villiers JG, de Villiers PA. A cross-sectional study of the acquisition of grammatical morphemes in child speech. J Psycholinguist Res 1973;2:267–278.

Foster R, Giddan J, Stark J. Assessment of Children's Language Comprehension. Palo Alto, CA: Consulting Psychologists Press, 1973.

Goldsworthy C. Multilevel Informal Language Inventory. Columbus, OH: Charles E. Merrill, 1982.

Hannah E, Gardner J. Preschool Language Screening Test. Northridge, CA: Joyce, 1974.

Hedrick D, Prather E, Tobin A. Sequenced Inventory of Communication Development. Seattle, WA: University of Washington Press, 1975.

Hopper R, Naremore RJ. Children's speech: a practical introduction to communication development. New York: Harper & Row, 1978.

Kamhi A, Nelson L. Early syntactic development: simple clauses and grammatical morphology. Top Lang Disord 1988;8(2):26–43.

Kirk S, McCarthy J, Winifred K. Illinois Test of Psycholinguistic Abilities. Urbana, IL: University of Illinois Press, 1968.

Klee T, Fitzgerald M. The relation between grammatical development and mean length of utterance in morphemes. J Child Lang 1985;12:251–269.

Klee T, Schaffer M, May S, et al. A comparison of the age-MLU relation in normal and specifically language-impaired preschool children. J Speech Hear Dis 1981;54:226–232.

Lahey M. Language disorders and language development. New York: Macmillan, 1988.

Lee L. Developmental sentence types: a method for comparing normal and deviant syntactic development. J Speech Hear Disord 1966;31:311–330.

Lee L. Northwestern Syntax Screening Test. Evanston, IL: Northwestern University Press, 1971.

Lee L. Developmental Sentence Analysis. Evanston, IL: Northwestern University Press, 1974.

Leonard L. Facilitating language skills in children with specific language impairment: a review. Appl Psycholinguist 1981;2:89–118.

Lund NJ, Duchan JF. Assessing children's language in naturalistic contexts. 2nd ed. Englewood Cliffs, NJ: Prentice-Hall, 1988.

Miller J. Assessing children's language behavior: a developmental process approach. In: Schiefelbusch R, ed. Bases of language intervention. Baltimore, MD: University Park Press, 1978; pp. 269–318.

Miller J. Assessing language production in children. Baltimore, MD: University Park Press, 1981.

Miller JF, Chapman RS. Length variables in sentence imitation. Lang Speech 1975;18:35–41.

Miller JF, Chapman RS. The relation between age and mean length of utterance in morphemes. Unpublished manuscript, University of Wisconsin-Madison, 1979.

Miller JF, Chapman RS. The relation between age and mean length of utterance in morphemes. J Speech Hear Res 1981;24:154–161.

Miller J, Yoder D. The Miller-Yoder Test of Grammatical Comprehension (Experimental Edition). Madison, WI: University of Wisconsin Bookstore, 1971.

Miller JF, Yoder DE. Miller-Yoder Language Comprehension Test (Clinical Edition). Baltimore, MD: University Park Press, 1984.

Nicolosi L, Harryman E, Kresheck J. Terminology of communication disorders: speech-language-hearing. 3rd ed. Baltimore, MD: Williams & Wilkins, 1989.

Overton T. Assessment in special education—an applied approach. New York: Macmillan, 1992.

Owens RE. Language development: an introduction. 2nd ed. Columbus, OH: Merrill, 1988.

Owens RE. Language disorders: a functional approach to assessment and intervention. New York: Macmillan, 1991.

Owens RE, Haney MJ, Giesow VE, et al. Language test content: a comparative study. Lang Speech Hear Serv Sch 1983;14(1):7–21.

Quigley S, Steinkamp M, Power D, Jones B. Test of Syntactic Abilities. Beaverton, OR: Dormac, 1978.

Retherford K. Guide to the analysis of language transcripts. Eau Claire, WI: Thinking Publications, 1993.

Shipley KG, Banis CJ. Teaching morphology developmentally. Tucson, AZ: Communication Skill Builders, 1981.

Shipley KG, Stone TA, Sue MB. Test for Examining Expressive Morphology (TEEM). Tucson, AZ: Communication Skill Builders, 1983.

Tager-Flusberg H. Putting words together: morphology and syntax in the preschool years. In: Berko-Gleason J, ed. The development of language. Columbus, OH: Merrill, 1989; pp. 135–166.

Tyack D, Gottsleben R. Language sampling, analysis and training. Palo Alto, CA: Consulting Psychologists Press, 1974.

Young EC, Perachio JJ. The Patterned Elicitation Syntax Test. Tucson, AZ: Communication Skill Builders, 1983.

Zachman L, Huisingh R, Jorgensen C, Barrett M. Oral Language Sentence Imitation Screening Test. Moline, IL: LinguiSystems, 1977.

Zachman L, Huisingh R, Jorgensen C, Barrett M. Oral Language Sentence Imitation Diagnostic Inventory. Moline, IL: LinguiSystems, 1978.

Zimmerman IL, Steiner VG, Pond RE. Preschool Language Scale—3. San Antonio, TX: The Psychological Corporation, 1992.

CHAPTER 12

Early Sentence Transformations and the Development of Complex Syntactic Structures

Janet A. Norris

EXAMPLE

(1) This is George.

(2) He lived with his friend, the man with the yellow hat.

(3) He was a good little monkey, but he was always curious.

(4) This morning George was curious the moment he woke up, because he knew it was a special day.

(5) At breakfast George's friend said: "Today we are going to celebrate, because just three years ago this day I brought you home with me from the jungle.

(6) So tonight I'll take you to the animal show.

(7) But first I have a surprise for you."

Favorite storybooks of childhood such as *Curious George Rides a Bike* (Rey, 1952) are so familiar to us that we do not even think about the language that they contain. Consider the pronouns. *He* in the second sentence must be understood to refer to George in the first sentence. *He* in the third sentence also must refer back to George, and not the man mentioned at the end of sentence 2, because of the relationship of the word *he* to *little monkey* in that sentence. The characteristics of *good* and *curious* must be in-

terpreted in some opposite relationship to each other because of their connection within sentence 3 by the conjunction *but*.

Sentence 4, like many of the sentences in this passage, is really a composite of several sentences: It was morning; George was curious; George woke up; George knew something; It was a special day. To combine all of these individual ideas the author used one prepositional phrase; one subordinating relative clause modifying the object noun; one subordinating clause modifying the verb; one complex coordinating conjunction; one particle; numerous noun modifiers, including articles, demonstratives, and adjectives; the pronouns *he* and *it* to indicate cohesive reference to previously given information; and verb tense markers to indicate earlier occurring events and states. Sentence 5 is even more complex—examine it and see if you can determine how many clauses and phrases underlie its construction.

The passage is very complex linguistically, and yet children of 3 years of age understand and love to listen to stories such as this. By 5 years of age they have mastered and use most of these complex and compound sentence patterns in their own speech (Brown, 1973; Brown & Fraser, 1964). How do children progress from looking at the picture and perhaps saying, "A monkey" or "There man," to understanding the abstract ideas and the relationships held between these ideas that are expressed through the vocabulary, word order, and word endings in this passage? The answer to this is complex and not well understood, even after many years of research. We do know that it involves the inherent cognitive abilities of the child to learn and organize information that is encountered within the environment (Bates, Benigni, Bretherton, et al., 1977; Bruner, 1974, 1975; Morehead & Morehead, 1974; Piaget, 1950). We also know that other people influence this development and assist the child in attending to and talking about important or culturally significant information (Snow, 1984; Chalkey, 1982; Dore, 1986). We also know that humans are genetically endowed with the ability to allow symbols such as words to represent objects, actions, and abstractions and to use this symbolic ability to form links with the physical and social world (Lenneberg, 1967).

We also have a very good description of what children learn about language and how they use it during the time between 1 and 5 years of age. It is during this short period that most of the adult syntactic constructions and morphological forms that comprise grammatical sentences, as well as an impressive vocabulary, are acquired. The purpose of this chapter is to present a description of the path that children take in discovering how language works to communicate meaning, beginning with simple utterances of one or two words and progressing toward mastery of the complex sentences found within Curious George.

THE BEGINNINGS OF LANGUAGE

The period from birth to approximately 1½ years of age is one of rapid growth and development in all areas. During this time children show that they are beginning to make important discoveries about the physical and social world and are learning how to successfully function within this environment. At birth children begin with reflexive and undifferentiated responses to everything that is seen, heard, or touched, but by 1 to 4 months the child already shows recognition of familiar people and objects (Inhelder & Piaget, 1969; Mahler, Pine, & Bergman, 1975; Morehead & Morehead, 1974; Piaget, 1950). By 3 to 8 months the child actively works to control his or her own learning by using bodily movements and vocalizations to sustain interactions with people and by producing experiments with objects, consisting of banging, shaking, and manipulating, to discover properties of these interesting things (Bates et al, 1977; Snow, 1984; Piaget & Inhelder, 1958). By 7 to 12 months the child has definite ideas about people and objects and what they should be doing or how they are used. This results in the use of purposeful and recognizable behaviors, gestures, and communications to accomplish goals involving objects and people (Bates et al., 1977; Mahler, Pine, & Bergman, 1975; Morehead & Morehead, 1974; Nelson, 1985). In just 1 year the child has organized much information about the world, including its *content*, or what there is to think and communicate about; how to *function* in a manner that accomplishes goals and satisfies needs; and how to use *forms* of communication to express content or to meet functional needs (Bloom, 1970; Bloom & Lahey, 1978).

Around the first birthday these discoveries result in a remarkable qualitative advance. By 12 to 18 months these purposeful behaviors become truly intentional, and the child begins to manipulate people and objects to fit with the child's fairly knowledgeable view of the world (Bates et al., 1977; Bates, Bretherton, Shore, & McNew, 1983; Gopnic & Meltzoff, 1984). The child exhibits the correct use of most common objects such as cups and combs within daily routines and begins to pretend with these objects in play situations (Inhelder & Piaget, 1969; Nelson, 1985; Sachs, 1984). The child can coordinate people and objects at the same time, and so adults are specifically directed to attend to an object as the child attempts to share, request, comment on, reject, or direct the adult to help obtain it (Mahler, Pine, & Bergman, 1975; Dore, 1986). The child also has discovered that verbalizations are useful in this process and begins to produce a limited vocabulary of conventional words, as well as many long strings of inflected sound patterns that are coordinated with gestures and looking at people and objects. Pointing, reaching, grabbing, giving, and leading all clearly indicate the child's wants and needs to the adult (Bates et al., 1977; Bates et al., 1983; Cox, 1985).

However, many important things are happening that render this communication system, impressive as it is, unsatisfactory to the developing child. First of all, this type of communication is very limited to the here and now. Points, gestures, single words, and pretend actions with real objects all require that the surrounding environment provide a context for understanding the intended meaning (Bloom, 1970; Bloom & Lahey, 1978; Braunwald, 1978; Hoff-Ginsberg, 1985). Pointing and vocalizing only work to share meaning if the object or event to be referred to is present and recognizable to the listener. The use of a single word such as "cookie" is interpretable only when the context cues are there to support the intended meaning (such as an accompanying reach for "I want") (Bloom, 1970; Bloom & Lahey, 1978). But the child between 1 to 2 years of age is highly mobile, and the environment is expanding beyond the here and now. Many of the things that the child needs or wants to communicate about will not be in the immediate vicinity, and so a different method of communication begins to be required (Mahler, Pine, & Bergman, 1975; Nelson, 1985). Also, the explorations of the child result in finding a wide variety of new objects and activities to examine. These new events and objects are often discovered beyond the proximity of the mother or other primary caregiver. The child requires a method for communicating these new discoveries to keep the parent informed and involved in the child's life (Bruner, 1974, 1975; Mahler, Pine, & Bergman, 1975).

Another factor that limits the usefulness of early communications is that the child's ability to put *ideas* together is increasing (Bowerman, 1976; Leonard, 1976). The coordination of multiple ideas increases the probability that the people and objects that these ideas refer to may not be present at the same time in the same place. The child also will need a method for specifying the exact relationship between these ideas such as whether one thing happened along with, because of, near by, after, or instead of another thing (Bloom, Lahey, Hood, et al., 1980; Clark, 1971; Coker, 1978). Furthermore, the child's social world is expanding to include other children and adults that are involved in activities very different from the routine caregiving that made up most of the child's first year experiences (Mahler, Pine, & Bergman, 1975; Piaget, 1950; 1954). The more unfamiliar a listener is, the more conventional a speaker's communication system must be (Bruner, 1974, 1975; Snow, 1984). While the child's mother might understand the child's idiosyncratic or "baby" words for familiar objects, other people who are with the child less frequently will not have the background to understand what the child means unless the child uses words and word order that are close to the conventional language forms. Thus, as a child's cognitive abilities become more advanced, as the physical and social world becomes more complex, and as the physical distance and number of unshared events between the child and primary adult increases, a tool is definitely needed for sharing these new experiences.

The expanding physical and social environment, the increased cognitive ability to combine ideas into meaningful relationships, the emotional need to maintain shared knowledge with a primary caregiver, the greater range of people and needs that must be managed, and the prior successful use of verbal and nonverbal means of communication are just some of the factors that result in both a greater need for language to develop and a greater ability for this development to occur between 1 ½ to 5 years of age. Looking at the types of language behaviors that develop during this period can provide some insights into the level of knowledge and types of information that the child is noticing and communicating about during this developmental period. The integrated development of cognitive, social, communicative (semiotic), and sensorimotor functions is displayed for each of Brown's (1973) five stages using a profile termed the Situational-Discourse-Semantic: Development Model (Norris & Hoffman, 1997). This profile can provide a quick reference to the characteristics and achievements of each stage. The situational context profiles what children are able to do and talk about, including the objects, topic, and people involved in the situation. The discourse context profiles the characteristics of the interactions, including how long they last, how they are organized, and what functions they perform. The semantic context profiles what the child is able to focus on and represent in both mental schemas and in words that refer to these concepts and the relationships between concepts.

BROWN'S STAGES AS A FRAMEWORK FOR DEVELOPMENT

The stages of language development identified by Brown (1973) will be used to provide the framework for tracing a typical course for acquiring the language patterns of English. In particular, the acquisition of word order, or *syntax*, and the use of *morphemes* within sentences to communicate exact meanings will be examined. Brown mapped out this course of development by studying the language acquisition of three children, Adam, Eve, and Sarah. His findings have since been replicated with additional groups of children, with findings that replicated the order of acquisition reported by Brown (de Villiers & De Villiers 1973; Mervis & Johnson, 1987). What is remarkable about these studies is that, while there are individual differences in the rate and style of language learning, all children ac-

quire the same forms at approximately the same age level and in the same, unchanging, predictable order (Nelson, 1975). Even children with language delays and disorders follow this same predictable path, although at a slower rate of acquisition and often with less adeptness in usage (Greenwald & Leonard, 1979; Muma, 1978; Ryan, 1975; Share, 1975; Wiig & Semel, 1984).

Stage I: Specifying Meaning at One-and-a-Half (Table 12.1)

Because Brown was interested in identifying the acquisition of word order, his first stage (Stage I) is seen when the child begins to put two-word utterances together, rather than when first words are produced (Bloom, 1970; Brown, 1973). Most children exhibit this stage of language during the age range of 19 to 26 months (Brown & Fraser, 1964). At this age children have much information to express and many contexts where language must be used and learned to accommodate new experiences and demands encountered within their rapidly expanding world. The average utterance length, or Mean Length of Utterance (MLU), is 1.01 to 1.99 morphemes, meaning that the majority of the utterances will consist of one or two words (Miller, 1981; Miller & Chapman, 1981).

One area of knowledge that is of interest to the child is the world of objects. The child at 19 months has spent a considerable amount of time exploring, banging, stacking, opening, moving, throwing, and performing a myriad of other actions with and on objects of all sizes, shapes, and descriptions (Piaget, 1950, 1954; Piaget & Inhelder, 1958). Much of the child's play at this age involves putting objects in containers, building towers, putting shapes in form boards, scribbling with writing instruments on any available surface, and using objects for functional purposes such as eating with spoons or looking at books page by page (Clark, 1973; Fein & Rivkin, 1986; Jalongo, 1988). It is not surprising that the child has something to say about objects during this early stage of language development.

Table 12.1	*Brown's Stage I (19–24 months)*		
	SITUATIONAL Symbolic Displacement	DISCOURSE Sequential Organization	SEMANTIC Descriptive Reference
COGNITIVE	**Object Displacement** Perform pretend actions with own body, but requires life size props. Talk about own action, comment on changes within ongoing event. Meaning unclear outside of context.	**Event/Discourse** Short, isolated schema combined in temporal sequence, including short series of self-help and pretend for familiar actions (feed doll and put to bed).	**Perceptual** Perceptual actions including puts objects in container, builds towers, shapes in form boards. Adj+ N such as "big block", determiners this/that prepositions in/on in 2-word phrase.
SOCIAL	**Self/Other Displacement** Actively watches others in play but does not participate. Concept of self as individual, differentiates things belonging to self vs others.	**Interactional** Engages in short verbal dialogue exchanging information by asking & answering questions. Cooperates with adult in shared activities (dressing, reading).	**Functional** Associates objects with people who use them (put baby in bed). Use most familiar objects appropriately. Possessives by word order (mommy shoe), pronouns I/mine, main verbs.
SEMIOTIC	**Time/Space Displacement** Symbolic reference to objects/needs that are not in the immediate vicinity; Talk about whatever draws attention in the immediate environment. Can refer to objects or persons not present within very familiar context.	**Locutionary** Informative function emerges (sharing information about non-present objects: Where go? Puppy gone.) Follows and gives simple requests within familiar events (no eat, two truck).	**Convention** MLU 1.01–1.99; At least 250 unique syntactic types of 2-word combinations that express objects, actions, characteristics, states, locations, roles. Word order & intonation wh-question: What that? That me?
SENSORY-MOTOR	**Imitative Displacement** Imitation of novel action or word sequences and patterns not already in child's repertoire. Verge on imitating vertical line with crayon or pencil.	**Exocutionary** Begins to climb, jump, run, throw; Navigates sequences (up and down stairs with one hand held). CVCV and VCVC syllable shapes and clusters appear, but cluster reduction, weak syllable and final consonant deletion, metathesis.	**Modality** Initial consonants /b/t/ k/g/m/n/h/w/f/s/; Final /p/t/k/n/r/s/ Phonetically appropriate /p/b/t/d/k/g/ m/n/ng/h/w/; Gestures accompany words and communicate much of the meaning. Scribbling for pleasure, not representation, emphasis on circles.

Reprinted with permission from Norris JA, Hoffman PR. (1997). The SDS: Development model of integrated functioning. (Presentation handout).

Objects, People, and Their Properties

Knowledge about objects can be roughly divided into two types of information. The first type involves information about the object itself, including its overall identity and its specific properties, or *perceptual* knowledge. The second type involves information about the *function* of objects, or how they are used (Clark, 1973; Piaget, 1954). The child's understanding of object identity is demonstrated through the early acquisition of a large vocabulary of nouns that name familiar objects (Barrett, 1978; Carey, 1978; Dollaghan, 1985). Nouns make up the largest syntactic class of the first 50 words used by most children (Stoel-Gammon & Cooper, 1984), and children ask adults for the names of things and spend time simply naming objects. But children also demonstrate that they notice things *about* objects (Mervis, 1987). They may notice or comment on the familiarity of the object, the number of objects, the location of the object, or some of the characteristics of the objects (Gopnic & Meltzoff, 1984; Leonard, 1976; Nelson, 1975). Their use of nouns in utterances often expresses these types of meanings (Bloom, 1970).

Children at this stage also are knowledgeable about people. At birth children do not have a concept of themselves as being separate from the environment or other people, a state Piaget (1950, 1954) refers to as *egocentrism* and Mahler and his colleagues (1975) refer to as *normal autism*. However, by 18 months of age the child has begun to form a concept of self as an individual, who is separate from and increasingly independent of an adult caregiver. Separation and independence result in the need for different names or labels to refer to self and others. A means for marking other information about people such as specific attributes or ownership also is needed (Bloom, 1970; Bloom & Lahey, 1978; Gopnic & Meltzoff, 1984). This growing knowledge of objects and people is often expressed through the use of *noun phrases*.

Articles. For example, during this first stage children use the article *a* with nouns. Articles provide speakers with a syntactic device for creating names that are more specific than the general class of the object. *Dog* is a general class of animal with a particular appearance. *A dog* indicates a specific instance of that class. It is used during Stage I as a marker to name or make reference to an actual instance of that category of object (Brown, 1973; Brown & Fraser, 1964; Emslie & Stevenson, 1981). In adult English the article *a* is also used when the referent is specific to the speaker but not the listener ("I saw a dog in my yard"), or when a single case is not specific to either the speaker or listener ("Lets go buy a dog"). This usage is more difficult and does not appear until much later in development (Brown, 1973; Emslie & Stevenson, 1981).

Pronouns. Pronouns are not used extensively during Stage I. They are relatively complex, serving many syntactic and semantic roles, and therefore are mastered gradually. Pronouns indicate many things about the referent such as whether it is the speaker (I, me, mine) or someone else. They frequently identify the gender of the referent (he versus she) or the number of people or objects referred to (he, it versus they). They indicate whether the referent is a participant in the conversation or a nonparticipant (I, you versus he, them), and the role of the person (the subject, object, or possessor). They suggest whether or not the referent is a person (she versus it) (Brown, 1973; C. Chomsky, 1969; N. Chomsky, 1969). They also indicate that the identity of the person or thing is already known to the listener and therefore does not have to be identified by name. This property of pronouns is related to *cohesion*, and the use of pronouns is one of the devices used in English to indicate to the listener that the speaker is referring to someone or something that has already been stated or that is obvious in context (Halliday & Hasan, 1976). Thus, if a speaker says "The dog was small. The dog scared me," potential ambiguity exists, and the listener must determine whether the speaker is referring to one dog, which is both small and which scared someone, or whether they are separate dogs. By using pronouns as a cohesive tie ("The dog was small. It scared me."), it is clear that both statements refer to the same dog.

The first pronouns to appear, often in Brown's Stage I, are *I* and *mine* (Brown, 1973; Clark, 1978). There are many reasons for their emergence as the first pronouns. Children of this age are still very egocentric in their view of the world and understand most things from their own perspective. These pronouns also are used to fulfill a conversational role rather than to refer cohesively to information that has been stated earlier (Brener, 1983; Charney, 1980). They do not require the child to code gender or number of participants. Subjective pronouns in general (including *I*) are used before objective pronouns (*me*), suggesting that the child understands the role of a person as an agent of action or change, rather than as the recipient of such events (Baron & Kraiser, 1975).

Noun Modifiers. Children at this stage specify other things about objects. They communicate who has general rights (mommy shoe) or temporary ownership (mommy coffee) of something, thus using word order to express *possessives* in their two-word noun phrases (Brown, 1973; Golinkoff & Markessini, 1980). Children direct others to focus on an object of interest by indicating which object they mean relative to a near or distant location using the *determiners* "this" versus "that" (Brown & Bellugi, 1964; de Villiers & de Villiers, 1974). They also use a variety of *adjectives* to indicate something about an object that they consider to be significant such as "broken" or "dirty" (Bartlett, 1977; Clark, 1973; Eilers, Oller, & Ellington, 1974; Richards, 1980). The ability to talk about properties of an object at this stage is limited to contexts where reference is made to only the object itself (Clark, 1975); that is, the use of articles, possessives, demonstratives, and adjectives occurs only when noun phrases are produced alone and not when a noun is combined with a verb or other syntactic

class. The ability to coordinate information about the characteristics of the object with information about the function or action of the object in one sentence does not develop until later (Brown & Bellugi, 1964; Ingram, 1972).

People and Objects in Action

This does not mean that children in Brown's Stage I fail to attend to or communicate about the actions or states related to people or objects. We indicated above that children know and express information about people and objects themselves, including their names and their properties. But children also use language to express their understanding of the second type of knowledge about people and objects, or *functional knowledge.* Functional knowledge is related to understanding what things do, or the state that things are in (Clark, 1973, 1979). Children from birth have been busy doing things—performing many actions on objects, observing changing states of objects, and experiencing many states of pleasure and discomfort. By this stage of development they have a good grasp of the function of many things within their environment and can use them appropriately (Clark, 1973; Inhelder & Piaget, 1969; Piaget & Inhelder, 1958). Children eat with spoons and dishes during real and pretend eating routines, and they attempt to use most familiar objects in appropriate ways during bath, bed time, dressing, and other everyday routines (Fein & Rivkin, 1986; Nelson, 1985). They imitate the actions of adults and other children when they encounter unfamiliar objects (Piaget, 1950, 1954). And they talk about these actions and states in many types of utterances, some of which include *verbs.*

Main Verbs.   Main verbs refer to specific actions or states such as sitting, eating, liking, or making. The child has a fairly large vocabulary of verbs during this stage and uses them in many constructions, although they are more difficult to learn than nouns for many children (Bloom, 1974; Dollaghan, 1985; Johnson, Toms-Bronowski, & Pittelman, 1982; Naigles,

1990). *Transitive* clauses are the most common and refer to someone/something engaged in some activity with/to someone/something (I eat bread). The verb requires a direct object. Verbs such as *love, hate, give, show, make,* or *know* are always intransitive. Other clauses are *intransitive*, or simply state the action or activity, and make use of verbs such as *swim, fall, eat,* or *run.* Many verbs can be used in both types of clauses (Hubbell, 1988). A few verbs do not actually express any action or event, but rather a state of being. They include verbs such as *seem, become, feel,* or *looks,* as in "It looks good" (Shatz, Wellman, & Silber, 1983). Most of the verbs used by children in Stage I occur in two-word constructions, and they are not inflected with any tense markers, except an occasional -ing ending (Brown, 1973; Cazden, 1968). The auxiliary verb (am, is, are, was, were) that accompanies the present or past progressive -ing ending in adult grammar is not used by children at this point in development, resulting in utterances such as "he eating" rather than "he is eating" (Brown, 1973; de Villiers & de Villiers, 1973).

Copula Verbs.   Another type of verb that does not express any action or event is called the *copula*. In these constructions, the only thing that is in the verb position is some form of the verb *to be* such as *am, is, are, was,* or *were* (Chomsky, 1965, 1969). These are different from the present progressive constructions. The copula verbs do not accompany any main verb, but rather they function as the only verb within the sentence (Chomsky, 1965; Hubbell, 1988). They equate one idea with another such as "The dog is hungry." The sentence order could be reversed—"Hungry is the dog"—without changing the meaning. This is not true of auxiliaries. Reversing "The dog is eating the bone" to create "The bone is eating the dog" does not result in equivalent ideas! Children at Stage I of development equate ideas through word order, but omit the copula, resulting in utterances such as "Dog hungry" (Bloom, 1970; Chapman & Miller, 1975; Klima & Bellugi, 1966).

Noticing Changes and Differences

Most of the things that children talk about exist or happen, but children also notice changes in objects or events, or differences from an expected state. One way of talking about change or difference is through the use of negation (Bellugi, 1967; Pea, 1979). During Stage I the words *no* and *not* are used interchangeably, either to precede a noun or a verb as in "No cookie" or "No eat" or following a noun phrase as in "Mommy no." Generally, three uses of negation occur. Often the first to appear is *nonexistence,* where some object does not exist or is not seen in a context where the child expects it to be. The words *gone* or *all gone* may also be used to express this observation. *Rejection* is the next use to emerge in sentences. This occurs when some object is rejected or when the event that is happening (or is about to happen) is opposed by the child (Brown, 1973; Bloom, 1970; Leonard, Wilcox, Fulmer, & Davis, 1978). The rejection may involve what the child does not want to do or have ("No night night") or what the child does not want others to do ("No daddy sit"). Rejection is the first type of negation to be expressed nonverbally through head shakes, pushing away, or fussing, and the child continues to use these nonverbal means even after the syntactic capability emerges. A third use of negatives to appear in Stage I is *denial,* or disagreeing with the truth value of a statement made by someone else (Brown, 1973; Clancy, 1985). Often this involves the identity of an object, as in "no truck" when the actual object was a car.

Gaining Information

Children are naturally curious and want to know much about their world, including the names for things, what people and objects are doing, where things are, or where they are going. One way of gaining information is by asking questions. Three general forms of questions are used in English. The first type of question assumes a *yes/no response* and in adult language frequently begins with an auxiliary verb such as "Are you tired?"; "Is that a doggie?"; or "Do you want a cookie?" Children in Brown's Stage

I of development accomplish this type of questioning by using rising intonation at the end of the utterance such as "That doggie^" or "Want cookie^" (Klima & Bellugi, 1966). A second type of question is produced in the form of a statement to which a *tag* is added, for purposes of eliciting agreement or confirmation. In adult language the tag is stated in opposition to the statement such as "He's cute, *isn't* he?" or "Its not funny, *is* it?" (Dennis, Sugar, & Whitaker, 1982; Hubbell, 1988). Young children produce approximations to tag questions when they say "It's a dog, right?" or "I'm going, OK?" They typically are not present at all during Brown's Stage I (Dennis, Sugar, & Whitaker, 1982; Reich, 1986).

A third question type requests a more complex answer, often of a specific nature. Adults accomplish this by asking *Wh- questions* such as "Why did you go there?" or "What is that thing?" A few Wh- questions are produced during Brown's Stage I, although they are limited to situations such as asking for names of objects ("What that?"; "What this?") (Klima & Bellugi, 1966), information about actions ("What do?"; "What dog [doing]?") (Ervin-Tripp, 1970), or locations ("Where kitty?"; "Where go?") (Wootten, Merkin, Hood, & Bloom, 1979). The questions are related to the immediate event or situation, rather than actions or events that happened at an earlier time or a different location (Klima & Bellugi, 1966; Tyack & Ingram, 1977). The question "Why?" may also be asked by children at this age. However, it is not intended as a request for a reason or an indication of causality. Rather, children learn that they can use this question as a conversational device and maintain a longer conversation with an adult by asking "Why?" during their turn (Tyack & Ingram, 1977).

Combining Ideas and Information

Children do not attend to things that are unchanging for very long. Rather, they are interested in how things change or what they can do or what can be done with them. It is not surprising that beginning word combinations refer to the actions performed by someone or something (agent-action), the actions that are done to someone or something (action-object), the place where an object or action was located or the direction in which it moved (action/object-locative), or a description or quality of something or someone (attribute-object) (Bloom & Lahey, 1978; Leonard, 1976). As children attend to combinations of people, objects, actions, characteristics, states, locations, and roles, then linguistic strategies for combining these ideas are needed. At the end of Stage I, as the MLU reaches 2.0, the utterances produced by the child exhibit at last 250 unique syntactic types (Bloom, Lightbown, & Hood, 1975; Chapman & Miller, 1975). Evidence suggest that children use word order to comprehend multiword utterances more complex than they can produce (Golinkoff & Hirsh-Pasek, 1995; Hirsh-Pasek & Golinkoff, 1993). Word order appears to provide clues about the meaning of words (Gleitman, 1990; Naigles, 1990), while at the same time understanding of word meaning helps children categorize words by syntactic categories (Bloom, 1990). We describe word order according to the syntactic phrases that exist within sentences.

Phrases.   Phrases and clauses are two types of word groups that can be used to combine ideas. *Phrases* are groups of words that cannot stand alone as sentences because they do not contain both a subject and a predicate (Hubbell, 1988). "In the house" does not tell who/what the subject is or what happened, but only the location. Simple sentences are made up of combinations of phrases in an NP (noun phrase) + VP (verb phrase) relationship such as

The dog loves bones.
NP   VP

Additional phrases can be embedded within the original sentence to combine further information into the relationship. These embedded phrases often are used as a substitute for a noun or as a modifier for a noun or verb. For example, a verb can be made to take the place of the noun in the sentence above by using an *infinitive* phrase to substitute for the noun (Chomsky, 1969; Hubbell, 1988).

The dog loves bones.
THE DOG LOVES *TO EAT*.

A phrase also may be used to modify a noun or a verb such as "The dog *in the house* loves bones" or "The dog loves bones *with some meat*" (here the prepositional phrases modify the noun), or "The dog loves bones *with a passion* (here the prepositional phrase modifies the verb). Particle phrases and gerund phrases can function to embed information in similar ways (Hubbell, 1988). At the end of Brown's Stage I the beginning of phrasal embedding is seen with the emergence of the prepositions *in* and *on*. They do not occur very frequently and appear in two-word combinations rather than complete phrases (Brown, 1973; Miller, 1981).

Clauses.   *Clauses* are groups of words that can stand alone because they contain both a subject and a predicate (Hubbell, 1988; Chomsky, 1969). "He is in the house" identifies the subject and states some fact about the subject. Simple sentences are composed of one clause, but sentences can have more than one clause. Two main clauses can be *conjoined* into a compound sentence such as "The dog ate the bone, and the cat licked the milk." Words such as *and, but, because*, or *if* are commonly used to combine main clauses. During Brown's Stage I, conjoining begins to emerge. Initially, the child simply lists objects that are to be conjoined such as "coat hat" or "cookie juice" (Brown, 1973). By Late Stage I the conjunction *and* appears and is used as an all- purpose word for combining ideas (Bloom, Lahey, Hood, et al., 1980).

Subordinating clauses are more complex and insert one clause inside of another such as "The dog that ate the bone is in the house." They function as nouns, adjectives, and adverbs that add information or support to the main clause. Their appearance is not seen until Stage IV (Bloom, Lifter, & Hafitz, 1980; Brown, 1973).

Clinical Implications and Applications

The language accomplishments described in Stage I are mastered by the majority of children who exhibit normal language development at or shortly after their second birthday. Unfortunately, however, not all children are able to easily acquire the words and word-order strategies that are used to express information about the world of objects, people, and events. For example, the language abilities among mentally retarded children are often delayed beyond expectations based on mental age alone, and language is often the child's most impaired developmental area, although the sequence and pattern of development parallels normal development (Greenwald & Leonard, 1979; Ryan, 1975; Share, 1975). Children also may exhibit a delay or difference together with a problem such as a hearing impairment, or they may demonstrate a specific language disorder in the absence of mental retardation or other observable handicap (Lahey, 1988). These children may not develop language at a level commensurate with their own potential for learning without special assistance or language intervention.

There are many approaches that have been used to provide language intervention. Some of these procedures specifically address syntax by identifying a discrete skill, such as Noun + Verb combinations or present progressive verb forms, and by teaching these skills through modeling and reinforcement. However, most recent intervention theories recognize that language acquisition is a constructive process and not a rotely learned set of skills. Ideas and intentions underlie utterances—children talk because they have something to say and a reason for saying it. Practice on grammatical forms and structures, or the form of the language alone, is empty (Lahey, 1988; MacDonald & Gillette, 1984; McLean, 1989; Norris & Hoffman, 1990; Scherer & Olswang, 1989; Warren & Bambara, 1989).

Intervention therefore must consist of an interactive process that allows children to discover, acquire, and use new language behaviors. Intervention must integrate language content, use, and form by providing developmentally appropriate experiences. The integration of the experience enables the child to code meaning and intention with various linguistic forms (Lahey, 1988; McLean, 1989; Norris & Damico, 1990; Norris & Hoffman, 1990; Warren & Bambara, 1989).

Interventionists can facilitate this integrated language learning process by establishing a stimulating and developmentally appropriate environment, adhering to developmental principles and sequences of language acquisition, and facilitating the use of communication to express meaning and to accomplish goals. For example, we know that at Stage I children are interested in objects, their properties, and actions that can be performed with or on them, particularly within the context of familiar, everyday routines and experiences. Providing children with real objects such as dolls, dishes, combs, or cars and modeling simple, single actions while talking about them ("Eat the cookie"; "All gone"; "No more!") can help the child learn what to attend to and how to talk about these events. The adult can provide opportunities for the child to be a collaborator in these communications by providing hesitations and pauses that invite a turn, talking about the child's actions or things within the child's focus of attention, expanding or revising utterances that are produced by the child, or asking the child to communicate some information to the dolls or another child (Lahey, 1988; McLean, 1989; Norris & Damico, 1990; Norris & Hoffman, 1990; Warren & Bambara, 1989). Whatever communicative attempts the child makes should be accepted as appropriate and interpreted as contextually meaningful. Children become communicators when they are successful at communicating and are free to attempt to use language without risk of failure.

Storybooks can be used as one context for language learning. At this stage, objects can be identified and talked about, as well as single actions such as pointing to the picture of Curious George and saying "George is eating"; "Eat George"; "Eat the cereal"; or "Its hot!"—thus providing many opportunities to use noun phrases with modifiers and to describe actions in simple utterances. Storybook reading also provides a natural context for many questions to be asked and for changes and differences to be expressed using negation (Jalongo, 1988; Norris & Damico, 1990).

Stage II: Learning to Use Grammatical Morphemes at Two (Table 12.2)

Development is rapid during the preschool years, both in the area of cognitive development, or what the child knows and understands about the world (Piaget, 1950, 1954), and in social development, or the roles and functions of people and objects and how to participate within events (Chalkey, 1982; Dore, 1986). Language development also changes remarkably fast. Stage II lasts only a short period—generally only about 3 months between the age range of 27 to 30 months. The most significant change is that the child begins to use morphemes to specify the same semantic relations that were communicated through word order alone during Stage I (Brown, 1973; Derwing & Baker, 1977). The average utterance length, or Mean Length of Utterance (MLU) is 2.00 to 2.49 morphemes, because many of the utterances now have word endings attached and consist of two or three words (Miller, 1981; Miller & Chapman, 1981). Although morphological development begins at this time, it is a highly complex system that continues to evolve even in adulthood. For example, many adults think of words such as "data" as singular and therefore incorrectly produce sentences such as "The data is interesting" (Koziol, 1973).

Objects, People, and Their Properties

Objects continue to be of great interest to children in Stage II. By 2 years of age the child has a large vocabulary for objects commonly encountered in daily routines, and many additional words are added daily

Table 12.2 *Brown's Stage II (27–30 months)*		
	SITUATIONAL Pre-op Logical Displacement	DISCOURSE Reactive causal Organization	SEMANTIC Attributive Reference
COGNITIVE	**Object Displacement** Attends to abstract symbols that suggest real objects (peg people, miniatures, drawing of head only). Language refers to own actions and consequences on status of others ("I feed baby. Baby all done.")	**Event/Discourse** Three or more related action sequences are embedded within longer perceptual property episodes of action with some temporal and causal links (get food, pour into pan, cook on stove, serve). Talk about action.	**Perceptual** Objects matched & sorted by one abstract (color, texture, size, shape). Comment on properties and location. Includes copula but no tense (I is big). Adj in object position (I want red truck).
SOCIAL	**Self/Other Displacement** Plays near others using same toys or materials and talks about actions or need from own perspective but not coordinated with the role of others within the inter-action.	**Interactional** Maintains extended verbal dialogue when adult responds contingent to child's topic. Asks questions but may not wait for answers. Peer inter-actions prevalent.	**Functional** Asks, watches and experiments to discover function of unfamiliar object or event. Relates two things to the same action (Want milk and cookie). Pronouns me, my, it.
SEMIOTIC	**Time/Space Displacement** Language used to recreate familiar objects or events in another time and location ("I drink juice" while pretending to pour juice); Follow pictured actions across time in a storybook.	**Locutionary** Interactions with peers involve requests, commands, protests, declarations, or comments about own actions. Tantrums and negativism common. Aware of consequences, react 'Oh-oh!'	**Convention** MLU 2.00–2.49; Use of morphemes to specify same semantic relations previously expressed in word order. A/the specify general vs specific, "my" possessive, main verb tense -ing, "no" precedes verb, use 'and'.
SENSORY-MOTOR	**Imitative Displacement** Imitates functional actions with new or familiar objects in a role other than child's own (tries to open door with keys, cooks).	**Excocutionary** Sequences of behaviors used to assert power, regulate others. Morphological markers add to syllable shape. Final clusters appear /ps/ /ts/.	**Modality** Initial consonants /**p**/b/t/**d**/k/g/m/n/h/ w/**j**/**l**/f/s/; Final /p/t/ **d**/k/**m**/n/**ng**/r/**f**/s/**sh**/ **ch**/. Phonetically appropriate: /p/b/t/ d/k/g/m/n/ng/h/w /**j**/**f**/. Communication less reliant on gestures.

Reprinted with permission from Norris JA, Hoffman PR. (1997). The SDS: Development model of integrated functioning (Presentation handout).

during this stage (Braunwald, 1978; Dollaghan, 1985; Stoel-Gammon & Cooper, 1984). The most significant difference between this stage and the previous one is the way in which the child begins to think about objects. Two years of age marks the beginning of logical and organized thought about objects and their properties, a stage Piaget (1950, 1954) calls *preoperational.* This logic is limited to properties or characteristics of objects that are closely tied to sensorimotor experience and that are static and irreversible. The child can consider an object from one perspective such as its size or its color, but not two simultaneously. However, the child is able to focus on the abstract property of the object rather than the object as a whole and spends much time engaged in activities such as matching and sorting objects according to perceptual similarities (Blank, Rose, & Berlin, 1978; Fein & Rivkin, 1986). Words such as *big* or words marking color or shape may be produced in the context of such activities (Bartlett, 1977; Gopnik & Mettzoff, 1987).

Articles. The articles *a* and *the* both are produced in Stage II, although there is wide variation in the age of acquisition among children (Warden, 1976) and the age at which mastery of various uses of articles is achieved. Naming continues to be the primary function of articles during Stage II, and the use of *a* versus *the* is frequently undifferentiated. A child at this stage may say "A dog" when referring to the first appearance of the character in her book. On successive pages the figure may be referred to as "the dog," communicating that for a temporary period (the duration of the storybook reading) "the dog" specifically meant only that character and not any other dog. Although many instances of use at this age are ambiguous, it is clear from Brown's data that children understand that differences exist between general and specific cases of an object and that they are using articles in many contexts for purposes of indicating the degree of specificity that they intend (Brown, 1973). It is not until 4 years of age that these two forms are used correctly in the majority of contexts (Warden, 1976).

While children may experience difficulty with specificity of determiner usage, they do not exhibit errors in grammatical use. Articles can occur in many sentence positions such as pre-verb (the baby crying), post-verb (see the baby), and post-preposition (on the baby). Young children use determiners only in correct grammatical positions, indicating that their syntactic categories for determiners are consistent with adult use (Ihns & Leonard, 1988).

Pronouns. The actual order of appearance of pronouns varies among children, as well as the tendency to use pronouns (Bloom, Lightbown, & Hood, 1975; Huxley, 1970). Some children produce them early and frequently, while other children use the noun to refer to people and things. A general order of pronoun acquisition is observed with the personal forms occurring before those referring to others, the subjective pronouns emerging prior to objective, and the use within conversational roles occurring before nonparticipant uses (Brener, 1983; Charney, 1980; Sharpless, 1974). During Stage I the child used pronouns to refer to himself or herself as the subject of a comment (I) or to indicate that something belonged to the child (mine). Stage II reflects further differentiation of personal roles. The child begins to use pronouns to refer to himself or herself as the object of a pronoun (me) such as "Give me cookie." However, subjective and objective roles are frequently confused, and sentences such as "Me eating" are common (Trantham & Pedersen, 1976; Waryas, 1973). Possession also begins to be marked with the pronoun *my* in the noun phrase such as "My shoe." The self is differentiated from other objects, and the pronoun *it* is used to talk about these things in both the subjective and objective case (Hass & Owens, 1985).

Noun Modifiers. Children continue to use word order and stress to mark *possession* during Stage II, although some children exhibit instances of the possessive *'s* at this age (de Villiers & de Villiers, 1973). Whereas adjectives were used to indicate number in Stage I (two truck, more cookie), the regular form of there-flects further differentiation of pe(Brown, 1973; Miller, 1981). Originally, it is used within familiar contexts or frequently used words, appearing in short phrases rather than sentences. A greater variety of *adjectives* is used, occurring frequently when noun phrases are used alone. Elaboration of noun phrases within sentences occur in the objective position (Mommy see *big truck*) but not yet the subjective position ("*Big truck* go fast") (Brown, 1973; Chapman, 1978; de Villiers & de Villiers, 1973).

People and Objects in Action

Children show an increasing focus on intentional actions and engage in a series of two or three actions related to the same event (Applebee, 1978; Fein & Rivkin, 1986; Piaget, 1954). These sequences are present in both play and storytelling. While each action may be intentional, the overall activity does not have a logical order or temporal sequence. Talk is related to whatever attracts the child's attention, without establishing relationships among the different events or elements within the events. This focus results in comments related to the child's own intentions and consequences (Kemper & Edwards, 1986). The child may use statements such as "Kitty in" or "Blanket go up" to refer to general plans or intentions directed at the items. The child is also aware of the consequences or results of these plans, producing statements such as "there!" when plans are successful; "Oh oh!" when they are not; and "More swing" when they want the plans repeated (Fein & Rivkin, 1986; Kemper & Edwards, 1986). While language in these examples is used to create a future before it happens, the future takes place in an immediate time frame (Mahler, Pine, & Bergman, 1975). Therefore the language that the child uses is embedded in the context of the here and now.

Main Verb. The child does begin to differentiate the relative status of the here and now in the verb phrase. During Stage II, the *main verb* is occasionally marked for simple present tense in utterances such as "Doggie eats" (Brown, 1973; Cazden, 1968). The child also begins to mark the status of actions or states according to whether the event is ongoing at the moment of the utterance, but is limited in its duration by inflecting the main verb with the *present progressive* -ing ending (Brown, 1973; de Villiers & de Villiers, 1973). However, the progressive form consists of two elements. One is the -ing verb ending, and the second includes a form of the auxiliary verb *to be*. The auxiliary form is complex, because it is represented differently depending on whether the noun is singular or plural, the time of the action, and the status or person of the noun referred to. A first-person singular present-tense sentence, "I am walking" is represented with a different form of the auxiliary than a first-person plural past-tense construction, "We were walking." The auxiliary *to be* can be represented as *am, is, are, was,* or *were* (Block & Kessel, 1980; Hubbell, 1988; Wells, 1979). It continues to be absent during Stage II.

Children are aware of the grammatical position of verbs at this age and probably use syntactic information to learn new verbs, a process called *syntactic bootstrapping.* For example, when the syntax of the sentence contains a directional preposition (to, across) verbs are likely to communicate action, whereas the verbs associated with relative clauses tend to reflect a mental state such as *think* or *know.* Children as young as 2 years are sensitive to this grammatical information and will interpret and use an unknown verb accordingly (Naigles, 1990).

Copula Verbs.   Unlike the auxiliary form of the *to be* verb, the copula does appear during Stage II (Brown, 1973; de Villiers & de Villiers, 1973). The child begins to produce utterances such as "I am big," where the copula serves as the only verb within the sentence. The child cannot yet coordinate the appropriate tense and number, so the actual form of the copula verb may not be in agreement with the noun ("I is big") (Brown, 1973).

Noticing Changes and Differences

While children were able to express many types of negation during Stage I, they accomplished this by using *no* or *not* with a statement. During Stage II the child begins to express negation syntactically, with the negative placed prior to the verb. Thus, while statements such as "No mommy eat cookie" were produced in Stage I, the same utterance would be produced "No eat cookie" in Stage II (Brown, 1973; Bellugi, 1967, Miller, 1981). The ability to place the negative next to the verb and to coordinate it with the subject is not present. The words *can't* and *don't* also begin to appear, but do not seem to be differentiated in meaning from each other or from *no* and *not* (Brown, Cazden, & Bellugi, 1969). They are probably learned as vocabulary words and not as contractions, since the positive counterparts *do* and *can* do not emerge until later.

Gaining Information

During State II children continue to seek information to yes/no questions by producing statements with rising intonation. But their ability to ask Wh- questions in sentences that contain subjects and predicates begins to emerge, resulting in sentences such as "What you do?" or "Where daddy going?" (Klima & Bellugi, 1966; Wootten, Merkin, Hood, & Bloom, 1979). Questions at this time are used in new situations and to acquire a wide variety of information and are not restricted to the few routines and types of questions that characterized Stage I. Children also respond to a wide variety of Wh- questions that are asked (Winzemer, 1980).

Combining Ideas and Information

The preoperational logic that emerges during this period is evidenced in the child's increasing realization that other people and objects are permanent and can be talked about even when they are absent from the immediate context. Language thus becomes truly representational, not only referring to present objects and ongoing events, but also standing for or creating objects or events when they are absent from a context (Morehead & Morehead, 1974). One result of this is an increased ability to play and pretend by representing familiar, daily experiences in detail. The child might gather items related to eating, pick up a pitcher, pour imaginary juice into a cup, and drink (Fein & Rivkin, 1986; Sachs, 1984). Language is used to sequence and specify these relational actions and states.

Phrases.   Stage II is characterized by the production of many short phrases and simple sentences. The prepositions *in* and *on* that occurred in two-word combinations earlier now occur in phrases such as "in that cup" or "lookie on the bed" (Brewer & Stone, 1975; Brown, 1973; Clark, 1973; Miller, 1981).

A form called the *semiauxiliary* also appears during this time, occurring before the main verb but without a noun phrase following it ("I gonna ride") (Brown, 1973; Lee, 1974; Menyuk, 1964). This form is related to a more complex structure in adult language, where two verbs are combined using the infinitive *to*, as in *want to go or have to sleep*. Children produce forms of one morpheme such as gonna, gotta, hafta, or wanna in order to communicate the same type of meaning before they have mastered the adult syntactic strategy (Bloom, Tackeff, & Lahey, 1984; Lee, 1974).

Clauses.   As early as 30 months, or the end of Stage II, many children begin combining phrases and sentences to express complex or compound propositions using *and* (Bloom et al., 1980; Cromer, 1968). It is used in contexts where two things are related to the same action such as "Want milk and cookie" or within familiar events.

Clinical Implications and Applications

Children at Stage II continue to focus on familiar routines and real objects, but now attention to short sequences of actions related to the same event should be facilitated. As the child produces a single action with toys such as feeding a doll with a spoon, the adult can add another element by suggesting another dish that can be used, or offering a toy stove to cook the food. Language can be modeled that includes modifiers ("Hot food") and negatives ("Don't touch it!") or that expresses a complete idea ("The pan is on the stove"). The adult can collaborate with the child to produce these longer utterances by expanding on the phrases initiated by the child; beginning an idea and hesitating to encourage the child to complete it; or prompting comments or other expressions by asking questions, gesturing, or suggesting information that can be talked about (Lahey, 1988; McLean, 1989; Norris & Damico, 1990; Norris & Hoffman, 1990; Warren & Bambara, 1989).

Because of the child's interest in pretending and curiosity about others, storybooks also provide an excellent context for intervention. The interrelationships between the objects on a single page can be examined and talked about, providing opportunities to use a wide variety of noun phrases, verb phrases, and simple descriptions of events. For example, the pictures from *Curious George* can be used to talk about what the characters are wearing, eating, and doing. At this stage the focus is not on the story, but rather the actions and interesting objects depicted (Norris & Damico, 1990)

Stage III: Conversing in Simple Sentences at Two-and-a-Half (Table 12.3)

As children near 3 years of age, many social and cognitive changes are occurring. Greater interest is shown toward other children, longer periods of time are devoted to a single activity, and sequences of actions are strung together related to the same event (Fein & Rivkin, 1986). During Stage III, from 31 to 34 months of age, the child begins to engage in long conversations with adults if adults assist by asking questions or pointing out things to comment about (Jalongo, 1988; Snow & Ferguson, 1977). This assistance is referred to as a "scaffold" by Bruner (1983), and it enables the child to produce longer sentences than the child could independently pro-

duce and to maintain a topic for an extended period (Brinton & Fujiki, 1984). The average utterance length, or Mean Length of Utterance (MLU) is 2.50 to 2.99 morphemes, with many simple, complete sentences of up to five words produced (Miller, 1981; Miller & Chapman, 1981). Parents help the child to increase sentence length by asking questions, pointing out things to comment on, modeling sentences that would work to communicate specific information, beginning a sentence and allowing the child to complete it, and providing other prompts during conversation and activities such as storybook reading (Brinton & Fujiki, 1984; Jalongo, 1988).

Objects, People, and Their Properties

By age 3 children have a vocabulary of over 1000 words for things that they have experienced (Braunwald, 1978; Dollaghan, 1985; Stoel-Gammon & Cooper, 1984). These include a wide variety of adjectives (Carey, 1978; Carey & Considine, 1973; Clark, 1973); labels for parts of objects; and concepts related to time (before, after, today) (Coker, 1978; French & Nelson, 1985), space (in, on, with, to) (Miller & Ervin-Tripp, 1964), and perspective (me, you, she, them) (Haas & Owens, 1985). The child increasingly shifts the focus away from whole objects viewed separately to the relationship between parts within the whole (Open my car *door*), or the relationships that unify unlike objects or events (*The boy* likes *the game*) (Blank, Berlin, & Rose, 1978).

The child continues to focus increasing attention on the people and events that are occurring at greater distances from himself or herself and that are less involved in daily caregiving (Mahler, Pine, & Bergman, 1975). Much time is spent playing near or next to other children, although it is not cooperative or interactive play and therefore not truly social (Fein & Rivkin, 1986; Piaget, 1954). The communications between the children mostly involve requests, commands, declarations of possession, or comments about the child's own activities or feelings. Play themes and representations show greater cultural and

Table 12.3	*Brown's Stage III (31–34 months)*		
	SITUATIONAL Pre-op logical Displacement	DISCOURSE Reactive causal Organization	SEMANTIC Attributive Reference
COGNITIVE	**Object Displacement** Establish context from words with minimal reliance on actual objects or people (Play with few props; follow action in pictures; report events that already occurred with emerging use of past tense, future can/will).	**Event/Discourse** Elaborated action sequences with details, causality, outcomes (baby cries and so feed, burp, wrap in blanket, rock to sleep). Discourse connected by cause; but, so, or, if: time; before, after.	**Perceptual** Can substitute objects if perceptual similarity (pen used for baby). Parts within wholes (Open my car *door*). Elaborated NP subject & object with attributes (number, color, texture, size), differential negative forms.
SOCIAL	**Self/Other Displacement** Stays near others in same activity but not social; language to others focuses on own actions and needs. Talks to characters during play ("Eat your food") followed by action.	**Interactional** Maintains an extended topic with adult scaffolding to increase sentence length and length of story; discourse devices used (cohesive use of the, you).	**Functional** Play themes and representations show cultural and world knowledge. The role of others taken in play that are less often experienced (doctor). Pronouns: gender (he/she his/her), number (we/them) sub/obj confused
SEMIOTIC	**Time/Space Displacement** Recreates experiences occurring at great distances in time and space from original event; talk about future actions if in immediate time timeframe ("I will get my car")	**Locutionary** Refer to own intention and the probability that future action will change present state, or implies change has occurred (It can break; It broked).	**Convention** MLU 2.50–2.99; 1000 words, many simple complete 5-word sentences with elaborated NP + VP. Tense -ed; modal can, will, won't; negative inserted; conjunc clauses; why, who?
SENSORY-MOTOR	**Imitative Displacement** Imitates actions for world events (zoo, dance), reenactments of events infrequently experienced. Draws lines, circles on imitation; scribbles have definite lines and forms.	**Exocutionary** Planned actions (walk backward, jumps down, forward, tip-toe, stand 1 foot). Initial clusters /fw/bw/kw/tr/sp/st/ **sn/sl/**. Final clusters /ps /ts/**ns/nch/nk/**.	**Modality** Initial consonant /p/b/t/d/k/g/m/n/w/r/ l/j/f/s/**sh**/h/**ch**/. Final /p/t/k/**b**/g/m/n/ng/r/ f/s/sh/**v**/**z**/ch/. Appropriate: /p/b/t/d/ k/g/m/n/ng/h/w//j/f/. Gestures merely embellish or emphasize meaning of words.

Reprinted with permission from Norris JA, Hoffman PR. (1997). The SDS: Development model of integrated functioning (Presentation handout).

world knowledge, consisting of reenactments of events that are infrequently experienced such as going to the zoo. These reenactments, as well as stories told by the child, include many details and events, but the sequences lack logical order (Applebee, 1978; Fein & Rivkin, 1986). Language becomes increasingly important as a tool for representing these experiences, which must be recreated at a time and location different from their original occurrence (Piaget, 1950, 1954). This is reflected in the production of complete sentences that specify both the subject and the predicate (Brown, 1973; de Villiers & de Villiers, 1973).

Articles. The articles *a* and *the* now appear in both the subject position ("A doggie eat") and the object position ("Doggie eat the bone"), although they are not always included or used appropriately in sentences (Brown & Bellugi, 1964; Emslie & Stevenson, 1981; Zehler & Brewer, 1982). Naming is no longer the primary function, as the child elaborates the noun phrases that occur within NP + VP sentences to include articles. As the child strings a series of ideas together that are all related to the same event, some cohesive use of *the* occurs to indicate that the object referred to in the present context is the same one that was introduced earlier (Maratsos, 1974; Warden, 1976).

Pronouns. The focus on people distanced from the child is evident in the pronouns that are produced during Stage III. Shortly after children learn to refer to themselves using pronouns, they begin to refer to another conversational participant as *you*. This self-versus-other distinction is next followed by a gender distinction, and the pronouns *he* versus *she* emerge. Finally, both the participant role and gender are coordinated, and children differentially use *I, you, he,* and *she* in most contexts (Brener, 1983; Charney, 1980; Sharpless, 1974). The differences between children who preferred to use nouns and those who produced pronouns frequently in Stage II are no longer apparent by the end of this stage (Bloom, Lightbown, & Hood, 1975).

Semantic relations such as possession that earlier were produced with possessive *-s* now are produced in pronominal forms, but not without confusion. The child may acquire *his* and *hers* during this stage, but may continue to add the possessive marker, resulting in sentences such as "This is hers baby" (Haas & Owens, 1985). Subjective/objective confusion also frequently occurs, but only among the pronouns that are overlapping in their semantic and phonological information. The child may substitute *he, him, his* or *she, her, hers* for each other within sentences, particularly as the child is learning new uses of pronouns (Bellugi-Klima, 1969). For example, pronouns used for naming (him) may be used in the subject position of a sentence as the child is learning to use pronouns syntactically such as "Him eating cookies" or "Her not nice." But pronoun confusion across classes (I for you) almost never occurs (Waryas, 1973). The child also begins to mark number in pronominal forms, producing utterances containing *we* and *them* during Stage III.

Noun Modifiers. During Stage II children begin to indicate number by using plurals. Number during Stage III is reflected in additional types of noun modifiers. Demonstratives are used not only to indicate a near-to-far distance from the speaker, but also to specify number, so that *this, these, those,* and *that* are differentially produced in the subject position of sentences (Charney, 1979; de Villiers & de Villiers, 1974). Quantifiers such as *some, a lot,* and *most* also are used within noun phrases. Adjectives that describe properties of objects such as general words marking size (big) or primary colors are used frequently to make comments or to specify needs, requests, and preferences (Bartlett, 1977; Gopnik & Meltzoff, 1987). Therefore, the subject noun phrase can be elaborated at this stage, as well as the object noun phrase (Brown & Bellugi, 1964). Both can contain many different elements, including articles, demonstratives, possessive nouns and pronouns, and adjectives (Miller, 1981).

People and Objects in Action

The sequences of related actions that are observed in play, daily routines, and storybook reading place greater importance on relative time frames. Related events either occur or can be considered in a number of temporal and logical relationships, including early versus later events, the duration of events, and probable future events (Applebee, 1978; French & Nelson, 1985). During Stage III a variety of grammatical strategies appear in the sentences produced by children that mark these relationships.

Main Verb. The child consistently produces verbs in all obligatory contexts within sentences, specifying the intended link between people, objects, states, and/or locations (Miller, 1981). The child's perspective also begins to displace from the immediate here and now. Comments frequently are related to events that already occurred, and this past status is marked with the regular past tense *-ed* (Brown, 1973). The child's strong interest in specifying time is exemplified by the overgeneralization of this morpheme to words that do not receive this marker in adult language. Children produce sentences such as "I eated all my cereal" or "I broked the doll" when they intend to refer to a completed action or earlier event (Berko, 1958).

Auxiliary Verb. During Stage III, the child begins to include both aspects of the auxiliary verb construction. The durative quality of continuing actions is marked by the -ing ending on main verbs and by the "to be" verb specifying the status of the noun (am, is, are), and the tense of the action (was, were) is present in the verb phrase (Brown, 1973; Tyack & Ingram, 1977). However, considerable difficulty is experienced coordinating these aspects of the verb, and many sentences are incorrectly marked for noun-verb agreement (They is playing) (Lee, 1974). The auxiliary *do* also begins to appear in statements (Wells, 1979). This auxiliary is primarily a syntactic marker, because it contributes little to the meaning of an utterance. It is grammatically important for the construction of negatives and questions in sentences when other auxiliaries are not present (Hubbell, 1988).

The intentional plans or actions that the child began to exhibit in Stage II are more sophisticated in Stage III, both in implementation and in linguistic specification (Kemper & Edwards, 1986). Two of the five *modal* verbs, *can* and *will*, appear in the auxiliary position of the verb phrase during this period to specify the intention and probability of future action ("I can do that"; "Mommy will help me") (Wells, 1979). Syntactically, a primary class of auxiliary verbs can precede the main verb, including *be*, *have*, and *do*, but a secondary class, called *modal verbs*, also can be used in the verb construction, either preceding the main verb (I will go) or one of the primary auxiliaries (I might have gone). These five modal verbs carry the tense of the sentence when they appear as the first verb in the auxiliary construction, and they consist of the present-tense and past-tense forms of will (would), shall (should), may (might), can (could), and must. They communicate aspects of future action and the conditions or certainty of the act (Hubbell, 1988).

Noticing Changes and Differences

Early in Stage III negation is produced through the interchangeable use of *no*, *not*, *don't*, and *can't*, resulting in statements such as "I can't know." The subject of the sentence frequently is omitted, following the pattern established in Stage II (Bellugi, 1967). However, late in Stage III *won't* appears, and shortly afterward the child begins to differentially use the negative forms (Brown, 1973; Brown et al., 1969). The negative also is inserted between the subject and the predicate consistently. These refinements in negative structure were considered by Brown (1973) to be one of the significant developments that distinguished Stage III from earlier stages.

Gaining Information

The patterns for asking yes/no questions with rising intonation and asking Wh-questions with subjects and predicates

(What kitty eat?) continue to be used in early Stage III. However, late in this stage the child begins to develop the auxiliary in questions (Klima & Bellugi, 1966). In the yes/no question form the auxiliary begins to be inverted as in adult forms, resulting in questions such as "Can he go?" instead of "He can go" with rising intonation, although both methods of question formation continue to be used (Bellugi, 1971). The primary and secondary auxiliary verbs also begin to appear within Wh-questions, although they are generally not inverted ("What that bug is?"; "Where him is going?"; "What that boy is doing?"). The most frequently produced Wh-questions include *what, what doing,* and *where,* but others also appear and are used infrequently during this stage, including *why, who,* and *how* (Kuczaj & Maratsos, 1975; Wootten, Merkin, Hood, & Bloom, 1979). *What, where,* and *who* appear early, probably because they are pronominal forms that stand in for the objects, people, or places that are unknown, and therefore are simple substitutions. *Why* and *how* are more difficult and reflect the child's emerging ability to consider intentionality and planning that was also observed in modal verb usage (Kemper & Edwards, 1986).

Combining Ideas and Information

Stage III is characterized by the ability to coordinate a wider variety of information within a sentence. Many new forms of syntactic complexity begin to emerge, and expansions of previous accomplishments are seen.

Phrases. Many types of phrases occur in the sentences produced by children in Stage III. Prepositional phrases containing *with, to, in,* and *on* frequently are used to modify the noun or the verb in the object position ("You go with me"; "I are going to the doctor"; "Put that hat on me") (Bangs, 1975; Menyuk, 1971; Morehead & Ingram, 1973). Particles appear either with the verb or separated from the verb within the sentence ("I dress up the baby" or "I dress the baby up") (Fraser, 1974). Therefore, by Stage III the child not only pro-

duces elaborated noun phrases and verb phrases within the basic sentence, but also embeds information into sentences using phrases.

Clauses. A variety of conjunctions appear during Stage III that are used to introduce a clause, but not to combine sentences or words within sentences. These include *but, so, or,* and *if,* although *and* continues to be the most frequently occurring and is used in place of others (Bloom et al., 1980; French & Nelson, 1985). They are used in familiar contexts and/or in response to questions or comments made by others.

EXAMPLE
Adult: Jimmy can't go with us.
Child: But I go.

The collections of related actions observed in play and storytelling also are apparent in the listing that occurs linguistically at this stage. Children begin a series of individual sentences with *and,* as in "And I eated the cookie"; "And it broked"; "And it have a raisin." This type of stringing is very common in the spontaneous speech of children between 2 and 5 years of age (Bloom et al., 1980). It appears to be a precursor to the use of relative clauses, a sophisticated linguistic means of embedding one clause into another (Ingram, 1989; Tavakolian, 1981). The difficulty of relative clauses is evidenced by the poor comprehension of these sentence types by children at this stage.

Clinical Implications and Applications

Children at Stage III should be helped to focus greater attention on details, rather than whole objects, and to sequence actions to create unified events. As the child reacts to the object as a whole, the adult can point out relevant aspects of the whole. For example, as the child feeds the doll, the adult can talk about body parts ("Open your mouth") or attributes of objects ("Pour the milk in the big cup"). Similarly, unified events can be facilitated, so that first the food is cooked, then the table is set, the meal is eaten, and the dishes cleaned. Less frequently experienced events such as eating in a restaurant and ordering food or paying a cashier can be incorporated. The verb tense markers and prepositional phrases that coordinate sequences of actions through changes in time and location can be modeled and incorporated into the expansions and cues produced in response to the child's utterances. The child's interest in other children can be facilitated by helping the child to formulate requests, comments, and protests in the course of this play (Lahey, 1988; McLean, 1989; Norris & Damico, 1990; Norris & Hoffman, 1990; Warren & Bambara, 1989).

Storybooks provide ideal contexts for learning about sequences of related actions. At this stage the actual story can be focused on, rather than individual actions or events. Completed actions depicted on old pages can be referred to in past tense, while events on new pages can be discussed in present tense. Predicting what will happen next provides opportunities to use the modals *can* and *will*, as well as conjunctions that combine related objects and events. Pronouns can be used to refer to the characters in the book, helping the child to establish the self/other distinction (Jalongo, 1988; Norris & Damico, 1990).

Stage IV: Creating Possibilities Through Words at Three (Table 12.4)

At 3 years of age children's ability to mentally represent their world results in a focus on imagining (Piaget & Inhelder, 1958). The child begins to view the world in terms of its possibilities, rather than only what exists in the here and now. Language becomes an increasingly important tool for functioning within the many social roles that the child takes on, both within real experiences and within imaginary play (Fein & Rivkin, 1986; Sachs, 1984). During Stage IV, from 35 to 40 months of age, the child begins to organize the world logically and acquires language to reflect this coordinated view (Foster, 1986). The average utterance length, or Mean Length of Utterance (MLU), is 3.00 to 3.99 morphemes, with three- to seven-word sentences produced that include complex constructions

(Miller, 1981; Miller & Chapman, 1981). All aspects of language, including semantics, pragmatics, syntax, and morphology, become more adultlike.

Objects, People, and Their Properties

The acquisition of new vocabulary words continues to occur very rapidly during this stage, and children learn words associated with events that they only observe without active or direct participation (Braunwald, 1978; Dollaghan, 1985; Stoel-Gammon & Cooper, 1984). They are particularly attracted to events that involve imagination and fantasy, those that bring both pleasure and fear (Fein & Rivkin, 1986; Inhelder & Piaget, 1958). Police officers, firefighters, super heroes, monsters, and warriors are of considerable interest, and children quickly learn vocabulary for entities associated with their favorite characters and/or occupations. They also have a strong interest in the perceptual attributes, or properties of objects. These concepts are continuing to develop and they have names for many colors, dimensions of size, spatial relations, shapes, textures, and so forth, although they are not always used accurately (Blank, Rose, & Berlin, 1978; Charlesworth, 1990). Words also appear that reflect desires, feelings, and thoughts, and the child can project these emotions to characters in play.

The roles performed by others provide the child with models of how to function with independence in the physical and cultural environment. The child's understanding of these roles is reflected in play and language. The child takes on roles and produces dialog consistent with those roles such as pretending to be a mother or father and talking to dolls in a manner consistent with those roles (Fein & Rivin, 1986). The child can switch roles, first talking to the doll and then talking for the doll. The family and the culture greatly influence the child's expectations and expression of roles during this time. Language is an important part of experiencing and responding to these roles (Westby, 1985).

The child is still dependent on context

Table 12.4 *Brown's Stage IV (35–40 months)*

	SITUATIONAL Decontextualized Displacement	DISCOURSE Abbreviated Plan Organization	SEMANTIC Interpretative Reference
COGNITIVE	**Object Displacement** Language decontextualizes and can be used to recount a personal experience; predict future events in real or imaginary situations based on present evidence (although logic may be faulty). Words support objects or toys in play.	**Event/Discourse** Elaborated sequences of plot-related events, but sequence is not well planned or goal oriented; talks about aspects of event throughout and coordinates ideas in space, perspective, or time across sentences.	**Perceptual** Interest in perceptual properties of objects is strong. Uses words that interpret distinctions (big-fat-tall vs little-short-thin). Interest in shapes, size, counting. Use blocks to make buildings or vehicles. Adj used in elaborated phrases (one little dog).
SOCIAL	**Self/Other Displacement** Plays with others in same activity but no coordinated goal (each paint) (associative). Talks about past and future possible acts (I'm gonna paint Barnie).	**Interactional** Takes turns with adults and peers in conversation; Can give reports on personal events as a near monologue. Takes other's perspective (I vs you).	**Functional** Language used for functioning within many social roles; switch role talking to and for doll in same event Words interpret desires, feelings, thoughts (I know, think, wish).
SEMIOTIC	**Time/Space Displacement** Language refers to things that are possible and future actions that could happen independent of actual experience. Demonstrations used to support meaning.	**Locutionary** A variety of utterances are used to report, entertain, show off, and regulate the actions of others. Embed subordinate clauses to ordinate ideas.	**Convention** MLU 3.00–3.99; adult-like talk; 3–7 word sentences include complex structures. Auxiliary verbs present but may have errors, used in neg. and questions. Past modals (would) Combine 2 clauses, embedding.
SENSORY-MOTOR	**Imitative Displacement** Imitates roles of others, producing dialogue consistent with less familiar and unexperienced roles (policeman, space traveler). New vocabulary learned without direct participation.	**Exocutionary** Bilateral coordination (rides trike, alternates feet upstairs) Walks backward, sideways, on tip toes, marches. Invents spellings with syllables.	**Modality** Decontextualized language requires greater phonemic accuracy: /p/b/t/d/k /g/m/n/ng/h/w/j/**r**/**l** /f/**s**/ occurs appropriately. Gestures represent action ("Like this" [demonstrates]).

Reprinted with permission from Norris JA, Hoffman PR. (1997). The SDS: Development model of integrated functioning (Presentation handout).

to provide reference and therefore requires props to play. However, the props can be abstract replicas of real objects, or simply objects that can stand for or represent the intended objects (Fein & Rivkin, 1986). The child can pretend that a piece of paper is a plate or that a chair is a horse to ride (Piaget, 1954). Toys such as blocks, which in previous stages were simply objects that could be stacked or sorted, now become buildings, animals, or vehicles in the child's imagination. Language is used to give them identity. Saying "This is my horse" causes the chair to become a horse for all participants. Play sessions, as well as stories told by the child, begin to have short sequences of causally and temporally ordered events within them, although they are not related to an overall coherent structure or plot (Applebee, 1978; Fein & Rivkin, 1986). The plot changes almost continuously because the process of doing is more important than the structure of the product to the child (Foster, 1986; Sachs, 1984).

Articles. The subject noun phrase at Stage IV always occurs when it is obligatory in a sentence, and the articles *a* and *the* are present and used appropriately (Ingram, 1972). Although a noun phrase is most frequently accompanied by only one element such as an article or a demonstrative or an adjective, some sentences are produced in which an elaborated noun phrase contains two elements such as an article + adjective + noun ("Give me the big block"; "I want a red color") (Ingram, 1971). Articles are used as cohesive devices to refer to previously identified referents (Bennett-Kaster, 1983).

Pronouns. Additional pronouns that mark distinctions such as inclusion and subject versus object role appear during Stage IV. *They* and *us*, which refer to multiple agents but contrast in the inclusion of the speaker and sentence position, are acquired (Ingram, 1972). Additional gender and role distinctions are marked through the use of *him, his,* and *hers* during this stage (Haas & Owens, 1985; Huxley, 1970). Confusion in the differential use of pronouns continues, and overgeneralization of regularities may occur. For example, after learning *hers* as a possessive marker, the child may use the *hims* as a parallel form (Trantham & Pedersen, 1976).

As children begin to recall events, tell stories, and play in longer sequences, pronouns used as cohesive devices become increasingly more frequent and important (Halliday & Hasan, 1976). The child does not always take the listener's perspective into consideration when making these reports and may use the pronoun as if the listener knows what it refers to without establishing the referent first. The child is able to take another speaker's perspective in regard to first- and second-person pronouns by 3 years (I versus you) but has more difficulty following third-person reference from another person's perspective (Tanz, 1980).

Noun Modifiers. Noun modifiers that draw comparisons between similar objects or that specify some salient feature continue to be added to noun phrases. Quantifiers, including *some, something, other, another,* and *more,* and numbers (children at this age can count three objects) appear during Stage IV (Charlesworth, 1990; Ingram, 1971). Adjectives that describe properties begin to reflect finer distinctions, so that *long* and *tall* may be used in place of a global *big* to describe a particular dimension of *big* (Bartlett, 1976; Carey & Considine, 1973). Adjectives occasionally are produced with other modifiers such as demonstratives ("Those funny clowns"), possessives ("My little baby"), or quantifiers ("Some more candy") (Ingram, 1972).

People and Objects in Action

The focus on possibilities, roles, imaginative thinking, and causality that begins to emerge during Stage IV continues to create both a need and a context for modulation in the time or states of action to be expressed. Events are viewed much less as loosely connected strings of actions, but are considered in relationship to each other. Aspects of the verb appear that reflect these relationships.

Main Verb. The past tense *-ed* form occurs with greater frequency to express completed action. It continues to be over-generalized, occurring on words that in earlier stages were produced correctly. For example, *went* may have been learned and produced early as a vocabulary word, as in "I went home" (Bellugi & Brown, 1964; Brown, 1973; Miller, 1981). During this stage the child is recognizing that the relative time frame of the same event can be modulated in time through verb inflection. Therefore, the relationship between *go* in the present tense versus the past tense is recognized, and the child produces sentences such as "I goed home" to indicate completed action or even "I wented home" (Brown & Bellugi, 1964).

Auxiliary   Verbs. Confusion   in noun-verb agreement with the many forms of the "to be" auxiliary continue, and this inappropriate marking is also evident in the copula (Erreich, 1980; Ingram & Tyack, 1979; Lee, 1974). The auxiliary *do* that was added to statements during Stage III now appears in questions and negatives as well (Klima & Bellugi, 1966; Miller, 1981; Wells, 1979). In negative sentences where the auxiliary expresses the past tense in adult speech, children occasionally doubly mark the verb phrase, resulting in sentences such as "I didn't breaked it" (Brown et al., 1969).

Possibility and intent are expressed with an increasing ability to use modals, and at least one form of past modal auxiliaries appear. *Could, would, should, must,* and *might* have all been observed in the language of children at this stage. The modals are used differentially in sentences to express such states as ability (can), permission (may), intent (will), possibility (might), and obligation (must) (Chapman, 1978; de Villiers & de Villiers, 1973). When the modal verb is used in the same verb phrase as the auxiliary *to be,* then the "be" verb remains in its unconjugated form, as in "I will *be going.*" Occasional appearances of this structure are observed in Stage IV (Miller, 1981).

Noticing Changes and Differences

The development of the negative within sentences continues to evolve during Stage IV as new forms and syntactic refinements occur. The use of *no* within a clause is replaced by *not* (Klima & Bellugi, 1966; Reich, 1986). This form is inserted between the subject and the predicate of the sentence, a syntactic placement that emerged late in Stage III. In this position the negative must be coordinated with the auxiliary verb, which itself is still developing, and many deviations from adult sentences occur (Erreich, 1980; Reich, 1986). Forms of the auxiliary *to be* are frequently omitted, but not always. Sentences such as "This not my car" or "I not crying" are produced, but at the same time utterances containing the auxiliary occur such as "That was not mine" or "I'm not going" (Miller, 1981; Reich, 1986). The contracted forms of the "be" auxiliary *isn't* and *aren't* appear by late Stage IV in sentences such as "That isn't yours" or "There aren't any colors" (Miller, 1981).

The positive forms of modal and auxiliary verbs that emerged, including *can, do, does, did,* and *will,* may be used with *not* in sentences, resulting in constructions such as "He can not go" or "I will not play." Many of these same verbs occur in their contracted forms of the negative, with *doesn't, didn't,* and *won't* appearing by late Stage IV (Brown, 1973). *Can't* and *don't,* which in Stage II were considered to be vocabulary words of one morpheme, now are analyzed as two morphemes, reflecting their grammatical status as true contractions.

Embedding negatives within sentences continues to cause confusion. The child experiences difficulty placing markers of tense and negation on the appropriate forms, resulting in deviations such as the double tense markings noted above ("I didn't did it," "I didn't catched it") and double negatives ("No one didn't see it") (Brown et al., 1969). The child also fails to make the *some* versus *any* distinction that occurs when affirmative sentences are made negative, producing utterances such as "I didn't see something" instead of "I didn't see anything" (Reich, 1986). The difficulties associated with negation are not specific to English. Children learning other languages such as French, German, and Italian have been observed to go through similar stages of acquisition and to produce similar patterns of errors (Antinucci & Volterra, 1975; deBoysson-Bardies, 1972; Grimm, 1973).

Gaining Information

The placement of the auxiliary verb at the beginning of yes/no questions that began at the end of Stage III continues to emerge in Stage IV (Bellugi, 1971). A greater variety of auxiliaries are produced in this inverted position, including forms of *to be* ("Am I big too?"); *do* ("Do you want a cookie?"); *can* ("Can I go with you?"); *will* ("Will the dog get hurt?"); and negative contractions ("Can't it go in there?") (Erreich, 1984; Ingram & Tyack, 1979; Klee, 1985; Kuczaj & Brannick, 1979). Rising intonation continues to be an alternative form for asking yes/no questions, but these questions are generally grammatically complete and produced similarly to those generated by adults ("You want to go out?"; "Want some juice?"; "Wanna play my game with me?") (Miller, 1981).

For many children the inversion of the auxiliary verb within *Wh-* constructions appears after its emergence in yes/no questions, or sometime during Stage IV (Ingram & Tyack, 1979; Klee, 1985). Other children do not show this lag and may even produce the inverted auxiliaries in *Wh-* questions first. However, by the end of Stage IV the inverted form does occur in the sentences produced by children, and their question formations are consistent with the basic adult form (Erreich, 1984; Ingram & Tyack, 1979; Klee, 1985; Kuczaj & Brannick, 1979). The correct sentence formations are observed for present tense forms of *to be* ("What is that?"); *do* ("Where do they sleep?"); *can* ("When can I talk to grandma?"); and *will* ("Why will it break?"). The child can ask a wide variety of question types, now frequently asking *who*, *why*, *how*, and adding *when* (Wootten,

Merkin, Hood, & Bloom, 1979). Confusions may exist when using *why*, *how*, and *when*, particularly regarding temporal aspects of these forms (Bloom, Merkin, & Wooten, 1982; Brown, 1968).

Combining Ideas and Information

The growth toward longer utterances and more adultlike language is dramatically evidenced in the child's ability to syntactically add and embed phrases and clauses to form complex sentences. Many of the true grammatical forms, the precursorers of which were seen at earlier stages, emerge during this stage, although it will be many years before they are fully mastered.

Phrases. The prepositions that children use within phrases reflect the position of an object compared with something else. The prepositions *up*, *at*, *under*, and *next to* appear during this stage (Bangs, 1975; Morehead & Ingram, 1973). The child also makes the *with* versus *for* distinction and produces sentences such as "Will you get the block for me?" Simple infinitives begin to be used by many children during Stage IV. They are embedded in the main clause of the sentence and often indicate the degree of intention or emotional response to an action by occurring with verbs such as *want*, *have*, *like*, and *need* (Miller, 1981). "I want to go to the store"; "I have to go to the store"; "I like to go to the store"; and "I need to go to the store" each communicate slightly different intentions or attitudes toward going. The entire phrase "to go to the store" is the infinitive phrase (Hubbell, 1988). During this stage the verb within the infinitive phrase shares the same noun as the main verb, or the subject noun of the sentence.

Clauses. The ability to actually combine two clauses and/or two phrases into a single sentence using conjunctions usually appears during Stage IV, although there are many reports of children producing these sentence types as young as 2½ years of age (Brown, 1973; Limber, 1973). There is no strict order of acquisition, with sentential coordination (two complete sentences such as "The boy walks" and "The boy runs") occurring at the same time as phrasal coordination (two phrases combined to share the same subject, as in "The boy *walks and runs*"). These sentence types do not seem to be directly related to each other in child language, with each exhibiting its own course of development (Bloom et al., 1980). The conjunction *and* appears first within conjoined constructions and is used to communicate a wide variety of semantic relationships between the two elements, including additive ("The kitty eats and the mouse runs"); temporal ("The kitty catches the mouse and eats him"); causal ("The kitty is hungry and he eats the mouse"); and adversative ("The kitty chases the mouse and he gets away") (Bloom et al., 1980; Brown, 1973; Limber, 1973).

Conjunctions that specify these relationships such as *then, because,* or *but* do not appear in complex sentences at this stage, although they are used to introduce a single clause (Bloom et al., 1980; Cromer, 1968; French & Nelson, 1985). *Because* is one conjunction that is added during this stage. It is frequently used alone, as when a child is asked a question and replies "Because" without actually giving a reason. It also may be attached to a single clause, as in "Because he ran fast." Children do not have a true sense of causality in their use of *because* at this stage. They either report one event that followed another or was the result of another as the cause (Why did you get scared? "Because I screamed"), or they answer the question as if they were asked "How do you know?", as in "Why did the kitty chase the mouse?"—"I saw the kitty's feet running" (Hood & Bloom, 1979; Inhelder & Piaget, 1969; McCabe & Peterson, 1985).

Embedding of subordinate clauses, or the insertion of one subject + predicate inside of another complete subject + predicate sentence, appears during Stage IV at about the same time as true infinitive embedding (Brown, 1973; Limber, 1973). One of the first to appear is the *object noun phrase complement*, where the clause takes the place of or is substituted for a noun

phrase. They follow the same basic pattern as simple sentences where there is a subject, a verb, and an object of the verb; however, in these constructions the object of the verb is itself a full subject + predicate clause (Limber, 1973; Menyuk, 1971). They generally occur with transitive verbs such as *think, know, wish, hope, forget,* or other states of cognition (Abbeduto & Rosenberg, 1985; Bloom, Rispoli, Gartner, & Hafitz, 1989). The ability to use this sentence type appears to be specific to the use of these verbs, indicating certainty/uncertainty, rather than a generalized grammatical rule. Consider these three sentences:

NP
I KNOW THE DOG.

Ob NP Cpl
I KNOW *THAT THE DOG IS HUNGRY.*

Ob NP Cpl
I KNOW THE DOG IS HUNGRY.

The complement allows for elaboration or specification of information about the noun. As the last sentence shows, the clause may or may not be marked by *that.*

A very similar construction also appears during this stage that embeds *Wh-* questions within statements, resulting in indirect questions. The first forms of these *embedded wh- questions* are *what, where,* and *when,* but *how, why,* or *if* also may appear infrequently (Garvey, 1975; Miller, 1981). Consider these sentences:

I know *the dog.*

I know *where the dog is.*

Look *how big the dog is.*

Remember *why the dog is there?*

Because this form of clausal embedding is developing at the same time as the inverted auxiliary in question forms, confusions may occur, resulting in sentences such as "I know where is the dog."

Clinical Implications and Applications

At Stage IV the adult should help the child to use language to create actions and events with minimal reliance on actual objects. During play, for example, pretend food can be prepared, or objects such as sticks or blocks can be used for needed materials by designating these things using words. Descriptions of these objects and materials can be incorporated into the play, including words for color, size, quantity, or texture. The child can be helped to take on the role of others such as pretending to be a chef in a restaurant and interacting with other children from that perspective. This type of play provides many opportunities for temporal terms to be used to sequence actions; for noun modifiers to be used to specify information about objects; and for various prepositional and verb phrases to be used to designate what each person could or should do, what each character needs or wants, and where actions or events are located or will be located. Opportunities for using conjunctions to sequence events or to begin to establish causality also naturally occur.

Storybooks can provide an excellent context for helping the child to sequence ideas and to use more complex sentences with greater independence. Through repeated readings of the same storybook, the child begins to internalize the plot and to learn how to talk about the events. By using the pictures to guide the storytelling, the child can begin to produce longer utterances and to establish cohesion across sentences. The adult can facilitate this independence by asking questions or requesting predictions, reminding the child of significant things in the picture, or prompting additional comments using relational terms such as "And then . . . "; "Because . . . "; or "Next to. . . . " The story can also be reenacted in play, either with toys or through drama, thus facilitating role taking (Lahey, 1988; McLean, 1989; Norris & Damico, 1990; Norris & Hoffman, 1990; Warren & Bambara, 1989).

Stage V: Expressing Complex Ideas Grammatically at Three-and-a-Half (Table 12.5)

Between ages 3 and 4 the child acquires most of the adult forms of sentences and begins to carry on conversations that maintain a topic and are very recognizable (Fos-

ter, 1986). The child's thinking becomes increasingly logical, although this logic is based very much on the perceptions of things, or what they look like, rather than on their function (Inhelder & Piaget, 1969; Piaget & Inhelder, 1958). Therefore, while the child shows the ability to reason and to predict future events based on the present evidence, this logic only considers some of the available information and focuses on one element at a time, leading to faulty conclusions and partial understanding. However, the ability to think logically during this stage, lasting from approximately 41 to 46 months of age, is reflected in the production of many compound and complex sentences that coordinate different events or ideas. The average utterance length, or Mean Length of Utterance (MLU), is 4.0 to 4.49 morphemes, with many coordinating and subordinating constructions used to produce lengthy sentences (Miller, 1981; Miller & Chapman, 1981).

Objects, People, and Their Properties

The number of words in a child's vocabulary surpasses 1500 by this stage (Braunwald, 1978; Dollaghan, 1985; Stoel-Gammon Cooper, 1984). Categorizing objects by some dimension such as "animals" or "red things" is a favorite activity as the child begins to focus on abstract properties of objects that make them the same and different, and words for these types of categories and concepts emerge (Blank, Rose, & Berlin, 1978; Fein & Rivkin, 1986; Inhelder & Piaget, 1969). Collecting and gathering are typical activities during this age as the child sorts experience into groups to impose some logical structure on the many things encountered. The ability to use language to symbolize experience is increasing and is highly observable in children's play. The objects no longer need to be physically present, but instead the child can create imaginary props and establish a context or scene using language alone (Fein & Rivkin, 1986; Sachs, 1984).

Children become aware of not only what they see or hear, but also what they think, and therefore more metacognitive

Table 12.5 *Brown's Stage V (41–46 months)*

	SITUATIONAL Decontextualized Displacement	DISCOURSE Abbreviated Plan Organization	SEMANTIC Interpretative Reference
COGNITIVE	**Object Displacement** Language decontextualizes and can be used to recount an event observed but not personally or directly experienced. Recounting understood by others who have some knowledge of the event.	**Event/Discourse** Elaborated sequences of plot-related events, with embedded episodes of plans, cause, end. Overall do not focus on a problem and plan to solve it, but some actions include a plan.	**Perceptual** Draws pictures to represent objects or events. Categorizes by same/different, dimensions (animals, red things). Perceptually based logic (more because its taller). Complex noun modifiers (four, big, blue, cars).
SOCIAL	**Self/Other Displacement** Cooperates with adults to achieve goals (bake cookies, simple chores) Takes on reciprocal roles in shared play, talking to and for characters. Assigns roles to other children, acts out roles using puppets.	**Interactional** Begins to adjust length of discourse to conform to the social context and participant expectations. Asks questions to find out how and why things are done or occur.	**Functional** Greater focus on future events and can infer possible actions (He might find a space man). Express facts, rules, beliefs, attitudes, emotions: Focus on function words (It *isn't* on, I *need to* go, *because* I *couldn't*.)
SEMIOTIC	**Time/Space Displacement** Language establishes the context by setting the scene and specifying the subjects and objects of an event, but often assumes shared information that listener may not have. Refers to possible and future actions. Emerging separate though vs action (I know . . .)	**Locutionary** Begins to differentiate between recountings of actual events vs fictional stories or fantasy. Reasoning emerges, resulting from integration of reporting, predicting, and projecting. Tease, warn, convey humor.	**Convention** MLU 4.0–4.49. Many compound and complex sentences, coordinating and subordinating clauses to relate complex events. Vocabulary surpasses 1500 words. Most verbs correctly inflected, contracted auxiliaries and negatives, gerunds.
SENSORY-MOTOR	**Imitative Displacement** Imitates complex actions and verbal expressions. Imitates pretend actions performed by super-heros and other fanciful figures.Uses imitation to draw complex figures.	**Exocutionary** Emerging maturity in locomotion including arm swing; runs smoothly, throws & catches. Uses many polysyllabic words (impossible, every-where); may have syllable simplifications.	**Modality** Phonemically appropriate /p/b/t/d/ k/g/m/n/ng/h/w/j/r/l /f/s/**z/sh/ch/** In most word positions. Errors: /v/dz/. Begins to recognize letters, pretend writing.

Reprinted with permission from Norris JA, Hoffman PR. (1997). The SDS: Development model of integrated functioning (Presentation handout).

words emerge such as *know, think, remember, pretend,* or *hope* (Abbeduto & Rosenberg, 1985). Less focus on the objects themselves and greater focus on the functions or interactions between people and actions lead to the emergence of abstract concepts such as *fair* or *happened.* The ability to sequence these interactions and to plan future actions is reflected in the acquisition of words such as *before, after, next, tomorrow,* and other terms of time and space (Carrow, 1973; Feagans, 1980). A greater number of words associated with people and their roles within the culture continue to emerge as the child's experience with the world expands beyond the family and the home (Fein & Rivkin, 1986).

Articles.   Articles continue to be used increasingly as cohesive ties, indicating when a general class of new information is being introduced, versus reference to already established information (Liles, 1985). As children's stories become longer or their reports of events acquire more detail, errors in cohesive reference occur. While the acquisition of cohesive reference has not been examined developmentally, analysis of stories told by children indicates that children use these ties correctly in simple contexts by 4 years and in relatively complex contexts by the time that they are 5 or 6 years of age (Liles, 1985; Norris & Bruning, 1988).

Pronouns.   The child continues to refine the "self" versus "other" distinction in the use of pronouns and indicates many conditions of the referent, including subject or object status, number, possession, and person. Inclusion of self is reflected in the use of *our, ours,* and the reflexive pronoun *myself* in which the subject and the object both refer to the same person (Bloom et al., 1975; Haas & Owens, 1985; Huxley, 1970). Reference to others appears in the use of *its, their, theirs,* and *yourself.* While these reflexive pronouns appear during this stage, errors in their use continue to occur (Wiig & Fleischmann, 1980).

Noun Modifiers.   The child's perceptual knowledge of objects and events continues to refine, and new words that describe weight (heavy, light), length (tall),

speed (fast), quantity (three, more), temperature (hot), volume (full, empty) and texture (soft) enter into the noun phrase (Charlesworth, 1990). The child begins to use a series of adjectives to modify the same noun, although the resulting string may not have the same order as that shown by adults (Richards, 1980). The child, like the adult, consistently places adjectives of size, shape, and length as the first adjective in a sequence, but after that may violate adult order, producing sentences such as "The big two blue cars is mine."

The child experiences difficulty using quantifiers such as *many, much,* and *few* (Gathercole, 1985). Some things such as cars are generally considered individually and are used with quantifiers such as *many* or *few.* Other things are considered as a mass or an undifferentiated group such as water or sand and are used with quantifiers such as *much* or *lots of.* The count/mass distinction appears very early in children's sentences, with primarily count nouns appearing in contexts that require count nouns (e.g., an X, another X) at 2 years (Gordon, 1988). More difficulty is experienced coordinating quantifiers with nouns, and children in this stage may fail to make the distinction, producing phrases such as "Give me a few sugars" or "I want one milk."

People and Objects in Action

The logical thought of this age leads to planning before action is taken and to hypothesizing about what would or could happen. Statements are made that reflect this logic, where the child expresses facts, rules, beliefs, attitudes, and emotions (Kemper & Edwards, 1986). The child also perceives the difference between an expected state or condition compared with what is said about it and therefore begins to tease, warn, and convey humor. Words are thus used to a great extent to indicate what *isn't* true or occurring during Stage V, rather than simply describing what *is* (Blank, Berlin, & Rose, 1978). Many new verbs enter the child's vocabulary to accommodate these abstract ideas and abilities.

Main Verbs. In addition to the increasing number of verbs acquired during this stage, the child also begins to inflect most of the verbs correctly within sentences. The regular and irregular past tense is used appropriately in most contexts, so that overgeneralizations such as *eated* rarely occur (Bellugi, 1964; Brown, 1973; Miller, 1981). The child is able to coordinate the noun and the verb in the simple present tense, differentially producing the third-person form "He eats" versus first person "I eat" (Cazden, 1968).

Auxiliary Verbs. While noun-verb agreement is attained for main verbs, children continue to experience difficulty mastering its use within the auxiliary verb phrase. However, several advances in the auxiliary system are seen. One of the most notable is the appearance of the contractible copula *be* (Miller, 1981). This is an option in English, where the copula verb can be contracted and attached to the noun. Examples include "I am happy," which contracts to become "I'm happy," or "He is in the house," which is expressed "He's in the house" in the contracted form. In contrast, the child does not yet use the contracted form of the "to be" auxiliary, as in sentences such as "He is throwing the ball" and "He's throwing the ball" (Brown, 1973; Miller, 1981).

Another advance is seen in the use of modals. Semiauxiliary complements such as *gonna*, *wanna*, or *hafta* now take noun phrases, resulting in the expression of complete ideas such as "I wanna eat *hot dogs*" (Miller, 1981). The ability to use the modal verb in the same verb phrase as the auxiliary is mastered, as in "I might *be staying* here," in both present- and past-tense forms. With this sentence type, the child can indicate the degree of certainty and the durative quality of an event (Chapman, 1978; Faegans, 1980). Additional conditions can also be expressed, as this construction also begins to appear in negative sentences.

Noticing Changes and Differences

The appearance of modal and auxiliary verbs within negative sentences during Stage IV occurs in contracted forms in Stage V (Brown, 1973; Miller, 1981). Thus the child is capable of producing sentences such as "He shouldn't be touching that." Similarly, the contracted negative is produced with auxiliary verbs, in both their present- and past-tense forms, as in "He wasn't in the kitchen" or "It isn't on the table." They also appear in past-tense modal constructions such as "I couldn't go with her" or "You shouldn't touch that." Generally, the contracted negatives that appear during this stage are *wasn't*, *weren't*, *couldn't*, *wouldn't*, and *shouldn't*, indicating that the child is able to consider the certainty of an action (permission, intent, or possibility), the time or duration of the event, and the status (rejection, denial, or nonrecurrence). Clearly, the child's thinking is becoming increasingly more logical and complex.

Gaining Information

By Stage V the inversion of the auxiliary verb in both yes/no questions and Wh- questions stabilizes (Ingram & Tyack, 1979; Klee, 1985; Kuczaj & Brannick, 1979). The child's question forms begin to reflect their interest in logical properties of objects, including *How much*, *How many*, or *Which* as in "Which one is bigger?" or "Which block is a circle?" (Wootten, Merkin, Hood, & Bloom, 1979). The developments observed in modal verb usage within negative constructions also appear in question forms. Contracted negatives in both their present- and past-tense forms are produced such as "Isn't he going, too?" or "Shouldn't the dog be in the house?"

The adult tag question, where the idea in the main clause is opposed within the tag ("He is going, *isn't* he?" or "He isn't going, *is* he?"), is used during Stage V (Brown & Hanlon, 1970). One reason for its late appearance is because of its relative semantic and syntactic complexity, involving negation, insertion, contractions, modal verbs and other more advanced constructions. Another reason for its late appearance is that these question forms are infrequently used (and apparently declining) in American English (Klee, 1985; Reich, 1986). Although it appears in Stage V, it is still not used by many children as late as 12 to 14 years of age (Dennis et al., 1982).

Combining Ideas and Information

The complex grammatical structures that emerged in Stage IV begin to appear in more sentence positions and with greater variety and frequency of use. More than one type of clause can be used within a single sentence, resulting in the expression of remarkably sophisticated ideas.

Phrases.   Advances in logical thought, including temporal and spatial knowledge are reflected in the prepositions that emerge in Stage V. The negative dimensions of previously used prepositions appear, including *down* (opposite pole of *up*) and *off* (opposite of *on*) (Brewer & Stone, 1975; Clark, 1973). The child begins to express relative distances or locations, as reflected in the use of *over*, *near*, and *by* (Morehead & Ingram, 1973). Coordination of both time and space are shown in the use of the preposition *through*, indicating that something is moving along a spatial distance during some continuing period of time (Cox, 1985). Groups or comparisons are expressed using the prepositions *of* and *like* (lots of dogs; dog like mine).

More complex methods of adding further information into the original sentence appear during Stage V. The infinitive phrase may be used with nouns that are different from the subject noun. Sentences such as "I got a card to give to grandma" appear, where *I* is the subject of the main verb *got*, but *card* is the subject of the infinitive phrase "to give to grandma" (Miller, 1981). Gerunds, or transformations of the use of a verb into a noun, are produced in sentences such as "I like swimming" (Hubbell, 1988). More than one of these embedded phrases may be used in the same sentence such as "I want *to go* (infinitive) *swimming* (gerund)" or "The baby is going *to start* (infinitive) *to cry* (infinitive).

Clauses.   While many children learned to use clausal conjoining early, others do not begin to use it until Stage V (Brown, 1973; Miller, 1981). A variety of conjunctions begin to appear in these complex sentences, including *then, and then, because, so, when, if, or, but,* and *while,* in no particular order (Cromer, 1968; French & Nelson, 1985). By Stage V most children are using between two and six of these different conjunctions (Cromer, 1968; Miller, 1981). The child's notion of causality begins to include the causes and consequences of the emotions of others, or psychological causality, but does not yet include true physical causality (Johnson & Chapman, 1980; Kemper & Edwards, 1986). Therefore, the child might give a reasonable motive as a cause for an action ("The dog bit him because he's mean"; "The kitty ate the mouse because he was hungry"), but fail to understand a physical cause ("The table broke because it has a broken leg" rather than "The table broke because the box was too heavy").

Mastery of subordinate clauses embedded into the object position of sentences continues to develop during Stage V (I think *that the clown is funny*), increasing in frequency of use (Miller, 1981). The child also begins to produce more complex relative clauses by attaching the subordinate clause to a noun with a relative pronoun. Relative pronouns can be words such as *who, which,* or *that* (Limber, 1973; Menyuk, 1969). The whole clause functions to *modify* the noun in the main clause, rather than to take the place of the noun. Consider these sentences:

NP
I know the dog.

Rel Cl
I know the dog that I want.

Rel Cl
I know the dog I want.

The relative clause allows for another complete idea (I want the dog) to be added to the main proposition of the sentence (I know the dog). As the last sentence shows, the clause may or may not be marked by a relative pronoun.

The embedded and conjoined phrases and clauses can be combined by the child during this stage, resulting in fairly sophisticated and complex sentences (Bloom et al., 1989; Bloom et al., 1980; Miller, 1981). The child produces sentences with two or more independent clauses conjoined ("If he bites him, he will get spanked"; "I found my key and then I could open my piggy bank), sentences containing both a conjoined and an embedded clause ("He was bad, *and* he wasn't supposed *to bite* that man's shoe"; "I know *that he was mean, because* he yelled at me"), and sentences containing more than one embedding ("I know *where the doll is that I want for my birthday*"; "Let's pretend *that we have to swim across the ocean*). Thus, by the end of Stage V, or shortly before the child's fourth birthday, most of the adult syntactic strategies for specifying information about people and objects, time and certainty of actions, and relationships between multiple events are produced (Brown, 1973). Elaborate noun phrases and verb phrases are seen, as well as complex and compound sentences. The child not only understands the language found in *Curious George*, but also is beginning to produce sentences that contain the complex linguistic structures.

Clinical Implications and Applications

At Stage V attention can be directed toward perceptual details within the context of play. For example, during real or pretend cooking activities, discussions can be conducted regarding the volume, weight, or quantity needed for various ingredients; the speed at which different actions such as stirring or beating need to be performed; and the relative size and shapes of containers and materials. Many spatial terms can be incorporated that reflect the relative distance of objects such as "Put the plate next to the cookie sheet" as the child begins to remove the cookies from the tray. Rather than directing the children to passively attend to these aspects of the situation, the adult can facilitate this type of language use by providing models and opportunities ("Jim's cookie is bigger than the one I made—tell us about your cookie"); by helping the children to verbally plan their actions before

they perform them ("What do we have to do with the cookies when they come out of the oven?"); and by placing the children in the role of group leader ("Its time to clean up—what should you tell the group to get them to get things washed and put away?"). The adult can be available to assist in these communications by providing cues and prompts, but the children should be provided the opportunities to formulate appropriate messages and to actively solve problems. Both the need and the opportunities for the types of language abilities that emerge during Stage V are thus provided.

A similar focus on problems, planning, expressing attitudes, describing relative spatial and temporal relationships between objects and events, and attending to the significance of perceptual characteristics of size, shape, speed, quantity, and so forth can occur within the context of storybook reading. The box that Curious George's surprise is in can be discussed and predictions can be made about what could fit into it or how George will like it. This type of interaction helps children to begin to use complex sentences, including relative clauses such as "I think that it's a . . . "; "George will get the present when . . . "; or "He will like it because . . . ." The changing events that are depicted on succeeding pages also provide opportunities to grasp spatial and temporal concepts such as "Before he opens it . . ." or "Tomorrow he will . . . ." The storybook further provides a context for the use of pronouns that refer to others ("Theirs was small") versus self ("I want a big one"), particularly if children are provided the opportunity to play or reenact experiences that parallel the ones in the book such as making and wrapping "surprises" for each other (Blank, Rose, & Berlin, 1978; Fein & Rivkin, 1986; Jalongo, 1988; Norris & Damico, 1990).

Above Stage V: Using Language to Create Context

As the child nears school age, most adult syntactic structures are produced, although some may be used infrequently, and full grammatical competence is not achieved until adolescence (Loban, 1976; Menyuk, 1971). During the school years, two periods of particular growth and refinement occur. Between 5 and 6 years, both the addition of new grammatical constructions and the sudden increase in infrequently used sentence type is seen, especially within noun phrases (O'Donnell, Griffin, & Norris, 1967). A similar increase in both type and frequency of grammatical constructions occurs between 10 and 14 years, particularly in the use of multiply embedded sentences that coordinate the nominals and predicates (recall the complex sentences from *Curious George*).

Not only the sentences used by the older child but also the discourse in which they are embedded exhibit sophisticated structure. At age 4 the child creates stories that have well-sequenced events all relating to the basic story. By 5 to 6 years the child tells true narratives with a distinct beginning; presentation of problem, goals, and attempts to resolve the problem; and a resolution (Applebee, 1978). Similarly, in conversation the child at 4 years can maintain the interaction and sustain a topic for an extended period, particularly when engaged in describing a present object or ongoing event, reenacting a familiar event in play, or engaged in problem solving (Schober-Peterson & Johnson, 1989). Speech also is modified to fit the needs of the listener or the social environment at 4 years (Guralnick & Paul-Brown, 1989). By age 5 the child is very aware of the listener's needs and will revise communications when breakdowns occur and use a variety of strategies to sustain the conversation (Brinton & Fujiki, 1984; Brinton, Fujiki, Loeb, & Winkler, 1986; Konefal & Fokes, 1984). By adolescence, syntax and word choice are modified to be appropriate to a context (Inhelder & Piaget, 1969; Palermo & Molfese, 1972). Different styles of speech are used in situations such as talking to strangers, participating in a meeting, talking with friends, conducting business, or engaging in a social function such as a dance or ball game (White, 1975).

The linguistic forms used in conversation and storytelling show agreement, not only within sentence boundaries but also across sentences. Pronouns, articles, and other aspects of language function to indicate which information is contained in previous sentences or which ideas are a continuation of the established topic. As the child tells stories or recounts events in conversation, language itself is used to set the scene, relate the actions, and describe the roles of participants. Thus language, or mental *symbols*, increasingly takes the place of physical objects and actions in the child's world (Inhelder & Piaget, 1969; Piaget, 1950, 1954). The child can talk about things that he or she previously had to do physically to understand. Thus the focus of language changes from "learning to talk" to "talking to learn" (Westby, 1985).

Objects, People, and Their Properties

The ability to represent experience through symbols leads to increasingly more logical thought, so that by 7 years the child begins to reorder, extend, subdivide, differentiate, or combine existing knowledge into new relationships or groupings. Prior to 7 years, when given a stimulus word, children typically give a syntagmatic response (given the word "cookie," they say "is good") (Brown & Berko, 1960). The older child is much more likely to give an answer that reflects a logical category such as "cake" or "something you eat" (Emerson & Gekoski, 1976). This ability to form categories based on abstract principles enables the child to think differently about the world and experiences (Nelson, 1985; Piaget, 1950).

One example of this new linguistic view of the world is the ability to use metaphors and other figurative language. Beginning at about age 4 and increasing throughout adolescence, children's ability to understand, explain, and use abstract metaphors increases (Glass, 1983). At age 4 short and conventional metaphors are used such as "cold as ice" or "small as a mouse." Children frequently invent inappropriate ones such as "tall as a string" or "soft as a rainbow." By age 7 the metaphor used are appropriate and include some elaborated endings such as "as big as a giant elephant that can't fit through the door." By age 11 many elaborated endings that embellish conventional sayings are used ("strong as an ox *pulling a wagon full of lead*"), and by adolescence metaphors become more poetic, aesthetic, and original, comparing between physical and psychological characteristics ("the bell made the sound of a happy child") (Gardner, Kircher, Winner, & Perkins, 1975).

Articles.   Articles continue to be used in longer and more complex contexts, although the definite form *the* is overused when referring to a general class of objects ("I want *the* [meaning *any*] kitty"), where adults would use the indefinite form *a* (Gordon, 1988). Forms other than *a* and *the* also begin to appear in connection with mass nouns, so that noun phrases such as "*some* milk" or "*any* sand" are produced by age 4. The demonstratives *this* and *that* are used differentially in context by age 7, functioning as demonstrative pronouns when used alone but as demonstrative articles when followed by a noun (Webb & Abrahmson, 1976).

Pronouns.   Pronouns are all mastered when used as subjects, objects, or possessives within a sentence prior to age 5, with the exception of reflexive pronouns such as *himself, herself,* and *themselves* (Haas & Owens, 1985). Their use as cohesive ties across sentence boundaries remains problematic until adolescence. By age 5 children recognize what information is requested through pronominalization in sentence sequences such as "Jane knew Jim was hungry. Who was hungry?" (C. Chomsky, 1969). The cohesive use across longer sentence sequences is often produced with ambiguity ("Bob and Steve were walking; *he* was tired") in narratives or other forms of extended discourse. Deictic contrasts change reference depending on who is speaking. In personal conversation, the child regards these deictic forms from his or her own perspective and generally uses them correctly by age 3. However, in contexts such as *Curious George,* these pronoun shifts must be considered from another speaker's perspective (Today *we* are going to celebrate, because just three years ago this day *I* brought you home with *me* from the jungle"). This type of deictic contrast is difficult for many children at age 7 (Brener, 1983; E. V. Clark, 1978; Westby, 1985).

Noun Modifiers.   Adjectives pertaining to perceptual attributes continue to be added by the older child. Words designating speed (*fast, slow*), height (*short*), width (*fat, thin*), position (*low*), and comparison (*different*) appear between 4 and 5 years of age. Comparisons are also designated by using the adjectival superlative suffix *-est* (*biggest, hottest*) at this time (Bangs, 1975; Carrow, 1973). Between 5 and 6 years the child begins to coordinate two characteristics such as size and color (*small, red*), an attribute sequence (*black and white*), and spatial-temporal terms (*first, last*). The adjectival comparative suffix *-er* also emerges at this age.

Nouns derived from other parts of speech begin to be produced late in the preschool years. The suffix *-er* is added to verbs, forming the name of a person who performs the verb, as in *hitter* (Carrow, 1973). Similarly, *man* is used to create words such as *fisherman* by 5½ years, and *-ist* (*bicyclist*) by 7 years. During the school-age years many additional derivational suffixes emerge to create nouns or adjectives within the noun phrase, including *-ful* (*helpful*), *-less* (*helpless*), *-ly* (*lovely*), *-ness* (*kindness*), *-al* (*accidental*), and *-ance* (*importance*) (Wiig & Semel, 1984).

People and Objects in Action

Children become increasingly sophisticated at referring not only to people, objects, and their properties, but also to their actions and states throughout the school years. They become more efficient in coding messages, using verbs and verb endings that state the informational and temporal relationships related to actions more explicitly. By the end of the preschool years children have acquired all of the necessary grammatical structures for expressing these relationships (Menyuk, 1963, 1964), but still lack facility in the use of language.

Between 5 and 7 years children frequently omit elements of the verb phrase that have been acquired and use others redundantly (Holden & MacGinitie, 1972). During the school years they gain efficiency, or the ability to coordinate a series of related actions in relative temporal frames, as in "I saw the dog. The dog was barking. The dog might bite. I was afraid" = "I was afraid the dog I saw barking might bite." They also continue to add new verbs or refine verb usage to reflect new concepts and reorganized perceptions gleaned from their experiences (Abkarian, 1988; E. V. Clark, 1983; Clark & Sengul, 1978; Nelson, 1974, 1985).

Main Verbs. Verbs with increasing semantic complexity are acquired with age. They are acquired along a continuum from generality to specificity (E. V. Clark, 1973), so that the child increasingly differentiates verbs such as *running* from *jogging* or *sprinting.* They also can be considered within a hierarchical relationship, so that *scrubbing, washing, scouring,* and *disinfecting* are all viewed as subcategories of *cleaning.* Many of the semantic relationships are expressed through syntactic means. The reverse of an action can be expressed through syntactic means by the use of a prefix ("He's packing the box"; "He's unpacking the box"); the use of a particle following the verb ("Climb up the ladder"; "Climb down the ladder") (Fraser, 1974); or the use of lexical opposites ("She threw the ball"; "She caught the ball") (Gentner, 1982). Children err by using one of these strategies with verbs that do not conform such as "She unvisited her grandma" (Boweran, 1981).

Some relationships between the subject and complement are difficult for school-age children and remain problematic for adults (Bowey, 1986). According to the minimum-distance principle (C. Chomsky, 1969), generally the first noun to the left of the complement is the subject ("Harry told *Sally to eat the squid*"). However, some verbs such as *promise* are exceptions to this principle and result in a different subject ("*Harry* promised Sally *to eat the squid*"). This *tell/promise* distinc-

tion is generally used correctly by 9 years, but the *ask/tell* contrast is not consistently used correctly until later (C. Chomsky, 1969; Kessel, 1970). This type of verb is problematic because it is deictic in nature, in that the meaning depends on who is speaking. Similarly, *bring/take* are difficult because not only the speaker but also the speaker's location relative to the destination of the action must be considered. Abkarian (1988) found that at 12 years this distinction was not fully made in all contexts or situations. Most main verbs are expressed in past tense using the -ed ending, but a small, frequently used group of irregular past-tense verbs are exceptions. These verbs are formed through a change in the internal vowel, and occasionally also the consonants, as in *bring-brought.* Children frequently regularize the past tense (bringed) or generate a vowel shift (brang). Many of these irregular forms are produced correctly by Stage V, but others are not learned until adolescence and are frequently produced incorrectly even in adulthood (Brown, 1973; de Villiers & de Villiers, 1973).

Several affixes can be used with verbs to modify their meaning, including *pre-* (*judge, prejudge*), *de-* (*throne, dethrone*), *re-* (*write, rewrite*), *a-* (*rise, arise*), *inter-* (*act, interact*), *mis-* (*spell, misspell*), *over-* (*work, overwork*), *trans-* (*plant, transplant*), or *un-* (*tie, untie*). These prefixes are restricted in the verbs that they can be affixed to, resulting in a gradual acquisition throughout the school years and frequent errors in usage (Wiig & Semel, 1984).

Auxiliary Verbs. Both the contractible auxiliary and the contractible copula, which appeared in Stage V, are mastered during the school years. The forms *is* and *are* ("He's talking" or "They're talking") are acquired before *am* (Trantham & Pedersen, 1976). Use with the pronoun *it* is more variable than use with names or animate pronouns (Brown, 1973). While the present tense of auxiliaries and modals is generally used correctly at the end of Stage V, the past-tense forms of these verbs, as well as the correct use of the main forms of *be (am, is, are,* *was, were),* continue to develop in correctness and efficiency of usage during the school years (Miller, 1981).

Modal verbs provide children with difficulty through adolescence. By 8 years of age children have established only a rudimentary system of modal meaning, differentially using *may* or *might* to represent *possible that* from the other modals. However, they do not consistently use the other modals to differentially represent prediction, obligation, ability, and intention. Even at 12 years of age the modal system is not isomorphic with the adult system (Coates, 1988).

The incorporation of the perfective aspect of the verb, consisting of *have + en,* occurs during the school years. The perfective aspect expresses a one-time, non-habitual action and may be used as a participle with the main verb, as in "I *have seen* the show" or I *had* eat*en* dinner," or it may occur along with the verbs ("I might *have* se*en* her"), or combinations of these structures ("I could have eaten" or "He might have been eating"). The tense is carried by the first verb within the series, a transformation that is difficult for children to master and that generally is not acquired before age 7 (Carrow, 1973).

Noticing Changes and Differences

Many of the semantic relationships involving negation are expressed syntactically. These expressions are not mastered until age 7 or beyond. Many of them require the coordination of negation with other concepts such as time or status. For example, *not* and *but* express exclusion, but the phrase "all . . . except" requires both inclusion and exclusion, while "no . . . instead" expresses exclusion and revision. "Don't . . . until" is temporal-conditional, while "neither . . . nor" involves exclusion by more than one dimension. *Without* requires exclusion of someone or something. These complex, syntactic means of expressing negation allow for more than one action or concept to be simultaneously considered in an adversative relationship (Carrow, 1973; Semel & Wiig, 1980).

The difficulty that children experience with negation is related to factors such as the distance of the negative word from the negated word or phrase and the complexity of the logical operation or thought required. Thus, "The dog is not big" is easier than "The dog is not under the bed in my room" or "Do not feed the dog that is big and wearing a red collar" (Wiig, Florence, Kutner, et al., 1977).

Gaining Information

Although most linguistic strategies for asking questions are acquired by Stage V, most of the requests produced are direct, stating specifically what the speaker wants. Indirect requests, or the use of questions to command, ask, forbid, and so forth, evolve with age. The first indirect requests appear prior to 3 years of age, but remain infrequent in use between 3 and 6 years (Garvey, 1975; Levin & Rubin, 1982). By age 7 the child is more adept at using indirect questions to gain compliance such as "Could you open the window?" or "Shouldn't you wait until Mom gets home?" At 7 years the child expects compliance to these requests, but by 8 years the child is more aware of the perspective of others and considers the request only a possibility, as in "Do you have a pencil I might borrow?" (Bock & Hornsby, 1981; Carrell, 1981; Ervin-Tripp & Gordon, 1986).

Some forms of indirect requests are stated positively ("Must you eat crackers in here?"), but convey cessation or negation, while others that are stated negatively ("Couldn't you go right now?") convey positive action (Clark & Chase, 1972; Leonard et al., 1978). Many of these forms are difficult for children, both in comprehension and production, until adolescence. They may respond to them with "Yes" or "No," failing to recognize the indirect request for action (Wiig & Semel, 1984).

Yes/no interrogative forms of questions also are formed by the older child using statements with rising intonation. Often these are preceded by a word or a phrase such as "I hope" or "I wonder" to indicate that it is a question, as in "I hope you can come over" or "I wish you had a bike."

Similarly, the tag question, infrequently produced by Stage V children, is used with increasing accuracy and frequency through adolescence (Clark & Clark, 1997).

Combining Ideas and Information

Syntactic growth involving the combining of phrases and clauses into complex grammatical structures continues until grade 12 or beyond (Hunt, 1964; Loban, 1976; Stotsky, 1987). When children cognitively are capable of forming logical and hierarchical links between ideas, coordinating multiple perspectives, and sequencing events temporally and causally, language is used as a means for organizing and expressing these relationships. In first grade approximately seven words are used in an average sentence, including an independent clause and its modifiers. By twelfth grade the average number of words produced increases to 12 (Loban, 1976). The number of dependent clauses increases correspondingly (O'Donnell et al., 1967). Thus, while grammatical structures continue to be added during the school years, the most significant change is that children become more adept at using syntax as a means of efficiently expressing complex ideas (Menyuk, 1964; Muma, 1978).

Phrases. Additional prepositions are acquired during the school years, as well as differential use. Those added include *beside, around, ahead of, behind, at the bottom of, beneath, on, within, before,* and *after* (Cromer, 1968; Johnston, 1984). The same preposition can function to communicate different meanings such as a spatial relationship ("at the beach"), a temporal relationship ("at one o'clock"), or an idiomatic use ("yelled at me") (Streng, 1972). The nine prepositions *at, by, for, on, from, in, to, of,* and *with* are the most frequently used, but they express approximately 250 possible meanings and functions. Most common prepositions may be used as idioms; the use of any particular one is not predictable according to any rule or pattern. Examples include "ran for office," "ran into her friend," or "ran through the script" (Streng, 1972).

Increasing precision in the use of prepositions continues into adulthood, particularly as the child is required to interpret location from the perspective of another person or object (Cox, 1985). Children tend to interpret and describe position relative to their own location, although there is an increasing ability between 5 and 9 years of age to interpret location from the viewpoint of the observer (Cox & Isard, 1990).

The infinitive phrase continues to be refined in its use. More complex infinitives appear first at the ends of sentences, including *wh-* infinitives ("I know how to make it work" or "Tell me where to find her house"). Unmarked infinitives, or those in which the infinitive *to* does not appear in the sentence, also are produced, as in "He can help [to] clean up the mess" (Bloom et al., 1984; Miller, 1981).

Phrases generated through the use of suffixes appear late in development. Gerunds, or the use of *-ing* to change a noun to a verb, develop as early as Stage V in the object position. They occur in additional sentence positions with increasing age. A later-developing derivational phrase is the participial phrase, with the suffixes *-ing, ed, -t, -en,* or an irregular form. Phrases such as *rising sun, lost hope, unbending rule,* and *wasted day* are examples of participial phrases. The frequency of use and the combinations of prepositional, infinitive, participial, and gerund phrases increase throughout the school years (Wiig & Semel, 1984).

Clauses. Clauses are used with increasing variety, accuracy, and complexity throughout adulthood. The variety of conjunctions used to combine clauses expands. Coordination of complete clauses occurs through the use of *nor, in addition to, and, but while,* and *or,* which emerged earlier. A greater number of subordinating conjunctions, or those used to establish a specific relationship between the clauses, appear throughout the school years. These include *since, in order that, as soon as, before, after, until, even though, unless,* and *although* (Lee, 1974; Menyuk, 1969).

In addition to conjoining clauses

within sentences, the school-age child develops syntactic devices for signaling logical relations between sentences. Adverbial devices, consisting of conjuncts (*still, as a result of, to conclude*), and disjuncts (*frankly, to be honest, perhaps, yet, however*) signal a logical relationship between separate sentences or convey the speaker's beliefs or perceptions regarding the content or information within the earlier sentence. The conjuncts *now, then, so,* and *though* are used by age 6, and both conjuncts and disjuncts are used by age 12, including *otherwise, anyway, therefore, however* (conjuncts), *really,* and *probably* (disjuncts) (Scott, 1984).

In addition to adverbial devices, school-age children also produce adverbial clauses, which are used to express aspects of location, distance, speed, time, and so forth. They subordinate two complete clauses such as "He put the box where he could find a place"; "We watched the baby while everyone else ate"; or "he yelled as loudly as he could" (Wiig & Semel, 1984).

Many different forms of relative clauses appear in sentences produced by older children, including sentences with multiple embeddings. The subordinating relative clauses that emerged in Stage V modify the object noun ("I know that he is here"). Relative clauses attached to the subject ("The man that I like lives in California") do not develop until after Stage V. This type of clause is also referred to as a center-embedded relative clause because it occupies a position between the subject and the predicate and thus interrupts the main clause. Another type that appears during the school years is the right-branched relative clause. This clause follows the main clause of the sentence and provides added meaning for the object or subject. Examples include "I gave the money to the man who drove up in the delivery truck" and "The dog ran away from the man who had owned him for 5 years" (Bloom et al., 1980; Menyuk, 1977; Wiig & Semel, 1984).

A series or relative clauses can be coordinated as in "The man who was from another town and had never been here be-fore but who knew my sister did not know my brother," or nested as in "The man who was in town asking for directions to the property he bought in the country doesn't know my brother" (Wiig & Semel, 1984).

Passive sentences are a rarely used sentence type in which the object of a verb or the recipient of an action is highlighted by placing it at the beginning of a sentence. Rather than saying, "The dog ate my homework," a passive construction would state, "My homework was eaten by the dog." Preschool-age children experience considerable difficulty in both comprehension and production of passive sentences, particularly when the nouns are semantically reversible (Horgan, 1978; Lempert, 1990). An example of a reversible type would be "The girl was teased by the boy." Children before the age of 5 are likely to produce this sentence when in fact the girl is the tormentor, and likewise they interpret these sentences incorrectly (Baldie, 1976; Bridges, 1980; Horgan, 1978).

The frequency, type, and correctness in use of passives increases with age. Four-year-old children produce more reversible passives, as well as truncated passives in which no agent is specified ("The homework was eaten" or "The girl was teased") (Bowey, 1982; Horgan, 1978). Lempert (1990) found children between 2 years, 10 months and 4 years, 7 months to be able to understand and produce the reversible passive more accurately than the nonreversible. Borer and Wexler (1987) consider the truncated passive to be grammatically different from the full passive in children's language, in that they are produced without the understanding that they are derived from the more complex full passive used by adults. Full passives, particularly the nonreversible passive, are produced by children between 7 1/2 and 8 years, and by 11 to 13 years more adultlike constructions are used that semantically differentiate between reversible and nonreversible passives using the prepositions *by* and *with*, respectively (Baldie, 1976; Horgan, 1978).

Clinical Implications and Applications

As the child enters school, interest in world knowledge increases, and the ability to participate socially and to cooperate within group activities becomes more important. The need for direct, perceptual experience is critical, particularly for children who are experiencing difficulty using symbols such as language to create concepts or events. The adult can help the child to grasp unfamiliar concepts such as "the jungle" from *Curious George*. Pictures of actual jungles and the animals, plants, insects, and people living within them can be discussed with comparisons drawn to other environments, including the child's community. Children can be helped to collaborate in small groups to explore a specific aspect of the jungle such as a river. Maps can be drawn, the uses of the river studied, and the importance of the river to animals considered. A field trip to a zoo can be planned and then implemented to observe the appearance, habits, and effects of the absence of a river on the jungle animals (Norris & Hoffman, 1995, 1996a, 1996b).

The experiences within these integrated explorations of a theme can be discussed orally and written about. Each of these activities provides many opportunities to use language, including complex sentences and syntactic devices to maintain ideas across sentences; to extend a topic; to consider the needs of the listener; to use terms such as locations and pronouns from shifting perspectives ("The tree was tall and so I saw him hiding behind the tree"); to use affixes to refer to the animals, actions, and states ("The hippo was a good swimmer, but he walked slowly on land"); to describe events using metaphors ("Tall as the tree"); and to accomplish many other language goals. Strategies such as making diagrams to organize ideas into categories or hierarchies (called semantic mappings, semantic webs, flow charting, or brainstorming) are very useful in this process (Jonassen, Beissner, & Yacci, 1993; Newman, 1985; Norris & Hoffman, 1993, 1996a, 1993b).

Books provide an excellent context for learning the many complex and subtle aspects of language that the school-age child encounters. The print provides a visual display of complex sentences, abstract ideas, and cohesive ties that connect ideas across sentences. By interactively reading stories, the adult can help the children understand how clauses interrelate, as in this example:

EXAMPLE
Adult: "How did George feel?"
Child reads: "George was curious."
Adult: "When was he curious?"
Child reads: "the moment he woke up."
Adult: "I wonder why he was curious?"
Child reads: "because he knew it was a special day."
Adult: "When did this special day start?"
Child reads: "This morning."

The child can also be shown how cohesive ties integrate information across text:

EXAMPLE
Adult: "But first *I*" (pointing to the pronoun in sentence 7)
"the man with the yellow hat" (pointing to the referent in sentence 2)
"I have a surprise for you" (pointing back to sentence 7).

Not only do these techniques facilitate language, but they have also been shown to improve reading ability, a problem common to children with language disorders (Badon, 1993; Hernandez, 1989; Michaelson, 1995; Norris 1991; Reichmuth, 1996).

ASSESSING GRAMMATICAL DEVELOPMENT

There are many purposes for examining the grammatical development of children, and many methods have been proposed for conducting these analyses. Researchers in particular are interested in analyzing the language of normally developing children to help us make new discoveries about how children accomplish this marvelous feat in such a short period. Researchers also examine the grammatical development of handicapped children to help determine whether they are demonstrating patterns of acquisition that are similar to those of normally developing children at a delayed rate, or whether there are important developmental differences. These insights help us to better plan and implement intervention for children at risk.

The same analytic procedures used by researchers are quite often used clinically to help determine the degree and pattern of impairment exhibited by children with language delays and disorders, or to assist in making the determination of whether a child is exhibiting a developmental difference that might require intervention. The predictable stages and acquisition order of syntactic and morphological aspects of language provide guidelines for assessing development, and therefore some measure of these abilities is usually included in the overall language assessment process.

Standardized Tests

One method of measuring grammatical development is through standardized testing. Standardized tests sample discrete morphological forms of grammatical structures by providing a specific set of instructions and stimuli such as pictures to elicit one particular response. This might be a comprehension-based response such as "Show me 'The boy *is* running,'" where the child is required to select the appropriate picture from a set of three that contrast according to whether the boy is getting ready to, is in the process of, or has completed running. Or it might be a production-based response such as a picture description ("Tell me what the boy is doing"), sentence imitation ("Say this sentence exactly as I say it—'The boy is running'"), or a sentence completion task ("The boy is getting ready to run. Now the boy ___ ___"). Many standardized tests for both preschool-age and school-age chil-

dren include a grammatical assessment as at least part of the test, and several are devoted specifically to syntactic measurement. Administration of this type of test results in a score, so that the child's performance can be compared to a set of norms to determine whether the child responded in a manner that is typical for his or her age.

Standardized tests have many limitations. They do not actually measure language, but only one type of language-related behavior (i.e., responding to a contrived task). Language itself occurs in a context for purposes of achieving goals and influencing the behaviors and beliefs of others. Most of the mental processes involved in contextualized language are eliminated in standardized testing such as choosing what is important to talk about, determining how much information is already shared or understood by the listener, selecting the words and word order to best communicate this information at an appropriate level for the needs of the listener, and embedding this message within the context of some larger discourse structure such as a conversation (Damico, 1991).

The ability to imitate a grammatical sentence, for example, tells the examiner very little about what a child does with language in a real-world situation. Furthermore, a score fails to provide any implications for intervention because it does not tell the examiner with what aspects of language the child experiences difficulty. Even if the individual items on a test are examined, they represent only a small sample of the linguistic abilities used by children, and basing an intervention program on these would result in providing a very narrow and impoverished experience with language.

Qualitative Assessments

Standardized tests are widely used throughout the educational system because of American culture's emphasis on making educational decisions and comparing children on the basis of test scores. They are also relatively quick to administer and to score. However, there has been an increasing movement away from reliance on standardized testing and toward more qualitative assessments of individual performance. Qualitative assessments analyze how a person actually behaves within a real context such as a classroom, at home, or when playing with peers. These nonstandardized procedures are flexible and allow the examiner to vary the situation and stimuli to fit the needs of the child or to gain information about changes in performance when conditions change. For example, the child may fail to use temporal markers to describe an event that happened earlier in the day, but may readily use them when talking about a similar ongoing situation. These comparisons can be used to help determine whether the child fails to produce temporal terms, or whether the initial failure to use them was more related to the difficult stimulus situation (James, 1989).

The same language sample elicited from a child can be subjected to a variety of different analyses, resulting in a profile of the quality of ideas expressed; types and diversity of words used; intelligibility of speech produced; amount of difficulty exhibited in formulating language; social appropriateness of the utterances; variety of requests, comments, or other intents expressed; overall structure and quality of the discourse; and syntactic complexity of the sentences used to express and communicate these ideas.

Mean Length of Utterance

Syntactic complexity can be measured in many ways. One overall index of grammatical development that is reasonably accurate up to an utterance length of four to five morphemes is the mean, or average, length of utterances (MLU) found in the language sample. The MLU is computed by adding up the number of morphemes for the entire sample and dividing it by the total number of utterances. Miller (1981) outlines detailed rules for counting morphemes, and Miller and Chapman (1981) have presented data on the relationship between chronological

age and MLU that can be useful, with certain cautions, in determining whether a child's MLU is significantly below age expectations. However, MLU provides only a gross measure of grammar because it does not indicate anything about specific forms or structures. It merely reflects the acquisition of these structures, because the MLU increases as morphemes such as verb tense markers, noun modifiers, and plurals are added.

The child's MLU has been used to place the child at one of Brown's five stages and then to compare the child's use of grammatical morphemes and sentence structures to those that typically are produced at that stage. However, Lund and Duchan (1988) argue that, since there is so much variability across children and the context in which the sample is elicited, the MLU does not accurately predict which forms and structures should appear in a given stage. Furthermore, beyond an MLU of 5 morphemes this index becomes even less accurate because children begin to use phrases, clauses, and grammatical options to add complexity, but may actually reduce sentence length.

Morphemes

The grammatical morphemes produced by the child can be examined by analyzing each utterance for the presence or absence of the morphemes in obligatory contexts, or places within a sentence where an adult speaker would use the form. Brown (1973) used a criterion of 90% correct use in obligatory contexts to place forms and structures within his five stages. It is considered clinically useful to consider a morpheme or structure mastered when it occurs with 80% correct use, and emerging if it occurs in 40 to 80% of obligatory contexts (James, 1989).

Syntax

A child's grammatical structures can be similarly analyzed. The noun phrases can be evaluated for the presence or absence of determiners, possessives, adjectives, and other modifiers. The verb phrases can be examined for the main verb and accompanying modal, progressive, and perfective elements, and adverbials or indirect objects. Other sentence components such as negatives, questions, conjoined and embedded phrases, and clauses can be analyzed. The structures that the child produces can be compared in terms of Brown's stages of development for young children or in terms of tables describing the percentage of occurrence of various clauses in the language of school-age children provided by researchers such as Loban (1976). Many commercial programs or published procedures for accomplishing this type of analysis are available, including computer-assisted programs.

The language sample also can be analyzed for information about the child's knowledge of relationships between sentences. For example, the use of pronouns, articles, conjunctions, and other syntactic classes can be examined across sentences to determine whether the child uses these devices to refer to previously established information or to refer to upcoming referents (Halliday & Hasan, 1976; Liles, 1985). Aspects of grammar are also useful in making judgments about the structure of different types of discourse such as conversation or storytelling.

CONCLUSION

Syntax is one perspective from which language can be viewed. It is one window into language acquisition and use, but in and of itself it is not language. Analysis of syntax can be useful in providing evidence of whether language advances are emerging, but these observable products of development are not the process by which development occurs. The process of acquiring language is complex and involves the interrelationships between a myriad of cognitive, social, and linguistic accomplishments. By learning all that we can about this process, we as professionals will have the best theoretical basis for understanding development and facilitating effective communication for all children.

REFERENCES

Abbeduto L, Rosenberg S. Children's knowledge of the presuppositions of *know* and other cognitive verbs. J Child Lang 1985;12:621–641.

Antinucci F, Volterra V. Lo sviluppo della negazione nel linguaggio infantile: un studio pragmatico. Lingua e Stile 1975;10:231–260. Cited in Clark & Clark, 1977, p. 315.

Applebee AN. The child's concept of story. Chicago: University Park Press, 1978.

Badon L. Comparison of contextualized versus decontextualized reading instruction in at-risk children. Unpublished doctoral dissertation, Louisiana State University, Baton Rouge, 1993.

Baldie B. The acquisition of the passive voice. J Child Lang 1976;3:331–348.

Bangs T. Vocabulary Comprehension Scale. Boston: Teaching Resources, 1975.

Baron J, Kaiser A. Semantic components in children's errors with pronouns. J Child Lang 1975;4:303–317.

Bartlett EJ. Sizing things up: the acquisition of the meaning of dimensional adjectives. J Child Lang 1976;3:205–219.

Bartlett EJ. Acquisition of the meaning of color terms. Paper presented to the Biennial Conference of the Society for Research in Child Development, New Orleans, 1977.

Barrett M. Lexical development and overextension in child language. J Child Lang 1978;5:205–219.

Bates E, Benigni L, Bretherton I, et al. From gesture to the first word: on cognitive and 'social prerequisites. In: Lewis M, Rosenblum L, eds. Interaction, conversation, and the development of language. New York: John Wiley, 1977.

Bates E, Bretherton I, Shore C, McNew S. Names, gestures and objects: the role of context in the emergence of symbols. In: Nelson K, ed. Children's language. Vol. 4. Hillsdale, NJ: Erlbaum, 1983.

Bellugi U. The acquisition of negation. Unpublished doctoral dissertation, Harvard University, 1967.

Bellugi U. Simplification in children's language. In: Huxley R, Ingram E, eds. Language acquisition: models and methods. New York: Academic Press, 1971.

Bellugi U, Brown R. The acquisition of language. Monogr Soc Res Child Dev 1964;29 (No. 92).

Bellugi-Klima U. Language acquisition. Paper presented at a symposium on cognitive studies and artificial intelligence research, University of Chicago, 1969.

Bennett-Kaster T. Noun phrases and coherence in children's narratives. J Child Lang 1983;10:135–149.

Berko J. The child's learning of English morphology. Word 1958;14:150–177.

Blank M, Rose S, Berlin L. The language of learning: the preschool years. New York: Grune & Stratton, 1978.

Block E, Kessel F. Determinants of the acquisition

order of grammatical morphemes: a re-analysis and re-interpretation. J Child Lang 1980;7:181–188.

Bloom L. Language development: form and function of emerging grammars. Cambridge, MA: MIT Press, 1970.

Bloom L. Talking, understanding, and thinking. In: Schiefelbusch R, Lloyd L, eds. Language perspectives: acquisition, retardation and intervention. Baltimore: University Park Press, 1974; pp. 285–312.

Bloom L, Lahey M. Language development and language disorders. New York: Wiley, 1978.

Bloom L, Lahey M, Hood L, et al. Complex sentences: acquisitions of syntactic connectors and the semantic relations they encode. J Child Lang 1980;7:235–262.

Bloom L, Lifter K, Hafitz J. Semantics of verbs and the development of verb inflection in child language. Language 1980;56:386–412.

Bloom L, Lightbown P, Hood L. Structure and variation in child language. Monogr Soc Res Child Dev 1975;40.

Bloom L, Merkin S, Wooten J. Wh questions: linguistic factors that contribute to the sequence of acquisition. Child Lang 1982;53:1084–1092.

Bloom L, Rispoli M, Gartner B, Hafitz J. Acquisition of complementation. J Child Lang 1989;15:101–120.

Bloom L, Tackeff J, Lahey M. Learning *to* in complement constructions. J Child Lang 1984;11:391–406.

Bloom P. Syntactic distinctions in child language. J Child Lang 1990;17:343–355.

Bock J, Hornsby M. The development of directives: how children ask and tell. J Child Lang 1981;8:151–164.

Borer H, Wexler K. The maturation of syntax. In: Roeper T, Williams E, eds. Parameter setting. Dordrecht, Holland: Reidel, 1987.

Bowerman M. Semantic factors in the acquisition of rules for word use and sentence construction. In: Morehead D, Morehead A, eds. Normal and deficient child language. Baltimore: University Park Press, 1976; pp. 99–179.

Bowerman M. The child's expression of meaning: expanding relationships among lexicon, syntax and morphology. Paper presented at the New York Academy of Science Conference on Native Language and Foreign Language Acquisition, 1981.

Bowey J. The structural processing of truncated passive in children and adults. J Psycholinguist Res 1982;11:417–436.

Bowey J. Syntactic awareness and verbal performance from preschool to fifth grade. J Psycholinguist Res 1986;15:417–436.

Braunwald SR. Context, word and meaning: towards a communicational analysis of lexical acquisition. In: Lock A, ed. Action, gesture, and symbol: the emergence of language. New York: Academic Press, 1978.

Brener R. Learning the deictic meaning of third person pronouns. J Psycholinguist Res 1983; 12:235–262.

Brewer W, Stone J. Acquisition of spatial antonym pairs. J Exp Child Psychol 1975;19:299–307.

Bridges A. SVD comprehension strategies reconsidered: the evidence of individual patterns of response. J Child Lang 1980;7:89–104.

Brinton B, Fujiki M. Development of topic manipulation skills in discourse. J Speech Hear Res 1984;27:350–358.

Brinton B, Fujiki M, Loeb D, Winkler E. Development of conversational repair strategies in response to requests for clarification. J Speech Hear Res 1986;29:75–81.

Brown RW. The development of wh- questions in child speech. J Verbal Learn Verbal Behav 1968;7:279–290.

Brown RW. A first language: the early stages. Cambridge, MA: Harvard University Press, 1973.

Brown RW, Berko J. Word association and the acquisition of grammars. Child Dev 1960;31:1–14.

Brown R, Bellugi U. Three processes in the child's acquisition of syntax. Harvard Educ Rev 1964; 34:133–151.

Brown R, Cazden C, Bellugi U. The child's grammar from I to III. In: Hill J, ed. Minnesota Symposia on Child Psychology. Vol. 2. Minneapolis: University of Minnesota Press, 1969.

Brown R, Fraser C. The acquisition of syntax. In: Bellugi U, Brown R, eds. The acquisition of language. Monogr Soc Res Child Dev 1964;92.

Brown R, Hanlon C. Derivational complexity and order of acquisition. In: Hayes J, ed. Cognition and the development of language. New York: Wiley, 1970; pp. 11–59.

Bruner JS. In search of mind. New York: Harper & Row, 1983.

Bruner JS. From communication to language: a psychological perspective. Cognition 1975;3:255–287.

Carey S. The child as word learner. In: Halle M, Bresnan J, Miller G, eds. Linguistic theory and psychological reality. Cambridge, MA: MIT Press, 1978.

Carey S, Considine T. The domain of comparative adjectives. Unpublished paper. Cambridge, MA: MIT, 1973. Cited in de Villiers & de Villiers, 1978; p. 137.

Carrell P. Children's understanding of indirect requests: comparing child and adult comprehension. J Child Lang 1981;8:329–345.

Carrow E. Test of auditory comprehension of language. Austin, TX: Urban Research Group, 1973.

Cazden C. The acquisition of noun and verb inflections. Child Dev 1968;39:433–438.

Chalkey M. The emergence of language as a social skill. In: Kuczaj S, ed. Language development: Vol. 2. Language, thought and culture. Hillsdale, NJ: Erlbaum, 1982.

Chapman RS. Comprehension strategies in children. In: Kavanaugh J, Strange W, eds. Speech and language in the laboratory school and clinic. Cambridge, MA: MIT Press, 1978; pp. 308–327.

Chapman RS, Miller JF. Word order in early two- and three-word utterances: does production precede comprehension? J Speech Hear Res 1975;18:355–371.

Charlesworth R. Math & science for young children. New York: Delmar, 1990.

Charney R. The comprehension of "here" and "there." J Child Lang 1979;6:69–80.

Charney R. Speech roles and the development of personal pronouns. J Child Lang 1980;7:509–528.

Chomsky C. The acquisition of syntax in children from 5 to 10. Cambridge, MA: MIT Press, 1969.

Chomsky N. Aspects of the theory of syntax. Cambridge, MA: MIT Press, 1965.

Chomsky N. Deep structure, surface structure, and semantic interpretation. Bloomington: Indiana University Linguistics Club, 1969.

Clancy P. Acquisition of Japanese. In: Slobin D, ed. The cross-linguistic study of language acquisition. Hillsdale, NJ; Erlbaum, 1985.

Clark EV. On the acquisition of the meaning of "before" and "after." J Verbal Learn Verbal Behav 1971;10:266–275.

Clark EV. What's in a word? On the child's acquisition of semantics in his first language. In: Moore TE, ed. Cognitive development and the acquisition of language. New York: Academic Press, 1973; pp. 65–110.

Clark EV. Knowledge, context and strategy in the acquisition of meaning. In: Dato DP, ed. Georgetown University Round Table on Language and Linguistics, 1975. Washington, DC: Georgetown University Press, 1975; pp. 77–98.

Clark EV. From gesture to word: on the natural history of deixis in language acquisition. In: Bruner J, Garton A, eds. Human growth and development. Oxford: Oxford University Press, 1978.

Clark EV. Building a vocabulary: words for objects, actions and relations. In: Fletcher P, Garman M, eds. Language acquisition. Cambridge, England: Cambridge University Press, 1979.

Clark EV. Meaning and concepts. In: Mussen P, ed. Handbook of child psychology. Vol. 3. New York: Wiley, 1983.

Clark EV, Sengul C. Strategies in the acquisition of deixis. J Child Lang 1978;5:457–475.

Clark HH, Chase W. On the process of comparing sentences against pictures. Cognit Psychol 1972;3:472–517.

Clark HH, Clark EV. Psychology and language: an introduction to psycholinguistics. New York: Harcourt Brace Jovanovich, 1977.

Coates J. The acquisition of the meanings of modality in children aged eight and twelve. J Child Lang 1988;15:425–434.

Coker P. Syntactic and semantic factors in the acquisition of "before" and "after." J Child Lang 1978;5:261–277.

Cox M. The child's point of view: cognitive and linguistic development. Brighton, England: Harvester Press, 1985.

Cox MV, Isard S. Children's deictic and nondeictic interpretations of the spatial locatives in front of and behind. J Child Lang 1990;17:481–488.

Cox M, Richardson J. How do children describe spatial relationships? J Child Lang 1985;12:611–620.

Cromer RF. The development of temporal reference during the acquisition of language. Ph.D. dissertation. Cambridge, MA: Harvard University, 1968. Cited in Bowerman, 1979.

Damico JS. Descriptive assessment of communicative ability in limited English proficient students. In: Hamayan EV, Damico JS, eds. Limiting bias in the assessment of bilingual students. Austin, TX: Pro-ed, 1991; pp. 157–217.

deBoysson-Bardies B. L'etude de la negation: aspects syntaxiques et lexicaux. Ph.D. dissertation. L'University de Paris, 1972. Cited in Bloom & Lahey, 1978.

Dennis M, Sugar J, Whitaker H. The acquisition of tag questions. Child Dev 1982;53:1254–1257.

Derwing BV, Baker WJ. The psychological basis for morphologic rules. In: MacNamara J, ed. Language learning and thought. New York: Academic Press, 1977.

de Villiers JG, de Villiers PA. A cross-sectional study of the acquisition of grammatical morphemes. J Psycholinguist Res 1973;2:267–278.

de Villiers PA, de Villiers JG. On this, that and the other: nonegocentrism in very young children. J Exp Child Psychol 1974;18:388–447.

de Villiers JG. Form and force interactions: the development of negatives and questions. In: Schiefelbusch R, Picker J, eds. The acquisition of communicative competence. Baltimore: University Park Press, 1984; pp 193–236.

de Villiers JG, de Villiers PA. Early language. Cambridge, MA: Harvard University Press, 1979.

Dollaghen CA. Child meets word: "fast mapping" in preschool children. J Speech Hear Res 1985; 28:499–454.

Dore J. The development of conversational competence. In: Schiefelbusch R, ed. Language competence: assessment and intervention. San Diego: College Hill, 1986; pp 3–60.

Eilers RE, Oller DK, Ellington J. The acquisition of word meaning for dimensional adjectives: the long and short of it. J Child Lang 1974;1:195–204.

Emerson HF, Gekoski WL. Interactive and categorical grouping strategies and the syntagmatic-paradigmatic shift. Child Dev 1976;47:1116–1125.

Emslie HC, Stevenson RJ. Preschool children's use of the articles in definite and indefinite referring expressions. J Child Lang 1981;8:313–328.

Erreich A. Learning how to ask: pattern of inversion in yes/no and wh- questions. J Child Lang 1984;11:579–592.

Ervin-Tripp SM. Discourse agreement: how children answer questions. In: Hayes J, ed. Cognition and the development of language. New York: Wiley, 1970.

Ervin-Tripp SM, Gordon DP. The development of requests. In: Schiefelbusch R, ed. Language competence: assessment and intervention. San Diego: College-Hill, 1986; pp. 61–96.

Feagans L. Children's understanding of some temporal terms denoting order, duration, and simultaneity. J Psycholinguist Res 1980;9:41–57.

Fein F, Rivkin M. The young child at play: reviews of research. Vol. 4. Washington DC: National Association for the Education of Young Children, 1986.

Foster SH. Learning topic management in the preschool years. J Child Lang 1986;13:231–250.

Fraser B. The verb-particle combination in English. Tokyo: Taishukan, 1974.

French LA, Nelson K. Young children's knowledge of relational terms: some *ifs, ors,* and *buts.* New York: Springer-Verlag, 1985.

Gardner H, Kircher M, Winner E, Perkins D. Children's metaphoric productions and preferences. J Child Lang 1975;2:125–141.

Garvey C. Requests and responses in children's speech. J Child Lang 1975;2:41–63.

Gathercole V. "Me has too much hard questions": The acquisitions of the linguistic mass-count distinction in much and many. J Child Lang 1985;12:395–415.

Glass AL. The comprehension of idioms. J Psycholinguist Res 1983;12:429–442.

Gleitman LR. The structural sources of verb meanings. Lang Acquisit 1990;1:3–55.

Golinkoff RM, Hirsh-Pasek K. Reinterpreting children's sentence comprehension: toward a new framework. In: Fletcher P, MacWhinney B, eds. The handbook of child language. Oxford: Blackwell, 1995; pp. 430–461.

Golinkoff RM, Markessini J. "Mommy sock": the child's understanding of possession as expressed in two-noun phrases. J Child Lang 1980;7:119–136.

Gordon P. Count/mass category acquisition: distributional distinctions in children's speech. J Child Lang 1998;15:109–128.

Gopnic A, Meltzoff A. Semantic and cognitive development in 15–21 month-old children. J Child Dev 1984;11:495–513.

Gopnic A, Meltzoff A. The development of categorization in the second year and its relation to other cognitive and linguistic developments. Child Dev 1987;53:1523–1531.

Greenwald P, Leonard L. Communicative and sensorimotor development of Down's syndrome children. Am J Ment Defic 1979;84:296–303.

Grimm H. Strukturanalytische Untersuchung der Kindersprache. Bern: Verlag-Huber, 1973. Cited in H. Clark & Clark, 1977.

Guralnick MJ, Paul-Brown D. Peer-related communicative competence of preschool children: developmental and adaptive characteristics. J Speech Hear Res 1989;232:930–943.

Haas A, Owens R. Preschoolers' pronoun strategies: you and me make us. Paper presented at the American Speech-Language-Hearing Association annual convention, 1985.

Halliday MAK, Hasan R. Cohesion in English. London: Longman Group, 1976.

Hernandez S.N. Effects of Communicative Reading Strategies on the literacy behaviors of third grade poor readers. Unpublished doctoral dissertation, Louisiana State University, 1989.

Hirsh-Pasek K, Golinkoff RM. Skeletal supports for grammatical learning: what the infant brings to the language learning task. In: Roves-Collioer

CK, ed. Advances in infancy research. Vol. 10. Norwood, NJ: Ablex, 1993.

Hoff-Ginsberg E. Some contributions of mothers' speech to their children's syntactic growth. J Child Lang 1985;12:267–385.

Holden M, MacGinitie W. Children's conceptions of word boundaries in speech and print. J Educ Psychol 1972;63:551–557.

Hood L, Bloom L. What, when, and how about why: a longitudinal study of early expressions of causality. Monogr Soc Res Child Dev 1979;44.

Horgan D. The development of the full passive. J Child Lang 1978;5:65–80.

Hubbell RD. A handbook of English grammar and language sampling. Englewood Cliffs, NJ: Prentice-Hall, 1988.

Hunt KW. Grammatical structure written at three grade levels. Champaign, IL: National Council of Teachers of English, 1964.

Huxley R. The development of the correct use of subject personal pronouns in two children. In: Flores d'Arcais G, Levelt W, eds. Advances in psycholinguistics. Amsterdam: North-Holland, 1970.

Ihns M, Leonard LB. Syntactic categories in early child language: some additional data. J Child Lang 1988;15:673–678.

Ingram D. Transitivity in child language. Language 1971;47:888–910.

Ingram D. The development of phrase structure rules. Lang Learn 1972;22:65–77.

Ingram D. First language acquisition: method, description, and explanation. New York: Cambridge University Press, 1989.

Ingram D, Tyack DL. Inversion of subject NP and Aux in children's questions. J Psycholinguist Res 1979;8:333–341.

Inhelder B, Piaget J. The early growth of logic in the child. New York: Norton, 1969.

Jalongo MR. Young children and picture books: Literature from infancy to six. Washington DC: National Association for the Education of Young Children, 1988.

James S. Assessing children with language disorders. In: Bernstein DK, Tiegerman E, eds. Language and communication disorders in children. 2nd ed. Columbus, OH: Merrill, 1989; pp. 157–207.

Johnson D, Toms-Bronowski S, Pittelman S. Vocabulary development. Volta Rev 1982;84(5):11–24.

Johnson HL, Chapman RS. Children's judgment and recall of causal connectives: a developmental study of "because," "so," and "and." J Psycholinguist Res 1980;9:243–260.

Johnson J. Acquisition of locative meanings: behind and in front of. J Child Lang 1984;11:407–422.

Jonassen DH, Beissner K, Yacci M. Structural knowledge: techniques for representing, conveying, and acquiring structural knowledge. Hillsdale, NJ: Lawrence Erlbaum, 1993.

Kemper S, Edwards LC. Children's expression of causality and their construction of narratives. Top Lang Disord 1986;7:11–20.

Kessel FS. The role of syntax in children's comprehension from ages six to twelve. Monogr Soc Res Child Dev 1970;35:6.

Klee T. Role of inversion in children's question development. J Speech Hear Res 1985;28:225–232.

Klima ES, Bellugi U. Syntactic regularities in the speech of children. In: Lyons J, Wales RJ, eds. Psycholinguistic paper. Edinburgh: Edinburgh University Press, 1966; pp. 183–208.

Konefal JA, Fokes J. Linguistic analysis of children's conversational repairs. J Psycholinguist Res 1984;13:1–11.

Koziol SM. The development of noun plural rules during the primary grades. Res Teach Engl 1973;7:30–50.

Kuczaj SA, Brannick N. Children's use of Wh question modal auxiliary placement rule. J Exp Child Psychol 1979;28:43–67.

Kuczaj SA, Maratsos MP. On the acquisition of front, back, and side. Child Dev 1975;46:202–210.

Lahey M. Language disorders and language development. New York: Macmillan, 1988.

Lee LL. Developmental sentence analysis. Evanston, IL: Northwestern University Press, 1974.

Lempert H. Acquisition of passives: the role of patient animacy, salience, and lexical accessibility. J Child Lang 1990;17:677–696.

Lenneberg EH. Biological foundations of language. New York: Wiley, 1967.

Leonard LB. Meaning in child language. New York: Grune & Stratton, 1976.

Leonard LB, Wilcox J, Fulmer K, Davis A. Understanding indirect requests: an investigation of children's comprehension of pragmatic meanings. J Speech Hear Res 1978;21:528–537.

Levin EA, Rubin KH. Getting others to do what you want them to: the development of children's requestive strategies. In: Nelson K, ed. Children's language. Vol. 4. Hillsdale, NJ: Lawrence Erlbaum, 1983.

Liles BZ. Cohesion in the narratives of normal and language disordered children. J Speech Hear Disord 1985;25:123–133.

Limber J. The genesis of complex sentences. In: Moore T, ed. Cognitive development and the acquisition of language. New York: Academic Press, 1973.

Loban WD. Language development: kindergarten through grade twelve. Urbana, IL: National Council of Teachers of English, 1976.

Lund NJ, Duchan JF. Assessing children's language in naturalistic contexts. 2nd ed. Englewood Cliffs, NJ: Prentice Hall, 1988.

MacDonald JD, Gillette Y. Conversation engineering: a pragmatic approach to early social competence. Semin Speech Lang 1984;5:171–183.

Mahler MS, Pine F, Bergman A. The psychological birth of the human infant. New York: Basic Books, 1975.

Maratsos M. When is a high thing the big one? Dev Psychol 1974;10:367–375.

McCabe A, Peterson C. A naturalistic study of the production of causal connectives by children. J Child Lang 1985;12:145–159.

McLean JE. A language-communication intervention model. In: Bernstein DK, Tiegerman E, eds. Language and communication disorders in children. 2nd ed. Columbus, OH: Merrill, 1989; pp. 208–228.

Menyuk P. Syntactic structures in the language of children. Child Dev 1963;34:533–546.

Menyuk P. Syntactic rules used by children from preschool through first grade. Child Dev 1964; 35:533–546.

Menyuk P. Sentences children use. Cambridge, MA: MIT Press, 1969.

Menyuk P. The acquisition and development of language. Englewood Cliffs, NJ: Prentice-Hall, 1971.

Menyuk P. Language and maturation. Cambridge, MA: MIT Press, 1977.

Mervis CB. Child-base object categories and early lexical development. In: Neisser U, ed. Concepts and conceptual development: ecological and intellectual factors in categorization. Cambridge, England: Cambridge University Press, 1987.

Mervis CB, Johnson J. Acquisition of the plural morpheme: a case study. Paper presented at the Twelfth Annual Boston University Conference on Language Development, Boston, MA, 1987 (October).

Michaelson M. The efficacy of Communicative Reading Strategies with low-achieving beginning readers. Unpublished doctoral dissertation, Louisiana State University, Baton Rouge, 1995.

Miller JF. Assessing language production in children. Baltimore: University Park Press, 1981.

Miller JF, Chapman RS. The relation between age and mean length of utterance in morphemes. J Speech Hear Res 1981;24:154–161.

Miller WR, Ervin-Tripp SM. The development of grammar in child language. In: Bellugi U, Brown R, eds. The acquisition of language: Monogr Soc Res Child Dev 1973;92:9–34.

Morehead DM, Ingram D. Development of base syntax in normal and linguistically deviant children. J Speech Hear Res 1973;16:330–352.

Morehead DM, Morehead AE. From signal to sign: a Piagetian view of thought and language during the first two years. In: Schiefelbusch R, Lloyd L, eds. Language perspectives: acquisition, retardation, and intervention. Baltimore: University Park Press, 1974; pp. 153–191.

Muma J. Language acquisition handbook. Englewood Cliffs, NJ: Prentice-Hall, 1978.

Naigles L. Children use syntax to learn verb meanings. J Child Lang 1990;17:357–374.

Nelson K. Concept, word, and sentence: interrelations in acquisition and development. Psychol Rev 1974;81:267–285.

Nelson K. Individual differences in early semantic and syntax development. In: Aaronson D, Rieber RW, eds. Developmental psycholinguistics and communication disorders. New York: Academic Science, 1975.

Nelson K. Making sense: the acquisition of shared meaning. New York: Academic Press, 1985.

Newman JM. Whole language: theory in use. Portsmouth, NH: Heinemann Press, 1985.

Norris JA. Providing language remediation in the classroom: an integrated language-to-reading intervention method. Lang Speech Hear Serv Sch 1989;20:205–219.

Norris JA. From frog to prince: using written language as a context for language learning. Top Lang Disord 1991;12(1):1–6.

Norris JA, Bruning RH. Cohesion in the narratives of good and poor readers. J Speech Hear Disord 1988;3:418–424.

Norris JA, Damico JS. Whole language in theory and practice: implications for language intervention. Lang Speech Hear Serv Sch 1990;21:212–220.

Norris JA, Hoffman PR. Language intervention within naturalistic environments. Lang Speech Hear Serv Sch 1990;21:72–84.

Norris JA, Hoffman PR. Whole language intervention for school-age children. San Diego, CA: Singular, 1993.

Norris JA, Hoffman PR. Storybook centered themes: an inclusive whole language approach. Tucson, AZ: Communication Skill Builders, 1995.

Norris JA, Hoffman PR. Storybook-centered lesson plans—Topical Unit 3: me and my world. Tucson, AZ: Communication Skill Builders, 1996.

Norris JA, Hoffman PR. Storybook-centered lesson plans—Topical Unit 4: spring and the environment. Tucson, AZ: Communication Skill Builders, 1996.

O'Donnell RC, Griffin WJ, Norris RC. Syntax of kindergarten and elementary school children: a transformational analysis. Urbana, Il: National Council of Teachers of English, 1967.

Palermo DS, Molfese DL. Language acquisition from age five onward. Psychol Bull 1972;78:409–428.

Pea RD. The development of negation in early child language. In: Olson D, ed. The social foundations of language and thought: Essays in honor of Jerome S. Bruner. New York: Norton, 1979.

Piaget J. The psychology of intelligence. London: Routledge & Kegan Paul, 1950.

Piaget J. The construction of reality in the child. New York: Basic Books, 1954.

Piaget J, Inhelder B. The growth of logical thinking from childhood to adolescence. New York: Basic Books, 1958.

Rey HA. Curious George rides a bike. Boston: Houghton Mifflin, 1952.

Reich P. Language development. Englewood Cliffs, NJ: Prentice-Hall, 1986.

Reichmuth S. The effects of Communicative Reading Strategies on reading fluency and comprehension in adult literacy learning. Unpublished doctoral dissertation, Louisiana State University, Baton Rouge, 1996.

Richards MM. Adjective ordering in the language of young children: an experimental investigation. J Child Lang 1980;6:253–277.

Ryan J. Mental subnormality and language development. In: Lenneberg EH, Lenneberg E, eds. Foundations in language development. Vol. 2. New York: Academic Press, 1975.

Sachs J. Children's play and communicative development. In: Schiefelbusch RL, Pickar J, eds. The acquisition of communicative competence. Baltimore: University Park Press, 1984; pp. 109–140.

Scherer NJ, Olswang LB. Role of mothers' expansions in stimulating children's language production. J Speech Hear Res 1984;27:387–395.

Schober-Peterson D, Johnson CJ. Conversational topics of 4-year-olds. J Speech Hear Res 1989; 32:857–870.

Scott CM. Adverbial connectivity in conversations of children 6 to 12. J Child Lang 1984;11:423–452.

Semel EM, Wiig EH. Clinical evaluation of language functions. Columbus, OH: Merrill, 1980.

Share J. Developmental progress in Down's syndrome. In: Koch R, de la Cruz F, eds. Down's syndrome. New York: Bruner Mazel, 1975.

Sharpless E. Children's acquisition of personal pronouns. Unpublished doctoral dissertation, Columbia University, 1974.

Shatz M, Wellman H, Silber F. The acquisition of mental verbs: a systematic investigation of the first reference to mental state. Cognition 1983; 14:301–321.

Snow CE. Parent-child interaction and the development of communicative ability. In: Schiefelbusch RL, Pickar J, eds. The acquisition of communicative competence. Baltimore: University Park Press, 1984; pp. 69–108.

Snow C, Ferguson C. Talking to children: language input and acquisition. New York: Cambridge University Press, 1977.

Stoel-Gammon C, Cooper J. Patterns of early lexical and phonological development. J Child Lang 1984;11:247–271.

Stotsky S. Teaching the vocabulary of academic discourse. In: Enos T, ed. A sourcebook for basic writing teachers. New York: Random House, 1987; pp. 328–347.

Streng A. Syntax, speech, and hearing: applied linguistics for teachers of children with language and hearing disabilities. New York: Grune & Stratton, 1972.

Tanz C. Studies in the acquisition of deictic terms. Cambridge, England: Cambridge University Press, 1980.

Tavakolian SL. The conjoined-clause analysis of relative clauses. In: Tavakolian SL, ed. Language acquisition and linguistic theory. Cambridge, MA: MIT Press, 1981.

Trantham C, Pedersen J. Normal language development. Baltimore: Williams & Wilkins, 1976.

Tyack DL, Ingram D. Children's production and comprehension of questions. J Child Lang 1977; 4:211–224.

Warden DA. The influence of context on children's use of identifying expressions and references. Br J Psychol 1976;67:101–112.

Warren SF, Bambara LM. An experimental analysis

of milieu language intervention: teaching the action-object form. J Speech Hear Disord 1989; 54:448–461.

Waryas CL. Psycholinguistic research in language intervention programming: the pronoun system. J Psycholinguist Res 1973;2:221–237.

Webb PA, Abrahamson AA. Stages of egocentrism in children's use of "this" and "that": a different point of view. J Child Lang 1976;3:349–367.

Wells G. Learning and using the auxiliary verb in English. In: Lee V, ed. Language development. New York: Wiley, 1979.

Westby CE. Learning to talk—talking to learn: oral-literate language differences. In: Simon C, ed. Communication skills and classroom success: therapy methodologies for language-learning disabled students. San Diego: College-Hill, 1985; pp. 181–218.

White B. Critical influence in the origins of competence. Merrill-Palmer Q 1975;22:243–266.

Wiig EH, Fleischmann N. Knowledge of pronominalization, reflexivization, and relativization by learning disabled college students. J Learn Disabil 1980;13:571–576.

Wiig EH, Florence DP, Kutner SM, et al. Perception and interpretation of explicit negations by learning disabled children and adolescents. Percept Motor Skills 1977;44:1251–1257.

Wiig EH, Semel EM. Language assessment and intervention for the learning disabled. Columbus, OH: Bell & Howell, 1984.

Winzemer JA. A lexical-expectation model for children's comprehension of wh-questions. Paper presented at the 5th Annual Boston University Conference on Language Development, October 1980.

Wootten J, Merkin S, Hood L, Bloom L. Wh-questions: linguistic evidence to explain the sequence of acquisition. Paper presented at the biennial meeting of the Society for Research in Child Development, 1979.

Zehler AM, Brewer WF. Sequence and principles in article system use: an examination of "a," "the," and "null" acquisition. Child Dev 1982;53:1268–1274.

CHAPTER 13

Communicative Refinement in School Age and Adolescence

Carol E. Westby

In the preschool years children learn to talk, but as they move into school, they talk to learn. In academic tasks language is used in the service of thought. Compared with language during preschool years, language during the school years requires an increased variety of language functions, greater variety of discourse styles and organization, more abstract vocabulary, more complex syntax, and the ability to reflect on all these aspects of language. This chapter will discuss major aspects of language development during the school years, particularly those that are related to academic success. The effects of deficits in these areas on students' performance will be described, suggestions will be given for evaluating these language abilities, and paradigms for intervention will be presented.

LEARNING TO DO SCHOOL

Understanding the development of language during the school years requires that we understand both what students bring to the language-learning tasks in the school curricula and the nature or requirements of the tasks. For a child to be successful in school, the language of academic lessons must be within the student's *zone of proximal development* (ZPD), which refers to the difference between a child's "actual developmental level as determined by independent problem solving" and his or her "potential development as determined through problem solving under adult guidance or in collaboration with more capable peers" (Vygotsky, 1978, p. 86). Working within the zone of proximal development requires that teachers and speech-language pathologists use a dual approach to language assessment and intervention. A dual approach has both inside-out and outside-in components. In assessment the inside-out component involves analysis of children's language skills; the outside-in component involves analysis of the academic content of the curriculum and expectations regarding how the content is accessed. In intervention the inside-out component involves strategies to increase the child's language skills; the outside-in component involves modification of the curriculum in terms of the content or the way the content is presented.

Students must be able to participate effectively in a range of school lessons—listening to teachers' lectures, contributing to class discussions or small group projects, and reading and writing independently. Lessons can be defined as the products of interactions among teachers and students with texts and materials (Green, Weade, & Graham, 1986). For students' answers to be considered correct, the answers must be right in both academic content and social form (Mehan, 1979). To function in school lessons, teachers and students draw simultaneously on two sets of procedural knowledge—knowledge of the academic task structure and of the social participation structure (Erickson, 1982). Figure 13.1 presents the structure of lessons. As teachers present academic content, they are simultaneously signaling how the lesson is to be accomplished. Students must be able to comprehend the academic aspects of the lesson and know the social

rules for how to participate in the lesson. Intrapersonal and interpersonal factors contribute to development of the academic and social components of successful lessons (Green, Weade, & Graham, 1988). The intrapersonal factors are the personal frames of reference that students bring to lessons (Frederiksen, 1981; Green & Harker, 1982; Tannen, 1979). These intrapersonal frames are determined by cultural experiences and individual skills and preferences and consist of sets of expectations for learning derived from past experiences, knowledge, perceptions, emotions, values, cultural assumptions, and abilities. The intrapersonal frames of children from culturally/linguistically diverse backgrounds may be different from those of mainstream children.

As teachers and students interact during lessons, they construct lesson-specific

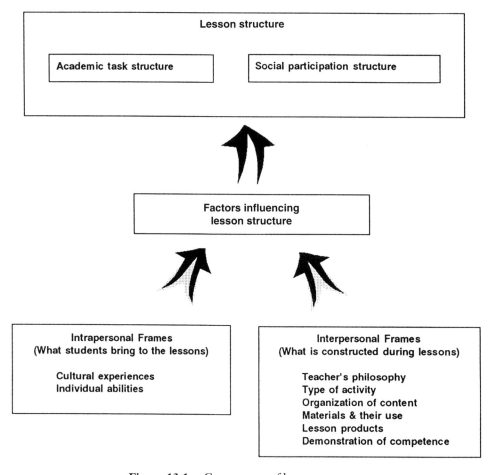

Figure 13.1.   Components of lesson structure.

frames of reference that influence what students will do and what they will come to know in the developing lesson. These frames are part of the interpersonal context of lessons (Green, Harker, & Golden, 1986). These interpersonal frames relate to the ways the teacher organizes the content, the teacher's educational philosophy, the materials that are used, what students are to do with the materials, and how the students will show competence in the lesson.

Students and teachers must develop a common set of frames or scripts for lessons. When teachers and students interpret frames differently, students will not learn what the teachers intend for them to learn, and teachers are likely to make negative judgments regarding the students' abilities to perform the lesson. Students with learning disabilities and students from culturally/ linguistically different environments are likely to experience difficulties learning the lesson and classroom frames or scripts. Adequate evaluation of students should take both an inside-out approach (what are the student's cognitive and linguistic processing abilities and disabilities) and an outside-in approach (what are the classroom scripts and other environmental influences on learning) (Nelson, 1992). At this time there is considerable information about ways in which children's cognitive and linguistic abilities develop that can be used in the inside-out aspects of student evaluation. There is less information on how environmental scripts and expectations may change over time—information that is essential for the outside-in aspect of student evaluation.

EXTENDING LANGUAGE FUNCTIONS FOR THOUGHT

Newspaper articles and television specials are expressing concern about the poor literacy and thinking skills of students in the United States. In the 1990s and for the new millennium, literacy involves more than being able to read printed words. Although the media pro-

claims the high illiteracy rate in the country, more people than ever before are able to read print. The problem is not one of being able to read print, but in being be able to comprehend and think about what is read. The demand for increasing literacy skills is not a demand for more people to be able to read words, but a demand for greater language skills in the service of thought. The focus of education now and for the future should be on *critical literacy*—the literate use of language to problem solve and communicate (Calfee, 1994). Today the literate person is expected to be able to read a wide variety of topics with understanding, identify barriers to understanding, and use the information gained for creative thinking and effective problem solving (Ellsworth, 1994). Critical literacy requires the acquisition of new language functions used to express more abstract content in a wider variety of linguistic structures. The specific nature of this critical literacy (and the language and thinking that underlie it) is not the same across all components of the school curriculum or all social situations. To understand the language-learning needs of school-age students, we must first understand the variety of language functions essential for mastering the school curricula and then the oral-interactive strategies that are used to access the curricula and the nature of the content and structure of the content of the various language functions or academic domains.

Language Genres

All social and academic activities involve communication, and communication involves the use of language to share meaning with someone for some purpose. These meanings and functions may be organized in different ways called *genres*. Each genre uses distinct vocabulary, syntactic structures, and text organization (Black, 1985; Grabe, 1987; Graesser & Goodman, 1985; Kieras, 1985). As children mature, these communication genres grow increasingly complex along two dimensions, the rhetorical (who is talked to) and the referential (what is talked about). Moffett (1968) proposed a school language arts curriculum reflecting a "universe of discourse genres" (Table 13.1). Along the rhetorical dimension, children initially communicate to one person at a time, a person they know well. Gradually, they communicate with more than one person at a time and with people they know less well or may not know at all. It is easier to talk with familiar people because one shares unspoken knowledge with a familiar person; consequently, one can use simple syntax and nonspecific vocabulary when communicating. It is easier to talk with one person rather than a group, because one can more easily track the topic of the conversation and take a turn in the communication. It is especially difficult to communicate in writing to persons one does not know, because one does not know what information the readers possess and how they will interpret the print. Without face-to-face interaction, writers cannot correct possible readers' misinterpretations; writers must therefore attempt to put themselves into the minds of their readers, anticipating what they know and do not know.

Along the referential dimension, children's early communication serves to meet their needs in the immediate situation. Gradually, they begin talking about past and future experiences, then generalizing about these experiences, and eventually theorizing about them. At each ref-

erential level the student is increasingly distant from contextual cues. At early levels one can generally see what one is talking about. When children narrate, they reflect on past or future experiences. After repeated experiences they can develop general principles, and later still they use these generalizations to hypothesize about possible future relationships. All aspects of the rhetorical and referential language dimensions should be a part of a language arts curriculum.

Children acquire language for social functions of requesting, commanding, and recording by 2 to 3 years of age. By age 3 they also begin to produce narratives. Narrative language is particularly important for success in the early school years. The majority of texts used in kindergarten through third grade are in a narrative format. Children learn to read by reading narratives, and math and science activities are often presented in narrative formats. There are a variety of narrative types (Heath, 1986a, 1986b):

1. *Recounts:* These generally occur when an adult requests that a child talk about something the adult and child have shared together, for example, the mother who says, *"Tell Daddy about our visit to the zoo today,"* or the teacher who asks *"Tell me what we discussed in history class."* Adults generally support children's recounting by asking scaffolding questions. *"What did the gorilla do? What did you do when the bird landed on you? Who rode the camel?"* or

Table 13.1 *Universe of Discourse*

Rhetorical Dimension	Discourse Type	Referential Dimension
Talking to a familiar person	Conversation	Requesting objects or actions in immediate environment; asking for information
Talking to a less familiar person or several persons	Pretend play or drama	Recording—talking about what one is doing
Talking to a group	Narrative	Reporting past or future experiences
Publication for an unknown audience	Exposition	Generalizing from experience
	Argumentation	Theorizing from generalizations

"What event are we studying?" "Who was president at the time?"

2. *Eventcasts:* Eventcasting is talking about what one is doing as it is being done; it is talking aloud to oneself. Older children and adults may eventcast to help them manage difficult tasks, for example, *"What do I have to do today, let's see . . . I need to study for tomorrow's test, then work on my math assignment."* Mainstream families frequently eventcast when they present children with new, unfamiliar activities, for example, *"You've got a blue and yellow puzzle piece with a straight edge, now you're looking for another piece with blue and yellow."*

3. *Accounts:* Accounts are narratives about a personal experience that are offered by a speaker to listeners who are unfamiliar with the experience. For example, a child may have visited the zoo with his class. In the evening he excitedly tells his parents, who were not on the outing, about his experiences. Because the parents did not participate in the experience, they cannot provide the type of scaffolding support they provide for recounts. The child must organize the account with little or no assistance from listeners.

4. *Stories:* Stories refer to narratives that the teller has not experienced. Generally, stories are of the "once upon a time" variety, but they can also include biographical stories.

Schools rely heavily on recounts, eventcasts, and stories. In most testing situations students are expected to recount something that has been taught. In science, art, and activity based-language programs, children are expected to produce a running eventcast of their activities. Opportunities for accounts occur less frequently in the academic school environment than at home or on the playground. Stories are the primary texts in the early grades. Mainstream children come to school with an awareness that stories have a beginning in which something disruptive or challenging happens to the characters, a middle in which characters react to what has happened, and an ending that returns the characters to some

sense of equilibrium. Children from non-mainstream backgrounds may come to school with little or no experience with stories of this type, with recounts, or with eventcasts.

By late elementary school, students must master expository texts that require greater abstraction and generalization than narratives. They must be able to discuss not only one experience of a vacation (a narrative), but the characteristics of vacations in general (an exposition); they must be able to talk about not only their dog at home (a narrative), but dogs in general and dogs in relationship to other animals (an exposition). By middle school/high school, students must engage in argumentative or persuasive texts. These are texts that take the generalized principles of expository texts and reason from them in systematic, logical ways. Science texts require students to predict outcomes of chemical reactions or to explain what type of machine would be the most efficient to use in a particular situation. Social studies texts require students to consider information on the United States' involvement in World War I, World War II, Korea, and Vietnam and to hypothesize reasons for our involvement in the 1990 Mideast crisis and how the people of the nation will respond.

Traditional educational curriculum has followed this Moffett's model, introducing reading and academic content through narratives, and only later moving to exposition and argumentation/persuasion. Recent research has shown, however, that even preschool children are capable of some types of exposition and persuasion (Axia, 1996; Snow & Kurland, 1996). Increasingly, children in elementary school are being asked to write in expository and persuasive genres, in addition to narrative genres (Burkhalter,1995; Newkirk, 1989; Temple, Nathan, Temple, & Burris, 1993; Tompkins, 1994).

Levels of Thought

The language genres of school require that children use language for increasingly abstract functions. The early language functions of the young child are focused on meeting immediate needs. Children request objects they want, command people to do things for them (up, come, out, help), or they show objects they have. They talk about only what they see in the environment. Their language is tied to their perceptions. Eventually, they talk about people and events seen in the past or that will be seen in the future, and later still they talk about ideas that cannot be seen.

Language Functions

The ability to use language for other than need-meeting purposes is critical for the academic tasks required by schools. Tough (1979) noted that, in addition to use of language for need-meeting purposes, preschool children from mainstream environments also used language to direct (including monitoring one's own and others' behavior), to report, to predict what was going to happen, to project into thoughts and feelings of others, and to reason. In addition, they could use all of these functions in imaginary play. Table 13.2 gives examples of each of these functions.

Many of these language functions require that the child move beyond what is perceptually obvious. One cannot see what happened in the past or what will happen in the future; one cannot see the thoughts and feelings of others—they must be inferred; and one often cannot see reasons behind events. Tough (1979) reported that children from lower socioeconomic environments used language for self-maintaining purposes twice as frequently as middle socioeconomic level children, but they used language for directing, reporting, predicting, projecting, and reasoning from three to nine times less frequently than middle socioeconomic level children.

Degrees of Abstraction

Language used in school requires students to distance from perception. Blank, Berlin, and Rose (1978) proposed a hier-

archy of language based on the distance between perception and language, that is, the distance between what is seen and what is talked about. Each level requires increasingly more abstract use of language. Table 13.3 presents the four levels they proposed.

At the first level there is a little distance between children's language and their perception. As the demand for abstraction increases, the distance between language and perception increases so that at the highest levels, children are required to evaluate their perceptions and arrive at judgements that go beyond the specific information given.

Bloom (1956) recommended a hierarchy of language-thinking levels that should be part of a school curriculum. No particular ages were placed on these levels, but even in the elementary school, all levels may be required depending on the content of the course and the expectations of the teachers. Each level requires the information and skills of the previous level. Young children may only be required to show that they recognize and comprehend information. As students progress through school, however, they are expected to be able to analyze, synthesize, and evaluate information. Table 13.4 explains the levels and the types of cue words that signal the tasks at each level.

Students must be able to do more than memorize and repeat information. They must be able to use language to think. They are expected to comprehend and use these language genres and levels in both oral and written language activities. How do students access these genres in the educational setting, and how are these thinking skills manifested in the oral interactions and academic tasks of school-age students?

ORAL INTERACTIVE DISCOURSE

Oral interactive discourse is not new to school-age children. The rules and the structure of the interactions, however, may change in school. Infants and tod-

Table 13.2 *Language Functions*

Function	Examples
Self-maintaining	
1. Referring to needs and wants	I want a cookie Gimme a hug.
2. Protection of self and self interests	Give it to me, it's mine. I was asked to do that, not you.
3. Justifying behavior	I hit him cause he broke my crayons It's mine! I asked first.
4. Criticizing others	You don't know how to paint. She can't stay in the lines.
5. Threatening	I'll tell the teacher if you don't give it to me.
Directing	
1. Monitoring one's own actions	I'm doing a good job. I'm almost done.
2. Directing one's own actions	I can't make this piece fit. Turn it around there.
3. Directing actions of others	Pour the sugar in the bowl. Now mix it up.
4. Collaborating with others	I'll hold the paper and you tape it.
Reporting	
1. Labeling components of a scene	There's a monster and some houses. The people are walking up the mountain.
2. Referring to details (attributes)	My puppet's got long black hair and a big hat.
3. Referring to incidents	The fireman showed us how to put on the mask and oxygen tank.
4. Referring to a sequence of events	We went to the zoo, and we saw lots of animals. We had a picnic, and then we watched a bird show.
5. Making comparisons	Your puppet's bigger than mine.
6. Recognizing related aspects	My alarm clock didn't go off, so I was late to school
7. Making an analysis using several of the above features	There are three suitcases—two green ones and one blue one. The blue one's too big to fit on the cart.
8. Recognizing main idea or theme	It's a story about a little girl that got lost.
Logical reasoning	
1. Explaining a process	When you break your arm, they put something on it like a bandage and plaster, all over.
2. Recognizing causal relationships	The house caught on fire, so I called 911 for the firemen to come.

Table 13.2 *Language Functions—continued*

Function	Examples
3. Recognizing problems and solutions	I tried to stick it together, but I didn't have enough glue, so I used tape.
4. Justifying judgements and actions	I'm being real careful so I don't knock the blocks down.
5. Reflecting on events and drawing conclusions	We have to play in the gym today cause it's cold and windy outside.
6. Recognizing principles	Only the pieces with iron in them will be attracted to the magnets.
Predicting	
1. Anticipating/forecasting events	We're going to the West Mesa tomorrow. We'll walk down into J volcano and collect lava rocks.
2. Anticipating details of events	The road to the volcano will be very rough, and the bus will have to go real slow.
3. Anticipating a sequence of events	We'll pick up sack lunches in the cafeteria, then we'll get on the bus. When we get to the volcano, we'll have a picnic. Then we'll climb into the volcano.
4. Anticipating problems and solutions	The bus driver will take a spare tire in case a tire gets cut on the rocks.
5. Anticipating and recognizing alternative courses of actions	If the bus doesn't come, then the teacher can take us in her van.
6. Predicting consequences of actions or events	We'll get a really good rock collection, and we can enter it in the science fair.
Projecting	
1. Projecting into the experience of others	The doctor isn't sure what to do to make her better.
2. Projecting into feelings of others	I think the astronauts worry that a shuttle will explode again. They want NASA to do thorough inspections to make sure the shuttle's safe.
3. Projecting into reactions of others	The king won't let the prince marry the princess unless he kills the dragon that has been destroying the countryside.
4. Projecting into situation never experienced	I'm going to the Space Academy at Huntsville. I'll be kinda scared cause I have to go by myself and I've never been on a plane before. I'll be really excited.

dlers engage in interactive discourse. They take turns with the individual with whom they are communicating. They listen to what is being said, and they re-spond. They initiate a communication and expect a response. In school students are expected to participate in class discussions and work cooperatively in groups.

Table 13.3 *Levels of Language Abstraction*

Level	Description	Examples
I: Matching perception	Reporting and responding to perceptually obvious material in the environment	What's this called? Find one like this.
II: Selective analysis of perception	Reporting and responding to perceptual information that is less salient	What color is the ball? What size are the apples? How are these puppets different?
III: Reordering perception	Using language to restructure perceptual information and inhibit predisposing responses	Tell me what happened at the zoo? Which of these are not farm animals?
IV: Reasoning about perception	Using language to predict, explain, theorize, and reason about relationships	Why did the cookies burn? What will we have to do to make this gingerbread house?

Table 13.4 *Bloom's Taxonomy*

Taxonomy level	Objective	Cue Words
Knowledge (facts, rote memory)	Show how you know by:	list, tell, identify, label, locate, recognize
Translation and interpretation	Show that you understand by:	explain, illustrate, describe, summarize, interpret, expand, convert, measure, translate, restate
Application (use what you know)	Show that you can use what is learned by:	demonstrate, apply, use, construct, find solutions, collect information, perform, solve, choose appropriate procedures
Analysis (take apart to solve problem)	Show that you can pick out the most important points presented or solve the problem	analyze, debate, differentiate, organize, determine, distinguish, take apart, figure out, solve
Synthesis (put together in a new way)	Show that you can combine concepts to create an original idea by:	create, design, develop a plan, produce, synthesize, compile
Evaluation (make a value judgement based on criteria)	Show that you can judge and evaluate ideas, information, procedures, and solutions based on your own stated criteria	judge, rate, compare, decide, evaluate, conclude, appraise (with reasons given)

Adapted from Tonjes MJ, Zintz MV. Teaching reading thinking study skills in content classrooms. Dubuque, IA: Wm. C. Brown, 1987.

At the same time that they are expected to increase their abilities to work in groups, they are also expected to work independently in reading and writing activities. Although the bases of discourse are established early, as children mature, these discourse skills must be refined. Children must become more sensitive to their listeners, and they must be sensitive to ways of managing the conversation. They must be able to maintain the topic of conversation by adding relevant comments and making repairs when communication breaks down.

Perspective Taking

Communicating effectively in oral interactive discourse requires social knowledge and, in particular, being sensitive to the needs of the listener, requires the development of perspective taking. When communication breaks down, it is generally because the speaker has made inappropriate assumptions about the listener. How effective children are in adapting their language to the listener's needs reflects not only their linguistic-pragmatic skills, but also their perspective-taking skills (Geller, 1989). Normal children's ability to take another person's perspective is evident by ages 3 to 4. This is not, however, an all-or-none phenomena. Perspective taking has a long developmental course. Geller (1989) proposed three types of perspective taking that affect children's communicative behaviors.

1. Perceptual perspective taking, which involves children's inferences about another person's perceptual experiences—the child's ability to determine what another person sees and how it is seen when the other person is in a different location than the child.

2. Cognitive perspective taking, which involves the child's inferences about other peoples' thoughts, feelings, beliefs, and/or intentions (the theory of mind discussed in the chapter on social-emotional bases of communication). Cognitive perspective taking requires that children make judgements about the internal psychological states of another person.

3. Linguistic perspective taking, which involves the ability to modify the form, content, and/or use of language in relation to the listeners' needs.

Aspects of perceptual perspective taking develop during the preschool years. A child can determine how another person sees a card in front of her. If shown two sides of a card and the card is held between the child and another person, the child can identify what the other person is seeing. Also the child can play with a visual display and hide a figure from the sight of two other figures.

Linguistic perspective taking also begins to develop during the preschool years. Children will use shorter sentences when talking to a younger child than to an older child (Shatz & Gelman, 1973). In play they can take on the role language of others, modifying their voices, vocabulary, and syntax to sound like a small child one minute, a parent the next, and a firefighter the next (Westby, 1988).

Cognitive perspective taking develops during the school years. In first and second grade typically developing children begin participating in barrier games that require them to describe an object or design to a naive listener so that the listener can replicate the child's design or identify the object. They can also infer another child's strategy in a card or board game. In mid to late elementary school, children can tell stories from the perspectives of multiple characters. Hence, they enjoy telling the story of the three pigs from the point of view of a misunderstood wolf. With greater perceptual and cognitive perspective-taking abilities, children develop greater abilities to modify their speech to different listeners and for different purposes. They will retell the story of a movie differently to a person who has seen the movie versus someone who has not seen it. By early adolescence students can consider the points of view of others in formulating persuasive discourse. For example, when asking for the family car, they consider the parents' possible objections and address these objections in their request.

Hey Dad, can I borrow the car. I have to go to the library to work on a paper for history (must be important; parents support activities that lead to good grades). I'll be back by 11:00—earlier if it starts to snow (parents worry if students stay out late or if they are driving in bad weather). I won't stop at Gary's house (parents don't trust Gary). I'll fill the tank on the way home (parents are complaining about the cost of gas). If you'd like, I'll wash and wax the car on Saturday (this will make them think I'm appreciative).

Cognitive perspective taking shows marked development during the preadolescent and adolescent years. At this time children develop an understanding of abstract traits such as intelligence, they begin to analyze social situations, and they use language to code personality traits and social situations (Case, 1985). Cognitive perspective taking requires that students be able to integrate multiple sources of information. As students develop, they are expected to integrate more and more pieces of information simultaneously. The ability to engage in cognitive perspective-taking reasoning enables students to communicate effectively with a wide variety of people.

Between ages 9 to 11 students can verbally characterize people based on their responses in a social situation, for example, when given the following situation:

Jack needed a new book for school, so he went into the store and joined the line to pick one up. There was only one book left for each person in the line. While he was counting his money, someone grabbed the last book that should have gone to him. As the other person went to pay for the book, Jack left the store. What type of person is Jack (Case, 1985, p.225)?

In characterizing Jack, students must not only focus on Jack's unwillingness to engage in confrontation, but also on his right to the book. Considering both of these pieces of information, students might characterize Jack as "shy" or as "someone who won't stand up for his rights."

Between ages 11 to 13 students develop the ability to analyze and integrate information from more than one social situation. Consider the following item:

Lisa wanted a new dress for a dance. She heard about a half-price sale at a local store, so she decided to go. At the sale Lisa found a nice dress and joined the line of people waiting to be served. Lisa laid the dress on the counter, and while she was counting her money, another customer grabbed the dress. As the other person was checking the dress, Lisa left the store. That afternoon when she arrived home, Lisa found that a person had taken her gardening tools and was using them. What do you think Lisa did (Case, 1985, p. 226)?

This item requires that students analyze two separate situations (waiting in line and tools being taken), perceive how the second situation is like the first, and then conclude that Lisa's behavior will be similar.

Between ages 13 to 15 students develop the understanding that an individual can have multiple traits or feelings that impact on a situation, and all these traits and feelings must be taken into account in determining how a person will respond. Consider the following example:

When Robert was visiting the computer fair, he became very interested in one of the latest models. While waiting to get information on the display model, Robert noticed that several people had been served before him. He told the salesman that he had been waiting for some time and would like to be served. Later that afternoon, as Robert was entering the school, he saw a student carrying a large cardboard box having problems opening the door. Robert offered his assistance by opening the door so that the student could get in. He then went to his class and found an older student sitting in his seat. What do you think Robert did (Case, 1985, p. 227)?

To respond to this task, students must analyze three situations (asking for service, helping carry a box, finding someone in his seat). In the first situation they might conclude that Robert is assertive; and in the second situation that he is considerate. The third situation contains elements of both of the other situations. Therefore they conclude that Robert will claim his seat, but will do so in a polite way.

By ages 15 to 18 students are not only able to recognize the multiple attributes of an individual, but also to acknowledge extenuating circumstances that may result in a person not responding in his or her usual manner. Note the following example:

> *Cathy was waiting in line to get her skates sharpened, and just as her turn came up, they announced that the shop was closing. Cathy told the people at the shop that she had been waiting a long time and she wanted her skates sharpened before they closed the shop. After skating she went over to see her friend. Late in the afternoon she remembered that she had to be home because relatives were coming, so she excused herself and started to leave when her friend asked her for help in finishing an assignment. Cathy helped her friend with the homework and then left for home. On her way home she slipped and ruined her favorite pants. When she got off the bus, a person approached her asking for directions. What do you think Cathy did (Case, 1985, p. 228)?*

Based on the first two situations, students would judge Cathy as being assertive and helpful. Yet they recognize that an unpleasant event coupled with being late, might result in her not responding in her usual way. Consequently, in this particular instance, Cathy may not be helpful.

As students develop perspective-taking skills, they are better able to predict the behavior of others and modify their own behavior and interactions as necessary to accomplish their goals.

Conversational Management

Being able to engage in perspective taking is essential, but not sufficient for successful conversation in school. Students must also manage conversation. What is involved in managing conversations? Students must know how to take

their turn. They must either maintain the topic of conversation or shade the topic to another topic they wish to discuss. They must not abruptly shift the topic to one of their own interest. If the conversation breaks down, students must know who is responsible—has the speaker failed to be explicit or has the listener failed to understand—and they must work to repair the breakdown.

As children mature, they become more successful in maintaining a conversational topic. Preschool children tend to maintain topics by repeating information previously provided (Brinton & Fujiki, 1984, 1989):

EXAMPLE
Speaker 1:   No lost letters
Speaker 2:   The alphabet
Speaker 1:   Good! (responding to Speaker 2). There's no lost letters. Look, there's no lost letters.
Speaker 2:   Alphabet (Britton & Fujiki, 1984, p. 354).

Older children also use repetition, but in addition, they maintain a topic by adding new information:

EXAMPLE
Speaker 1:   Look, I've got a new dress.
Speaker 2:   Oh, yeah, It's really pretty.
Speaker 1:   I found it on sale.
Speaker 2:   It's hard to find a dress that nice on sale (Britton & Fujiki, 1989, p. 50).

The number of conversational topics maintained increases slightly between ages 5 and 9 and considerably more between ages 9 and adult.

Preschool children can be aware of communication breakdowns and will respond when a listener requests further information, usually repeating what they had just said:

EXAMPLE
Anna took my doll.
Huh?
Anna took my doll.

They have difficulty, however, with repeated requests, often giving either irrelevant responses or saying they don't know:

EXAMPLE
There's a girl chasing a dog.
Huh?
There's a girl chasing a dog?
What?
A dog ate somebody's shoe (Britton, Fujiki, Loeb, & Winkler, 1986, p.78).

Between ages 7 to 10 year, children seldom give inappropriate responses to requests for clarification. Compared with preschool children, they are more likely to add information when asked for clarification:

EXAMPLE
The dog is swimming.
Huh?
The dog is swimming in the water.

By age 9 children provide conversational repairs by defining terms or offering background context:

EXAMPLE
They're on a teeter-totter.
Huh?
They're on a teeter-totter, something that one person sits on one side and you go up and down on it.

or

EXAMPLE
He's on a stool getting cookies.
Huh?
There's a family in a kitchen. There's a boy. He's on a stool getting cookies (Britton, Fujiki, Loeb, & Winkler, 1981, p. 78).

To participate in classroom discussion with teachers and peers, it is essential that students be alert to conversational breakdowns, that they be able to signal when they have not comprehended, and that they be able to repair the breakdowns. By late elementary school these conversational skills are in place for normally developing students.

LANGUAGE FOR LITERACY

A major language development during the school years is the development of literacy skills—reading and writing of extended texts. Comprehension and production of extended texts requires that students use their pragmatic, semantic, syntactic, and phonology skills in more complex ways. They must also have additional language skills and knowledge to succeed with academic tasks. Figure 13.2 shows the language knowledges involved in comprehending and producing literate texts. The lines linking each of the knowledges indicate that all knowledges are interrelated and affect one another (Lesgold & Perfetti, 1981; Marzano, Hagerty, Valencia, & DiStefano, 1987).

Schools use a more formal *literate language style* than the oral interactive language of the home or playground (Westby, 1984, 1985). Written language is not simply oral language written down. Written language uses a more explicit vocabulary and complex syntax. Semantic information must be integrated into larger units or *content schemas.* Students must understand relationships among semantic elements. For example, not only must they understand what a spider is—its characteristics—but also what is does, where it lives, its relationship to other arachnids, its relationship to insects, the relationship of arachnids and insects to other animals, and so forth. The information in these content schemas is presented in systematically organized patterns called *text structures or text grammars* (Anderson & Pearson, 1984; Meyer & Rice, 1984). Reading and writing require *metalinguistic abilities*, that is, conscious awareness of language. Students must be able to separate words from the speech stream, segment words into sounds, and match phonemic sounds with grapheme symbols (Adams, 1990; Clay, 1985; Temple, Nathan, Temple, & Burris, 1993). Students must use *metacognitive planning and monitoring abil-*

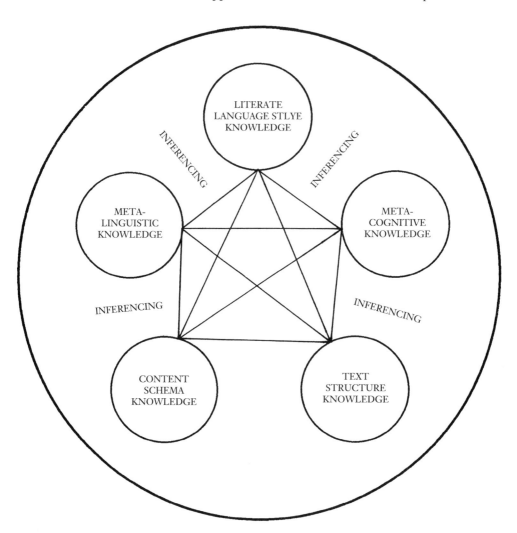

Figure 13.2. Language knowledges for literate texts.

ities to determine if they are comprehending oral and written information. They must use metacognitive strategies when they have failed to comprehend and when they are presented with complex learning tasks (Baker & Brown, 1984). All of these knowledges must be integrated and drawn on to make appropriate *inferences and predictions* (Wallach & Miller, 1989). A strength in one knowledge area may compensate for a weakness in another area. For example, a student with weak metalinguistic skills may be able to use content knowledge to predict words; a student weak in content schemas may use metacognitive strategies to gain additional schema knowledge.

Literate Language Style

Reading and writing require a language style that differs from oral-interactive language in vocabulary, syntax, and organization. Literate language generally requires more explicit vocabulary, more complex syntax, and a topic-centered organization. In an oral style speakers may use nonspecific language (pronouns and words such as *that, this, here, there, stuff, things*), and short sentences. Ideas may be strung together in an associative style, with one idea leading to another, but with little or no relationship among all the ideas. In oral language speakers may rely on prosody and intonation to carry much of the meaning rather than the vocabulary and syntax. For example, "What a GREAT movie!" said with higher pitch and stress on GREAT implies that the viewers thoroughly enjoyed the movies; whereas, "What a great movie" said with a lower pitch on "great" and falling inflection at the end implies that the movie was terrible. When the speakers have both seen the movie, there is seldom the need to explain the basis for their judgements.

In the literate style speakers and writers must use explicit vocabulary and complex syntax that makes the interrelationships between elements of the text explicit. When an adult and child are looking at a picture in a book together, it is understandable to them if one says:

EXAMPLE
He hit him. He ran away.

Without the context of the picture, however, these sentences make no sense. One does not know who did the hitting, who ran away, and why he ran. To understand what happened when no pictures are available, one may need to say or write:

EXAMPLE
The boy who stole the bike hit the boy who was watching. Then the boy who saw the bike being stolen swiftly ran away because he was not strong enough to fight back.

Written language makes greater use of a variety of conjunctions (in addition to the conjunctions *and*, *then*, and *cause* used in oral conversation, words such as but, therefore, however, meanwhile, nevertheless, in addition, in so far as, etc.); adverbs (*swiftly*, *angrily*, *smoothly*); adverbial clauses (*When I finish my homework*, I can watch TV); and relative clauses (The clever fox, *who tricked the coyote into holding up the mesa*, trotted off with the money). In the early school years the vocabulary and syntax of children's oral language is in advance of their reading and writing abilities. By late elementary school, however, the print that children read is more complex than their oral language and begins

to influence the vocabulary and syntax they use in their oral language (Miller & Gildea, 1987).

The function of pronominal reference changes in literate texts. Preschool children understand pronouns in conversational discourse and use them deictically to point out something in the immediate context (e.g., *Here he is, she's running, he's biting him*). In these instances, pronouns refer to an extralinguistic referent—an object or a picture. In school texts pronominal reference must be used in its discourse function, that is, to refer to elements within the discourse, rather than in the external environment. Compare the preschool child's story about a picture with that of a fourth-grade student:

EXAMPLE
Preschool Child: And he's up there. And here they come. He's gonna throw that. They're gonna get him. They'll burn him with the fire.
Fourth-Grade Student: Once there was a village in the mountains. No one really knows for sure. And there was a monkeylike creature who lived on top of the mountain and would get rocks and boulders and throw them down at the village. But finally one day the people got mad so they're climbing up the mountain to get rid of the monkey creature. But the monkey creature got a boulder and he threw it down at the people. He missed some, but he hit some of them. And the men finally got up the mountain. Then the men stopped. "We shouldn't kill the creature. He's only doing what he's supposed to do. Maybe we can become friends with him." And they became best friends forever.

The preschool child uses pronouns and deictics (*he, they, here, there, that*) that are understandable only when one is looking at the picture. The fourth-grade child first introduces places (*village, mountain*) and characters (*monkey, people*) with nouns, then refers to them with pronouns. He reintroduces the noun referents as necessary to make the text clear to listeners. Effective oral and written production of extended discourse and successful reading comprehension requires the ability to use the cohesive principles of conjunctive relations and pronominal reference (Chapman, 1983; Irwin, 1986).

Content Schema

Content schema represents the child's organization of knowledge about a given topic or domain. Content schemas include semantic knowledge, as well as cognitive knowledge of spatial, temporal, and causal relationships. One can have schemas for scenes (houses, jungles, schools), events (birthday parties, camping trips), or concepts/ideas (government, energy). A schema for a school might include classrooms, chalkboards, desks, chairs, books, teachers, principal, gym, and restrooms. A schema for a birthday party would include a person having a birthday, gifts, ice cream, cake, playing games, blowing out candles, and singing happy birthday. Event schemas might also include the scripts, or what would be said by people engaging in the event. A schema for energy might include sources of energy, location of energy sources, how energy is produced, pollution created by energy generation, and so forth.

Semantic development during the school years involves the addition of more abstract words to the lexicon; refinement and decontextualization of word meanings already in the lexicon; ability to define words; development of multiple word meanings, including understanding of figurative words, metaphors, and idioms; and perhaps most importantly, the development of an organized semantic network whose related words become closely associated (Nelson, 1985; Pease, Gleason, & Pan, 1989). Understanding children's schema content development during the school years provides insight into children's reading comprehension abilities. A major aspect of semantic development during the school years is the establishment of semantic networks or interrelationships among words in the lexicon. Words are related to one another through superordinate and subordinate relation-

ships and through spatial, temporal, and cause-effect relationships. Because of spreading semantic networks, students recognize that robins and canaries are types of birds; birds are related to snakes and dogs because they are all animals; birds are related to planes, bees, and kites because they all fly; birds are related to pillows because they both have feathers; birds and fish are related because they both eat worms; and birds and leaves are related because they are both found in trees.

As students develop these content schema networks, they acquire new vocabulary. Children with large vocabularies are more efficient in using the context of printed language to identify words in texts (Nelson, 1988). As children's semantic knowledge increases during the school years, they grow in their ability to rely less on environmental cues and more on textual cues to process information. When a word is first acquired, its comprehension may be tied to the context in which it is used (French & Nelson, 1987). For example, a young student may comprehend the teacher's instructions, "*Before you leave for gym, turn in your math paper,*" but not recognize the sequence of events in a story that says, "*Before the fox left for Acoma, he asked the coyote for all his money.*" Students are familiar with the context of turning in math assignments before gym class, but not with the interactions of foxes and coyotes. Slowly, during the school years, students break free of the attachment of words to specific, concrete contexts and develop the ability to rely only on linguistic context for understanding and determining meaning.

Children's approach to defining words changes from preschool to adolescence (Wiig & Secord, 1985). When asked to define words, preschool children typically respond by stating a function or by producing an associated response (e.g., "What is a ring?" response: *"what you wear"* or *"people steal rings"*). Elementary-school children give synonyms and categorical responses (a ring is jewelry). Synonyms and categorical responses reflect the enlarging semantic webs among words. Adolescents give abstract, dictionary definitions, for example, *"A circular band, made of metal, perhaps with jewels, that is worn on the finger."*

Text Grammars

The content of texts is organized or structured in systematic ways. This structure is called a text grammar. Students who are able to recognize text structures exhibit better comprehension (Fitzgerald, 1989; Slater & Graves, 1989). Narrative text grammars have been extensively studied. The structure of narratives is dependent on their content (Mandler & Johnson, 1977; Stein & Glenn, 1979). Nearly all narratives in Western cultures have the same content and structure (Westby, 1994). All narratives involve the same basic content—characters, their goals, and their attempts to achieve these goals. Figure 13.3 depicts the common narrative structure. Narratives in Western cultures have the following components:

Setting
Describes the characters and the social, physical, or temporal context in which the story happens.

Initiating event
A natural occurrence (e.g., earthquake, tornado), an activity of a character (e.g., stealing, threat), the perception of an event (hearing thunder), or changes in physiologic state (hunger, pain) that trigger a response in characters.

Internal response
The emotional state of the character in response to the initiating event.

Plan
A character's strategy for obtaining a goal.

Attempt
A series of actions intentionally carried out by the character in an effort to achieve a goal.

Consequence
The success or failure of the character in achieving a goal.

Resolution
The character's feelings, thoughts, or actions in response to the consequences of attaining or not attaining a goal.

Ending
A statement announcing the conclusion of the story, summarizing the story, or stating a moral or general principle.

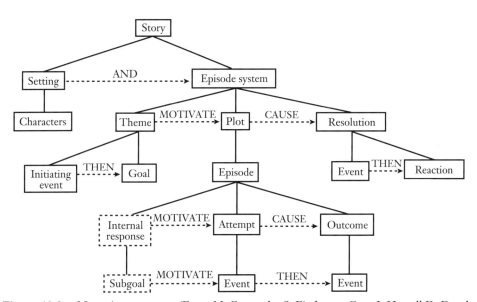

Figure 13.3. Narrative structure. (From McConaughy S, Fitzhenry-Coor I, Howell D. Developmental differences in schemata for story comprehension. In: Nelson K, ed. Children's language. Vol. 4. Hillsdale, NJ: Erlbaum, 1983.)

At a minimum, a true narrative episode must contain the following (Stein, 1979):

1. Some reference to the motivation or purpose of the character's behavior (of an initiating event or an internal response)

2. An overt goal directed action (an attempt)

3. The attainment or nonattainment of the goal (a direct consequence)

The following story is a well-structured story written by a 7-year-old girl. The story contains all the components expected in a good story.

EXAMPLE

Setting: Once there was a witch who lived in a haunted house. She had a cat named Edgar. And the witch's name was Witchie.

Initiating event: One day they were stirring their brew with a broom. While they were stirring their brew someone ringed the doorbell. She had run away from her mother and father, and she was looking for a place to stay. The witch say come in. Then she said hahaha to the little girl.

Internal response: And the little girl was scared that the witch would cast a spal on her.

Plan: She knew she had to get away.

Attempt: She was trying to get out,

Consequence: but she couldn't.

Additional setting: Then finally one of the windows were open.

Attempt: So she jumped out the window

Consequence: and found her way home.

Resolution: And did'nt come back.

Ending: The end.

As early as 2½ years children who have heard stories will respond to requests to produce a story. Table 13.5 lists the narrative content and narrative structure associated with mainstream children's ages.

Narrative language skills in kindergarten and early elementary are better predictors of literacy skills in later elementary schools than are measures of vocabulary or syntactic skills (Bishop & Edmundson, 1987; Feagans & Applebaum, 1986). The curriculum of schools requires

Table 13.5 *Progression of Narrative Development*	
Content	Structure
Preschool	
Ability to describe	Isolated description: Child labels or describes objects, characters, surroundings, and ongoing actions; no interrelationships among the elements mentioned
Awareness that animate beings act and inanimate objects are acted upon	Action sequence: Child lists actions that may be chronologically related based on perception (child is not necessarily aware of temporal sequence); no interrelationships among characters; characters act independently of each other; story may have a central character or a central theme (actions that each character does)
Awareness of physical cause-effect relationships; awareness of linear time for familiar sequences	Reaction sequence: Beginning of chaining—one activity or event automatically causes other changes, but with no planning involved (e.g., a storm damages a bird's wings, the bird can't fly, so the bird crashes)

Table 13.5   *Progression of Narrative Development—continued*

Content	Structure
Early elementary school	
Awareness of psychological causality for primary emotions (happy, mad, sad, scared, surprises, disgusted), i.e., awareness of situations that cause these emotions and what one might do because of these emotions (child loses teddy bear—child sad—child cries—child searches for bear); some perspective taking for characters; scriptal knowledge of common characters (wolves are bad and eat pigs; princes are good and save princesses from dragons)	Goal-directed episode: Centering and chaining are present, i.e., story has a central character who engages in a series of temporally or causally related activities; stories describe goals or intentions of characters, but planning must be inferred; can apply story grammar analysis to stories—stories have at least components of initiating event, response, and consequence
Further development of psychological causality (cognitive emotions, e.g., jealousy, guilt, shame, embarrassment); further development of perspective taking—awareness of interaction of character attributes with story elements of setting and events that enables child to comprehend/predict novel behaviors of characters; understanding of longer time frames (days, weeks); meta-awareness of the need to plan and how to plan; understanding of the need to justify plans	Complete episode: Goals and intentions of characters described with some evidence of planning; story has at least an initiating event (problem), internal response (character's reaction to the problem), plan, attempt (carrying out the plan), and consequence
Late elementary school	
Ability to perceive character change/growth (i.e., understanding that character attributes change over course of story as a result of events); ability to detect deception or trickery and to deceive or trick; awareness of time cycles (seasons, years); beginning awareness of multiple meanings for words and literal versus figurative meanings	Elaborated stories: Stories may be elaborated in the following ways. The list represents a developmental sequence:
	1. Multiple episodes: story has more than one "chapter" with each chapter having at least the minimal story grammar elements
	2. Complex episodes: A single episode that includes an obstacle to achieving a goal; involves multiple plans or multiple attempts because initial plans and attempts are not successful
	3. Embedded episodes: One episode is embedded within another; first episode is suspended, a second episode is introduced, then storyteller returns to and completes the first episode

that students comprehend and produce the story elements in a complete episode by third to forth grade. Normally developing children from mainstream backgrounds who have been exposed to stories have this ability. Children who exhibit poor reading comprehension have been shown to have deficits in their oral narrative skills (Cain, 1996). Once the basic complete episode story structure is acquired, it is elaborated by including obstacles resulting in multiple attempts and consequences, sequences of episodes, and episodes embedded within episodes. Stories from Native American and some Asian cultures, however, may not follow this same text structure, and students from some cultures may have little or no opportunity to hear or practice producing narratives before entering school (Heath, 1986a, 1986b; Hsu, 1981; Scollon & Scollon, 1981; Westby, 1994; Worth & Adair, 1972).

Expository Text Grammars

Compared with narrative texts, less is known about the development of comprehension and production of expository texts. Expository texts have a greater variety of structures than narrative texts because they are about a greater variety of ideas, different structures best fitting each idea. Not only do different texts have different structures, but also within any text may be several different structures. For narrative texts, readers need only acquire a single basic narrative episode structure that is tied to the content. The structure of expository texts is not tied to content. The same content may be presented in multiple text structures. To comprehend expository texts, students must acquire a variety of text structures and be able to switch between these structures within a single text. Each paragraph in a text may have a different structure and several structures may be embedded in long paragraphs.

As children progress through school, more of the curriculum is presented in an expository format. By junior high school all the curriculum, with the exception of language arts, is presented in an expository format. Figure 13.4 diagrams the common expository structures.

Table 13.6 presents the major types of expository texts, their functions, and key words that signal the type of expository text. To comprehend expository texts, students must comprehend these words, recognize that these words signal text organization, and then use knowledge of these structures to recognize the relationship among the concepts presented.

Students from fourth grade through college increasingly develop their ability to use expository text structure to facilitate

comprehension and recall (Slater & Graves, 1989). Research regarding which expository text structure results in the best memory for text content had yielded mixed results, perhaps because certain structures are more suitable for certain content, situations, and readers (Horowitz, 1987; Maria, 1990). In general, there is a tendency for descriptive and enumerative structures to be the most difficult to remember for students of all ages. Comparison/contrast texts may be descriptive or enumerative, but the comparison/contrast structure appears to facilitate comprehension and retrieval of the factual information presented. Sequential/procedural texts have some similarity to narrative structures and are an early recognized structure. Problem-solution and cause-effect structures tend to be the last to be acquired and may not be used well until high school.

Over 30 states currently require writing assessments of students in several genres or text structures. The National Assessment of Educational Progress (NAEP, 1994) conducts periodic assessment of students' reading, writing, mathematics, and science achievement. NAEP presented a developmental hierarchy of content/structural characteristics for two types of expository texts—informative and persuasive (Table 13.7).

Metacognitive Skills

The importance of metacognition in social, language, and literacy skills has received increased attention in recent years (Meltzer, 1993; Pressley & Woloshyn, 1995). Metacognition refers to the knowledge that learners have about their learning systems and the decisions learners makes about how to act on information coming into the learning systems. Brown (1981) cited two types of metacognition: (1) knowledge about cognition, which includes conscious access to one's own cognitive operations and reflections about those of others and (2) regulation of cognition, which involves planning and control of actions, including checking, monitoring, testing, revising, and evaluating. Knowledge about cognition allows learn-

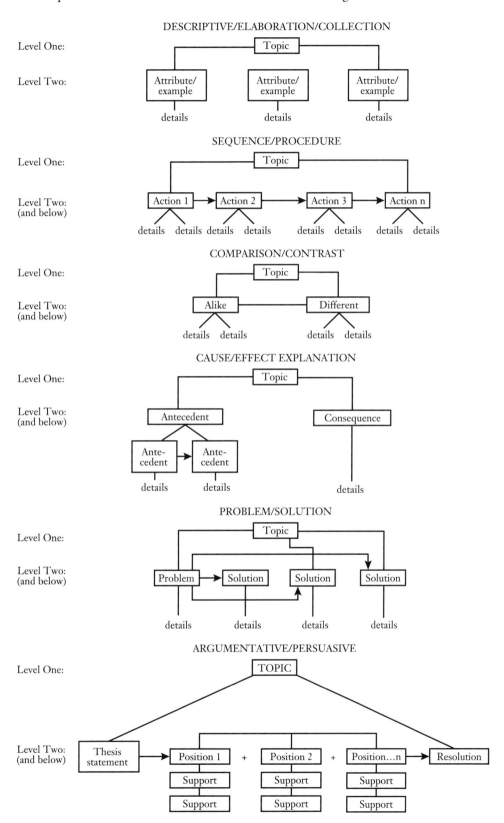

Figure 13.4. Expository text structures. (Adapted from Richgels D, McGee D, Lomax R, Sheard C. Awareness of four text structures: effects of recall of expository text. Read Res Q 1987;22:177–196.)

Table 13.6 *Characteristics of Expository Texts*

Text Pattern	Text Function	Key Words
Description	The text tells what something is	Is called, can be defined as, is, can be interpreted as, is explained as, refers to, is a procedure for, is someone who, means
Collection/enumeration	The text gives a list of things that are related to the topic	An example is, for instance, another, next, finally, such as, to illustrate
Sequence/procedure	The text tells what happened or how to do something or make something	First, next, then, second, third, following this step, finally, subsequently, from here . . . to, eventually, before, after
Comparison/contrast	The text shows how two things are the same or different	Different, same, alike, similar, although, however, on the other hand, contrasted with, compared with, rather than, but, yet, still, instead of
Cause/effect explanation	The text gives reasons for why something happened	Because, since, reasons, then, therefore, for this reason, results, effects, consequently, so, in order to, thus, depends on, influences, is a function of, produces, leads to, affects, hence
Problem/solution	The text states a problem and offers solutions to the problem	A problem is, a solution is

ers to state what they know and do not know, how they learn, and what they will remember—although this knowledge may not be accurate. This type of metacognition is relatively late in developing. Generally, students begin to report this awareness in third grade.

The second type of metacognition, regulation of cognition, consists of self-regulatory mechanisms used by learners while attempting activities. Children begin as early as 3½ years to regulate themselves by using language (self-talk) to control and monitor their behavior (Luria, 1982). These metacognitive behaviors are unstable (the students may use them on some occasions and not on others), rarely stateable (the students can do many things they cannot describe in words), and relatively

independent of a student's age. Even 4 year olds may be capable of planning their next move, checking on the effectiveness of their strategies, and revising their strategies when they have not worked (Duell, 1986).

As children move through school, they are expected to take increased responsibility for their own behavior and learning. To do so, they must use language to guide their behavior and evaluate their success or lack of success. In first grade, teachers carefully control both the children's behavior and presentation of learning activities. By third grade, teachers expect students to know the rules of school and to comply with the rules without reminders; they are expected to have internalized the rules and follow them even when the

Table 13.7 *NAEP Scoring Guides*

	Informative	Persuasive
1.	Listing: Lists pieces of information or ideas all on the same topic, but does not relate them. A range of information/ideas is presented.	Opinion: Statement of opinion, but no reasons are given to support the opinion, or the reasons given are inconsistent or unrelated to the opinion.
2.	Attempted discussion: Includes several pieces of information and some range of information. In part of the paper, an attempt is made to relate some of the information (in a sentence or two), but relationships are not clearly established because ideas are incomplete or under-developed (the amount of explanation and details is limited).	Extended opinion: states opinion and gives reasons to support the opinion, but the reasons are not explained or the explanations given are incoherent.
3.	Undeveloped discussion: Includes a broad range of information and attempts to relate some pieces of information. The relationships are somewhat established, but not completely. The ideas are confused, contradictory, out of sequence, illogical, or undeveloped.	Partially developed argument: States opinion and gives reasons to support the opinion, plus attempts to develop the opinion with further explanation. However, the explanations are given but not developed or elaborated. May give a brief reference to the opposite point of view.
4.	Discussion: Includes a broad range of information and, in at least one section, clearly relates the information using rhetorical devices (such as temporal order, classification, comparison/contrast, cause and effect, problem/solution, goals/resolution, predications, speculations, suppositions, drawing conclusions, point of view, ranking, exemplification).	Developed argument: States opinion, gives reasons to support the opinion, plus explanations, with at least one explanation developed through the use of rhetorical devices (such as sequence of events, cause and effect, comparison/contrast, classification, problem/solution, point of view, drawing conclusions). May contain a brief summary of the opposite point of view.
5.	Partially developed discussion: Includes a broad range of information and establishes more than one kind of relationship using rhetorical devices, such as those listed above. Information and relationships are well developed, with explanations and supporting details. Paragraphs are well formed but the paper lacks an overriding sense of purpose and cohesion.	Partially developed refutation: States opinion, gives reasons to support opinion, explanations, plus attempts to discuss and/or refute the opposite point of view. Contains an adequate summary of the opposite point of view.
6.	Developed discussion: Includes a broad range of information and establishes more than one kind of relationship using rhetorical devices, such as those listed above. Information and relationships are explained and supported. The paper has a coherent sense of purpose and audience, and is free from grammatical problems. An overt organizational structure is used (such as the traditional essay format).	Developed refutation: States opinion, gives reasons to support opinion, explanations, plus a discussion and/or refutation of opposing point of view. Refutation is clear and explicit—summarizes opposite point of view and discusses why it is limited or incorrect.

teacher is not present. Although the students are working somewhat more independently, the teacher still carefully organizes and monitors learning activities. By fifth grade, students are expected to manage both their behavior and learning. They must be able to organize and complete a project with minimal support from the teacher (Westby, 1997).

Metacognitive abilities involving knowing about knowing require that children develop a theory of mind. A theory of mind includes five elements (Wellman, 1985):

1. *Existence*. Student must know that thoughts and mental states exist and are not the same as external events. This involves realizing that one can think about something and talk about something. Furthermore, what one thinks may not be what one says. One may say, "My, what a pretty ring you have," while thinking "That's the gaudiest ring I've ever seen."

2. *Distinct processes*. There are many types of thought processes that one can engage in: knowing, remembering, forgetting, guessing, dreaming, hypothesizing, et cetera.

3. *Integration*. Although there are many different mental acts, all mental processes are also similar and related. One cannot remember or forget unless one knew something in the first place. One guesses when one cannot know. One hypothesizes when one knows some general principles.

4. *Variables*. Many factors affect how well the mind performs the various mental acts. Familiar content is easier to remember than unfamiliar content; short lists are easier to remember than long lists. One is more likely to find learning difficult when one does not feel well or when one has many other concerns.

5. *Cognitive monitoring*. Finally, students are often able to read their own mental states or monitor their ongoing cognitive processes. They know when then know and do not know; they know if they are likely to forget something; and they know what will help them remember or not remember.

A theory of mind begins to develop during the preschool years. The development of metacognitive verbs (*know, forget, remember, guess, doubt, infer, hypothesize, conclude, assume*) are critical for children's learning and participation in school activities. Wellman (1985) reported that the words *know, forget, remember,* and *guess* develop between ages 3 and 7 years. To carry out teachers' instructions, children must know if they understand what is expected, and they must ask questions or ask for assistance if they do not know. They must know if they have the necessary information or if they are guessing. They also must remember what they have been told to do and be aware if they have forgotten what they were told. Without this active awareness of knowing, remembering, forgetting, and guessing, children will not function independently.

Jenkins (1979) proposed a tetrahedral model to account for the metacognitive processes that students use in monitoring their learning of materials. Four components are involved:

1. The characteristics of the learner, that is, what learners know about themselves—about their present knowledge, what is hard and what is easy for them, what they like and what they do not like.

2. The nature of the materials to be learned. This includes the learners' awareness of the organizational structure of the texts and the types of facts and content information that will appear in texts.

3. The criterial task, that is, what is to be the end product of the learning. For example, is the student to retell the story, complete a multiple-choice test or essay test, or teach the material to someone else?

4. Learning strategies at one's disposal, that is, can one reread, does one know how to outline or make semantic maps of the material, does one use visual imagery to remember the information, and so forth.

Knowledge of cognition begins to develop when children are aware of their knowledge or lack of knowledge. A great deal of the literature related to knowledge of cognition has focused on metamemory, that is, awareness of variables that make remembering difficult and what one can do to facilitate memory. A general developmental trend emerges in the use of memory strategies (Kail & Hagen, 1982):

1. Five and six year olds show little or no awareness of what to do when they are asked to remember or little ability to judge what they will be able to remember.

2. A transitional stage emerges between 7 to 10 years of age, when strategies begin to appear but are related to the specific strategy and the context in which it is to be used. When asked to learn a list of items, 7 year olds are beginning to name the items as they look at them (Appel, Cooper, McCarrell, et al., 1972), they can be trained to rehearse the item names to facilitate memory, and they are aware that familiar items are easier to remember (Kreutzer, Leonard, & Flavell, 1975). They cannot, however, predict what they will remember, nor do they develop or use strategies spontaneously.

3. Mature strategy use begins at age 10 and will continue to develop through adulthood. Ten year olds spontaneously rehearse information they are expected to learn, and they employ chunking strategies with the information (i.e., looking for relationships among the items to be remembered). Students begin to take notes or underline sections of a passage as they study (Brown & Smiley, 1978). As they do so, they isolate the crucial ideas in a passage and begin to devote less attention to less critical information.

Using knowledge about cognition clearly requires a wide variety of language skills, and the ability to use knowledge about cognition increases students learning of more language.

Metalinguistic Skills

The term metalinguistics refers to the ability to reflect on language or to use language to talk about language. It involves the ability to focus on the form of language in and of itself, rather than merely as a ve-

hicle for conveying meaning. Metalinguistic studies have encompassed six areas: (1) repairing communication breakdowns, (2) adjusting language to the listener, (3) making judgements of language content and form, (4) analyzing language into linguistic units, (5) understanding rhymes, puns, and riddles, and (6) understanding and producing figurative language (Kamhi, 1987).

Preschool children are able to make repairs when communication breaks down and to adjust their language content and structure to their listeners (Shatz & Gelman, 1973). The remaining metalinguistic abilities develop during the school years. The literature suggests that children cannot make explicit, out-of-context judgments about linguistic form until age 4, and frequently not until ages 7 or 8 (Hakes, 1980, 1982; Smith & Tager-Flusberg, 1982).

Phonological Awareness

Phonological awareness has been defined as awareness of "the ways in which words and syllables can be divided into small units" (Goswami & Bryant, 1990, p. 2). It refers to rhyme knowledge, syllable and sound segmentation, sound manipulation, and sound blending.

Analyzing language into linguistic units is considered essential in learning to read (Adams, 1990). Children must develop a word consciousness. Word consciousness involves awareness of the arbitrary nature of words and the fact that words are separate from the things they represent. This knowledge enhances reading development because it fosters the child's realization that words and their properties (word length, sounds) can be isolated from the meaning denoted by the word. For example, the child becomes aware that the words *train* and *snake* are short words even though they refer to long objects.

Many preschool children are able to segment sentences into words. Children demonstrate early awareness that language consists of individual words in a number of ways. In playing with language they may repeat sentence frames, substituting one word for another:

EXAMPLE
Dog ran away with spoon
Dog ran away with dog.
Dog ran away with dish (van Kleeck & Bryant, 1984).

Studies have shown that the awareness of word boundaries is a significant predictor of reading achievement in first graders (Evans, Taylor, & Blum, 1979; McNinch, 1974). Segmentation skills develop in a hierarchical manner. First, children are most successful in segmenting content words (nouns and verbs) and only later in segmenting functions words (articles, conjunctions, prepositions) (Papandropoulou & Sinclair, 1974).

The ability to segment sentences develops before the ability to segment words into syllables and sounds, which are phonologic awareness tasks. Phonologic awareness tasks tend to develop in the following sequence:

Syllable segmentation (hot/dog; ba/na/na)

Rhyme recognition (Do cat and hat rhyme? top and tip? What rhymes with fish?—dish or ball)

Blending of sounds (What is /b/ /æ/ /t/?)

Sound segmentation (What is the first sound in home? the last sound in goat?)

Sound manipulation (Say meat without the /m/.)

Syllable segmentation and rhyme recognition develop during the preschool years; blending and sound segmentation in kindergarten and first grade; and sound manipulation in second grade. Segmentation ability has been widely studied in its relationship to reading. Rhyme recognition in preschool predicts emergent literacy in kindergarten; sound segmentation ability in kindergarten predicts reading in first and second grade (Goswami & Bryant, 1990). Ability to segment phonemically facilitates early reading, and at the same time, reading appears to increase the

ability to segment phonemically (Ehri, 1979; Stackhouse, 1997; Stanovich, 1986).

Closely related to the ability of phonemic segmentation is the development of knowledge of sound-symbol association. Children from highly literate environments frequently acquire some awareness of sound-symbol relationships during the preschool years and will engage in spontaneous writing using invented spelling. Children match the way they produce the phonemes of the language with the way they say the letters of the alphabet. For many letters there is a letter-sound match. For example when saying B /bi/, F / ɛf/, S/ ɛs/, L / ɛl/ the child produces the phoneme when saying the letter name. Hence, when asked to write "baby" or "soap" the child can easily produce "babe" or "sop" by relying on this letter-sound correspondence.

Multiple-Word Meanings and Figurative Language

Figurative language refers to language that is used in nonliteral ways. Development of multiple-word meanings and figurative language is an aspect of both semantic development and metalinguistic development. Children who comprehend and appropriately use multiple-word meanings and figurative language demonstrate an awareness that language is an arbitrary code. Such an awareness is a metalinguisitic skill (Kamhi, 1987). Figurative language includes similes, metaphors, idioms, and proverbs. Idioms are expressions such as "*It's raining cats and dogs*" or "*break the ice*" that have fixed or conventional meanings that cannot be determined from the literal meanings of the words (Nippold, 1985). A metaphor is a term that is likened to another term because of some shared features, as in the phrases "*evening of life*" or "*she is the sunshine of my life.*" A simile is similar to a metaphor, but makes the relationship explicit, for example, "*Her eyes sparkle like diamonds.*" Proverbs are short statements that express well-known truths. They may offer encouragement (e.g., "*It's always darkest before the dawn*"), or advice ("*A bird in the hand is worth two in the bush*"), warn of danger ("*When the wolf shows his teeth, he isn't laughing*"), or comment on events ("*A new broom sweeps clean*") (Nippold, 1988).

Some multiple-meaning words refer to specific concrete objects or actions (e.g., lie on the river *bank;* put your money in the *bank; bank* the car on the sharp turn,) as well as to figurative meanings (don't *bank* on it). Some multiple meaning words may refer to both physical and psychologic attributes (a *sharp* knife and a *sharp* manager; a *crooked* nail and a *crooked* accountant). Preschool children understand only the physical meaning of words such as *sweet, sharp, crooked, soft, hard, warm, cold, bright,* or *deep.* By ages 7 to 8 they begin to comprehend the psychological meanings of these words; by ages 9 to 10 they begin to be able to explain the relationship between the physical and psychological terms; and by 13 to 14 years they can give adultlike explanations (e.g., "he's hard like a rock cause you can't move him or change him") (Wiig, 1989). A similar pattern of development occurs with similes, metaphors, and idioms. Comprehension of proverbs is somewhat more difficult than the other types of figurative speech. In fact, children show little or no comprehension of proverbs before adolescence (Douglas & Peel, 1979; Richardson & Church, 1959).

Appreciation of jokes and riddles also requires metalinguistic abilities. Jokes and riddles involve linguistic ambiguity that can occur at any of four levels (Schultz & Pilon, 1973; Schultz & Horibe, 1974):

EXAMPLE
Lexical ambiguity
Order! Order in the court!
Ham and cheese on rye, please, Your Honor.

EXAMPLE
Phonologic ambiguity
Waiter, what's this?
That's bean soup, ma'am.

I'm not interested in what it's been, I'm asking what it is now.

EXAMPLE
Surface-structure ambiguity
Tell me how long cows should be milked.
They should be milked the same as short ones, of course.

EXAMPLE
Deep-structure ambiguity
Call me a cab.
You're a cab.

The 6- to 8-year-old period is a transition time in beginning to perceive the incongruity in jokes and riddles. Phonologic ambiguity is the first form of linguistic ambiguity to be considered funny by a child, beginning at ages 6 or 7. Appreciation of lexical ambiguity soon follows. Jokes and riddles based on surface and deep-structure ambiguity are seldom understood by children until ages 11 or 12.

Inferencing and Predicting

Comprehension involves more than reading the words of a text. One must also read between the lines to comprehend what is read. The ability to make inferences and predictions is dependent on all the other knowledges. Inferencing/predicting is a natural part of the comprehension process. Inferences can be categorized as pragmatic or logical. Pragmatic inferences involve bringing one's world knowledge to the text. If we read,"After check-in, the bellhop helped us carry out luggage to our room," we would infer that we are in a hotel. If we read,"In the morning, the trees were uprooted and some homes had lost their roofs," we might infer that there had been a violent windstorm (or tornado or hurricane). These inferences are not based on information within the text itself, but on world knowledge that the listener or reader possesses. Logical inferences use only the information in the text. For example, if a text states the following:

> All mammals are warm-blooded and nurse their young. A teledu is a mammal. What can you say about a teledu?

we can logically infer that a teledu is warm-blooded and nurses its young, even though it is unlikely that we have ever seen a teledu. Narrative texts tend to rely more on pragmatic inferences, and expository texts require greater use of logical inferences. Even preschool children will make appropriate pragmatic inferences. Making logical inferences is generally more difficult, but is required of students by junior-high age.

CHARACTERISTICS OF STUDENTS WITH LANGUAGE-LEARNING DISABILITIES

The school-age population with language-learning disabilities is heterogenous. There are multiple etiologies for their disabilities, and multiple manifestations of their disabilities. Some students exhibit deficits in all aspects of oral and written communication, while other students exhibit difficulty in only one or two areas. Generally, students who exhibit oral language deficits will exhibit written language deficits. It is possible, however, for students to appear to have normal oral language skills, yet exhibit difficulty in literate language. In fact, the language basis of learning disabilities has often been overlooked in students who did not exhibit obvious oral language deficits.

Oral Interactive Discourse Disabilities

Students with language-learning disabilities are likely to exhibit a variety of pragmatic or oral interactive discourse difficulties in establishing friendships and participating in social and academic classroom interactions (Donahue, 1994; Fujiki, Brinton, & Todd, 1996; Gallagher, 1993). Many of the criteria used to identify students with ADHD reflect pragmatic dysfunction (e.g., difficulty awaiting turns, talking excessively, interrupting

others, not listening to what is being said, and blurting out answers to questions before they are completed) (American Psychiatric Association, 1993). Children with ADHD have also been shown to have less knowledge about social skills and appropriate behavior with others (Grenell, Glass, & Katz, 1987). They seem to lack self-talk, which is critical to the control and organization of interpersonal behavior. As a consequence, they do not read essential verbal, nonverbal, and situational cues or make decisions based on that evidence in accordance with social expectations (Whalen & Henker, 1985).

Students with language-learning disabilities and those with ADHD may exhibit difficulty in getting turns in a conversation, initiating topics, maintaining topics, giving turns to others, responding to requests for conversational repair, and requesting repairs from others (Brinton & Fujiki, 1989; Donahue, Pearl, & Bryan, 1983). Students with language-learning disabilities may not persist in initiation attempts long enough to get a turn. Once they do get a turn, they may have difficulty initiating topics within turns (Fey & Leonard, 1983). They may not make their topics clear, and they may fail to use connective devices that link their contributions to previous information. Consequently, others cannot maintain the topics initiated by students with language-learning disabilities (Dollaghan & Miller, 1986; Schneider, 1982). Students with language-learning disabilities may participate in the topics initiated by others, but fail to initiate their own topics. Because they may have limited content schema knowledge, they may have a limited number of topics they can discuss and may have difficulty in determining what topics can or should be discussed in a particular situation (Bedrosian, 1988).

Some students may not relinquish turns to others. They may not use questions, intonation contours, or pauses effectively to allow others to join the conversation (Roth & Spekman, 1984). Some students may monopolize the conversation, ignoring communicative attempts of their partners. Such children may ramble from one topic to another; others may repeat information on a single topic. Some of these students appear to attempt to maintain the floor because they have some awareness that they will not understand what others will talk about.

With regard to topic maintenance, students with language-learning diabilities may have difficulty adding new, relevant information to topic sequences. They may be passive conversationalists, relying on back-channel responses (uh huh, yeh, oh) to maintain their role in the conversation, rather than contributing new, meaningful information (Fey, 1986). Such students may also have difficulty following conversations where the topic change is fairly rapid, and, consequently, their contributions appear inappropriate. School-age students with language-learning disabilities are more likely to make more competitive and negative/rejective comments to their peers and fewer helpful and considerate comments compared to students without learning disabilities (Smiley & Bryan, 1983a; 1983b). They lack persuasiveness in peer interactions, produce unassertive messages, and ask fewer open-ended questions than their normal peers (Wiig, 1984).

Deficits in oral interactive skills will prevent students with language-learning disabilities from effectively participating in classroom discussions and group projects. Reduced or inappropriate participation can result in limiting their access to necessary information. As a consequence, they fall even further behind their peers without learning disabilities. Donahue (1994) proposed three profiles for students who exhibit deficits in oral interactive discourse. Students with a *newcomer* profile appear to have little or no awareness of the classroom social scripts. They are confused by activities and have no effective strategies for becoming involved in either social or academic activities. Although they may have been in the classroom for some time, they are very slow to pick up on the cues that signal expected behavior such as flipping the lights to be-

come quiet, raising hands to get a turn, or line leaders to go to lunch or recess.

Students with an *immigrant* profile appear to operate on a different set of rules from others in the class. Students with language-learning disabilities may exhibit an immigrant profile because they may receive many services outside the regular-education classroom. As a consequence, they may be learning different rules in another context, and they are missing experiences within the regular-education classroom. Even within the regular-education classroom, the teacher may not have the same expectations for students with learning disabilities. As a consequence, the students may be engaged differently. For example, in an effort to encourage a child's participation, the teacher may respond to a student's off-topic remark given without hand-raising. Although this may be a way to bring the student into the discussion, it can inhibit the student's learning the rules that in a discussion students are expected to raise their hands and offer information on the topic of the discussion.

Students with an *imposter* profile attempt to hide their difficulties. These students may be quite aware of the rules for interaction and classroom expectation. They believe, however, that they do not have the skill to participate effectively so they attempt to hide their difficulties. They may not participate in activities they consider difficult, or they may participate in a different way. For example, they are more likely to acquiesce to others opinions and less likely to disagree because attempting to negate a partner's opinion requires greater linguistic and negotiation skills (Donahue & Prescott, 1988).

Literate Language Disabilities
Deficits in Literate Style and Metalinguistics
Literate language is generally more decontextualized, and hence more abstract than oral interactive language. Consequently, students who have difficulty with oral interactive language will almost always have difficulty with literate lan-

guage. Students who appeared to have been "cured" of speech and/or language delays and disorders during the preschool years will frequently present with language-based academic learning disabilities during the school years (Bashir & Scavuzzo, 1992). For some students the difficulties are manifested when they must segment words into phonemes and break the phoneme-grapheme code. Children identified as dyslexic have particular difficulty breaking the phoneme-grapheme code. Success with this early stage of reading, however, is no guarantee for future success. Indeed, some children, termed hyperlexic, can "read" anything put before them, yet have no comprehension of what they read (Aram, 1997). Hyperlexia has been associated with autistic-like behaviors and hydocephalus.

By third grade the focus of literacy activities shifts from segmentation and breaking the code to comprehension. Students who continue to have poor segmentation abilities may continue to focus all their attention on breaking the print code. They may be unaware that the purpose of reading is to gain meaning, or their decoding may be so slow that they cannot integrate the content information they read (Clay, 1973; Johns & Ellis, 1976; Reid, 1966). At this point students with syntactic and semantic deficits or limited content schema and text grammar knowledges who were successful code breakers begin to exhibit academic difficulties (if they had not done so earlier). Students with poor reading comprehension have been shown to have poorer syntactic skills (Vogel, 1974; Stothard & Hulme, 1996) and less mature oral narratives than nondisabled learners (Cain, 1996). They tell shorter, less complete, less organized stories; comprehend and remember less of stories; and make fewer inferences about stories (Feagans & Short, 1984; Graybeal, 1981; Hensen, 1978; Liles, 1985, 1987; Merritt & Liles, 1987; Roth & Spekman, 1986; Weaver & Dickinson, 1979; Westby, 1984; Westby, Van Dongen, & Maggart, 1989). Students with poor semantic, syntactic, and metalin-

guistic skills have difficulty accessing the information in print. Their inability to access literate language can result in a magnification of their language disabilities as they move through school.

Numerous studies have shown that students with language-learning disabilities experience difficulty producing and understanding figurative language (Lee & Kamhi, 1985; Nippold & Fey, 1983). Delays in comprehending jokes and riddles that are popular in elementary school can increase students' difficulties in participating in peer-group communication. Students who exhibit poor reading comprehension despite good decoding skills have more difficulty explaining riddles than good readers (Yuill, 1996). There are a number of explanations for why students with language-learning disabilities exhibit difficulty with figurative language: (1) they may have less exposure to figurative language (particularly in print); (2) they may fail to monitor their comprehension, and hence they do not recognize the discrepancy between the literal meaning of an utterance and the context in which it is used; and/or (3) they may not be able to employ the inferencing skills necessary to interpret the metaphor, simile, or idiom (Milosky, 1994).

Problems With Content Schemas and Inferencing

Students with language-learning disabilities exhibit a variety of deficits with content schemas. They may have fewer and less elaborated schemas than normally developing children. Because reading is critical to content schema acquisition in school, students with reading difficulties fall farther and farther behind in acquisition of schema knowledge. Not only must students have content schemas, but they also must be able to select appropriate schemas readily and effortlessly. Students with language-learning disabilities may exhibit difficulty retrieving appropriate schemas and may not be aware of when they have selected the wrong schema. Students must know when to maintain or change content schemas as they read. As students read, they must decide whether the information they are reading supports the schema they have selected. If it does, then they continue to process the information in accordance with the selected schema. If it does not, then they need to search for another schema. For example, if students read the words "Running a Successful Race" in a title, they may retrieve a schema for an Olympic race. As they read, however, they do not encounter the information they expected about athletes; instead, they find themselves reading about politicians. They must then switch their schema from Olympic racing to political campaigns. Students with poor decoding skills may direct all their attention to the decoding process and ignore processing of content. Students with semantic and syntactic deficits may not comprehend the relationships among elements of the text necessary to determine the schema content (Pearson & Spiro, 1980).

Much information important to the content schemas is unstated in actual texts. Speakers or writers assume that listeners and readers have certain prior knowledge, and they assume that listeners and readers will be able to "read between the lines" or make the necessary inferences. Students with language-learning disabilities do less well than non-LLD students in answering both literal and inferential questions, but they experience markedly more difficulty in answering inferential questions (Oakhill & Yuill, 1996, p. 72), for example,

EXAMPLE

Linda was playing with her new doll in front of the house. Suddenly she heard a strange noise coming from under the bushes. It was the flapping of wings. Tears come to Linda's eyes because she did not know what to do. She ran inside and got a shoe box from the cupboard. Then Linda looked inside her desk until she found eight sheets of yellow paper and some scissors. When she had finished, she put the little pieces of paper in the box. Linda gently picked up the helpless creature and

took it with her. Her teacher knew what to do.

Literal questions:
What was Linda doing when she heard the strange noise?
What color was the paper?

Inference questions:
What creature was making noise?
What did Linda do with the paper before she put it in the box?

Students may have difficulty making inferences for several reasons: (1) they may not have the necessary content schema knowledge, (2) they may have difficulty accessing relevant content schema knowledge and integrating it with what is in the text because of processing limitations, (3) or they may focus on getting the literal meaning from the text and may not realize that inferences are necessary.

Metacognitive Deficits

If students exhibit language deficits in the areas discussed so far, they will likely also experience metacognitive monitoring deficits. It is possible, however, for students to have adequate skills in these other areas, yet exhibit difficulty planning their behavior and oral and written productions, monitoring their comprehension, and generating and employing strategies for learning and remembering. In general, students with language-learning disabilities show little evidence of using effective strategies to meet task demands (Schumaker & Deshler, 1984; Torgensen, 1977a, 1977b). Some students do not possess the oral language necessary for planning behavior; others have little awareness that mental acts exist; others may have the necessary language and awareness of mental acts, but cannot generate strategies to facilitate their performance; and still others may be able to generate strategies, but be uncertain of when to use them.

Current work with persons with attention-deficit-hyperactivity disorder (ADHD) implies that a primary component of ADHD is a metacognitive deficit, rather than an attentional deficit. Barkley (1990) defined ADHD as consisting of "developmental deficiencies in the regulation and maintenance of behavior by rules and consequences." These metacognitive deficiencies "give rise to problems with inhibiting, initiating, or sustaining responses to tasks or stimuli and adhering to rules or instructions, particularly in situations where consequences for such behavior are delayed, weak, or nonexistent" (p. 71). Metacognitive deficiencies affect both the social and academic behavior of students with ADHD. Although children with ADHD are more likely to talk more than normal children, especially during spontaneous conversation (Barkley, Cunningham, & Karlsson, 1983; Zentall, 1989), they do not monitor their communication, and when confronted with a task in which they must plan, organize, and generate speech in response to specific task demands, they are likely to talk less, to be more dysfluent, and to produce less cohesive and coherent language (Hamlett, Pelligrini, & Conners, 1987). They frequently demonstrate deficits in study behavior that depends on monitoring of one's knowledge (O'Neill & Douglas, 1991). Students with ADHD study for less time, expend less effort, and use strategies that adults rate as less effective.

As children progress through school they are expected to become more responsible for their own learning. They must be able to monitor their comprehension of texts and take appropriate actions when they are not comprehending by rereading, checking for additional information, or asking for assistance. They must determine the goals of assignments, gather information necessary to complete assignments, organize the information into a product, and evaluate the product. All of these steps require metacognitive processing. Students with metacognitive deficits will likely fall farther behind because they will not be acquiring the vocabulary, content schemas, and text-structure knowledge at the rate of other students.

ASSESSMENT STRATEGIES

Knowing the patterns of normal language development and the curricular requirements of the classroom provides the bases for assessing students who may exhibit language-learning disabilities. Assessment should involve both inside-out and outside-in approaches (Nelson, 1992). The assessment should consider what skills the student brings to the activities (the inside-out component) and the language requirements of the social and academic activities (the outside-in approach). This section presents some strategies for obtaining language behaviors from students that can be compared with what is known about normal development and school demands.

Assessing Language Functions and Levels of Thought

Students' use of language functions can be evaluated by collecting and analyzing language samples in several contexts using a system of analysis such as that proposed by Tough (1979). Collecting and analyzing language samples is a time-consuming activity. When time does not permit such a detailed analysis, the examiner can prepare a checklist with the major Tough categories (self-maintaining, directing, reporting, predicting, projecting, and reasoning) and code the behavior as it is observed.

Blank, Rose, and Berlin (1978) developed the *Preschool Language Assessment Instrument* to assess preschool children's abilities to comprehend and use language at several levels of abstraction. Although the test was developed for preschool children, it can often be used throughout elementary school with children who have significant language impairments. For other students, the examiner can use the framework presented by Blank and her colleagues and develop questions to assess each level using material from the students' classroom. A similar approach can be used to assess the levels of thought proposed by Bloom (1956). Table 13.8 presents questions based on Bloom's taxonomy that were

Table 13.8   Sample Questions for Curriculum-Based Assessment Using Bloom's Taxonomy

Level	Definition	Language Arts Examples	Science Examples	Social Studies Examples
Knowledge	Memorizes and repeats information presented; answers simple questions	What was the little girl's name in *Charlotte's Web?* Where did Templeton the rat live?	What kind of rock is made of mud and clay pressed together?	Where did the Alaskan oil spill occur? What company owned the boat that caused the spill?
Comprehension	Demonstrates understanding by paraphrasing or stating it in another form.	What was the story about? Tell me the story you just heard.	Explain how metamorphic rock is produced.	Describe how the Alaskan oil spill occurred.
Application	Uses information, rules, methods, or principles in new but similar situations	Charlotte and Wilbur are friends. How can friends help each other?	(After a discussion of the characteristics of granite) What could we use granite for?	What are some other ways that the wildlife could have been rescued?
Analysis	Identifies components gives reasons, identifies problems	How did Wilbur change over the course of the story?	How are limestone, shale, and sandstone alike?	What types of problems were caused by the spill?
Synthesis	Abstracts from previously learned knowledge to generate new solutions to problems	What would have happened if Templeton hadn't found words for Charlotte to weave in her web?	How would the world be different if there were no volcanoes?	What kinds of problems would occur if there were a chemical spill in our town?
Evaluation	Compares alternatives, states opinions, justifies responses	Which character do you like best in this story and why?	If you were commissioned to create a monument, what type of rock would you use and why?	Discuss who should be responsible for the cleanup and why they should be responsible?

asked about a third-grade language arts lesson and science lesson and a high school social studies lesson.

Assessing Discourse Turns and Topics

Brinton and Fujiki (1989) proposed a list of screening questions to evaluate a student with possible turn-taking and topic-manipulation problems:

1. Does the child seem hesitant to talk in interactions with peers as well as adults?

2. Does the child seem overly intimidated by other speakers? For example, does he give up turns or topics easily if interrupted?

3. Does the child often interrupt other speakers so that they are not allowed to finish sentences and messages?

4. Does the child frequently respond to questions with single-word or stereotypic utterances?

5. Does the child seem to produce a high proportion of back-channel responses in conversation with peers and an adult?

6. Does the child often change the topic in response to a question? (Do not count instances where the child may be avoiding answering, such as in response to "Who broke this?")

7. Does the child often introduce topics without properly introducing referents? Look for utterances such as "He took my pajamas again" in situations where the listener would not know who "he" is.

8. Does the child rarely contribute to topics that are introduced by others?

9. Does the child often continue with a topic even when another speaker has introduced a different topic?

10. Does the child seem to perseverate on certain topics?

11. Does the child seem to have difficulty grasping the big picture in conversation and instead focus on tangential aspects of topics?

12. Does the child seem to have difficulty making relevant contributions to interactions?

13. Does the child often seem to be one step behind the conversation? For ex-ample, does the child tend to respond to questions late or continue with topics that others have left?

14. Do other children seem to have difficulty following this child in interaction (Brinton & Fujiki, 1989, p. 121)?

15. When talking with this child, do you do an inordinate amount of work to make the interaction successful?

Damico and Oller (1985) provided a discourse screening system called *Spotting Language Problems.* The speech-language pathologist observers a student for 2 to 5 minutes in a least four different situations (e.g., playground, reading group, committee activities, etc.). Using a 1 to 5 point scale the clinician rates the child in the following areas:

1. Linguistic nonfluency: student repeats or makes unusual pauses or hesitations.

2. Revisions: student makes many false starts, interrupts himself/herself, and starts over.

3. Delays before responding: student pauses for 2 seconds or more before responding to a question or other verbal stimuli.

4. Use of nonspecific vocabulary: student uses pronouns or other terms such as *this, there, thing,* and *stuff* when the listener has no way of knowing what the child is referring to.

5. Inappropriate responses: the student's utterances do not seem to follow naturally what has been said or asked previously by someone else.

6. Poor topic maintenance: Student changes topics so suddenly that the listener is apt to get lost.

7. Need for repetition: repetition is often required before the child will understand a question or comment that is not apparently difficult.

A student who performs poorly on these screening assessments should receive a more comprehensive evaluation. Interviewing students can provide a means of differentiating students who reflect the newcomer, immigrant, and imposter profiles. Students can be asked questions that explore their knowledge of the classroom scripts (Morine-Dershimer, 1985), for example:

EXAMPLE
When the teacher wants us to be quiet, she _____.
When we finish our work, the teacher says _____.
When I want to ask the teacher something, I _____.
If I know the answer to a question, I _____.
If I don't know the answer to a question, I _____.
If I need help, I _____.
When I finish my work, I can _____.

The evaluator needs to determine if students know the classroom scripts but choose to select their own strategies for participating (imposter profile); have some awareness of school scripts but have different experiences or expectations of them (immigrant profile); or are unaware of classroom scripts and how to respond to them (newcomer profile).

Assessing Metalinguistic Skills for Emergent Literacy

Children from mainstream backgrounds enter school with some knowledge of literacy. Even though they may not be reading and writing, they know something about the conventions of reading and writing. Preliteracy skills can be assessed both informally and formally.

van Kleeck (1984) proposed informal interview questions that could be used to assess students' word referent awareness:

1. *Interview questions:*
    a. Tell me a long word. Why is it long?
    b. Tell be a short word. Why is it short?
    c. Tell me a difficult word. Why is it difficult?
    d. Tell me an easy word. Why is it easy?
    e. I'm going to say some sentences and I want you to tell me how many words are in each. (1) The cat climbed the tree. How many words? What are they? (2) Six

children are playing. How many words? What are they?
2. *Word identification:* I'm going to say some things and I want you to tell me whether or not they are words. If the child says no, ask why.

house	bink	a
cat	the	my
mup	boy	ptib
and		

3. *Word length versus referent length:* I'm going to say some words and I want you to tell me if they are long words or short words. Then I want you to tell me why.

crocodile (long word; long referent)
spaghetti (long word; long referent)
train (short word; long referent)
fly (short word, small referent)
banana (long word; long referent)
hose (short word; long referent)
toe (short word; small referent)

Several formal, published tests are available for assessing metaphonologic awareness. The *Test of Awareness of Language Segments* (Sawyer, 1987) provides a means of assessing some metalinguistic skills that underlie the ability to break the phoneme-grapheme code necessary for spelling. Children listen to short sentences and are asked to use blocks to represent the words in the sentence. Then they are asked to indicate the number of words in sentences, the number of syllables in words, and finally the number of phonemes in words. The *Test of Phonological Awareness* (Torgesen & Bryant, 19941) has students mark pictures that begin or end with similar sounds. The *Lindamood Auditory Conceptualization Test* (Lindamood & Lindamood, 1979) requires more refined discrimination, segmentation, and sequential auditory skills. Again using blocks, the child indicates the number of phonemes in nonsense syllables and then the number of phonemes in nonsense words and then must reorder the sequence of phonemes.

Several formal tests are available that assess children's familiarity with print. The *Test of Early Reading Ability-2 (TERA)* (Reid, Hresko, & Hammill, 1981) evaluates a child's skills in (1) finding meaning in print by identifying environmental print such as store logos and identification of words in context, (2) reciting the alphabet and recognizing letters, words, and sentences, (3) knowledge of print conventions such as identification of the top and bottom of a book and the progression of print on a page. Using the *Concepts about Print Test* (Clay, 1979), an adult shares a book with a child and asks questions about parts of a book, what is read (print not pictures), progression of print on a page, orientation of print on a page, and identification of a letter, a word, punctuation marks, and capital and lower-case letters.

Assessing Syntactic Development

Most formal, published tests of syntactic development have ceilings around 8 years of age. Analysis of students' oral and written narrative and expository texts probably provides the best ways of assessing the syntactic development of school-age students. T-unit analysis is sometimes used as a measure of syntactic development during the school years. A T-unit is a minimal terminal unit that consists of an independent clause and any development clauses that are attached to it (Hunt, 1975). Although mean T-unit length tends to increase during the school years, the overlap from grade to grade is too great to use mean t-unit length as a clear measure of syntactic delay. It is, however, helpful to note the ratio of dependent to independent clauses, the variety of dependent clauses, and the variety of connectives that are used. The following are types of dependent clauses:

EXAMPLE
Adverbial: *While the boy was sleeping,* the frog climbed out of the jar.

Adjective (relative): The woman *who was eating the salad* found a frog in her food.

Noun: The little frog didn't understand why *the big frog wanted to get rid of him.*

Independent clauses are connected by words such as:

EXAMPLE

and	however
but	meanwhile
besides	or
instead	then
therefore	

Dependent clauses are connected by words such as:

EXAMPLE

after	though
although	till
as	until
as if	unless
as long as	when
as though	whenever
because	whereas
before	while
even if	if
even though	if only
since	in order that
so that	

or Relative Pronouns such as

who	what
that	whatever

By late elementary school, students should be using a variety of dependent clauses and connectives.

Students may have the competence to use a variety of connective and dependent clauses, but fail to do so spontaneously. Sentence-combining activities can provide a mechanism for evaluating students' abilities to produce more complex sentences (Strong, 1986). Students are given several related sentences and asked to combine them into a single sentence, for example:

EXAMPLE
Jerod was working hard on his test.
Michelle slipped him a note.
Jerod unfolded the paper carefully.
He didn't want his teacher to see.

Possible response: Jerod was hard at work on his test when Michelle slipped him a note, which he carefully unfolded because he didn't want his teacher to see.

The *Test of Written Language 3* (Hammill & Larsen, 1996) for students from second through twelfth grade contains a sentence-combining subtest.

Assessing Content Schemas

Children's knowledge of narrative content can easily be assessed by asking them to relate the story in wordless picture books. Many of the books by Mercer Mayer (e.g., *One Frog Too Many; A Boy, a Dog, and a Frog; Frog Goes to Dinner; A Boy, a Dog, a Frog, and a Friend*) are particularly useful for this purpose because they include all the elements of complete or complex episodes. For evaluation, select wordless picture books with content that should be familiar to the children based on what is known of their cultural background. The goal is to understand what the students understand about relationships (temporal, physical, and cause-effect) between people, objects, and events in the world, that is, to evaluate a student's ability to interpret the literal action in a picture, to make judgement's about physical and psychologic causality, to make judgements about a character's internal thoughts and feelings and external behavior (e.g., is there a disjunction—is the character being deceitful), and to logically reason from present to future situations using information about physical causality and attributes or traits of the characters that affect their motivational, intentional, and psychological behavior. The student is told, "Tell me the story that happened in this book. Make it the best story you can." If the student is hesitant to respond or has difficulty organizing extended verbal responses, the examiner can ask questions that focus on the relationships. The questions fall into four categories (Tough, 1979):

1. *Reporting:* What was the boy doing here? What happened here? Tell me about this picture.

2. *Projective:* What is the boy saying to the big frog? What is the frog thinking? How does the boy feel?

3. *Reasoning:* Why is the frog thinking that? Why does the boy feel angry? Why did the big frog bite the little frog? Why did the tree fall down?

4. *Predicting:* What will happen next? What will the big frog do now?

If the student responds to these questions or is able to tell the story without assistance, ask yourself the following questions:

1. Does the student simply label/describe pictures or does he/she interpret pictures; that is, does the child use information in the pictures to generate schemas that go beyond the details of the pictures. For example, if a picture shows a boy carrying a pole, a bucket, and a net, does the student simply say, *"The boy has a pole, and a bucket, and a net"* or does he infer, *"The boy's going fishing."* If a picture shows a boy holding a sword and wearing a three-cornered hat, does the child say, *"The boy's got a hat on and he's got a sword,"* or does he say, *"The boy's playing pirate."*

2. Does the child indicate awareness of temporal relationships in stories? Does the child use temporal markers or conjunctions that indicate time relationships, for example, *just, already, always, before, after, while, then, when, now, as soon as?*

3. Does the child recognize emotional feelings of the characters? What words does he/she use to describe the feelings?

4. Does the child explain relationships between characters' emotions and events in the story by using words such as *because, so, therefore?*

5. Does the child recognize the theme or reason for the characters' goal-directed behaviors? Does the child explicitly state the story theme?

The teacher or speech-language pathologist can also assess students' content knowledge by engaging them in semantic webbing activities on a topic or theme. Words or themes can be selected from the students' textbooks. The teacher writes the word or theme on the chalkboard and asks students to generate ideas related to the word or theme. As the students give suggestions, the teacher requests information regarding the relationships among the words and ideas they suggest. Students' contributions of reasonably related concepts to a semantic web are a measure of their semantic skills, particularly those required by expository texts. Children who are able to develop extensive webs on a topic are more likely to be able to follow a topic of conversation or theme in a text.

The Prereading Plan (PreP) (Langer, 1981) is another method for determining the content knowledge a student possesses on a topic and how that knowledge is organized. It enables the teacher or speech-language pathologist to know the language the students use to express the knowledge they have about the topic and what additional background information the adult will need to teach on a particular topic. There are three steps to the procedure:

Teacher	Students
1. Tell me everything you think of when you hear . . .	Students access prior knowledge and free associate, saying anything they think of related to the topic
2. What made you think of . . .	Students reflect on their thought processes and organization of knowledge—they explain why they said what they did
3. Do you want to add to or change your first responses	Students reformulate and refine their comments

The nature of students' responses gives insight into their levels of knowledge:

Much Knowledge	Some Knowledge	Little Knowledge
1. Superordinate concept—higher-class category	1. Examples—appropriate class, but more specific	1. Associations—tangential cognitive links
2. Definitions—precise meaning	2. Attributes—subordinate to larger concept	2. Morphemes—smallest units of meaning
3. Analogies—substitution of comparison for literal concept	3. Defining characteristics—defines a major aspect of the concept	3. Sound alikes—similar phonemic units
		4. First-hand experiences—tangential responses based on experience
		5. No apparent knowledge

Assessing Text Grammars

Children's narrative text grammars can be evaluated by asking students to produce a story without a stimulus or from stimuli with minimal structure such as a poster picture or a set of dolls or action figures. The students' stories can then be analyzed like the child's story discussed earlier; or analysis of narrative level can be done more quickly by using the binary decision tree in Figure 13.5. To use this decision tree, read through a student's story, then ask the following questions:

1. "Does the story have a temporally related sequence of events?" If it does not, then the story is an isolated description.

2. If the story does have a temporally related sequence of events, then ask, "Does the story have a causally related sequence of events?" If it has a temporally related sequence of events, but does not have a causally related sequence of events, then the story is an action sequence.

3. If the story does have a causally related sequence of events, then ask, "Does the story imply goal-directed behavior?" If the story has a causally related sequence of events, but does not imply goal-directed behavior, then the story is a reactive sequence.

4. If the story does imply goal-directed behavior then ask, "Is planning or intentional behavior made explicit?" If the story implies goal-directed behavior, but does not make the planning of this behavior explicit, then the story is a goal-directed episode.

5. If the story does make the planning or intentional behavior explicit, then ask, "Is the story elaborated by having multiple attempts or consequences, multiple episodes, or embedded episodes, or is the story told from the point of view of more than one character?" If the story does make intentional behavior explicit, but is not elaborated, then the story is a complete episode.

6. If the story is elaborated, how is it elaborated? Is one aspect of the story elaborated? For example, is there an obstacle in the attempt path and multiple attempts. Does the story have multiple episodes—are they sequential or embedded? Is the story told from the perspective of more than one character?

A variety of expository text structures can be elicited with the following activities:

1. *Sequential-procedural:* "Tell me how to make. . . . (something familiar, e.g., lemonade, peanut butter sandwich)

2. *Cause-effect:* "Tell me what would happen if. . . . (children didn't have to go to school, children could go to bed whenever they wanted to, there were no required classes and students could choose only the classes they want to take, et cetera).

3. *Problem-solution:* The landfill is nearly full, and the city does not know what to do. What can the city do about all the trash and garbage that people are throwing away?

4. *Persuasion:* "You have chores to do, but you don't want to do them. How would you convince your parents to get out of doing chores."

At this time there is no agreed on developmental hierarchy for expository texts. For written informative and persuasive texts, the NAEP scoring hierarchy can be used to determine a developmental level. One can also compare the child's expository productions with the expository tasks required in the classroom.

Assessing Metacognitive Strategies

If students are to use metacognitive monitoring and study strategies, they must be aware that mental acts exist. Wellman (1985) proposed some simple tasks to assess children's understanding of *know, remember, forget,* and *guess:*

Task 1: Knowing-remembering condition. Children see an item hidden in one of two containers. Then after a brief delay, the children are asked to find the item. At that point, they are asked, "Did you know where the item was? Did you guess where the item was? Did you remember where the item was?"

Task 2: Guessing condition: Children do not see where the item is hidden and cannot know where it is, but must make a choice between two containers. They are asked, "Did you know where the item was? Did you guess? Did your remember where the item was? Did you forget where it was? Why do you say you guessed?"

Task 3: Forgetting condition. Children watch a toy character who sees his coat put in one of two closets, and they are asked, "Does he know here his coat is? Why do you say he knows?" Later the character comes back looking for his coat and looks in the wrong closet. The children are asked, "Did he know where his coat was? Did he remember? Did he forget? Why do you say he forgot?

The ability to use metacognitive strategies becomes critical for success in junior high school. Interviewing junior and senior high school students can provide insight into their metacognitive awareness of the reading comprehension process. The

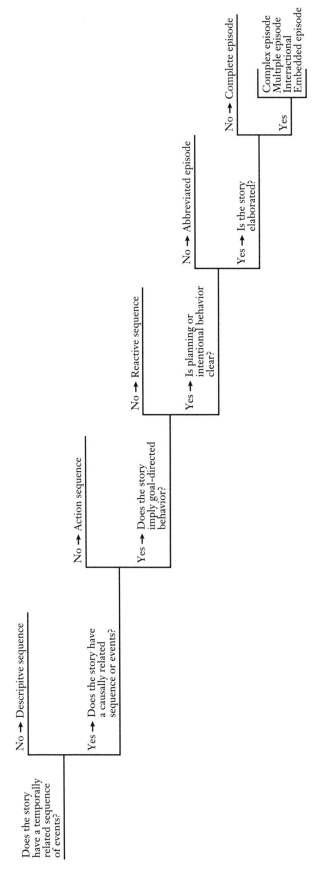

Figure 13.5. Binary decision tree for story grammar structure. (Modified from Stein N, Policastro M. The concept of story: a comparison between children's and teacher's viewpoints. In: Mandl H, Stein N, Trabasso T, eds. Learning and comprehension of text. Hillsdale, NJ: Erlbaum, 1984.)

following questions are useful (Wixson, Boskey, Yochum, & Alverman, 1984):

1. What is the most important reason for reading this kind of material? Why does your teacher want you to read this book?

2. How good are you at reading this kind of material? How do you know?

3. What do you have to do to get a good grade in _____?

4. If the teacher told you to remember the information in this chapter, what would be the best way to do this? Have you ever tried_____?

5. If your teacher told you to find the answers to questions in this book, what would be the best way to do this? Why? Have you ever tried_____?

6. What is the hardest part about answering questions like the ones in this book? Does that make you do anything differently?

Determination of school-age students' language-learning needs for social and academic success requires assessment of their oral interactive language abilities; the language functions and genres they effectively use; the style, structure, and complexity of their language patterns; their content knowledge, metalinguistic skills, and metacognitive awareness and strategies. With this information, one can plan an intervention program.

INTERVENTION STRATEGIES

Components of Literacy Learning

Language and literacy learning in academic settings have several components (Lee & Fradd, 1997) (Table 13.9). Intervention strategies must assure that students *know* the necessary academic vocabulary and content knowledge for the curriculum. They must have the social knowledge and skills necessary to *do* the curriculum; that is, they must be able to participate in reading groups, class discussions, science projects, and other class activities. Just having the vocabulary, content schema knowledge, and social skills is not, however, sufficient for critical literacy. Students must also be able to *talk* in liter-

ate ways; they must know the academic genre styles—the types of sentence structures and text organizations that are used to convey information. In addition, to be successful with critical literacy, they must be able to carry out oral and written discourse at multiple levels of abstraction. They must be able to use literate discourse for thinking and problem solving. Intervention strategies must facilitate students' knowing, doing, and talking. Speech-language pathologists and educators must recognize that students' knowing, doing, and talking are affected by their attitudes about their own abilities and about school and by their cultural experiences with how things are done in school.

Paradigms for Intervention

The ways we teach knowing, doing, and talking have been changing. The field of speech-language pathology is experiencing a series of paradigm shifts. A paradigm represents a model or framework with which we approach a task. These paradigm shifts are changing the ways in which language intervention programs are provided. We are moving as follows:

1. *From a model of quantitative methodology to a model of qualitative methodology.* Rather than focusing only on what children are doing and how much they are doing it, we are focusing on the quality of their performance. Thus we consider not only the words, sentence structures, and language functions children can produce, but also how effectively they use all these aspects of language in communicative interactions.

2. *From a discrete-point, decontextualized testing and treatment model to an integrative, descriptive, naturalistic assessment and treatment model.* Although we continue to use standardized tests that rely on assessment of discrete components of language (testing vocabulary, syntax, morphology), we realize that information gained from these sources may tell us very little about what a child actually does and that being able to perform an activity in the shelter of a therapy room does not guarantee the ability to perform

Table 13.9 *Components of Academic Literacy*

Knowing (vocabulary and knowledge)

- Building on prior knowledge
- Using appropriate vocabulary
- Understanding concepts and relationships in content schemas

Doing (inquiry and process)

- Engaging in inquiry
- Using relevant strategies

Talking (discourse and communication)

- Participating in extended social and academic discourse
- Appropriating the academic discourse style
- Using multiple representational formats and multiple levels of abstraction

Attitudes and values

- Manifesting generic values and attitudes
- Appropriating culturally mediated values and attitudes

World view

- Recognizing ways of knowing

the activity in other contexts. Hence, the child is evaluated in a variety of natural contexts, and intervention is provided within these contexts.

3. *From a client-centered model to a social-systems model of intervention. In the past we have located all of the disability within the client.* Now we are considering the interaction of the client with the environment and how the environment inhibits or facilitates a student's performance. The student may not be the only individual who must change. In some instances the student's difficulties may lie in the school curriculum, the texts that are used, or the interaction patterns of the classroom—not in the student. In such instances changes are made in the curriculum, rather than to the student.

4. *From a model that focused only on spoken words and sentences to a model that includes literacy and thought.* The role of the speech-language pathologist has often been assumed to be limited to oral speech and language. We are now aware that the content of the academic curriculum is language, whether it is oral or written. Literacy is now seen as a natural extension of language development. Speech-language pathologists have as much a role in facilitating reading and writing as they do in facilitating oral language.

5. *From a model that implied that working with individuals in one-on-one situations was the ideal service to a model that maintains that for some students and some language needs working within the classroom is the ideal.* In the past speech-language pathologists used primarily an "expert" model. The speech-language pathologist was the one who possessed all the knowledge and skills necessary to treat the language-impaired student. Children were withdrawn from classrooms, "treated" for speech and language problems, and sent back to the classroom. More and more, however, speech-language pathologists and classroom teachers are using the "collaborative consultation" model in which professionals work together to understand the needs of the child and to develop intervention strategies, many of which are carried out within the classroom.

6. *From an exclusive, skill-based model to a skill-based plus strategy-based model.* For a long time we believed that if children had the necessary skills, they would use them. Attention to skill development alone is not sufficient for students with language-learning disabilities. They must also develop the strategies to know when and how to use their skills. Hence, increasing attention is being given to teaching learning strategies.

7. *From a model of normality-based language development in white, mainstream children to a model of normality that recognizes the cultural variations in language development.* Most of the data available on language development are based on language development in children from white, middle-class homes. The demographics of the nation are changing. Soon one-third of the nation will be from traditional minority groups. In many cities and in some states, these minorities are already in the majority. Consequently, we must broaden our base of understanding language development. We must understand that not all children develop language in the same ways, and we must understand how variations in language development impact on students' school performance.

These paradigm shifts in speech-language pathology reflect the shifts that have been occurring in regular and special education. In the last 10 years educational philosophy has shifted from what has been termed the behavioral or reductionistic paradigm to the holistic/constructivist paradigm (Poplin, 1988a, 1988b). The reductionist paradigm breaks ideas, concepts, and skills into smaller units and relies on direct teaching of the skills. The holistic paradigm maintains that students construct knowledge through naturalistic experiences and that they do not require explicit teaching of skills. Goodman (1986), a major advocate for the holistic paradigm, proposed that language is easy to learn when:

It's real and natural.
It's whole.
It's sensible.
It's interesting.
It's relevant.
It belongs to the learner.
It's part of a real event.
It has social utility.
It has purpose for the learner.
The learner chooses to learn it.
It's accessible to the learner.
The learner has power to use it.

This holistic paradigm has been widely adopted in schools in the whole language approach to reading and the process approach to writing in which children learn to read by reading and learn to write by writing. With the rise of holistic/constructivist teaching approaches, reductionistic approaches have fallen into disrepute. It has become unfashionable to directly teach phonologic awareness, sentence structures, writing conventions, and so forth.

Intervention Procedures

One cannot argue with many of the tenets of the holistic/constructivist paradigm. Language is indeed more than the sum of its parts. Just knowing vocabulary, concepts, sentence patterns, and sound-symbol relationships does not ensure that a child can use this knowledge in extended oral and written activities. The meaning of discourses does not lie only in the discourse. The meaning must be constructed by integrating prior knowledge (or content schema knowledge) with information in the discourse. Furthermore, children do require meaningful, enjoyable experiences if they are to learn how to use language and want to use language.

One cannot, however, assume that simply providing students with language-learning disabilities with meaningful language experiences will result in their acquiring the necessary communication abilities and strategies. If this were the case, they would not be language-learning disabled. Students with language-learning disabilities can benefit from whole language approaches that expose them to quality children's literature and provide them with authentic opportunities to write. Many of these students, however, will require additional explicit instruction in aspects of language. The *genre movement* in Australia has recommended explicitly teaching students the rules of the literacy game within the context of authentic reading and writing activities (Cope & Kalantzis, 1993). Students are given opportunities to write authentic narrative, persuasive, informative, descriptive, explanatory, and procedural texts. Teachers, however, model the texts, teach the types of sentence structures and text organization needed for each type of text, provide opportunities for students to jointly construct texts, and support students in writing their own texts.

To optimize a student's benefiting from naturalistic language contexts, one must know the students' current language abilities, present activities that are within the students' zone of proximal development, and assist students in mastering the material by providing supportive scaffolding. In conversational activities adults model appropriate language functions, requests for clarification, conversational repairs, literate language style, and metacognitive monitoring. Students practice these aspects of language while working on group projects. Throughout all school activities—art, science, social studies, language arts, math, and gym—adults are alert to the language functions and levels of language abstraction that students are using, and they make statements and ask questions to assist students in using more diverse functions and higher levels of thought. When necessary, adults should also explicitly teach the information necessary to complete activities successfully.

Students with language-learning disabilities frequently require explicit teaching in phonological awareness to learn to break the print code (Adams, 1990). They benefit from activities such as the *say-it-and-move-it* segmentation activity in which they move a disk from the top half to the bottom half of a sheet to represent sounds in one-, two-, and three-phoneme words; sound categorization activities involving grouping words on the basis of shared beginning or ending sounds; and matching letter names to phonemes (Blachman, 1994).

Well-structured, interesting narrative and expository texts are used for reading. Ideally, the texts are selected according to the students' narrative and expository abilities. Adults read to students, as well as have students read to them. Before reading activities, adults prepare students for the content material that will be presented by hypothesizing what the story may be about based on the title and cover picture (making inferences) or by discussing what the students know about the topic (their content schema). During or following reading, adults assist students in recall by using scaffolding questions based on the content/structure of the texts. For complete episode narrative texts, such scaffolding questions might include the following:

EXAMPLE
What was the problem in the story? or What did _____ want? (goal)
    Why did _____ do? (initiating event or internal response)
    What did _____ think/feel to cause _____? (internal response)
    What did _____ want to do then? (plan)
    How did the story end? (consequence)
    How did _____ feel in the end? (reaction)

As students develop the ability to talk about texts, adults can reduce the scaffolding support.

From the beginning of school, students and adults write. They write meaningful messages or notes to each other, then personal stories, and then fictional stories and expository texts. Initially, the focus is on communicating a message, and the use of invented spelling is permitted and encouraged. As students deal with writing and reading for meaning, the necessary metalinguistic skills are discussed—what are words, how do you "sound out" words, what letters go with what sounds, and how and why do you use punctuation. Use of particular syntactic structures can be facilitated by choosing stories or other texts that emphasize particular structures. Adults can also provide supportive scaffolds to facilitate the style of literate discourse by revoicing students' statements (O'Connor & Michaels, 1996). By revoicing a student's contribution, the adult adds material, deletes material, or uses different lexicalizations to teach, clarify, highlight, or reframe aspects of the student's utterance in relation to the desired academic content. For example, if in retelling a story a student says:

EXAMPLE

Max was riding his bike. He hit a snail. The snail's shell broke. The snail cried. Max gave the snail a nut. The snail still cried.

The adult may respond,

EXAMPLE

So, what you're saying is that while Max was riding his bike he hit a snail and broke it's shell. Max tried to help the snail by giving him a nut for a shell, but the snail didn't like it.

The adult takes what the student has said, gives the student credit for his or her ideas, and then revoices the ideas into a more literate discourse style. Revoicing socializes students into particular intellectual and speaking practices by placing them in the roles entailed by the speech activity or the group discussion.

As students are able to produce extended texts, adults can also explicitly discuss the structure of different types of texts and have students identify parts of texts such as the setting, initiating event, plan, attempts, consequence, and resolution of a narrative, or the topic sentences and supporting statements for an informational text.

Throughout all activities, adults should be modeling metacognitive strategies. They should talk aloud (eventcast) as they carry out activities. As they do so,

they not only let students hear a variety of language functions and structures, but they also let children hear how the task is to be accomplished, how the adult plans to approach the task, how he or she monitors performance, and what is done about success or lack of success. For example:

1. *Problem definition:* "What do I have to do? Let's see. . . ."
2. *Focusing attention and directing:* "Find step one . . . now find the piece shown in the picture. . . ."
3. *Self-reinforcement:* "Good, I found that piece."
4. *Self-evaluating coping skills and error correcting options:* "This is the wrong piece. I need to look more carefully." (Meichenbaum, 1977).

A similar strategy can be used during reading. The adult asks the students to read along silently and the adult reads the passage aloud and notes how he or she is thinking through the trouble spots. Davey (1983) suggests a number of points that can be made during this comprehension monitoring:

1. *Making predictions:* "From the title I think this will be about. . . ."
2. *Describing the pictures you are forming in your head about the information:* "I have a picture of this scene in my head, and this is what it looks like. . . ."
3. *Developing analogies:* Show how to link prior knowledge with new information in the text. "This reminds me of. . . ."
4. *Identifying confusing points:* Show how you monitor comprehension. "This doesn't make sense."
5. *Demonstrating fix-up strategies:* Show how you make sense of the passage. "I'd better reread this." "I'll read ahead and see if I can get some more information."

Language, both oral and written, can only be acquired by hearing and using language in meaningful, authentic contexts. For many students with language-learning disabilities, this authentic use of language must be supplemented with direct, explicit teaching about the elements of language—phonology, semantics, syntax, pragmatics, and discourse structure.

Direct teaching, however, should not be limited to isolated drills, but rather should be linked to meaningful activities. Language learning does not end at age 5, nor does it end in adolescence. Language learning is a lifelong process.

REFERENCES

Adams MJ. Beginning to read: thinking and learning and print. Cambridge, MA: MIT Press, 1990.

American Psychiatric Association. Diagnostic and statistical manual of mental disorders. 4th ed. Washington, DC:American Psychiatric Association 1993.

Anderson RC, Pearson PD. A schema-theoretic view of basic processes in reading. In: Pearson PD, ed. Handbook of reading research. New York: Longman, 1984; pp. 255–291.

Appel LF, Cooper RG, McCarrell N, et al. The development of the distinction between perceiving and memorizing. Child Dev 1972;43:1365–1381.

Aram D. Hyperlexia: reading without meaning in young children. Top Lang Disord 1997;17(3): 1–13.

Bake L, Brown AL. Metacognitive skills and reading. In: Pearson PD, ed. Handbook of Reading Research. New York: Longman, 1984; pp. 353–394.

Barkley RA. Attention deficit and hyperactivity disorder: a handbook for diagnosis and treatment. New York: Guilford Press, 1990.

Barkley RA, Cunningham CE, Karlsson J. The speech of hyperactive children and their mothers: comparisons with normal children and stimulant drug effects. J Learn Disabil 1983;16:105–110.

Bashir A, Scavuzzo A. Children with language disorders: natural history and academic success. J Learn Disabil 1992;25(1)53–65.

Bedrosian JL. Adults who are mildly to moderately mentally retarded: communicative performance, assessment and intervention. In: Calculator SN, Bedrosian JL, eds. Communication assessment and intervention for adults with mental retardation. San Diego: College-Hill, 1988; pp. 265–07.

Bishop DVM, Edmundson A. Language-impaired 4-year-olds: distinguishing transient from persistent impairment. J Speech Hear Disord 1987;52: 156–173.

Blachman BA. Early literacy acquisition. In: Wallach G, Butler K, eds. Language learning disabilities in school-age children and adolescents. New York: Macmillan, 1994; pp. 253–274.

Black J. An exposition on understanding expository text. In: Britton B, Black J, eds. Understanding expository text. Hillsdale, NJ: Erlbaum, 1985.

Blank M, Rose SA, Berlin LJ. The language of learning: the preschool years. New York: Grune & Stratton, 1978.

Bloom N. Taxonomy of educational objectives:

handbook 1, cognitive domain. New York: Longman, 1956.

Brinton B, Fujiki M. Development of topic manipulation skills in discourse. J Speech Hear Disord 1984;27:350–358.

Britton B, Fujiki M. Conversational management with language-impaired children. Rockville, MD: Aspen, 1989.

Britton B, Fujiki M, Loeb DF, Winkler E. Development of conversational repair strategies in response to requests for clarification. J Speech Hear Res 1986;29:75–81.

Brown AL. Metacognition: the development of selective attention strategies for learning from texts. In: Kamil ML, ed. Directions in reading: research and instruction. Washington, DC: National Reading Conference, 1981; pp. 21–43.

Brown AL, Smiley S. The development of strategies for studying texts. Child Dev 1978;49:1076–1088.

Burkhalter N. A Vygotski-based curriculum for teaching persuasive writing in the elementary grades. Lang Arts 1995;72:192–199.

Cain, K. Story knowledge and comprehension skill. In: Cornoldi C, Oakhill J, eds. Reading comprehension difficulties: processes and intervention. Mahwah, NJ: Erlbaum, 1996; pp. 167–192.

Calfee R. Critical literacy: reading and writing for a new millennium. In: Ellsworth NJ, Hedley CN, Baratta AN, eds. Literacy: a redefinition. Hillsdale, NJ: Erlbaum, 1994; pp. 19–38.

Case R. Intellectual development: birth to adulthood. New York: Academic Press, 1985.

Chapman J. Reading development and cohesion. Portsmouth, NH: Heineman, 1983.

Clay M. Reading: the patterning of complex behavior. Portsmouth, NH: Heinemann, 1973.

Clay M. Sand or stones. Portsmouth, NH: Heinemann, 1979.

Clay M. The early detection of reading difficulties. 3rd ed. Portsmouth, NH: Heinemann, 1985.

Cope B, Kalantzis M, eds. The power of literacy: a genre approach to teaching writing. Pittsburgh: University of Pittsburgh Press, 1993.

Damico J, Oller J. Spotting language problems. San Diego: Los Amigoes Research Associates, 1985.

Davey B. Think aloud: modeling the cognitive process of reading comprehension. J Read 1983;37: 104–112.

Dollaghan C, Miller J. Observational methods in the study of communicative competence. In: Schiefelbusch RL, ed. Language competence: assessment and intervention. San Diego: College-Hill, 1986; pp. 99–129.

Donahue M. Differences in classroom discourse styles and students with learning disabilities. In: Ripich DN, Creaghead NA, eds. School discourse problems. 2nd ed. San Diego: Singular, 1994; pp. 229–261.

Donahue M, Pearl R, Bryan T. Communicative competence in learning disabled children. In: Bialer H, Gadow K, eds. Advances in learning and behavioral disabilities. Vol. 2. Greenwich, CT: JAI Press, 1983.

Donahue M, Prescott B. Reading disabled children's conversational participation in dispute episodes with peers. First Lang 1988;8247–258.

Douglas JD, Peel B. The development of metaphor and proverb translation in children grades one through seven. J Educ Res 1979;73:116–119.

Duell OK. Metacognitive skills. In: Phye GD, Andre T, eds. Cognitive classroom learning: understanding, thinking, and problem solving. Orlando: Academic Press, 1986.

Ehri L. Linguistic insight: threshold of reading acquisition. In: Walker T, Mackinnon G, eds. Reading research: advances in research and theory. New York: Academic Press, 1979; pp. 63–114.

Ellsworth NJ. Critical thinking and literacy. In: Ellsworth NJ, Hedley CN, Baratta AN, eds. Literacy: a redefinition. Hillsdale, NJ: Erlbaum, 1994; pp. 91–108.

Evans M, Taylor N, Blum I. Children's written language awareness and its relation to reading acquisition. J Read Behav 1979;11:7–19.

Feagans L, Applebaum MI. Validation of language subtypes in learning disabled children. J Educ Psychol 1986;78:358–364.

Feagans L, Short E. Developmental differences in comprehension and production of narratives by reading disabled and normally achieving children. Child Dev 1984;55:1727–1736.

Fey M. Language Intervention with Young Children. San Diego: College-Hill, 1986.

Fey M, Leonard L. Pragmatic skills of children with specific language impairment. In: Gallagher TM, Prutting CA, eds. Pragmatic assessment and intervention issues in language. San Diego: College-Hill, 1983; pp. 65–82.

Fitzgerald J. Research on stories: implications for teachers. In: Muth KD, ed. Children's Comprehension of Text. Newark, DE: International Reading Association, 1989.

French L, Nelson K. Young children's knowledge of relational terms. New York: Springer-Verlag, 1985.

Fujiki M, Brinton B, Todd CM. Social skills of children with specific language impairment. Lang Speech Hear Serv Sch 1996;27:195–201.

Gallagher TM. Language skill and the development of social competence in school-age children. Lang Speech Hear Serv Sch 1993;24:199–205.

Geller E. The assessment of perspective-taking skills. Semin Speech Lang 1989;10:28–41.

Goodman K. What's whole in whole language. Portsmouth, NH: Heinemann, 1986.

Goswami U, Bryant PE. Phonologic skills and learning to read. Hillsdale, NJ: Erlbaum, 1990.

Grabe W. Contrastive rhetoric and text-type research. In: Connor U, Kaplan R, eds. Writing across cultures: analysis of L2 text. Reading, MA: Addison-Wesley, 1987.

Graybeal C. Memory for stories in language impaired children. Appl Psycholinguist 1981;2:269–283.

Graesser AC, Goodman SM. Implicit knowledge, questions answering, and the representation of expository text. In: Britton BK, Black JB, eds. Understanding expository text. Hillsdale, NJ: Erlbaum, 1985.

Hakes D. The development of metalinguistic abilities in children. New York: Springer-Verlag, 1980.

Hakes D. The development of metalinguistic abilities: what develops? In: Kuczaj S, ed. Language development: language, thought, and culture. Vol. 2. Hilldsale, NJ: Erlbaum, 1982.

Hamlett KW, Pelligrini DS, Conners CK. An investigation of executive processes in the problem-solving of attention deficit disorder-hyperactive children. J Pediatr Psychol 1987;12:227–240.

Hammill DD, Larsen SC. Test of written language. 3rd Ed. Austin, TX: Pro-ed, 1996.

Hansen C. Story retelling used with average and learning disabled readers as a measure of reading comprehension. Learn Disabil Q 1978;1:62–69.

Heath SB. Talking a cross-cultural look at narratives. Top Lang Disord 1986a;7:1:84–94.

Heath SB. Sociocultural contexts of language development. In: Beyond language. Los Angeles: Evaluation Dissemination and Assessment Center, 1986b.

Horowitz R. Rhetorical structure in discourse processing. In: Horowitz R, Samuels SJ, ed. Comprehending oral and written language. New York: Academic Press, 1987.

Hsu FLK. Americans and Chinese: passage to differences. Honolulu: University of Hawaii Press, 1981.

Hunt K. Grammatical structures written at three grade levels. Champaign, IL: NCTE Research Report 3, 1975.

Irwin JW. Understanding and teaching cohesion comprehension. Newark, DE: International Reading Association, 1986.

Jenkins J. Four points to remember: a tetrahedral model and memory experiments. In: Cermak LS, Craik FIK, eds. Levels and processing in human memory. Hillsdale, NJ: Erlbaum, 1979.

Johns J, Ellis D. Reading: children tell it like it is. Read World 1976;16:2:115–128.

Kail R, Hagen JW. Memory in childhood. In: Wolman BB, ed. Handbook of developmental psychology. Englewood Cliffs, NJ: Prentice-Hall, 1982; pp. 350–366.

Kamhi AG. Metalinguistic abilities in language-impaired children. Top Lang Disord 1987;7:2:1–12.

Kieras DE. Thematic processes in the comprehension of expository prose. In: Britton BK, Black JB, eds. Understanding expository text. Hillsdale, NJ: Erlbaum, 1985.

Kreutzer MA, Leonard C, Flavell HH. An interview study of children's knowledge about memory. Monogr Soc Res Child Dev 1975;40.

Langer J. From theory to practice: a prereading play. J Read 1981;25:152–156.

Lee O, Fradd SH. Science for all: including students from non-English language backgrounds. Paper presented at the American Educational Research Association Convention, Chicago, IL, 1997.

Lee R, Kamhi A. Verbal metaphor performance in learning disabled children. Paper presented at the meeting of the American Speech-Language-Hearing Association, Washington, DC, 1985 (November).

Lesgold AM, Perfetti CA, eds. Interactive Processes in reading. Hillsdale, NJ: Erlbaum, 1981.

Liles B. Cohesion in the narratives of normal and language disordered children. J Speech Hear Res 1985;28:123–133.

Liles B. Episode organization and cohesive conjunctions in narratives of children with and without language disorder. J Speech Hear Res 1987;30: 185–196.

Lindamood C, Lindamood P. Lindamood Auditory Conceptualization Test. Allen, TX: DLM Teaching Resources, 1979.

Luria AR. Language and cognition. New York: Wiley, 1982.

Mandler JM, Johnson NS. Remembrance of things parsed: story structure and recall. Cognit Psychol 1977;9:111–151.

Maria K. Reading comprehension instruction: issues and strategies. Parkton, MD: York Press, 1990.

Marzano RJ, Hagerty PJ, Valencia SW, DiStefano PP. Reading diagnosis and instruction. Englewood Cliffs, NJ: Prentice-Hall, 1987.

McNinch G. Awareness of aural and visual word boundary within a sample of first graders. Percept Motor Skills 1974;38:13–28.

Meichenbaum D. Cognitive behavior modification: an integrative approach. New York: Plenum, 1977.

Meltzer LJ, ed. Strategy assessment and instruction for students with learning disabilities. Austin, TX: Pro-Ed, 1993.

Merritt D, Liles B. Story grammar ability in children with and without language disorder: story generation, story retelling, and story comprehension. J Speech Hear Res 1987;30:539–552.

Miller GA, Gildea PM. How children learn words. Sci Am 1987;257:94–99.

Milosky LM. Nonliteral language abilities: seeing the forest for the trees. In: Wallach GP, Butler KG, eds. Language learning disabilities in school-age children. New York: Macmillan, 1994; pp. 275–303.

Moffett J. The universe of discourse. Boston: Houghton Mifflin, 1968.

Morine-Dershimer G. Talking, listening and learning in elementary school classrooms. New York: Longman, 1985.

Myer B, Rice GE. The structure of text. In: Pearson PD, ed. Handbook of reading research. New York: Longman, 1984; pp. 319–351.

NAEP 1992: Writing report card. Office of Educational Research and Improvement, U.S. Department of Education, 1994.

Nelson K. Making sense: the acquisition of shared meaning. New York: Academic Press, 1985.

Nelson N. Reading and writing. In: Nippold M, ed. Later language development. Boston: College-Hill, 1988; pp. 95–125.

Nelson NW. Targets of curriculum-based language assessment. In: Secord W, Damico JS, eds. Best practices in school speech-language pathology. Austin: The Psychologic Corporation, 1992; pp. 73–85.

Newkirk T. More than stories: the range of children's writing. Portsmouth, NH: Heinemann, 1989.

Nippold M, Fey S. Metaphoric understanding in preadolescents having a history of language acquisition difficulties. Lang Speech Hear Serv Sch 1983;14–171–181.

Oakhill J, Yuill N. Higher order factors in comprehension disability: processes and remediation. In: Cornoldi C, Oakhill J, eds. Reading comprehension difficulties: processes and intervention. Mahwah, NJ: Erlbaum, 1996; pp. 69–92.

O'Connor MC, Michaels S. Shifting participant frameworks: orchestrating thinking practices in group discussion. In: Hicks D, ed. Discourse, learning, and schooling. New York: Cambridge University Press; 1996; pp. 63–103.

O'Neil ME, Douglas VI. Study strategies and story recall in attention deficit disorder and reading disability. J Abn Child Psychol 1991;19:671–692.

Papandropoulou I, Sinclair H. What is a word? Experimental study of children's ideas on grammar. Hum Dev 1974;17:241–258.

Pease DM, Gleason JB, Pan BA. Gaining meaning: semantic development. In: Gleason JB, ed. The development of language. 2nd ed. Columbus: Merrill, 1989; pp. 101–134.

Poplin M. The reductionistic fallacy in learning disabilities: replicating the past by reducing the present. J Learn Disabil 1988a;21:389–401.

Poplin M. Holistic/constructivist principles of the teaching/learning process. J Learn Disabil 1988b; 21:401–417.

Pressley M, Woloshyn V. Cognitive strategy instruction that really improves children's academic performance. Cambridge, MA: Brookline Books, 1995.

Reid D, Hresko W, Hammill D. The Test of Early Reading Ability. Austin, TX: Pro-Ed, 1981.

Richardson C, Church J. A developmental analysis of proverb interpretations. J Genet Psychol 1959; 94:169–179.

Richgels D, McGee D, Lomax R, Sheard C. Awareness of four text structures: effects of recall of expository text. Read Res Q 1987;22:177–196.

Roth FP, Spekman NJ. Assessing the pragmatic abilities of children. Part II. Guidelines, considerations, and specific evaluation procedures. J Speech Hear Disord 1984;49:12–17.

Sawyer D. Test of Awareness of Language Segments. Rockville, MD: Aspen, 1987.

Scollon R, Scollon SBK. Narrative, literacy and face in interethnic communication. Norwood, NJ: Ablex, 1981.

Schneider P. Formal operations skills vs. explanation. Psycholinguistic Newsletter (Northwestern University) 1982;8:16–23.

Schumaker JB, Deshler DD. Setting demand variables: a major factor in program planning for the LD adolescent. Top Lang Disord 1984;4(2):22–40.

Shatz M, Gelman R. The development of communication skills: modification of speech of young children as a function of the listener. Monogr Soc Res Child Dev 1973;38:1–37.

Shultz TR, Horibe F. Development of the appreciation of verbal jokes. Dev Psychol 1974;10:13–20.

Shultz TR, Pilon R. Development of the ability to detect linguistic ambiguity. Child Dev 1973;44:728–733.

Slater WH, Graves MF. Research on expository text: implications for teachers. In: Muth KD, ed. Children's comprehension of text. Newark, DE: International Reading Association, 1989.

Smiley A, Bryan T. Learning Disabled boy's problem solving and social interaction during raft building. Chicago: Chicago Institute for the Study of Learning Disabilities, 1983a.

Smiley A, Bryan T. Learning disabled junior high school boys' motor performance and trust during obstacle course activities. Chicago: Chicago Institute for the Study of Learning Disabilities, 1983b.

Smith C, Tager-Flusberg H. Metalinguistic awareness and language development. J Exp Child Psychol 1982;34:449–468.

Snow CE, Kurland BF. Sticking to the point: talk about magnets as a context for engaging in scientific discourse. In: Hicks D, ed. Discourse, learning, and schooling. New York: Cambridge University Press, 1996.

Stackhouse J. Phonologic awareness: connecting speech and literacy problems. In: Hodson BW, Edwards ML, eds. Perspectives in applied phonology. San Diego: Singular, 1997; pp. 157–196.

Stanovich K. Matthew effects in reading: some consequences of individual differences in the acquisition of reading. Read Res Q 1986;21:360–407.

Stein NL. How children understand stories. In: Katz L, ed. Current topics in early childhood education. Vol. 2. Norwood, NJ: Ablex, 1979.

Stein N, Glenn C. An analysis of story comprehension in elementary school children. In: Freedle R, ed. New directions in discourse processing. II. Norwood, NJ: Ablex, 1979.

Stein N, Policastro M. The concept of story: a comparison between children's and teacher's viewpoints. In: Mandl H, Stein N, Trabasso T, eds. Learning and comprehension of text. Hillsdale, NJ: Erlbaum, 1984.

Stothard SE, Hulme C. A comparison of reading comprehension and decoding difficulties in children. In: Cornoldi C, Oakhill J, eds. Reading comprehension difficulties: processes and intervention. Mahwah, NJ: Erlbaum, 1996; pp. 93–112.

Strong W. Creative approaches to sentence combining. Urbana, IL: National Council of Teachers of English, 1986.

Temple C, Nathan R, Temple F, Burris N. The beginnings of writing. Boston: Allyn & Bacon, 1993.

Tompkins GE. Teaching writing: balancing process and product. New York: Macmillan, 1994.

Tonjes MJ, Zintz MV. Teaching reading thinking study skills in content classrooms. Dubuque, IA: Wm. C. Brown, 1987.

Torgesen JK. The role of nonspecific factors in the task performance of learning disabled children: a theoretical assessment. J Learn Disabil 1977a;10:27–34.

Torgesen JK. Memorization processes in reading-disabled children. J Educ Psychol 1977b;69:571–578.

Togesen JK. The test of phonological awareness. Austin, TX: Pro-ed, 1994.

Tough J. The development of meaning. New York: Wiley, 1977.

Tough J. Talk for teaching and learning. Portsmouth, NH: Heinemann, 1979.

van Kleeck A. Assessment and intervention: Does "meta" matter? In: Wallach GP, Butler KG, eds. Language learning disabilities in school-age children. Baltimore: Williams & Wilkins, 1984.

van Kleeck A, Bryant D. Learning that language is arbitrary: evidence from early lexical changes. Paper presented at the meeting of the American Speech-Language-Hearing Association. San Francisco, 1984 (November).

Vogel SA. Syntactic abilities in normal and dyslexic children. J Learn Disabil 1974;7:103–109.

Vygotsky LS. Mind in society. Cambridge MA: Harvard University Press, 1978.

Wallach G, Miller L. Language intervention and academic success. Boston: College-Hill, 1989.

Weaver P, Dickinson D. Story comprehension and recall in dyslexic students. Bull Orton Soc 1979;28:157–171.

Wellman HM. The origins of metacognition. In: Forrest-Presley DL, MacKinnon GE, Waller TG, eds. Metacognition, cognition, and human performance. New York: Academic Press, 1985.

Westby CE. The development of narrative language abilities. In: Wallach GP, Butler KG, eds. Language learning disabilities in school-age children. Baltimore: Williams & Wilkins, 1984.

Westby CE. From learning to talk to talking to learn: oral-literate language differences. In: Simon C, ed. Communication skills and classroom success: therapy methodologies for language-leaning diabled students. San Diego: College-Hill, 1985.

Westby CE. Children's play: reflections of social competence. Semin Speech Lang 1988;9:1–14.

Westby CE. Assessing and facilitating text comprehension. In: Kamhi A, Catts H, eds. Reading disabilities: a developmental language perspective. Boston: College-Hill, 1989; pp. 199–259.

Westby CE. The effects of culture on genre, structure, and style of oral and written texts. In: Wallach G, Butler K, eds. Language Learning disabilities in school-age children and adolescents. New York: Macmillan, 1994; pp. 180–218.

Westby CE. There's more to passing than knowing

the answers. Lang Speech Hear Serv Sch 1997;28: 274–287.

Westby CE, Van Dongen R, Maggart Z. Assessing narrative competence. Semin Speech Lang 1989; 19:63–76.

Wiig E. Language disabilities in adolescents: a question of cognitive strategies. Top Lang Disord 1984;4:2:41–58.

Wiig E. Steps to language competence. San Antonio: The Psychologic Corporation, 1989.

Wiig E, Secord W. Test of Language Competence. New York: The Psychologic Corporation, 1985.

Wixson K, Boskey A, Yochum M, Alverman D. An interview for assessing students' perceptions of classroom reading tasks. Read Teach 1986;37: 104–112.

Worth S, Adair J. Through Navajo eyes. Bloomington, IN: University of Indiana Press, 1972.

Yuill N. A funny thing happened on the way to the classroom: jokes, riddles, and metalinguistic awareness in understanding and improving poor comprehension in children. In: Cornoldi C, Oakhill J, eds. Reading comprehension difficulties: processes and intervention. Mahwah, NJ: Erlbaum, 1996; pp.193–220.

Zentall SS. Self-control training with hyperactive and impulsive children. In: Hughes JN, Hall RJ, eds. Handbook of cognitive behavioral approaches in educational settings. New York: Guilford, 1989; pp. 305–346.

Variability and Individual Differences in Communication Development

The first two sections of this book have provided a basis for understanding the foundations of communication development and its chronology as revealed by the extant literature. Over the past 30 years, when examining the information we have assembled on communication development, authorities have noted that significant degrees of variation exist in the process. Though early researchers were content to define *common patterns* in communication development that could generally describe the "average" child, more recent investigations have begun to look for subgroups and sources of individual variation. Part III addresses variability in the communication development process.

Chapter 14 examines cultural differences in communication development. Because communication is intimately related to culture, there is a good chance that there may be cultural differences in the order, environment, or even mechanisms of communication development.

The bulk of the research literature on communication development has focused almost exclusively on white, middle-class American or British children. The literature on cultural differences in communication development not only is relevant to us clinically because the world is progressively become more culturally diverse, but it also applied directly to many theoretical aspects of communication development.

Chapter 15 considers the individual patterns of development found in the mainly white, middle class children studies over the past 30 years. These individual differences also have clinical and theoretical relevance. Finally, we still have a long way to go before fully understanding communication development. There are many areas of future research that will provide insight into this complex and interesting process. We challenge you, the researchers of tomorrow, to get involved in the study of communication development and its clinical applications.

Ethnic and Cultural Differences in Communication Development

William O. Haynes and Brian B. Shulman

Traditionally, the study of communication development in the English language has largely focused on mainstream children who are typically from white, middle socioeconomic class families. Many investigations utilizing both longitudinal and cross-sectional methodologies have given us a fairly accurate picture of how these mainstream children develop semantically, syntactically, morphologically, phonologically, and pragmatically. We have attempted to detail the results of these studies in the prior sections of the present volume. It would, however, be a gross misrepresentation of the communication development process if we were to leave students with the impression that *all* children learning English develop in a similar fashion. As we indicate in Chapter 15, subgroups of communication development in the form of individual patterns of language acquisition have been found even in the studies of mainstream children. While there is a general progression to communication development that is followed by most children, there is also considerable heterogeneity in the paths that youngsters follow in learning to communicate, and these patterns can be found in all areas of language.

The past emphasis on communication development in mainstream children has been instructive; however, it has not adequately addressed the process of acquiring English shown in nonmainstream youngsters. The cultural makeup of the United States is rapidly changing. In fact, recent projections suggest that by the year 2050, ". . . the average U.S. resident, as defined by Census statistics, will trace his or her descent to Africa, Asia, the Hispanic world, the Pacific Islands, Arabia—almost anywhere but White Europe" (*Time Magazine*, 4/9/90, "The Changing Colors of America: Beyond the Melting Pot"). We know that high birth and immigration rates among "nonmainstream" groups such as Hispanics, Asians, and African-Americans are increasing, while the white population is showing no substantive increases. In view of the rapidly changing cultural makeup of the United States, any discussion of communication development must address the influence of cultural differences.

One might wonder why cultural diversity may have an impact on communication development. First, language is an inseparable part of culture. Each cultural group has distinct patterns of communication both within the group itself and when group members speak English. Certain cultures represented in the United States may speak a language that is totally different from English (e.g., Spanish, Chinese), which could impact on how the English language is first learned and later spoken by a child. On the other hand, a cultural group may speak a *dialect* of English (e.g., African-American English, Southern English, Eastern New England English) that is for the most part similar to the "Standard" version of the language. A dialect is a "variety of a national language" (Taylor, 1986, p.386) that is shared by a particular speech community for purposes of interaction. Even though the differences in dialect speakers may be less dramatic than the influence of a foreign language, these features may have an impact on how English is learned and spoken by a child. Thus, because children from different cultures learn English in dramatically different linguistic environments, their communication development may deviate from the acquisition patterns we typically associate with mainstream children. To determine if this is true, it is important to report the results of studies that deal with communication development in nonmainstream children and to define any similarities and differences in the development of language. A major difficulty, however, is that research on communication development in the varied cultures of America is only in its beginning stages. Initial research concentrated on defining the linguistic structural differences between Standard English and the languages spoken by cultural groups (Wolfram & Fasold, 1974). Much is known about the specific linguistic characteristics of Hispanic English and African-American English as they compare with Standard English communication. However, we know far less about specific effects of the many Asian, Native American, and Pacific Island languages on learning to speak English. It is clear that different first languages could have varied effects on English as it is spoken by members of specific cultural groups. It is im-

portant to point out that an awareness of the *features* that characterize a person's communication pattern (e.g., the features of Hispanic English) is different from a knowledge of patterns of communication *development* in specific cultural groups. Thus, we know there are specific features that differentiate English spoken by various cultural groups in the United States from what has been called "Standard English." We do not know, however, if the versions of English spoken by these cultural groups *develop* in the same manner as that acquired by the white, middle-class children who comprise the bulk of the communication development literature. A determination of developmental patterns in different cultural groups is important for several reasons. First, knowledge of different developmental patterns will contribute to theoretical formulations about language acquisition (see Chapter 3). Second, the information regarding communication development is used clinically in assessment and for the selection of intervention targets. If it is determined that children from diverse cultures exhibit different patterns of development or timetables of acquisition, there would be significant clinical implications regarding if and when to enroll a child in treatment. If parents from different cultures engage in "nonmainstream" patterns of interaction and language stimulation with their children, professionals need to be aware of this as they deal with families in assessment and treatment.

IMPLICATIONS OF BILINGUAL AND BIDIALECTAL ENVIRONMENTS FOR COMMUNICATION DEVELOPMENT

Whether a child is developing English communication in a bilingual or a bidialectal environment, he or she faces the task of learning the features of two linguistic systems. One could ask a variety of questions about this process. Does the learning of two languages affect the rate of acquisition of both systems? Do children make developmental errors the same way in both languages? It is useful to separate acquisition of two languages into two major categories, *simultaneous acquisition* and *successive acquisition* (Owens, 1996). Simultaneous acquisition of languages refers to learning two languages at the same time, typically prior to age 3. Successive acquisition is the learning of one language prior to age 3 and later acquiring another language usually in the context of school or social experiences. Clearly, different processes are involved in simultaneous versus successive acquisition.

Interestingly, there are reports indicating that children learning two languages simultaneously tend to acquire both languages at a normal rate (Dulay, Hernandez-Chavez, & Burt, 1978; Doyle, Champagne, & Segalowitz, 1978; Padilla & Lindholm, 1976). In fact, Owens (1996, p. 420) indicates that ". . . in spite of the bilingual linguistic load, the child acquires both languages at a comparable rate to that of monolingual children. . . . The degree of dissimilarity between the two languages does not appear to affect the rate of acquisition. The key to development is the consistent use of the two languages within their primary use environments." The patterns of acquisition in both languages tend to progress from grammatically simple to complex. Most of the interference of one language with another is due to differences in syntactic organization rather than semantic influences (Slobin, 1973). According to Albert and Obler (1978), the child becomes genuinely bilingual by about age 7.

In successive acquisition there are parallels to first language learning in that simple structures are learned first followed by more complex sentence arrangements (Dulay & Burt, 1974). When the child makes errors in the second language, there are similarities to the types of errors found in first language learning (Venable, 1974).

Expertise with a language, whether learned simultaneously or successively, depends in large measure on the amount of use and practice of the linguistic system. Most linguistic use by bilingual or bidialectal speakers is highly situational in nature with each language used in specific contexts (e.g., home, work, school) largely due to pragmatic considerations involving interactants and levels of formality. The exception is the use of *code switching* in which semantic elements from one language are included in another, and in cases where the syntactic systems of two codes are similar, even sentence structures are transferred from one language into another (McClure, 1981; Poplack, 1981; Huerta-Macias, 1981). Code switching occurs largely due to pragmatic considerations involving interactants, conversational conventions (e.g., stylistic devices), and levels of formality (e.g., interviews versus informal talking).

Whether a child learns English in a bilingual or bidialectal environment, he or she will learn to use both linguistic systems with varying degrees of facility. As mentioned previously, the language that is used the most will probably be the most well developed. If the home environment speaks largely the native language or dialect as opposed to the standard version of English, the child will have more experience with this particular code. If the parents speak mostly Standard English in the home, the child will have more expertise with this linguistic system. As the child reaches school age, he or she is faced with a curriculum that is based on a standard English model. That is, most literacy experiences in learning how to read, spell, and write are geared for the Standard English speaker. Learning to read, spell, and write a linguistic code that differs from the spoken language a child has the most facility with may present difficulties for some children. Also, a child may enter a school environment in which the staff have no appreciation of linguistic diversity and its relation to culture. In this case a child may be treated as speaking an "impoverished form" of English and given negative feedback on his or her communication skills. Historically, a disproportionate number of nonmainstream students have been enrolled in speech and language treatment. Many of these children did not exhibit legitimate communication disorders but only dialectal variations. Currently, legal and legislative developments have helped to ensure nondiscriminatory testing and enrollment of children in treatment (Taylor, 1986). Thus it can be seen that a child who learns to communicate with two linguistic systems may develop in a different language environment, may follow a different timetable or path of acquisition compared with mainstream children, and may have differing experiences in learning literacy skills both before and after school entrance. The present chapter will review selected literature in an attempt to clarify the issues in this important area.

AFRICAN-AMERICAN AND HISPANIC CULTURES AS EXAMPLES OF BIDIALECTAL AND BILINGUAL COMMUNICATION DEVELOPMENT

Language variations abound in the United States. There are variations in language as a product of ethnicity, race, region, peer group, and first language community (Taylor, 1986). For example, the two largest racial/ethnic groups in the United States who have distinct dialects that differ from Standard English are African-Americans and Hispanics. Other groups who came from Asia and the Pacific Islands speak languages such as Mandarin, Cantonese, Taiwanese, Hakka, Tagalog, Ilocano, Japanese, Korean, Vietnamese, Khmer, Lao, Hmong, Mien, Chamorro, Samoan, and Hindi (Cheng, 1989). According to Saville-Troike (1986), nearly one-fourth of Navajo children on reservations in the Southwest are learning the Navajo language as their mother tongue and English as a second language.

The present chapter will focus on African-American and Hispanic English development for several reasons. First, these groups comprise the two largest populations of nonmainstream speakers in the United States. Second, most of the available literature has concentrated on these groups. Less information is presently available on the development of

English spoken by Asian and Native American children. Third, the two groups represent good examples of communication development in a *bilingual* population (Hispanics) and a *bidialectal* group (African-Americans). It is clear that this chapter cannot cover all available information on every dialect spoken in the United States, but a focus on African-American and Hispanic English can act as a model for later expositions of other dialects as pertinent research emerges. It is important for speech-language pathologists to become familiar with dialects spoken in their geographic areas, not only in terms of the features of the dialects as spoken by adult language users, but also the *development* of English in children raised in bilingual or bidialectal environments.

COMMUNICATION DEVELOPMENT IN AFRICAN-AMERICAN CHILDREN: PRELIMINARY DATA OVERVIEW

It is important to make clear from the outset that not all African-American children come from bidialectal households. Many of these youngsters are Standard English speakers or regional dialect speakers (e.g., Eastern Seaboard English). Most research suggests that African-American children from lower socioeconomic classes have an increased likelihood of speaking African-American English. Dillard (1972) has estimated that African-American English is used by as many as 80% of African-Americans. We should view dialect use in any culture as being on a continuum. On one end of the scale are speakers who incorporate every possible feature of the dialect into their communication. On the other end are people who only use a few features of the dialect. Thus some speakers exhibit a "heavy" dialect, while others may only demonstrate a hint of dialectal variation. Tables 14.1 and 14.2 from Owens (1996) illustrate the features of African-American English reported by linguists. We must remember that some African-Americans do not use any of these features and that dialect

Table 14.1   *Phonemic Contrasts Between Black English (BE) and Standard American English (SAE)*

SAE Phonemes	Position in Word		
	Initial	Medial	Final[a]
/p/		Unaspirated /p/	Unaspirated /p/
/n/			Reliance on preceding nasalized vowel
/w/	Omitted in specific words (*l'as, too!*)		
/b/		Unreleased /b/	Unreleased /b/
/g/		Unreleased /g/	Unreleased /g/
/k/		Unaspirated /k/	Unaspirated /k/
/d/	Omitted in specific words (*l'on't know*)	Unreleased /d/	Unreleased /d/
/n/		/n/	/n/
/t/		Unaspirated /t/	Unaspirated /t/
/l/		Omitted before labial consonants (*help-hep*)	"uh" following a vowel (*Bill-Biuh*)
/r/		Omitted or /ə/	Omitted or prolonged vowel or glide
/θ/	Unaspirated /t/ or /f/ between vowels	Unaspirated /t/ or /f/	Unaspirated /t/ or /f/ (*bath-baf*)
/v/	Sometimes /b/	/b/ before /m/ and /n/	Sometimes /b/
/ð/	/d/	/d/ or /v/ between vowels	/d/, /v/, /f/
/z/		Omitted or replaced by /d/ before nasal sound (*wasn't-wud'n*)	

Blends

/str/ becomes /skr/

/ʃr/ becomes /str/

/θr/ becomes /θ/

/pr/ becomes /p/

/br/ becomes /b/

/kr/ becomes /k/

/gr/ becomes /g/

Final Consonant Clusters (second consonant omitted when these clusters occur at the end of a word)

/sk/   /nd/   /sp/

/ft/   /ld/   /dʒ d/

/st/   /sd/   /nt/

Reprinted with permission from Owens R. Language development: an introduction. New York: Merrill, 1996. Data drawn from Fasold R, Wolfram W. Some linguistic features of Negro dialect. In: Fasold R, Shuy R, eds. Teaching standard English in the inner city. Washington, D.C.: Center for Applied Linguistics, 1970.
[a]Note weakening of final consonants.

Table 14.2 *Grammatical Contrasts Between Black English (BE and Standard American English (SAE)*

BE Grammatical Structure	SAE Grammatical Structure
Possessive -'s	
Nonobligatory where word position expresses possession Get *mother* coat. It *be* mother's.	Obligatory regardless of position Get *mother's* coat. It's *mother's*.
Plural -s	
Nonobligatory with numerical quantifier He got ten *dollar*. Look at the *cats*.	Obligatory regardless of numerical quantifier He has ten *dollars*. Look at the *cats*.
Regular past -ed	
Nonobligatory, reduced as consonant cluster Yesterday, I *walk* to school.	Obligatory Yesterday, I walk*ed* to school.
Irregular Past	
Case by case, some verbs inflected, others not. I *see* him last week.	All irregular verbs inflected I *saw* him last week.
Regular Present Tense Third Person Singular -s	
Nonobligatory She *eat* too much.	Obligatory She *eats* too much.
Irregular Present Tense Third Person Singular -s	
Nonobligatory He *do* my job.	Obligatory He *does* my job.
Indefinite an	
Use of indefinite *a*. He ride in *a* airplane.	Use of *an* before nouns beginning with a vowel He rode in *an* airplane.
Pronouns	
Pronominal apposition: pronoun immediately follows noun Momma *she* mad. She . . .	Pronoun used elsewhere in sentence or in other sentence; not in apposition Momma *is* mad. She . . .
Future Tense	
More frequent use of *be going to* (gonna) I *be going to* dance tonight. I *gonna* dance tonight. Omit *will* preceding *be* I *be* home later.	More frequent use of *will* I *will* dance tonight. I *am going to* dance tonight. Obligatory use of *will* I *will* (I'll) *be* home later.
Negation	
Triple negative *Nobody don't never* like me. Use of *ain't* I *ain't* going.	Absence of triple negative *No* one ever likes me. *Ain't* is unacceptable form *I'm not* going.

Table 14.2 *Grammatical Contrasts Between Black English (BE and Standard American English (SAE)—continued*

Modals

Double modals for such forms as *might, could,* and *should*
    I *might could* go.
	Single modal use
	    I *might be able to* go.

Questions

Same form for direct and indirect
    What *it is?*
    Do you know what *it is?*
	Different forms for direct and indirect
	    What *is it?*
	    Do you know what *it is?*

Relative Pronouns

Nonobligatory in most cases
    He the one stole it.
    It the one you like.
	Nonobligatory with *that* only
	    He's the one *who* stole it.
	    It's the one *(that)* you like.

Conditional If

Use of *do* for conditional *if*
    I ask *did* she go.
	Use of *If*
	    I asked *if* she went.

Perfect Construction

Been used for action in the distant past
    He *been* gone.
	Been not used
	    He left a long time ago.

Copula

Nonobligatory when contractible
 	
    He sick.
	Obligatory in contractible and uncontractible forms
	    He's sick.

Habitual or General State

Marked with uninflected *be*
    She be workin'.
	Nonuse of *be;* verb inflected
	    She's *working* now.

Reprinted with permission from Owens R. Language development: and introduction. New York: Merrill, 1996. Data drawn from Fasold R, Wolfman W. Some linguistic features of Negro dialect. In: Fasold R, Shuy R, eds. Teaching standard English in the inner city. Washington D.C.: Center for Applied Linguistics, 1970.

speakers, as mentioned above, incorporate varied numbers of features.

African-Americans represented about 12% of the United States population in 1988, although they are more heavily concentrated in most major inner-city areas and in the southeast United States where they comprise about 21% of the population. The culture is characterized by a rich heritage that incorporates a very strong sense of family, community, and culture. Elders are respected as having wisdom and insight. Education is important to African-American families as a means of realizing one's full potential. Most African-Americans value religion as a source of inspiration and sustenance through difficult times. Communication is valued in the African-American culture (Genovese, 1974; Willis, 1992), and one's facility with language is a significant contributor to prestige. There is also a downside associated with the African-American culture. As a group they have experienced slavery, oppression, and discrimination for centuries, and, in spite of this, they have made contributions that have shaped the nation. There are almost four times as many African-American families below the poverty level as compared with whites. While there is a strong sense of family in African-American Culture, about 43% of families live in homes where there is no father. Also, African-Americans hold significantly fewer managerial positions as compared with whites (Willis, 1990). African-Americans also lead whites in such dismal statistics as males killed in homicides, heart disease, infant mortality, low birth weight, and nutritional deficiency (DHHS, 1985). While this brief sketch cannot hope to capture the richness of an entire culture, it does point out several important aspects that relate to communication development. First, there is a strong sense of family and even in homes with absent fathers, the mother, siblings, grandparents, and extended family participate in child-rearing tasks. Second, communication is a valued trait, and thus a disorder of language is especially penalizing. Third, a disproportionate number of African-American children are at risk for language delay due to conditions such as prematurity, low birth weight, and poor prenatal care. Fourth, since such a large percentage of the African-American population is in the lower socioeconomic strata, it is often difficult for researchers to disentangle the effects of social class from cultural practices.

While research on language development in white children began in the early 1900s, studies on linguistic acquisition in African-American children did not begin in earnest until the 1970s. Only a decade ago a major review of the research on language development in African-American children focused on less than 15 investigations, the bulk of which were unpublished doctoral dissertations and papers presented at various conventions (Stockman, 1986). Thus it can be seen that we are still in the beginning stages of understanding how African-American children acquire communication skills. Further, with an absence of adequate developmental data on African-American children, diagnosticians are at a loss for normative data to use in making assessment decisions. Unfortunately, our most widely used normative data on something as basic as Mean Length of Utterance (MLU) are still based on a limited sample of white, middle-class children (Miller & Chapman, 1981).

CARETAKER-CHILD INTERACTION

Earlier in Chapter 5 we discussed caretaker-child interaction and its relationship to communication development. As was mentioned in that chapter, the majority of information on how parents and children interact was based on studies of "mainstream" families. Of these mainstream caretaker-child dyads, most of the groups studied were from middle-class backgrounds.

Research has demonstrated cultural differences in caretaker-child interactions, play, and parenting styles. For example, Fogul, Toda, and Kawai (1988) found that Japanese mothers used more nonverbal stimulation and touching than their American counterparts. In a study by Bornstein, Toda, Azuma, et al. (1990) American mothers tended to focus on objects the child was attending to during interactions, while Japanese mothers encouraged face-to-face contact instead of emphasizing objects. Similarly, Bornstein, Tal, and Tamis-Lemonda (1991) found that both French and Japanese mothers showed lower rates of object stimulation than American mothers. American infants attended to the environment more than the French infants during interactions. Bornstein, Tal, and Tamis-Lemonda (1991) found American toddlers to have higher productive and receptive vocabularies as compared with Japanese children, which is consistent with the finding that American mothers use more labels and descriptions of objects than Japanese mothers. Among the Kugu-Nganychara, an Aboriginal tribe of the Cape York Peninsula in Australia, adults communicate with each other through their children. The child is exposed to adult language, but is not viewed as an independent communicative partner (Schieffelin, 1985). Many cultures use sibling caregivers, and the mothers only give limited care to the infant. For instance, the Kikuyu group in Eastern Africa and the Gusii of Kenya make heavy use of sibling caregivers (Leiderman & Leiderman, 1974; Rogoff & Gardner, 1984; Kermoian, 1982; LeVine & LeVine, 1966). This pattern has also been noted in Western Samoa. Further, Samoan mothers may not regard their children as "conversational" partners until after 6 months of age (Ochs, 1988). The studies cited above suggest cultural differences in caretaker-child interaction that may have an effect on the development of a first language in children. The research certainly shows that the patterns of caretaker-child interaction differ from the one described in the "mainstream" literature.

Young (1970) studied 46 African-American families in southern Georgia and found that children were in an almost exclusively "human" environment. The child is cared for by many family members and sleeps in the same bed with the parents. Object exploration is not emphasized, but rather, face-to-face contact is encouraged. This style is similar to that reported in the Japanese and French cultures mentioned above. Heath (1983) examined African-American and white, lower-class families in two different towns named Trackton and Roadville in the Carolina Piedmont. She was interested in communication development, among other things, in the African-American children from Trackton as compared with the white children from Roadville. Like Young (1970), Heath found the emphasis on face-to-face communication rather than an attention to objects during joint referencing in the African-American community. She also reported that parents in Trackton do not treat their infants as communicators early on in development, and thus they are not directly spoken to as much as reported in the mainstream literature. The African-American child's initial forays into communication are imitative in nature. Conversely, the parents of white children in Roadville exhibit all the language stimulation and "conversational" characteristics reported for mainstream caretakers in terms of slowing speech rate, reducing complexity, and engaging in turn-taking with their children. Heath also reported more of an emphasis on objects as opposed to the human, face-to-face emphasis found in the children of Trackton. Heath found that despite the differences in language learning environments, the children of Trackton and Roadville learned to talk at about the same time.

Anderson-Yockel and Haynes (1994) studied lower socioeconomic class African-American and white children between the ages of 1 and 2 years during a joint book reading task with their mothers. Many similarities were found between the groups; however, the white mothers asked significantly more WH and Y/N questions than African-American mothers. This agrees with the observations of Heath (1983) in her ethnographic research. Saunders and Haynes (1994) failed to find differences in questioning behavior during joint book-reading in middle-socioeconomic-class African-American and white groups, so there may be an interaction between culture and SES on this variable.

THE FIRST LEXICON

Little information is available on the development of vocabulary in children from a variety of cultures. Heath (1982), however, has reported that the African-American children from Trackton referred to above tended to exhibit what Nelson (1973) called "expressive" as opposed to "referential" speech. As explained in Chapter 15, referential speech is comprised of a high percentage of nominals, while expressive speech is made up of mainly personal-social and other grammatical categories. Recall that the African-American parents tended to emphasize face-to-face interaction while minimizing object naming, and the opposite was true of the parents of white children in Roadville. These differing inter-action styles may have had an effect on the development of the first lexicons of the children in the cultural groups. More re-search is needed to determine if this is a widespread pattern.

SEMANTIC RELATIONS

In 1973 Roger Brown found a rela-tively small of semantic relations that characterized early combinatorial utter-ances of children representing a number of different languages. Brown's (1973) analysis "reveals the fact that Stage I ut-terances, in all the languages for which studies exist, concentrate on the same set of meanings . . . (p. 173)." It would be no surprise, then, if African-American chil-dren also exhibited a similar set of early word combinations found in speakers of Standard English and a variety of foreign languages. The few studies on African-American children, in fact, bear this out (Blake, 1984; Steffensen, 1974; Stock-man, 1984; Stockman & Vaughn-Cooke, 1982). After reviewing this literature, Stockman (1986, p. 147) stated: "Black children acquire language for coding the same early domains of meaning as those acquired by SE speaking children. . . The number of semantic categories repre-sented increases with age. The semantic categories of action and existence are among the earliest ones acquired, whereas categories underlying multiproposition such as coordination or causality are among the latest acquired." It is logical that Stage I developments are similar cross-culturally since they appear to be based, at least in part, on cognitive attain-ments in the early sensorimotor period, which are grossly comparable in different cultural groups (Brown, 1973). Also, most features of African-American English in-volve grammatical morphemes typically acquired by Standard English speakers in Brown's Stage II after the early semantic relations have been established. While later research may reveal some subtle dif-ferences in Stage I for African-American children, the studies available at the pres-ent time suggest patterns similar to a va-riety of cultures in early communication.

SYNTAX/MORPHOLOGY

The differences between Standard English and African-American English span all areas of language; however, the ef-fects of dialect are perhaps the greatest in the areas of syntax and morphology. Con-sonant cluster reduction rules in African-American dialect operate in such a manner as to delete most bound morphemes due to morphophonemic rules. For example, the cluster reduction rule eliminates the fi-nal consonant in clusters where both members of the blend are either voiced or voiceless (e.g., ca**ts**, do**gz**), but not in clus-ters where the members differ in their voicing component (e.g., be**lt**, gu**lf**). Al-most all bound morphemes are attached using a rule that states that the inflection must be similar in voicing to the final con-sonant in the word. Thus most bound morphemes that attach single sounds to words ending in consonants are elimi-nated in dialect speakers who incorporate all features of their dialect. Specifically, possessive -s, plural -s, regular past -ed, and third-person singular -s (regular & ir-regular) could all be eliminated. Other syntactic variations include double nega-tion, pronominal apposition, no interrog-ative reversal on some questions, zero cop-ula in contractible contexts, and use of "be" as a habitual marker. While these fea-tures could occur in a mature speaker of African-American English, little informa-tion is available on children's development of syntax/morphology. We do know that until about age 2.5 to 3.0, MLU increases at rates similar to Standard English-speak-ing children (Blake, 1974; Stockman, 1986). Some time between ages 2.5 and 7, African-American children go through a process of learning dialect-specific rules for phonology, morphology, and syntax. These rules are at least as complex as those learned by Standard English speakers with regard to morphology. For example, it is not enough to simply state that African-American English speakers "omit the copula when contractible in Standard English." Research has continued to show that use of the copula is highly variable and context dependent in both adult and child speakers of African-American dialect (Wyatt, 1991, 1996; Labov, 1969; Steffensen, 1974). For instance, use of the copula tends to be more obligatory in forms such as first-person singular, past tense, emphatic contexts, and final clauses.

PHONOLOGY

As mentioned above, one predominant phonological difference in African-American English is the consonant cluster reduction rule. While this rule is a phonological difference, it can appear on the surface as a morphological difference since many bound morphemes are attached as single consonants (e.g., ha**ts**). Another phonological difference that has a significant impact on utterances is the production of final singleton consonants. Certain final singleton consonants are either deleted or at least weakened in some African-American English speakers. Much of the research on African-American English has been gathered on adolescent or adult speakers, and we are just beginning to know about how children develop aspects such as final consonants. For instance, research on adult speakers does not widely report final singleton deletions with the exception of final /b/, /d/ and /g/ weakening or unreleased productions of these sounds. There are also some reports of deletion of final nasal sounds with concurrent nasalization of the preceding vowel (Fasold & Wolfram, 1970). On the other hand, many speech-language pathologists in public school settings have noted that young dialect speakers between the ages of 4 and 9 tend to delete or weaken final consonants. In Standard English speakers, Ingram (1976) suggests that the final consonant deletion process tends to disappear in mainstream children by about age 3. Several studies have shown that African-American children appear to be on a different timetable for the development of final singletons

(Seymour & Seymour, 1981; Haynes & Moran, 1989; McCallion, Ford, & Haynes, 1982) with deletion/weakening of certain voiced stops (/b/, /d/ & /g/) and some fricatives (/s/, /v/ & /th/) persisting until third grade.

We know that there are developmental changes in the phonology of African-American English, as well as regional variations. Certainly, far more similarities than differences exist between the phonologies of African-American English and Standard English. The phonemic inventories are basically the same, and most differences appear to be in distribution and frequency of phoneme use in certain contexts (Stockman, 1996). Most differences appear in the medial and final positions, and phoneme differences from Standard English are rule governed.

PRAGMATICS

One aspect of pragmatics that has been studied in African-American children is the acquisition of communicative functions. Several investigations (Bridgeforth, 1984; Blake, 1984) have shown that these children develop communicative intents in an additive fashion with the numbers of functions increasing with age as in Standard English-speaking subjects (Stockman, 1986). The specific intents developed are similar to those found in mainstream children and involve informatives, requesting, regulation, imaginative, affective, participative, and attentive functions. Westby, in Chapter 8, reports the results of Heath (1983), who stated that ". . . early language functions of African-American children in the Carolina Piedmont included bossing, cussing, fussing, begging, and comforting—not the early communicative functions reported for mainstream children." Little is presently known about the development of communicative functions in African-American children from various social classes. Most research to date (Wetherby, Cain, Yonclas, & Walker, 1988) has focused on mainstream children. Without more detailed study of African-American children, normative data will be less useful to clinicians serving multicultural populations.

Pragmatics involves the use of language in a communicative context. Research on African-American children has shown that youngsters as young as 3 years have begun to incorporate dialect-specific rules into their communication. It has also been noted that by age 4 there is an increase in the use of African-American English features, especially in lower socioeconomic class groups (Blake, 1984; Steffensen, 1974; Stockman, 1984; Stockman & Vaughn-Cooke, 1982; Stockman, 1986). As the child becomes older and more aware of social aspects of communication, there is also an increase in style shifting between extreme versions of the dialect (typically with peers and family) and utterances that incorporate more features of Standard English.

Many researchers have studied narratives produced by African-American children and have found that narratives vary with culture and elicitation tasks (Hester, 1996). This variation is present both between and within cultures. For example, some researchers have characterized narratives of African-American children as reflecting an "oral" as opposed to "literate" style. Oral style incorporates more personal anecdotes without an overriding theme and more use of prosodic cues instead of structural semantic/syntactic forms to attain cohesion. Literate style is more thematic and uses syntactic forms to facilitate cohesion. These narratives sound more like the language used in books to tell stories. In actuality, Hester (1994) found that African-American children's narrative style changed along the oral-literate continuum as they produced narratives with differing elicitation tasks and engaged in style shifting. Narrative development is very complex and must take into account cultural, cognitive, social, and linguistic development.

A FINAL NOTE

Much more research is needed to understand the impact of the African-Amer-

ican culture on language acquisition in children. We have significant gaps in areas such as development of comprehension, lexical acquisition, complex utterance development, metalinguistic development, phonological acquisition, and narrative development, just to name a few. Even more data are required before we know exactly how to deal with this population in language assessment and treatment. Almost all of our current language tests are developed and scored using Standard English models. While some normative samples include African-Americans, no attempt has been made to discern patterns of cultural bias or socioeconomic bias in these tests. It is not enough to include nonmainstream subjects in the standardization samples in the proportions similar to the U. S. Census (e.g., 12%). This does not help when testing in the inner cities and rural South where the percentages of African-American students may be triple these census figures. We need more data for use in nonstandardized testing (e.g., MLU, vocabulary size, type-token ratio, percent consonants correct, measures of conversational performance, etc.). We also need more information on the effects of bidialectal language development and the acquisition of varied literacy skills, including reading, spelling, and other academic areas.

There is currently an emphasis on multicultural issues in education, communication disorders, and the behavioral sciences. We can expect research in this area to proliferate in the next decade, which will give us both a broader and deeper understanding of the communication development process.

COMMUNICATION DEVELOPMENT IN HISPANIC CHILDREN: PRELIMINARY DATA

Population Description: Defining "Hispanic"

Hispanic individuals represent many diverse cultural and ethnic backgrounds. In the United States, the Hispanic population is linguistically heterogeneous. Some may be monolingual Spanish speakers, while others are monolingual English speakers (Garcia, in press). More specifically, some Hispanic people have been reported to be descendants of Native Indians, while others have been direct off-spring from Spanish and European cultures (Melville, 1987). While still other Hispanic individuals represent African-American, Asian, and white heritages, Langdon (1992) reports that the greatest majority of Hispanic individuals represent Indian and European backgrounds.

Langdon (1992) further reports that prior to 1970, the Hispanic population was not represented in the U.S. Census data as a separate cultural orientation but rather as a representative portion of the general population. Moreover, the term "Hispanic" was seldom used prior to the 1970s. Since this time, however, a significant number of Hispanics has arrived in the United States representing different residency statuses, including naturalized citizens, refugees, citizens by birth, "green card" recipients, and illegal aliens (Trevino, 1987).

Population Distribution: Prevalence and Subgroups

In the 1990 U.S. Census, Hispanics made up approximately 9% of the total population, with African-Americans, Asians, and Native Americans comprising 12%, 5%, and 1%, respectively (Taylor, 1992). In its Current Population Report of 1990, the U. S. Census Bureau subdi-vided the Hispanic population into five distinct subgroups: Mexicans, Puerto Ricans, Cubans, Central and South Americans, and Other Hispanics. As illustrated in Figure 14.1, Mexicans represent the largest portion of the Hispanic popula-tion with Cubans representing the small-est percentage. The subgroup identified as "Other Hispanics" is defined as those individuals who report that their geo-graphic or familial origins were in Spain or that they are descendants of families who have been in the Unites States for one of several generations (Langdon, 1992). Approximately 55% of the total Hispanic population reside in the states of California (34%) and Texas (21%). Sig-nificant numbers of Hispanic individuals also maintain residency in the states of

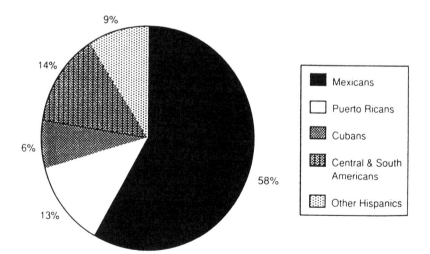

Figure 14.1.   Percentage of each Hispanic subgroup. (Note that percentages are rounded up.) (From Langdon HW, ed. The Hispanic population: facts and figures. In: Hispanic children and adults with communication disorders: assessment and intervention. Gaithersburg, MD: Aspen, 1992, p. 26; and from The Hispanic population in the United States, current population reports. Washington, DC: Bureau of the Cen-sus, 1990.)

New York, Florida, Illinois, Arizona, New Jersey, New Mexico, and Colorado.

In further describing the Hispanic population and its five subgroups, Langdon (1992) asserts: "not only do characteristics such as age, family size, income, education, occupation, and health care utilization often differ between the Hispanic group as a whole and the rest of the United States non-Hispanic population, but also they may differ among the various subgroups" (p. 27). Langdon (1992) provides an extensive discussion of these six characteristics.

The following section describes Hispanic children's development of communication/language skills. In keeping with the communication development information provided thus far in previous sections of this text, various connections will be offered. That is, attempts will be made to associate developmental information relative to syntax, semantics, and pragmatics to delineate substantive similarities and differences relative to the development of Hispanic communication/language.

Development of Syntax and Morphology

The literature on communicative development in Hispanic children has focused primarily on the acquisition of syntactic and morphologic skills (Brisk, 1972, 1974, 1976; Dale, 1980; Dato, 1975; Fantini, 1982; Gonzalez, 1978; Kernan & Blount, 1966; Kvaal, Shipstead-Cox, Nevitt et al., 1988; Linares, Orama, & Sanders, 1977; Merino, 1983). Merino (1992) provides rationale for the interest in studying Spanish syntax and morphology. Since morphology and syntax are the two language components that have been researched the most relative to language acquisition in English and other languages, these data are readily available for comparison. Data corresponding to the acquisition of syntactic and morphologic markers in English can be used to compare similar acquisition in Spanish. Dulay, Hernandez-Chavez, and Burt (1978) further substantiate this case by stating

that syntactic and morphologic skills are less likely to be affected by dialectal and stylistic variation. This notion has most recently been challenged by individuals who have examined language proficiency from a pragmatic, communicative perspective (Hamayan, 1974; Hamayan & Damico, 1991).

According to Garcia (1983), the development of language by Hispanic children in the United States cannot be understood without an analysis of the data represented by the "Spanish/ English interface within the specific linguistic/social/ psychological context of development." Such data include the notion that the two languages develop simultaneously (Garcia, 1983). Furthermore, the two languages may intermingle morphologically and syntactically (Huerta, 1977; Zentella, 1978; Valdes-Fallis, 1979). They may also develop differentially as a function of differential contextual support (Garcia, Maez, & Gonzalez, 1981; Gonzalez & Maez, 1981; Berdan & Garcia, 1985).

In further describing the interface between the acquisition of Spanish and English, Berdan and Garcia (1985) offer the following developmental progression:

1. Spanish is spoken exclusively while English is being acquired. English speech is avoided.

2. English is used when necessary and with effort. English utterances are short, rarely as long as a clause.

3. English is used as a concession to the situation, but under duress. When difficulty is encountered, the speaker switches to Spanish and maintains that language as long as possible.

4. English can be used more extensively with switching in and out of Spanish (i.e., code-switching) according to involvement in what the speaker is saying, playing against self-monitoring to maintain English.

5. Preference, especially in public and peer situations, shifts toward English, according to the preferences and abilities of the perceived majority in the situation.

6. Overreaction may set in with suppression of Spanish except when Spanish is absolutely necessary. Dual-lingual behavior may occur. Merino (1992) also offers a cogent discussion about the similarities and differences between the Spanish and English languages.

Merino (1992) further notes that the language development research on Hispanic children, while occurring over the last 20 years, is very limited. Moreover, she describes that the majority of Spanish language acquisition research is characterized as either longitudinal or cross-sectional. Longitudinal studies involve following individuals as they mature or age and observing changes in their behaviors or characteristics over time. Cross-sectional research, however, involves the selection of individuals from various age groups. In turn, differences between the behaviors or characteristics of the different groups are described (Ventry & Schiavetti, 1986). Inherent strengths and weaknesses of each type of research design have been described in the literature (Campbell & Stanley, 1963; Hulley & Cummings, 1988; Ventry & Schiavetti, 1986).

A number of diary (Vivas, 1979; Belendez, 1980; Eisenberg, 1982; Pardo, 1984) and cross-sectional studies (Kernan & Blount, 1966; Burt, Dulay, & Hernandez-Chavez, 1975; Brisk, 1976; Linares, Orama, & Sanders, 1977; Merino, 1982; Kvaal, Shipstead-Cox, Nevitt, et al., 1988; Perez-Pereira, 1989) relative to the acquisition of Spanish syntax and morphology have been described by Merino (1992). Merino (1992) notes that universal patterns of syntactic and morphological development may be more easily identified from cross-sectional research paradigms than from diary studies. The major advantage of the former type of research is that data are obtained from a larger sample of subjects at one particular point in time. Merino (1992) elaborates on this concept by stating that "the underlying assumption of a cross-sectional study is that specific language features used by older children indicate the development of language in younger children" (p. 72).

With specific reference to the chronological ages at which Hispanic children comprehend and use certain syntactic and morphological structures, Table 14.3 illustrates these data, which are based in part on the results of the studies referenced above in addition to others referenced within the table.

While Merino (1992) notes the difficulty in establishing specific ages for the development of these syntactic and morphologic structures, she provides general statements about which structures are used prior to and after the age of 6 years. Table 14.4 lists these structures.

In examining the development of English syntax and morphology (i.e., Chapters 10, 11, and 12), one should attempt to understand how such structures are acquired by Hispanic speakers who use English as a secondary language. Table 14.5 provides a sampling of syntactic and morphologic changes that have been observed in Hispanic speakers' use of English.

Semantic and Pragmatic Development

According to Meara (1980), there has been a lack of sufficient research into the development of semantic skills in Hispanic children. Studies relative to the lexical (vocabulary) acquisition have primarily focused on methods for *teaching* vocabulary rather than on the developmental process by which words are learned (Langdon & Merino, 1992). More research is warranted to explain the acquisition of semantic skills in Hispanic children.

As stated earlier in this text, pragmatics refers to the use of language in context (Bates, 1976). Its framework rests in the notion that children should be able to use language to signify basic communicative needs in the form of speech acts (Austin, 1962; Searle, 1969). Furthermore, these communicative intents are used during discourse to maintain and change topic, take conversational turns, request clarification, and reject or deny, among others. A child's ability to effectively engage in the dynamics of conversational interac-

Table 14.3 *Age of Acquisition of Selected Spanish Grammatical Features*

Feature	Age of Acquisition (Years and Months)	Investigator
Noun Phrase		
Short plural /s/	4:0	Merino (1982)
	5:0	Dale (1980)
	5:0–7:0	Kernan & Blount (1966)
	7:1–9:0	Gudeman (1981)
Long plural /es/	4:0	Merino (1982)
	8:0	Dale (1980)
	11:0–12:0	Kernan & Blount (1966)
Gender (noun adjective)	4:0	Merino (1982)
	6:0	G. González (1975)
Gender (direct object pronoun)	5:0	Brisk (1972, 1974)
	5:0–7:0	Merino (1982)
Verb Phrase		
Number	4:0–5:0	Merino (1982)
	5:0	Dale (1980)
	5:0–7:0	Kernan & Blount (1966)
	7:1–9:0	Gudeman (1981)
Progressive	2:0–2.6	G. González (1970, 1972)
	3:0	Cohen (1980)
	4:0	Merino (1982)
Regular preterite	2:0–2.6	G. González (1970, 1972)
	3:0	Cohen (1980)
	4:0	Merino (1982)
	5:0	Dale (1980)
	7:1–9:0	Gudeman (1981)
	11:0–12:0	Kernan & Blount (1966)
Irregular preterite	4:0–5:0	Merino (1982)
	11:0–12:0	Kernan & Blount (1966)
Present perfect	4:0	Merino (1982)
	6:0	G. González (1975)
	11:0–12:0	Kernan & Blount (1966)
Present subjunctive	4:0	R. J. Blake (1980)
	4:0	G. González (1975)
	4:0	Cohen (1980)
	4:0	Merino (1982)
Optative	4:0	Merino (1982)
Purposive	5:0–6:0	Merino (1982)
Word Order		
Active	4:0	Merino (1982)
	5:0–6:0	Gudeman (1981)
Passive	5:5–8:3	Echeverria (1975)
	7:0–8:0	Merino (1985)
	12:4; Adults	Gudeman (1981)

Table 14.3 *Age of Acquisition of Selected Spanish Grammatical Features—cont'd*

Feature	Age of Acquisition (Years and Months)	Investigator
Indirect object	7:0–8:0	Merino (1972, 1974)
	9:0–12:4	Gudeman (1982)
Conditional (yes/no)		
	5:0	Brisk (1972, 1974)
	6:0	G. González (1975)
	6:0	Merino (1982)

Reprinted with permission from Merino BJ. Acquisition of syntactic and phonologic features in Spanish. In: Langdon HW, ed. Hispanic children and adults with communication disorders: assessment and intervention. Gaithersburg, MD: Aspen, 1992.

tion contributes to his communicative competence. Communicative competence refers to an individual's ability to effectively communicate an intentional message to alter the listener's attitudes, beliefs, and/or behaviors (Nicolosi, Harryman, & Kresheck, 1989). Moreover, communicative competence is contingent on the child's ability to appropriately interact with a variety of conversational partners about a variety of topics. Syntactic, morphologic, and lexical performance also contribute to one's communicative competence. It is important to remember

Table 14.4 *Development of Spanish Syntactic and Morphologic Structures Before and After Age 6*

	Example
Before Age 6	
Number in noun phrase (short plural)	gato-gatos (cat-cats)
Number in verb phrase	las ranas saltan (the frogs jump)
Gender in noun adjective	la camisa blanco (the white shirt)
Preterite	la rana saltó (the frog jumped)
Irregular past tense	ella lo trajo (she brought it)
Present progressive	está saltanado (he/she/it is jumping)
Subjunctive (optative form)	quiere que coma (he/she wants him/her to eat)
Subjunctive (purposive form)	abra la puerta para que entre (open the door so he/she can get in)
After Age 6	
Subjunctive (adjective/adverbial phrase)	no hay cosa que sirva (there isn't a thing that would be useful)
Conditional	si el tren no fuera, no cabria (if the train wasn't big enough, it/he/she wouldn't fit)

Adapted from Merino BJ. Acquisition of syntactic and phonologic features in Spanish. In: Langdon HW, ed Hispanic children and adults with communication disorders: assessment and intervention. Gaithersburg, MD: Aspen, 1992.

Table 14.5   Grammatical Contrasts Between Hispanic English and Standard American English (SAE)

SAE Grammatical Structure	Hispanic English Variation
Possessive *'s*	Use postnoun modifier; article used with body parts
This is my mother's coat.	This is the coat *of my mother.*
I cut my hand.	I cut *the* hand.
Plural *-s*	Nonobligatory
The boys are funny.	The boy are funny.
Regular past *-ed*	Nonobligatory
She walked to school.	She walk to school.
Regular third person *-s*	Nonobligatory
Juan runs very fast.	Juan run very fast.
Articles	Nonobligatory
Father is a policeman.	Father is policeman.
Subject pronouns	Omitted when the subject has been identified in the previous sentence
Mother is mad. She is very angry.	Mother is mad. Is very angry.
Future tense (*going to*)	Use of *go* + *to*
I am going to eat later.	I *go to eat* later.
Negation	Use of *no* before the verb
She is not happy.	She *no* is happy.
Questions	No verb inversion
Is Maria happy?	*Maria* is happy?
Copula	Occasional use of *have*
I am ten years old.	I *have* ten years.
Negative imperatives	*No* used for *don't*
Don't throw the book.	*No* throw the book.
Do insertion	Nonobligatory in questions
Do you want some?	You want some?
Comparatives	Use of longer form (*more*)
He is faster.	He is *more* faster.

Adapted from Owens, RE. Language Development: Merrill Publishing Company, 1988.

than a very young child could be communicatively competent with a minimal development of linguistic skills.

Research pertaining to pragmatic development in Hispanic children is also minimal. Peters-Johnson (in press) attributes this to the fact that such research has been insensitive to the interaction of some sociocultural factors that impact language variation. Since much of the literature describes pragmatic development within homogeneous groups, little attention has been provided to heterogeneous and/or nonmainstream groups of children from multicultural backgrounds. An investigation by Barrenechea and Schmitt (1989) studied the development of seven language functions (i.e., labeling, description, informative, affirmation/negation, repetition/revision, requesting, and personal) and three discourse behaviors (i.e., topic introduction, establishment, and maintenance) in 18 Spanish-speaking preschool children. Results indicated that the preschoolers had exhibited communicative competence in the use of the seven functions and three discourse behaviors. The authors suggested that future research focus on the development of these ten features in a larger sample of Hispanic children to derive similarities and individual differences. Such research would, in turn, determine the degree of variability across age groups and define more specifically the "developmental pattern of the pragmatic features studies" (p. 365).

Similar to the notions raised above relative to semantic development in Hispanic children, more research is needed to describe pragmatic development in these children as well. To date, it appears that speech-language pathologists who evaluate the semantic and pragmatic skills of Hispanic children are at a significant disadvantage in that they can only rely on the existing normative semantic and pragmatic data currently documented in the literature. Such data are not sensitive to cultural diversity.

What we know is that pragmatic skills progress through a developmental hierarchy and that pragmatic development co-occurs with social, cognitive, and linguistic development. What we do not know is what the subtle differences are among and between multicultural populations (Peters-Johnson, in press).

Development of Phonology

In addition to clearly documented syntactic and morphologic differences in the English of Hispanic children, there are also data available that describe the development of phonology in these children (Anderson & Smith, 1987; Gonzalez, 1981). It is important to note that there are some observable differences between the English and Spanish languages' sound systems. Perhaps the major difference is the fact that certain English consonants (e.g., /th/ and /z/) and vowels (e.g., /I/ and /ae/) are not present in the Spanish language. Furthermore, when Hispanic

speakers produce these sounds, they are often substituted for other sounds and/or distorted.

Eblen (in press) describes three general phonological processes observed in Spanish-speaking children that have also been observed in English-speaking children. These include consonant cluster reduction, stopping, and assimilation (see Ingram, 1976, for specific definitions). In commenting on Hispanic children's speech sound acquisition process, Eblen (in press) asserts that one should be cautious in trying to assign chronologic ages for Spanish sound acquisition until more significant published data are available similar to those documented by Templin (1957), Poole (1934), and Prather, Hedrick, and Kern (1975) relative to English speech sound production. Furthermore, professionals should consider individual variation in Spanish-speaking children's phonologic development (Macken, 1978; Macken & Ferguson, 1981).

Clinical Applications

This chapter has described communicative development in African-American and Hispanic populations of children as a framework for understanding that developmental language differences occur cross-culturally. Speech-language pathologists have observed increased numbers of children from multicultural backgrounds who require clinical services (i.e., assessment and/or intervention).

Historically, language assessment has involved the analysis of language by breaking it down into its component parts of syntax/morphology, semantics, and pragmatics. This *discrete point* or *modular* perspective on assessment has been documented by Acevedo (1986) and Mattes and Omark (1984). Moreover, language deficits are described based on omitted language forms or structures. Standardized test instruments are primarily used in this assessment methodology, which assumes that language functions independently and has no direct interaction with context, cognitive ability, experience, or learning potential (Damico, 1991). This perspective has received much criticism because it lacks linguistic realism and authenticity, has poor psychometric strength, has inherent and unavoidable bias, and lacks construct validity (see Hamayan & Damico, 1991, for an extensive discussion of these assessment issues). Figure 14.2 illustrates the major constructs of this approach.

In contrast to the discrete point approach, the *synergistic* or *descriptive* approach assesses all aspects of language as it relates to the *communication* process. It recognizes that language exists only as an integrated whole and that communication is highly influenced by context, cognitive ability, experience, and learning potential. Moreover, assessment is conducted using naturalistic methodologies and observation. Data are analyzed to determine if the child's language is purposeful, contextually appropriate, and functional. The overall goal of this approach attempts to determine how *proficient* the child is as a communicator. Figure 14.3 illustrates the major constructs of the descriptive approach.

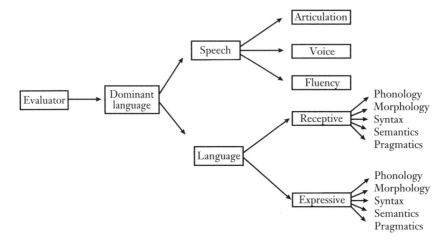

Figure 14.2.   Discrete point assessment process.
(From Damico JS. Descriptive assessment of communicative ability in limited English proficient students. In: Hamayan EV, Damico JS, eds. Limiting bias in the assessment of bilingual students. Austin, TX: Pro-ed, 1991; p. 163.)

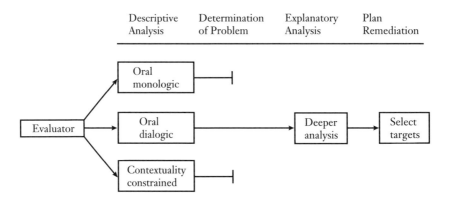

Figure 14.3.   Descriptive assessment process.
(From Damico JS. Descriptive assessment of communicative ability in limited English proficient students. In: Hamayan EV, Damico JS, eds. Limiting bias in the assessment of bilingual students. Austin, TX: Pro-ed, 1991; p. 163.)

In describing the language/communicative proficiency of children from multicultural backgrounds, it behooves the speech-language pathologist to consider these different assessment perspectives. Damico (1991) states the following:

> Pragmatic and naturalistic description enable more valid and reliable assessment that is both effective in describing communication problems in the domain of focus and in differentiating between language and cultural differences versus language impairment. Culturally and linguistically diverse students need not be victims of the system of communicative assessment; rather, they can benefit from the testing process and the appropriate remediation that it generates (1991, pp. 204–205).

REFERENCES

Acevedo MA. Assessment instruments for minorities. In: Bess FH, Clark BS, Mitchell HR, eds. Concerns for minority groups in communication disorders. (American Speech-Language-Hearing Association Reports 16), Rockville, MD: American Speech-Language-Hearing Association, 1986.

Albert M, Obler L. The bilingual brain. New York: Academic Press, 1978.

Anderson R, Smith BL. Phonological development of two-year-old monolingual Puerto Rican Spanish-speaking children. J Child Lang 1987;14: 57–78.

Anderson-Yockel J, Haynes W. Joint book reading strategies in working-class African-American and White mother-toddler dyads. J Speech Hear Res 1994;37(3):583–593.

Austin J. How to do things with words. Cambridge: Harvard University Press, 1962.

Barrenechea IL, Schmitt JF. Selected pragmatic features in Spanish-speaking preschool children. J Psycholinguist Res 1989;18:353–367.

Bates E. Language and context: the acquisition of pragmatics. New York: Academic Press, 1976.

Belendez P. Repetitions and the acquisition of the Spanish verb system. Unpublished doctoral dissertation. Harvard University, Cambridge, MA, 1980.

Berdan R, Garcia M. Discourse-sensitive measurement of language development in bilingual children. In: Garcia E, Padilla R, eds. Advances in bilingual education research. Tucson, AZ: University of Arizona Press, 1985.

Blake I. Language development in working-class Black children: an examination of form, content and use. Unpublished doctoral dissertation. Columbia University, NY, 1984.

Blake RJ. The acquisition of mood selection among Spanish-speaking children: ages 4–12. Unpublished doctoral dissertation. University of Texas, Austin, 1980.

Bornstein M, Toda S, Azuma H, et al. Mother and infant activity and interaction in Japan and the United States. II. A comparative microanalysis of naturalistic exchanges focused on the organization of infant attention. Int J Behav Dev 1990; 13(3):289–308.

Bornstein M, Tal J, Tamis-Lemonda C. Parenting in cross-cultural perspective: the United States, France and Japan. In: Bornstein M, ed. Cultural approaches to parenting. Hillsdale, NJ: Lawrence Erlbaum, 1991.

Bridgeforth C. The development of language functions among Black children from working-class families. Paper presented at the pre-session of the 35th Annual Georgetown University Round Table on language and Linguistics. Georgetown University, Washington, DC, 1984.

Brisk ME. A preliminary study of the syntax of five-year-old Spanish speakers in New Mexico. Int J Sociol Lang 1974;2:69–78.

Brisk ME. The Spanish syntax of the preschool Spanish-American: the case of New Mexican five-year-old children. Unpublished doctoral dissertation. University of New Mexico Albuquerque, 1972.

Brisk ME. The acquisition of Spanish gender by first-grade Spanish-speaking children. In: Keller GD, Teshner RV, Viera S, eds. Bilingualism in the bicentennial and beyond. Jamaica, NY: Bilingual Review Press, 1976; pp. 143–160.

Brown R. A first language: the early stages. Cambridge, MA: Harvard University Press, 1973.

Cheng L. Service delivery to Asian/Pacific LEP children: a cross-cultural framework. Top Lang Disord 1989;9(3):1–11.

Burt M, Dulay H, Hernandez-Chavez E. The bilingual syntax measure. San Francisco, CA: Harcourt Brace Jovanovich, 1975.

Campbell DT, Stanley JC. Experimental and quasi-experimental designs for research. Chicago, IL: Rand McNally College Publishing, 1963.

Cohen AD. The sequential order of acquisition of Spanish verb tenses among Spanish-speaking children of age 3–7. Unpublished doctoral dissertation. University of San Francisco, 1980.

Dale P. Acquisition of English and Spanish morphological rules by bilinguals. Unpublished doctoral dissertation. University of Florida, Gainesville, 1980.

Damico JS. Descriptive assessment of communicative ability in limited English proficient students. In: Hamayan EV, Damico JS, eds. Limiting bias in the assessment of bilingual students. Austin, TX: Pro-ed, 1991.

Dato DP. On psycholinguistic universals in children's learning of Spanish. In: Dato D, ed. Developmental psycholinguistics: theory and applications. Washington, DC: Georgetown University Press, 1975.

Dillard J. Black English. New York, NY: Random House, 1972.

Doyle A, Champagne M, Segalowitz N. Some issues in the assessment of linguistic consequences of early bilingualism. In: Paradis M, ed. Aspects of bilingualism. Columbia, SC: Hornbean Press, 1978.

Dulay H, Hernandez-Chavez E, Burt M. The process of becoming bilingual. In: Singh S, Lynch J, eds. Diagnostic procedures in hearing, language and speech. Baltimore: University Park Press, 1978.

Dulay H, Burt M. Errors and strategies in child second language acquisition. TESOL Q 1974;8:129–138.

Eblen RE. Some observations on the phonologic acquisition of Hispanic-American children. In: Cole L, Deal VR, eds. Communication disorders in multicultural populations. Rockville, MD: American Speech-Language-Hearing Association (in press).

Eisenberg AR. Language acquisition in cultural perspective: talk in three Mexican homes. Unpublished doctoral dissertation. University of California, Berkeley, 1982.

Fantini A. Language acquisition of the bilingual child: a sociolinguistic perspective. Brattleboro, VT: The Experimental Press, 1982.

Fasold R, Wolfram W. Some linguistic features of Negro dialect. In: Fasold R, Shuy R, eds. Teaching standard English in the inner city. Washington, D.C.: Center for Applied Linguistics, 1970.

Fogel A, Toda S, Kawai M. Mother-infant face-to-face interaction in Japan and the United States: a laboratory comparison using 3-month-old infants. Dev Psychol 1988;24:398–406.

Genovese E. Roll, Jordan, Roll: The world slaves made. New York: Pantheon Books, 1974.

Garcia E, Maez LF, Gonzalez G. A national study of Spanish/English bilingualism in young Hispanic children of the United States. Los Angeles, CA: National Dissemination and Assessment Center, California State University, July 1981.

Garcia E. Bilingualism in early childhood. Albuquerque, NM: University of New Mexico Press, 1983.

Garcia EE. The development of Spanish morphology and syntax among Hispanic children in the United States. In: Cole L, Deal VR, eds. Communication disorders in multicultural populations. Rockville, MD: American Speech-Language-Hearing Association (in press).

Gonzalez G. The acquisition of Spanish grammar by native Spanish speakers. Unpublished doctoral dissertation. University of Texas, Austin, 1970.

Gonzalez G. Analysis of Chicano Spanish and the problem of usage. Aztatlan 1972;3:223–231.

Gonzalez G. The acquisition of grammatical structures by Mexican-American children. In: Hernandez-Chavez E, Cohen AD, Beltramo AF, eds. El languaje de los Chicanos. Washington, DC: Center for Applied Linguistics, 1975.

Gonzalez G. The acquisition of Spanish grammar by native Spanish-speaking children. Rosslyn, VA: National Clearinghouse for Bilingual Education, 1978.

Gonzalez A. A descriptive study of phonologic development in normal-speaking Puerto Rican preschoolers. Unpublished doctoral dissertation. Pennsylvania State University, 1981.

Gonzalez G, Maez L. To switch or not to switch: the role of code-switching in the elementary bilingual classroom. In: Padilla R, ed. Ethnoperspectives in bilingual education. Ypsilanti, MI: Eastern Michigan University, 1981.

Hamayan E. Assessment of language proficiency of exceptional bilingual students: an integrative approach. Workshop on communicative disorders and language proficiency: assessment, intervention, and curriculum implementation. Los Alamitos, CA: National Center for Bilingual Research, 1974.

Hamayan EV, Damico JS. Limiting bias in the assessment of bilingual students. Austin, TX: Pro-ed, 1991.

Haynes W, Saunders D, Anderson-Yockel J. Cultural and socioeconomic differences in mother-toddler joint book reading. Paper presented at the convention of the American Speech-Language-Hearing Association, San Antonio, TX, 1994.

Haynes W, Moran M. A cross-sectional developmental study of final consonant production in Southern Black children from preschool through third grade. Lang Speech Hear Serv Sch 1989;20: 400–406.

Heath S. Ways with words: language, life and work in communities and classrooms. Cambridge, England: Cambridge University Press, 1983.

Hester E. Narratives of young African-American children. In: Kamhi A, Pollock K, Harris J, eds. Communication development and disorders in African-American children: research, assessment and intervention. Baltimore, MD: Paul H. Brookes, 1996.

Hester E. The relationship between narrative style, dialect and reading ability of African-American Children. Unpublished doctoral dissertation. University of Maryland, College Park, 1994.

Huerta, A. The acquisition of bilingualism: a code-switching approach. Sociolinguist Work Pap 1977;39:1–33.

Huerta-Macias A. Codeswitching: all in the family. In: Duran R, ed. Latino Language and communicative behavior. Norwood, NJ: Ablex, 1981.

Hulley SB, Cummings SR, eds. Designing clinical research. Baltimore, MD: Williams & Wilkins, 1988.

Ingram D. Phonological disability in children. New York: Elsevier, 1976.

Kermoian R. Infant attachment to mother and child caretaker in an East African community. Ph.D. dissertation. Stanford University, Stanford, CA, 1982.

LeVine R, LeVine B. Nyansango: a Gusii community in Kenya. New York: John Wiley, 1966.

Kernan K, Blount BG. The acquisition of Spanish

grammar by Mexican children. Anthropol Linguist 1966;8:1–14.

Kvaal J, Shipstead-Cox N, Nevitt S, et al. The acquisition of 10 Spanish morphemes by Spanish-speaking children. Lang Speech Hear Serv Sch 1978;19:384–394.

Labov W. Contraction, deletion and inherent variability of the English copula. Language 1969; 45:715–762.

Leiderman, P. & Leiderman, G. Affective and cognitive consequences of polymatric care in the east African highlands. In: Peck A, ed. Minnesota symposia on child psychology. Vol. 8. 1974.

Langdon HW, ed. The Hispanic population: facts and figures. In: Hispanic children and adults with communication disorders: assessment and intervention. Gaithersburg, MD: Aspen, 1992.

Langdon HW, Merino BJ. Acquisition and development of a second language in the Spanish speaker. In: Langdon HW, ed. Hispanic children and adults with communication disorders: assessment and treatment. Gaithersburg, MD: Aspen, 1992.

Linares T, Orama N, Sanders LJ. Evaluation of syntax of three-year-old Spanish-speaking Puerto Rican children. J Speech Hear Res 1977;20: 350–357.

Macken M, Ferguson CA. Phonological universals in language acquisition. In: Winitz H, ed. Native language and language acquisition. New York: Annals of the New York Academy of Sciences, 1981.

Macken MA. Permitted complexity in phonological development: one child's acquisition of Spanish consonants. Lingua 1978;44:219–253.

Mattes LJ, Omark DR. Speech and language assessment for the bilingual handicapped. Austin, TX: Pro-ed, 1984.

McCallion M, Ford M, Haynes W. A preliminary study of final consonant production in Black and White children from grades K-6. Paper presented at the convention of the Georgia Speech and Hearing Association. Savannah, Ga, 1982.

McClure F. Formal and functional aspects of the codeswitched discourse of bilingual children. In: Duran R, ed. Latino language and communicative behavior. Norwood, NJ: Ablex, 1981.

Meara P. Vocabulary acquisition: a neglected aspect of language learning. In: Kinsella V, ed. Surveys 1. New York: Cambridge University Press, 1980.

Melville MR. Hispanics: race, class or ethnicity? J Ethnic Studies 1987;16:67–83.

Merino BJ. Language development in normal and language handicapped Spanish-speaking children. Hispanic J Behav Sci 1983;5:379–400.

Merino BJ. Language development in Spanish as a first language: implications for assessment. Paper presented at the National Conference on the Exceptional Bilingual Child, Phoenix, AZ, 1982 (October/November).

Merino BJ. Acquisition of syntactic and phonological features in Spanish. In: Langdon HW, ed. Hispanic children and adults with communication

disorders: assessment and intervention. Gaithersburg, MD: Aspen, 1992.

Nelson K. Structure and strategy in learning to talk. Monogr Soc Res Child Dev 1973;38:11–56.

Nicolosi L, Harryman E, Kresheck J. Terminology of communication disorders: speech-language-hearing. 3rd ed. Baltimore, MD: Williams & Wilkins, 1989.

Ochs E. Culture and language development: language acquisition and language socialization in a Samoan village. Cambridge, England: Cambridge University Press, 1988.

Owens R. Language development: an introduction. New York: Merrill, 1992.

Padilla A, Lindholm K. Acquisition of bilingualism: a descriptive analysis of the linguistic structures of Spanish/English speaking children. In: Keller G, ed. Bilingualism in the bicentennial and beyond. New York: Bilingual Review Press, 1976.

Pardo E. Acquisition of the Spanish reflexive: a study of a child's overextended forms. Unpublished doctoral dissertation. Stanford University, 1984.

Perez-Pereira M. The acquisition of morphemes: some evidence from Spanish. J Psycholinguist Res 1989;18:289–311.

Peters-Johnson C. Pragmatic development: cross-cultural or universal? In: Cole L, Deal VR, eds. Communication disorders in multicultural populations. Rockville, MD: American Speech-Language-Hearing Association(in press).

Poole E. Genetic development of articulation of consonant sounds in speech. Element Engl Rev 1934;11:159–161.

Poplack S. Syntactic structure and social function of code switching. In: Duran R, ed. Latino language and communicative behavior. Norwood, NJ: Ablex, 1981.

Prather E, Hedrick D, Kern C. Articulation development in children aged two to four years. J Speech Hear Disord 1975;40:179–191.

Rogoff B, Gardner W. Adult guidance of cognitive development. In: Rogoff B, Lave J, eds. Everyday cognition. Cambridge, MA: Harvard University Press, 1984.

Saville-Troike M. Anthropological considerations in the study of communication. In: Taylor O, ed. Nature of Communication disorders in culturally and linguistically diverse populations. San Diego, CA: College-Hill Press, 1986.

Schieffelin B. The acquisition of Kaluli. In: Slobin D, ed. The crosslinguistic study of linguistic acquisition. Vol. 1. Hillsdale, NJ: Lawrence Erlbaum, 1985.

Searle J. Speech acts. New York: Cambridge University Press, 1969.

Seymour H, Seymour C. Black English and Standard American English contrasts in consonantal development of four- and five-year-old children. J Speech Hear Disord 1981;46:274–280.

Slobin D. Cognitive prerequisites for the development of grammar. In: Ferguson C, Slobin D, eds. Studies of child language development. New York: Holt, Rinehart & Winston, 1973.

Steffensen M. The Acquisition of Black English. Unpublished doctoral dissertation. University of Illinois, Evanston, 1974.

Stockman I. Language acquisition in culturally diverse populations: the Black child as a case study. In: Taylor O, ed. Nature of communication disorders in culturally and linguistically diverse populations. San Diego, CA: College-Hill Press, 1986.

Stockman I. The development of linguistic norms for nonmainstream populations. Paper presented at the National Conference on Concerns for Minority Groups in Communication Disorders. Vanderbilt University, 1984.

Stockman I, Vaughn-Cooke F. Semantic categories in the language of working class Black children. In: Johnson C, Thew C, eds. Proceedings of the second international child language conference. Vol. 1. 1982; pp. 312–327.

Stockman I. Phonological development and disorders in African-American children. In: Kamhi A, Pollock K, Harris J, eds. Communication development and disorders in African-American children: research, assessment and intervention. Baltimore, MD: Paul H. Brookes, 1996.

Taylor O. Language differences. In: Shames G, Wiig E, eds. Human communication disorders: an introduction. Columbus, OH: Merrill, 1986.

Templin M. Certain language skills in children: their development and interrelationships. Minneapolis, MN: University of Minnesota Press, 1957.

Trevino FM. Standardized terminology for Hispanic populations. Am J Public Health 1987;77:69–72.

US Department of Health and Human Services. Health status of minorities and low income groups (DHHD Publication No. HRS-P-DV 85–1). Washington, DC: US Government Printing Office, 1985.

Venable G. A study of second language learning in children. Unpublished masters thesis. McGill University, 1974.

Valdes-Fallis G. Language diversity in Chicano speech communities: implications for language teaching. Working Papers Sociolinguist 1979;54:209–229.

Ventry IM, Schiavetti N. Evaluating research in speech pathology and audiology. 2nd ed. New York: Macmillan, 1986.

Vivas D. Order of acquisition of Spanish grammatical morphemes: comparison to some cross-linguistic methodological problems. Kansas Working Papers Linguist 1979;4:77–105.

Wetherby A, Cain D, Yonclas D, Walker V. Analysis of intentional communication of normal children from the prelinguistic to the multiword stage. J Speech Hear Res 1988;31:240–252.

Willis W. Families with African-American roots. In: Lynch E, Hanson M, eds. Developing cross-cultural competence. Baltimore: Paul H. Brookes, 1992.

Wolfram W, Fasold R. The study of social dialects in American English. Englewood Cliffs, NJ: Prentice-Hall, 1974.

Wyatt T. Linguistic constraints on copula production in Black English child speech. Paper presented to the Convention of the American Speech-Language-Hearing Association, Atlanta, GA, 1991.

Wyatt T. Acquisition of the African-American English copula. In: Kamhi A, Pollock K, Harris J, eds. Communication development and disorders in African-American children: research, assessment and intervention. Baltimore, MD: Paul H. Brookes, 1996.

Young V. Family and childhood in a southern Negro community. Am Anthropol 1970;72:269–287.

Zentella M. Code-switching in elementary level Puerto Rican children. Working Papers Sociolinguist 1978;43:112–145.

CHAPTER 15

Individual Differences in the Acquisition of Communication and Directions for Future Research

William O. Haynes

There was once a question on a graduate comprehensive examination that read: "Discuss and provide research evidence for the notion that children acquire language in basically the same way, only differently." Many students would read this question over several times before the "lightbulb" went on in their heads and they could formulate an appropriate answer. This question could create a bit of "cognitive dissonance" in readers of the present text, because when you reach this chapter, you should be feeling some degree of security in your knowledge about the normal process of communication development. In fact, we have devoted many pages of this book to pointing out trends and similarities in the communication development process and trying to consolidate information so it would be retrievable and useful. It is ironic that after describing the consistencies in communication development, that we must end with a chapter that suggests that the process is fraught with individual differences. Just as you begin to feel some confidence in your knowledge of the communication development process, the exceptions and variations are introduced, and the rug is pulled out from beneath

you. So it is with many complex processes; they are never as simple and straightforward as they may initially seem. However, lest the reader think that we will totally obviate the work reported in the previous chapters, there are several mitigating considerations: (1) The research on individual differences in communication development is only in its infancy. There are not many reports of such differences in the literature. (2) The research in the individual-differences literature has been confined to only a handful of areas; therefore the specific idiosyncratic patterns are few in number. In this chapter we will talk about the importance of considering individual differences in communication development and discuss the major areas in which research has suggested differences occur among children. We will also talk about the clinical applications of the individual-differences literature. Finally, we will provide a brief overview of the general trends in research on communication development.

INDIVIDUAL DIFFERENCES

Most early textbooks on communication development would not have included a section on individual differences. In the early treatments of communication development, authorities were actively searching for *common* threads and trends so that the normal developmental progression could be described and fully understood. Often, children who did not exhibit the typical acquisition pattern were excluded from investigations or perhaps even thought to be disordered. Researchers did not want to find differences, only similarities. Since the early 1970s, however, reports have steadily appeared in the research literature that describe numbers of children who appear to demonstrate specific identifiable patterns in communication development. The numbers of children are significant enough to suggest that they do not simply represent random variations in language development, but actual developmental patterns worthy of scientific scrutiny. Even prior to the appearance of research reports, however, clinicians routinely heard anecdotal reports from parents, colleagues, relatives, and friends who knew of a child that "did not talk until he was almost two, and then he talked in 'phrases'." Another common report was of children who began talking using pronouns instead of nouns. We have always been confronted with anecdotes of children with rates of communication development that were impressively fast or slow. For example, we often think of the child producing his or her first word near 1 year of age. Yet, there are many reports of children who say their first word at 8 or 9 months and other studies showing normal children who do not talk until they are 16 months old. There are cases of children combining words when they are 14 or 15 months old or before, while some language development books suggest that a child is about 2 years old before word combinations appear. Prior to the emergence of the individual-differences research, clinicians would often dismiss these reports as unreliable or untrue. Today, the notion of individual differences cannot be ignored. There is no question that they exist, the only mystery is determining all the extant patterns and the true extent of variability in normal communication development. At any rate, individual differences have always been with us, in every aspect of child development.

Differences in the First Lexicon: Expressive Versus Referential

In 1973 a seminal investigation by Katherine Nelson introduced the notion that not all children in the single-word period learned the same types of lexical items. Nelson studied 18 children from the time they were 1 year old until they were over the age of 2 by taking both maternal diary data and language samples. An especially interesting part of her investigation concerned the point at which these children were about 19 months old and had attained a lexicon of about 50 different words. Nelson analyzed these initial vocabularies and found that the children could be roughly divided into two groups depending on the percentage of general nominals (generally, common nouns) in their lexicons. Children whose number of general nominals constituted over 50% of their total vocabulary were called "referential," and those with general nominals accounting for less than 50% of their lexicon were called "expressive." The expressive children used many personal-social words, and the referential children used many nouns. This pattern of high and low use of nominals by different children has been noted in many studies (Bloom, 1973; Dore, 1974; Starr, 1975; Peters, 1977; Horgan, 1978, 1979, 1981; Lieven, 1980; Dellacorte, Benedict, & Klein, 1983; Goldfield, 1986, 1987). Snyder, Bates, and Bretherton (1981) found the expressive-referential distinction in children well before they reached 50-word vocabularies. They could see the patterns as young as 13 months when the children studied had only 10 to 12 words in their lexicons.

It should be emphasized early in this section that the categories of expressive and referential should not be viewed dichotomously. Indeed, most authorities indicate that expressive and referential probably represent extreme points on a continuum as opposed to separate classifications or typologies of language-developing children (Nelson, 1981; Goldfield & Snow, 1989; Bates, Bretherton, & Snyder, 1988; Nelson, Baker, Denninger, et al., 1985).

As research began to focus on expressive and referential children, it was found that certain characteristics, in addition to lexical composition, were often observed in these cases. For instance, referential children were reported to develop language earlier and faster than expressive ones (Nelson, 1973; Ramer, 1976; Horgan, 1978, 1979). Snyder, Bates, and Bretherton (1981) examined children in the single-word period and compared those developing language at earlier ages (precocious) with those who were acquiring words at later ages. They found that the most precocious children were those with the highest percentage of common nouns in their first lexicons, and this held true for both comprehension and production vocabularies. Also, the referential children tended to use words in context-flexible ways. For example, their word use was not as context bound. They would use a word to refer to many exemplars of an object, instead of using a word infrequently in only a narrowly defined context (e.g., use of ball only to refer to one ball). Horgan (1981) found that precocious children used more nouns and object descriptions, while the slowly developing children tended to be more cautious and less "risk-taking." For example, the precocious children were more willing to use language even if they made errors, while the slower children were more reluctant to attempt language they may have not been familiar with.

Another characteristic found in expressive and referential children to different degrees is the tendency to imitate the speech of adults. The research in this area, however, seems to reveal inconsistent results. Nelson (1973) reported a relationship between imitation and the expressive style of language development in that expressive children tended to be better imi-

tators of caretaker utterances. This observation has also been reported by other researchers (Bloom, Hood, & Lightbown, 1974; Clark, 1974; Ferguson & Farwell, 1975). Conversely, some studies suggest that the referential child is the better imitator of parental utterances (Leonard, Schwartz, Folger, et al., 1979; Nelson et al., 1985). Bates, Bretherton, and Snyder (1988) point out that some of the disagreement in the literature may stem from differing ages of subjects in these studies and/or from the various uses of imitation in interactions. For example, imitation can fulfill a number of functions such as memory, conversational place-holding, or repeating for analysis of new lexical items. Also, elicited imitation is quite different than spontaneous imitation. More research is needed to determine specific relationships between expressive and referential styles and imitation.

Some studies have indicated that children with expressive and referential styles may even behave differently in play interactions. Initially, Nelson (1973) suggested that certain children tended to focus on people and social interactions (expressive) and others arranged their play routines around objects (referential). Rosenblatt (1977) found that children who used higher percentages of general nominals persisted in toy and object play, had a higher visual attention to toys, and participated less in social interactions as compared with expressive children. Wolf and Gardner (1979) noted two varieties of symbolic play in children they studied longitudinally. One group of children was called "patterners" who concentrated on object characteristics and arrangements. These children had a large proportion of nominals in their vocabularies. The other group of children was named "dramatists" and was characterized as preferring social interactions with people and using certain toys in social exchanges (e.g., puppets, telephones). This group had a lesser percentage of nominals in their lexicons. There is some question in the literature concerning the use of objects. Object play can involve manipulation of toys as an end in itself, but it can also play a role in facilitating social interactions. Goldfield and Snow (1989) suggest that we must consider not just the number of nominals in the child's lexicon, but how these words are used in social interactions. For example, object words can be used for the purpose of instigating and maintaining social interactions with caretakers. Perhaps the joint attention of parent and child on objects is more important than the persistence of a child in object play or the amount of social-versus-object play behavior. In fact, Goldfield (1985) found that referential children did not focus on object play for longer periods to the exclusion of social interaction, but tended to use objects to initiate social interactions. This has also been suggested by Ross, Nelson, Wetstone, and Tanouye (1980).

There has been some speculation regarding the influence of parental interactions on expressive and referential styles. For instance, Nelson (1973) suggested that maternal style may be related to expressive/referential modes of lexical development in that some mothers tended to emphasize play with objects and others focused more on social interactions during play. Similarly, Furrow and Nelson (1984) found communicative function differences between mothers of expressive versus referential children. For example, mothers of referential children used more references to objects during interactions and mothers of expressive children referred more often to people. This occurred especially in the early portions of language development and a similar finding was reported by Klein (1980). Dellacorte, Benedict, and Klein (1983) did not find a difference in the actual language used by mothers (e.g., number of nominals used), but they did find that mothers of referential children talked more and used more descriptions than mothers of expressive children. Mothers of expressive children tended to use more commands than mothers of expressive children. In Chapter 5 we discussed play routines engaged in by mothers and babies, and it was noted that many of these

interactions involved naming or labeling games (e.g., joint book reading, naming body parts or objects, etc.). Many authorities have suggested that these naming games may be especially prevalent in mothers of referential children (Brown, 1973; Nelson & Bonvillian, 1972; Dore, 1974; Goldfield & Snow, 1989). Goldfield and Snow (1989, p.313) point out an interesting observation:

> A good deal of children's referential language, for example, may originate in certain routinized naming games. . . . Nelson (1973) also observed that 28 percent of the first 50 words acquired by referential children referred to body parts, almost surely learned in this kind of routine, whereas none of the expressive children had acquired labels for parts of the body. Expressive children, on the other hand, learn many conventional social expressions (e.g., "hi," "bye," "please," "thank you," "let's go," and "oh dear") that typically mark events such as arrivals, departures, and exchanges. Mothers of children with more expressive speech tend to use many such stereotypical utterances.

As the research continues to develop on the expressive-referential modes of early language development, it will probably be revealed that both elements within the child and maternal styles interact in formulating these styles. In fact, Goldfield and Snow (1989, p. 314) report the following:

> Goldfield (1987) found that children's lexical differences were best predicted by a combination of child and caregiver variables. More referential language was acquired by children who more often used objects to elicit maternal attention and who had mothers who more often labeled and described toys. More expressive speech was acquired by children in dyads ranking low on these two measures. Children in mixed dyads (mother ranking high, child ranking low; child ranking high, mother ranking low) acquired a relatively balanced distribution of object labels and expressive speech.

More research is also needed to determine exactly how far these early styles of communication development extend into later periods of learning language.

Nominal and Pronominal Strategies

Nelson (1973) also noted that some children in her sample tended to use more pronouns than others. Some children used nouns to refer to people and objects, while others used more pronouns. The distinction between these groups has become known as nominal versus pronominal. The fact that some children exhibit a preference for either nouns or pronouns to refer to people and objects has been noted by many researchers (Peters, 1977; Branigan, 1977; Goldfield, 1982; Nelson, 1975, 1981; Bloom, Lightbown, & Hood, 1975). An interesting observation about the nominal-pronominal distinction is that it appears to be generally related to the referential-expressive styles of communication development. For example, Nelson (1975) found that expressive children exhibited a balance between nouns and pronouns in their early multiword combinations, while the referential children showed a clear preference for combining nominals.

A classic study by Bloom, Lightbown, and Hood (1975) examined the development of four children as their MLU progressed from 1.0 to 2.5. They found that all four children exhibited similar semantic knowledge (e.g., they talked about the same types of objects and events); however, the linguistic means of representing this knowledge differed among the subjects. Two children used a nominal system to refer to objects and events, and the other two children developed a pronominal system of reference. This means that nominal children constructed utterances using nouns (e.g., hit ball; Johnny go; want milk), and pronominal children used more pronouns (e.g., hit it; you go; want that). As these two groups of children were followed over time, it was noted that the two styles of reference began to change as the MLU approached 2.5. At the attainment of 2.5 MLU the nominal children tended to become progressively more pronominal, and the pronominal

children used significantly more nominals in their utterances. In other words, the children learned the alternate strategy as their communication development progressed.

There have been other characteristics that have been associated with nominal and pronominal styles. For instance, the pronominal children (who also tend to be expressive) have a higher incidence of using "phrases" as early as the single-word period. These children are reported to use multiword combinations such as "stop it," "I love you," or "Do it again." These multiword combinations are not thought of as generative by most authorities and are considered to be formulas or unanalyzed wholes having no real syntactic organization (Nelson et al., 1985; Nelson, 1973; Bates, Bretherton, & Snyder, 1988). The use of formulaic speech is rarely reported in children who are described as referential/nominal.

Another characteristic seen in pronominal children is their reported use of "dummy terms" to extend their utterance length. Many of these dummy terms were referred to in Chapter 9 where we referred to them as transitional phenomena (e.g., "Mommy wida"). Some authorities have suggested that pronominal children tend to rely more on limited scope formulas such as "more + X" or "that + X" more than nominal children (Braine, 1976; Bates, Bretherton, & Snyder 1988). This is related to the use of formulas since the child may be producing an utterance that he/she has not analyzed in terms of its component parts and how they fit together. Another related aspect seen in pronominal children is the frequently reported use of later developing grammatical morphemes during early periods of language development. For example, there have been many reports of pronominal children using function words such as articles, pronouns, auxiliary verbs, question forms, and prepositions (Brannigan, 1977; Horgan, 1978; Ramer, 1976; Nelson, 1975). All of the examples in this paragraph suggest that the pronominal/expressive child learns language by concentrating on larger units (e.g., phrases) rather than focusing on single categories like the referential/nominal child. The notion of larger units is also reflected in the fact that pronominal/expressive children are noted for using intonation patterns that suggest they are attempting to reproduce phrases or multiword utterances, while the referential/nominal child is not typically reported to produce utterances that have phraselike intonation contours (Dore, 1974; Peters, 1977). There have also been reports that pronominal/expressive children tend to be less intelligible due to phonological instability or deletions (Branigan, 1977; Ferguson & Farwell, 1975; Nelson, 1973; Peters, 1977).

In an effort to summarize and consolidate some of the information discussed above we refer to Table 15.1 taken from Bates et al. (1988). The table lists a combination of empirical findings coupled with more anecdotal claims of authorities found in the individual differences literature. Bates et al. (1988) suggest a "Two-Strand Theory," which implies that two basic patterns exist in the individual-differences literature that cut across all the language domains and have particular demographic characteristics. Not all authorities would agree with such a formulation (e.g., Wells, 1986), but Bates et al. (1988, p. 55) are clear on the tentative nature of their theory:

> But the apparent unit in [the] table . . . is still a matter of speculation. The Two-Strand claim rests on the results of many separate studies, most of them based on only a small subset of these many and disparate variables, usually with a small sample of children, studied over a relatively brief span of development. An adequate test of the theory requires a unified study, examining all (or most) of these factors in a single sample of children, across the relevant age range.

In fact, Bates et al. provided only partial support for a two-strand theory in a unified test of this hypothesis and suggest that ". . . . the total picture is much more complex (p. 273)." Table 15.1, however, does provide an interesting juxtaposition of existing data and speculation.

Hypotheses About Early Communication Development Styles

Researchers have used a variety of terms to refer to the children characterized in the preceding portion of this chapter. Some of the labels they use are shown in Table 15.2. Many language theorists have pondered the possible reasons for the communication styles listed above. Figure 15.1 from Wells (1986) depicts some of the pertinent areas that may relate to the development of individual differences. One of the better summaries of the explanations can be found in Bates, Bretherton, and Snyder (1988). Bates et al. (1988) review theories that break down into the following four areas: social explanations, linguistic explanations, neurologic explanations, and cognitive explanations. Some of these explanations have rather obvious and understandable connections to the two communication styles, while other theories are more arcane and require much reading in linguistic and information processing theory. Basically, however, it seems reasonable to suggest that some of the explanations rely on external influences, and other theories reflect internal tendencies. For instance, such variables as maternal interaction style, maternal linguistic input, and social class represent external factors that could influence a child toward becoming expressive or referential. We have mentioned some studies that suggest mothers of expressive and referential children may talk differently to them and might emphasize objects or social interactions in play. The present state of research, however, does not permit us to conclude that these environmental influences are responsible for the expressive/referential styles of communication development.

There are also internal influences such as the infant's innate temperamental makeup, hemispheric processing style (right or left brain), and cognitive style (analytic versus gestalt; part versus whole). We know that there are certain

Table 15.1   Individual Differences in Language Development: Summary of Claims in the Literature

Strand 1	Strand 2
Semantics	
High proportion of nouns in first 50 words	Low proportion of nouns in first 50 words
Single words in early speech	Formulae in early speech
Imitates object names	Unselective imitation
Greater variety within lexical categories	Less variety within lexical categories
Meaningful elements only	Use of "dummy" words
High adjective use	Low adjective use
Context-flexible use of names	Context-bound use of names
Rapid vocabulary growth	Slower vocabulary growth
Grammar	
Telegraphic in Stage I	Inflections and function words in Stage I
Refers to self and others by name in Stage I	Refers to self and others by pronoun in Stage I
Noun-phrase expansion	Verb phrase expansion
Morphological overgeneralization	Morphological undergeneralization
Consistent application of rules	Inconsistent application of rules
Novel combinations	Frozen forms
Imitation is behind spontaneous speech	Imitation is ahead of spontaneous speech
Fast learner	Slow learner
Pragmatics	
Object-oriented	Person-oriented
Declarative	Imperative
Low variety in speech acts	High variety in speech acts
Phonology	
Word-oriented	Intonation-oriented
High intelligibility	Low intelligibility
Segmental emphasis	Suprasegmental emphasis
Consistent pronunciation across word tokens	Variable pronunciation across word tokens
Demographic Variables	
Female	Male
Firstborn	Later-born
Higher SES	Lower SES

Reprinted with permission from Bates E, Bretherton I, Snyder L. From first words to grammar: individual differences and dissociable mechanisms. New York: Cambridge University Press, 1988.

| Table 15.2. Various Terms Used by Researchers to Describe "Expressive" and "Referential" Patterns of Development |||
Terms		Source
Expressive	Referential	Nelson (1973)
Intonation baby	Word baby	Dore (1974)
Synthesizer	Analyzer	Bloom et al. (1975)
Gestalt	Analytic	Peters (1977)
Dramatists	Patterners	Wolf and Gardner (1979)
Message oriented	Code oriented	Dore (1974)
Noun leavers	Noun lovers	Horgan (1978)
Pronominal	Nominal	Bloom et al. (1975)

children who appear to be more "social" from birth, and neonatal temperamental scales may show them to be different on such variables as approach/withdrawal or sociability. In Chapter 2 we reviewed much literature suggesting that the right and left hemispheres of the brain act as different types of information processors. The right hemisphere tends to be more gestalt and holistic, while the left is more analytic and segmental. The parallels are striking when one applies some of the neurologic-organization literature to expressive and referential styles of language development. Perhaps some children tend to process language more right hemispherically and thus attend to intonation patterns and formulas that are "wholes" or gestalts. Other children may process it more left hemispherically and attend to the segments (words and syllables) as opposed to the gestalt. It is inter-

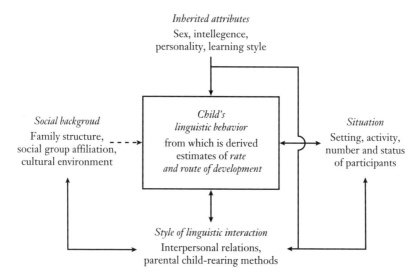

Figure 15.1. Types of variation. *Dashed arrow*, indirect influence; *solid arrow*, direct influence. (From Wells G. Variation in child language. In: Fletcher P, Garman N, eds. Language acquisition: studies in first language development. Cambridge, England: Cambridge University Press, 1986; p. 112.)

esting to speculate on the possible extent of various internal influences on early communication development style, but we must remember that at present no one knows with any certainty about these relationships.

Two other interesting parallels have been suggested, which relate to the expressive/referential styles of communication development. First, there have been reports that adults and children learning second languages tend to fall into categories that seem to fit the analytic/holistic notions. Hatch (1974) found people learning second languages to represent what he called "rule learners" (referential) and "data gatherers" (expressive). Fillmore (1979) also noted that some children learning a second language were adept at learning formulas and experimenting with syntax, while others were more rigid and tended to work on one construction at a time until it was learned well prior to use. These characteristics were reported earlier in the nominal/pronominal groups of children learning a first language. The fact that second-language learners persist in these strategies may also point to either internal mechanisms or the nature of language itself in accounting for individual differences in learning style. There have even been reports of children mastering different skills within their own language (e.g., reading) that show disparate styles of learning analogous to expressive/referential (Bussis, Chittenden, Amarel, and Klausner (1984). Another interesting parallel is the possible relationship between nominal/pronominal style and socioeconomic class. Bates, Bretherton, and Snyder (1988) indicate that there is some evidence that lower socioeconomic class and lower educational levels may be associated to a greater extent with the pronominal/expressive style of communication development. A similar suggestion was made by Nelson (1973). Sociolinguists have long noted that lower socioeconomic class members tend to use a restricted code as opposed to an elaborated code. While this is still speculative, it is interesting in terms of potential influences caretakers may have on their children's learning styles.

The Case of "Late Bloomers"

Children who reach the age of 2 years with significant delays in expressive language, despite normal cognitive, auditory, structural, and language comprehension abilities, have been the subject of much research. These children usually have less than a 50-word lexicon and no evidence of multiword combinations at age 2. Some authorities suggest that as many as 50% of these children will be at-risk for language delay persisting beyond their third birthday, while the other 50% may "catch up" and exhibit near-normal communication at age 3. This latter group has been called "late bloomers" or "late talkers." The existence of late bloomers raises a question about whether this pattern of language acquisition found in so many children by different researchers represents an individual difference in communication development. A series of studies suggests that there are some variables that can distinguish late bloomers from those children who will not grow out of their language delay (Thal & Tobias, 1992, 1994; Rescorla & Goossens, 1992; Paul & Jennings, 1992; Weismer, Branch, & Miller, 1994). Generally, the children whose language is likely to develop normally after age 3 have no family history of language impairment, higher frequency of communication acts, more mature syllable structure, larger phonetic inventories, high language comprehension scores, and higher levels of symbolic and combinatorial play. As more children fitting this pattern are identified clinically and through research, the "late bloomer" pattern may come to be viewed as one of many "normal tracks" of language development.

Phonetic and Phonological Variations

Earlier we made the point that children representing expressive and referential communication development styles are thought to differ in general intelligibility. The expressive child tends to be less intelligible than the referential child (Nelson, 1981; Peters, 1977; Branigan, 1977; Horgan, 1979, 1981; Ferguson, 1984; Ferguson & Farwell, 1975; Leonard, Newhoff, & Masalem, 1980). As Bates, Bretherton, and Snyder (1988) suggest, this does not necessarily mean that the expressive child is not adept at phonology, but could indicate that they are simply concentrating on different aspects of the communication signal such as intonation contours at higher linguistic levels. Also, since these children are prone to develop formulas, their length of utterance is greater than referential children who are concentrating on single-word production. It is well established that misarticulations tend to increase with added linguistic complexity and length (Panagos, Quine, & Klich, 1979; Haynes, Haynes, & Jackson, 1982). At any rate, there are individual variations in levels of intelligibility among children in development.

Researchers in phonology have also reported that children exhibit variations in the use of certain phonological processes. For instance, Ingram (1976, p. 31) discussed the process of reduplication (e.g., wawa for water; dada for daddy) and said, ". . . . children do vary in their use of it." That is, some children use the reduplication strategy often and others have little evidence of the process. This has also been reported by Ferguson, Peizer, and Weeks, 1973). Other researchers in the area of normal and deviant phonology have reported the existence of "idiosyncratic processes" or "phonological preferences" in the speech of individual children that, on the surface, appear to be random productions, yet when examined more closely are highly systematic (Ferguson, 1979; Weiner, 1981; Maxwell & Rockman, 1984). Ferguson (1979, p.191) discusses the individual variation associated with dialects and goes on to say the following:

> Some individual differences in phonology, however, are not of the dialectal type but are more clearly idiosyncratic and have such sources as accidents of language input, anatomical and physiological characteristics, different learning strategies and pho-

nological hypotheses, or personality characteristics. . . . The position I am assuming in this paper is that every user of a language variety develops over time his own inventory of phonetic elements, the phonological organization of them, and a set of processes applied to them, and this phonological development begins at or before birth and continues until death.

The term "idiosyncratic" in itself implies individual difference or variation. These individual differences are of interest to phonologists mainly because they are not the typical phonological alterations produced by most children. Some of these phonological productions are deviant; however, others may well be just infrequently occurring patterns of normal development. Interestingly, there has been an increasing number of case studies and articles in the literature and in convention presentations that purport to show an "unusual" phonological system in a child. As these reports continue to accrue, it is instructive that we are beginning to see repetitions of patterns previously noted, which makes one wonder if these idiosyncratic processes are really so unusual. As the research begins to report uncommon patterns more frequently, they may actually form various subgroups of phonological production that is not as idiosyncratic as we once had imagined.

Lest the reader think that the individual-differences literature is without controversy, we should point out here that this is not the case. For instance, Wells (1986) has suggested several methodological considerations in the individual-differences literature. First, he suggests that researchers may have difficulty obtaining reliable data. The samples obtained in any language research depend to a large extent on the presence of observers, identity of participants (parent versus experimenter), and the artificiality of the testing context. A child may not interact the same in a strange laboratory setting as he does at home in familiar surroundings. Most of the studies included children who were socially homogeneous, and this ignores the sociocultural aspects of variation. Another problem was the representativeness of the samples obtained. Most of the individual-difference studies have used small numbers of subjects, and we really have no idea about the size of these subgroups in the general population of children developing communication. Finally, there is often incomplete agreement on the quantification of linguistic data in terms of deciding what to count and the criteria used for deciding if a particular aspect of communication is acquired. All of these factors can cause variability in the results of studies and distortion in our theoretical formulations. Wells (1986, p. 117) states the following:

> Thus, if it is an essential prerequisite of work on variation in child language that the data for study should be obtained in such a way that they meet the criteria that have just been discussed, it must be concluded that there is as yet little or no research in this field that will support any confident generalization.

It is also instructive to remember that most researchers in the area of individual differences refer to a continuum on which children may exhibit more or less of the referential/nominal or expressive/pronominal characteristics. In fact, most children show evidence of both strategies to some extent. Bretherton, McNew, Snyder, and Bates (1983, p. 312) suggest, "many children balance both strategies; none use one to the exclusion of the other." It could very well be that these "styles" may vary situationally with different stimuli, tasks, and familiarity with participants. Evidently, all children have both capabilities, and they seem to appear in different proportions in the various studies that have been reported. Perhaps some of the individual differences reported in studies can be partially accounted for by methodological artifacts. Wells (1986, p. 139) comes to the following conclusion:

> . . . in many cases where such oppositions have been proposed the categories identified by the two ends of the continuum will both be required if the child is to develop as a normal language user. Both nouns and

pronouns are necessary in mature speech, as are the functional uses indicated by such terms as "expressive" and "referential." The same is true of the strategies labeled "analytic" and "holistic." Both are necessary if the child is to construct his language on the evidence of the speech addressed to him. Differences of these kinds between individuals, therefore, can only be relative: a matter of timing and emphasis rather than of presence or absence.

INDIVIDUAL DIFFERENCES IN THE LANGUAGE-IMPAIRED CHILD

If normal children exhibit individual variation in communication development, one can almost guarantee that language-impaired children will show such differences to an even greater extent. Muma (1986, p. 99) states: "Needless to say, individual differences are even greater in clinical populations such as language disorders, aphasia, mental retardation, and hearing impairment." The language-impaired population is an extremely heterogeneous group due to the wide variety of cognitive, social, linguistic, and physiological differences that may play a role in their disorder. They not only have the same tendencies that normally developing children show, but they also must compensate for a variety of differences in the processes that underlie language. It is not surprising then that researchers have found many patterns of language impairment in children. An early example of individual differences in language-impaired children was reported by Aram and Nation (1975). These researchers examined 47 children between the ages of 3 and 7 who were diagnosed as language disordered. The children were given tests that employed a variety of response modes, including imitation, comprehension, and spontaneous formulation of language. Each response mode was used to test a child's facility with semantic elements, syntax, and phonology. The test scores were then subjected to statistical analyses that delineated patterns of performance or subgroups of language-impaired children within the total population tested. Aram and Nation found that there were distinct subgroups of language impairment depending on the response mode and the type of linguistic element tested. For example, there were children who were performing well in comprehension and poorly in production. There was also the opposite pattern in which a group of children had strengths in production that they did not show in comprehension. There were other differences in terms of linguistic areas. For instance, one pattern of performance showed strength in phonology but low performance in other areas. Another pattern showed high imitative ability, but low abilities in spontaneous production. This study did not test pragmatics, but we know that some language-impaired children have strengths or weaknesses in this area as well. Chapman and Nation (1981) performed a similar study on educable mentally retarded children with language impairments and found similar patterns of individual difference. Wolfus, Moskovitch, and Kinsbourne (1980) studied 20 children between the ages of 4 and 7. After administering a variety of tests to the group these researchers also reported different types of language disorder. They concluded that the language-impaired children did not comprise a homogeneous population. One subgroup was termed "expressives" who had difficulty with syntactic production; however, their comprehension was within normal limits. Another group was "expressive-receptives" who had trouble in both areas. While we must be extremely cautious in the interpretation of the studies mentioned above in terms of specific typologies of language-impaired children, the main point is that they all found high individual variability in the population. Thus research supports the notion that individual differences are present in language-impaired children just as they are in normally developing youngsters.

LANGUAGE-IMPAIRED CHILDREN: ASSESSMENT APPLICATIONS

The obvious clinical assessment application of individual differences in the language-impaired population is that the speech-language pathologist must examine a variety of performance areas in these children. If a language-impaired child can have deficits in different modes of responding (imitation, comprehension, production), then the clinician must be certain to evaluate these avenues of language use. For instance, it would be important for a clinician to not omit comprehension testing with a language-impaired child and just perform a spontaneous language sample to determine language ability. It is possible that the child could be experiencing comprehension problems that might be overlooked if only production were evaluated. While some tests of language are based on imitation (Carrow, 1974; Zachman, Huisingh, Jorgensen, & Barrett, 1978), it is well known that reliance on imitation alone could grossly underestimate or overestimate a child's language ability. Thus the clinician must test language in a variety of response modes to be sure that individual variations in communication ability are evaluated.

A similar argument could be made for examining the various domains of language in a child with a linguistic impairment. For example, a child could have an almost normal vocabulary, but inadequate syntax. Another child's syntax might be relatively intact, but the phonological system may be deficient. There are children with quite normal vocabulary, syntax, and phonology who have abnormal pragmatic abilities. Thus it is important in an assessment to examine semantic, syntactic, phonological, and pragmatic areas of language because of individual differences in the adequacy of these domains in disordered children. In children who are nonverbal we must also be careful to note individual differences in cognitive abilities and social skills as these areas relate to communication.

Individual differences may be especially important in dealing with older children with language disorders. Many of these children have been diagnosed as learning disabled, and many learning disabilities have a basis in impaired abilities to deal with linguistic information. The learning-disabled child requires an extremely careful evaluation because, in addition to potential problems with all of the domains of language mentioned above, we must evaluate the child's ability to solve problems using language. These children may have difficulty with attending, listening to, remembering, and evaluating information presented in classrooms. The learning-disabled child may also demonstrate a variety of problems with producing language in such a way that the listener can understand the message. Some common problem areas include difficulties in sequencing and organization, producing an utterance that is specifically tailored for a particular listener and context, staying on a conversational topic, and knowing how to introduce a new topic of discussion. In addition to the possible problems with expression and comprehension of language, the older learning-disabled child may have difficulty using language especially for academic purposes. This requires strategies for organization, memorization, and retrieval of verbally presented information. Communication in the classroom also requires the child to use written language and gain information through reading as well as listening. Some of the classroom work involves metalinguistic skill and a knowledge of language so intimate that one can examine it as an object of study and manipulate it in various ways. Each language-learning disabled child in the schools may present a slightly different individual pattern of abilities and impairments. Some can listen, but not read well, while others have the opposite problem. There are children who have such difficulty with learning that they must consciously learn specific strategies or study skills to facilitate their academic progress. The diagnostician must be canny indeed to adequately describe the individual patterns of communication use in older, disordered children.

Another issue to be considered in assessment is the use of formal, standard-ized tests versus more descriptive, language sampling procedures. It has long been known that formal tests tend to obscure individual differences and highlight group similarity (Muma, 1973). When we give a language-impaired child a standardized test, we are not observing his individual differences, but rather seeing how he compares in performance with a normative sample. Most tests assume that children perform, react, and learn alike. If we consider individual differences present in normally developing children, it is clear that there are many ways to effectively process information, communicate, learn concepts, and behave in testing situations. Diagnosticians must always remember that individual differences, which may be important to consider in treatment, may be obscured by administrations of tests that reduce communication down to a handful of scores. This is why nonstandardized testing has gained popularity over the past 20 years and informal measures are preferred by clinicians for pointing the direction of intervention (Haynes & Pindzola, 1997).

Even normal children differ in terms of the ways they process linguistic information; however, language-impaired children represent an even more heterogeneous group because they have the normal individual differences plus the strategies they have developed to compensate for their impairments. This is a challenge for the speech-language pathologist in assessment.

LANGUAGE-IMPAIRED CHILDREN: TREATMENT APPLICATIONS

Perhaps the clearest treatment application of the individual differences in literature would be that it is not practical to develop programs that are highly generic for developing communication in language-impaired children. The notion that any child with a language impairment could be "plugged into" an existing program is rather naive. Since we know that each child with a language impairment has individual strengths and weaknesses, it is important to incorporate these into the treatment program. Each child with a language impairment will respond to differing types of cues from a clinician to elicit the appropriate language. One implication of the existence of individual differences and strategies in communication is that the clinician can choose to capitalize on the child's tendencies, as opposed to eradicating them. For example, a clinician might be teaching language to a child who tends to be socially oriented and appears to communicate most in the context of interacting with people. The clinician could easily say that this child needs to learn words for objects and try to make this child more referential in nature. This is not necessarily a positive way to increase the child's use of language and initiation of communicative interactions. The child may learn more language and increase his communication if the clinician understands that he may well have tendencies rather similar to normally developing, expressive and referential children. The important aspect of treatment would be to increase the child's communication attempts and initiations and expand the lexicon to allow the child to refer to features in the environment that are of interest to him or her. Interestingly, Weiss, Leonard, Rowan, and Chapman (1983) found that language-impaired children *do* exhibit expressive and referential patterns similar to those found in normally developing children. They noted that the normally developing children manifested the referential and expressive styles in silent play, as well as when they were verbalizing. For instance, the normally developing, referential children became more object oriented during silent play, and the expressives were more people oriented during these periods. In the language-impaired group the expressive and referential styles were manifested mainly during verbal interactions and not necessarily during silent play periods, suggesting that in the language-impaired population the style might be ".... best characterized as a language specific phenomenon rather than as a more general manner of dealing with the world (p. 161)." Weiss et al. (1983) suggest that it may be important to take into consideration a child's linguistic as well as play orientation in designing a treatment program. For example, they state the following (p. 161):

> Should our findings be replicated, it would appear that the child with a specific language impairment who exhibits a clearly referential style may be more likely to play with the objects used in therapy activities rather than with people who are present . . . one method of utilizing the style information would be to provide opportunities for the child to engage in object-related activities in therapy such as picture and object naming, possibly in an individual therapy setting and less probably in a group treatment situation . . . the expressive speaker might prefer experiential activities where role-playing tasks and routines are introduced. This child might find a group therapy situation best suited to his/her social-interaction orientation.

The researchers go on to say that while it may be important to take into account a child's style, it is also important that the clinician not neglect introducing material that represents the opposite style. They indicate that it could be "potentially detrimental" to language learning to persist in only one style.

While we have a long way to go in determining the optimal treatment uses of the individual differences literature, we know that it has important potential clinical impact. The more in tune we are with the child's idiosyncratic ways of processing information and learning, the greater will be our ability to customize our treatment offerings so maximum gains can take place.

DIRECTIONS FOR FUTURE RESEARCH

At the conclusion of almost every research report is a ubiquitous statement suggesting that further research is necessary. There is no area in communication development about which we do not need more information. Each area covered in the present text has avenues of research that have just begun to be traversed by scientists. We could easily reiterate the research needs in such areas as cognition, information processing, social development, affect, linguistics, child development, play, sociolinguistics, and many others. The knowledge base is especially lacking with regard to how these areas and others interact to affect communication development. Even if we had enough basic data on one of the above developmental areas, then we would certainly require more research on how to assess this behavior in the clinic and how to facilitate its growth in treatment. In the sections that follow, we will attempt to elucidate some of the general areas in communication development that represent gaps in the existing research and possible directions for further empirical development. The focus will be general as opposed to specific since some narrow areas of further research have already been mentioned in prior chapters.

Large Group Studies

Probably the most widely used norms on Mean Length of Utterance (MLU) are based on the performance of 123 largely middle-class children from a city in the Midwest (Miller & Chapman, 1981). These children represented ages between 18 months and 5 years, which means that some age levels had small numbers of subjects. These data were sorely needed for use in research in communication development and disorders. While the above study made a significant contribution, it is important that we obtain data from larger groups of children who represent different geographic areas and cultural groups (Wells, 1986; Hardy-Brown, 1983). If we are going to gain an appreciation of the variability in any aspect of communication development, we need to have more large-scale studies that provide mean and standard deviation data. The data on variability are used to determine if a child is significantly delayed in the development of communication or just representing the slower end of the acquisition contin-

uum. Studies using small samples are important in providing detailed descriptions of individual differences in development, which can then be validated by larger sample investigations as was done in the work on acquisition of grammatical morphemes. After the initial work of Brown (1973), who followed children's morphological development longitudinally, larger-scale studies confirmed the order of acquisition found in the smaller-sample work (DeVilliers & DeVilliers, 1973). Most of the individual differences discussed in the present chapter were initially uncovered by examining the behavior of individual children or small samples of children. The majority of investigators now affirm that unquestionably individual differences exist, and the primary emphasis now is to determine the causes of these variations in terms of social, cognitive, affective, and demographic variables. Statistical analysis is especially well suited to investigating the covariation of subject characteristics and environmental attributes to determine the possible multivariate influences on communication development. Small-sample designs are especially vulnerable to a variety of statistical errors that may make it impossible to detect relationships among variables or to find relations by chance if multiple procedures are used. Additionally, small sample sizes make it extremely difficult to replicate results from one study to another. Hardy-Brown (1983) makes an impressive case for the extreme variability and lack of replicability in the results of small-sample studies. For example, Hardy-Brown (1983, p. 616) states the following:

> The analysis of large numbers of interdependent behaviors within a single mother-child pair can provide excellent information about that pair and will contribute important guidelines concerning measurements within such dyads that can be translated into larger scale studies. We must not be lead to conclude prematurely, however, that interaction patterns documented for one or two mother-child pairs will necessarily characterize most other mother-child pairs.

She also advocates the use of twin and adoption experimental designs to disentangle the effects of genetic and environmental influences on individual differences in communication development.

Interactions of Variables in Communication Development

In studying any aspect of communication it is rare to find that the object of investigation is influenced by only one variable. For instance, the age-old "nature versus nurture" issue is typically resolved by authorities who indicate that there are clear influences from both directions. We know that the genetic makeup of a child as well as the environment play major roles in the development of almost all phenomena we study. There are many types of interactions that can take place in development. First, one domain of development can affect another. We know that motor skill, for instance, has an impact on the development of social behavior (moving toward others), cognitive development (manipulation of objects), and language development (articulating sounds). A second way to look at this is also from the point of view that various internal and external influences affect motor skill development. For instance, there are neurological as well as structural changes that take place within the body that allow for more sophisticated movement patterns, but also the environment provides a variety of objects and obstacles that facilitate practice in motor skills. While early studies in communication development often focused on the development of single aspects of communication, more recent research has considered the multiple developments during periods of growth and how these acquisitions relate to one another. Other research is dedicated to uncovering the multiple internal and external influences on communication development such as the combined effect of temperament, language stimulation, and cognition on a specific aspect of language acquisition. More research is needed before we understand the influence of one domain on another and the impact of genetic and environmental factors on communication development. This is exactly the kind of research that is beginning to emerge.

Individual Differences Research

As mentioned above, we have just begun to identify individual differences in communication development. Individual case studies followed by a re-analysis of subjects showing variability in large-sample investigations may unearth more patterns or subgroups of development in cognition, language, and social growth. Since there is research in progress around the world, it would be ideal if scientists would make available specific data on their subjects to data consortiums or provide access to aspects of their data through other means to interested researchers. Unfortunately, the information obtained from most studies is only a small proportion of the possible knowledge that could be gleaned from multiple analyses of the same data. These heterometric procedures could examine data for a variety of issues. For instance, the same mother-child dyads could be examined for play, language models, child language production, phonology, nonverbal communication, affect, and many other aspects related to communicative development. Also, if similar methodologies were used in several studies, the data might be combined to create a larger number of subjects for large-scale statistical analyses. Work has already begun on collective use of data in a number of fields including communication development.

Ethnic and Cultural Variations

For decades sociolinguists have reported language differences among members of various ethnic and cultural groups. These communication differences span all domains of language, including semantics, syntax, morphology, phonology, and pragmatics. While we are aware of cultural differences, we know almost nothing about the *development* of communication in most of these diverse ethnic or cultural groups. These data would be important not only for basic knowledge about how communication develops, but also for use in assessment decisions. For example, young children who are developing Black English are often compared with middle-class, white, Midwestern subjects by using normative data that were generated from the latter group. This occurs because there are few large-scale studies available that included substantial subgroups of minority populations, and there are also no major research reports on the communication development of exclusively minority subjects. Speech-language pathologists must deal with a difficult task in terms of differential diagnosis when confronted with minority children. There are not only the dialectal variations associated with social classes and geographic regions, but also the many ethnic languages that abound in the United States. We have a great deal of information about the characteristics of adult speakers of various dialects, but little data regarding how children gradually develop the features of these varieties of language. Research on the development of these dialects will make the evaluation of minority children an easier task and reduce the cultural bias that exists in our current modes of testing.

Applied Clinical Research

When research questions are asked that directly deal with assessment and treatment of a communication disorder, it is in the province of applied research. More "basic" research has been cited throughout the present text that describes the nature of language and its development. However, we are in need of more research that focuses on valid and reliable ways to measure the phenomena of communication development for use in clinical assessment and measuring treatment progress. When a researcher asks about the effectiveness of treatment methods or attempts to compare methods for efficiency and impact, or if a study focuses on the interjudge reliability of a number of assessment methods, it constitutes applied clinical research. We need more research on the efficacy of early interven-

tion, the ways that communication behaviors generalize to nontreatment environments, or the generalization that occurs when one aspect of language is trained and a second, untrained feature improves spontaneously. Other issues might concern the characteristics of particular, language-impaired children as they relate to specific types of treatment. In other words, do certain subgroups of language-impaired children respond to one type of treatment better than another? Another area could be clinician characteristics and how they affect child performance. Research on parental involvement and the impact of the home environment on response to treatment or development of language impairments is one more area where gaps exist. We could name many other aspects of assessment and treatment that could be explored in the next decade, but the point is that the research has begun in multiple areas, and as the communication development literature grows, so too will the applied clinical research. As soon as researchers find new aspects of development, or better understand the old aspects, other scientists are applying the information to clinical work.

REFERENCES

Aram D, Nation J. Patterns of language behavior in children with developmental language disorders. J Speech Hear Res 1975;18:229–241.

Bates E, Bretherton I, Snyder L. From first words to grammar: individual differences and dissociable mechanisms. New York: Cambridge University Press, 1988.

Bloom L. One word at a time: the use of single word utterances before syntax. The Hague: Mouton, 1973.

Bloom L, Hood L, Lightbown L. Imitation in language development: if, when and why? Cognit Psychol 1974;6:380–420.

Bloom L, Lightbown L, Hood L. Structure and variation in child language. Monogr Soc Res Child Dev 1975;40:Serial No. 160.

Braine M. Children's first word combinations. Monogr Soc Res Child Dev 1976;41:1, Serial No. 164.

Branigan G. If this kid is in the one word stage, so how come he's saying whole sentences? Paper presented at the Second Annual Boston University Conference on Language Development, Boston, 1977.

Brown R. A first language: the early stages. Cambridge, MA: Harvard University Press, 1973.

Bretherton I, McNew S, Snyder L, Bates E. Individual differences at 20 months: analytic and holistic strategies in language acquisition. J Child Lang 1983;10:293–320.

Bussis A, Chittenden E, Amarel M, Klausner E. Inquiry into meaning: an investigation of learning to read. Hillsdale, NJ: Erlbaum, 1984.

Carrow E. Carrow-elicited language inventory. Austin, TX: Learning Concepts, 1974.

Chapman D, Nation J. Patterns of language performance in educable mentally retarded children. J Commun Disord 1981;14:245–254.

Clark R. Performing without competence. J Child Lang 1977;1:1–10.

Dellacorte M, Benedict H, Klein D. The relationship of pragmatic dimensions of mothers' speech to the referential-expressive distinction. J Child Lang 1983;10:35–44.

Dore J. A pragmatic description of early language development. J Psycholinguist Res 1974;4:423–430.

DeVilliers J, DeVilliers P. A cross-sectional study of the acquisition of grammatical morphemes in child speech. J Psycholinguist Res 1973;2:267–278.

Ferguson C, Farwell C. Words and sounds in early language acquisition. Language 1975;51:419–439.

Ferguson C. From babbling to speech. Invited address to the International Conference on Infant Studies, New York, 1984.

Ferguson C, Peizer D, Weeks T. Model-and-replica phonological grammar of a child's first words. Lingua 1973;31:35–65.

Ferguson C. Phonology as an individual access system: some data from language acquisition. In: Fillmore C, Kempler D, Wang W, eds. Individual differences in language ability and language behavior. New York: Academic Press, 1979.

Fillmore L. Individual differences in second language acquisition. In: Fillmore C, Kempler D, Wang W, eds. Individual differences in language ability and language behavior. New York: Academic Press, 1979.

Furrow D, Nelson K. Environmental correlates of individual differences in language acquisition. J Child Lang 1984;11:523–534.

Goldfield B. Intra-individual variation: patterns of nominal and pronominal combinations. Paper presented at the seventh annual Boston University Conference on Language Development, Boston, 1982.

Goldfield B. Referential and expressive language: a study of two mother-child dyads. First Lang 1986;6:119–131.

Goldfield B. The contributions of child and caregiver to referential and expressive language. Appl Psycholinguist 1987;8:267–280.

Goldfield B, Snow C. Individual differences in language acquisition. In: Gleason J, ed. The development of language. Columbus, OH: Merrill, 1989.

Hardy-Brown K. Universals and individual differences: disentangling two approaches to the study of language acquisition. Dev Psychol 1983;19:610–624.

Hatch E. Second language learning-universals? Work Pap Bilingual 1974;3:1–18.

Haynes W, Haynes M, Jackson J. The effects of phonetic context and linguistic complexity on /s/ misarticulation in children. J Commun Disord 1982;15:287–297.

Horgan D. How to answer questions when you've got nothing to say. J Child Lang 1978;5:159–165.

Horgan D. Nouns: Love 'em or leave 'em. Address to the New York Academy of Sciences, New York, 1979.

Horgan D. Rate of language acquisition and noun emphasis. J Psycholinguist Res 1981;10:629–640.

Ingram D. Phonological disability in children. New York: Elsevier, 1976.

Klein D. Expressive and referential communication in children's early language development: the relationship to mother's communicative styles. Unpublished doctoral dissertation. Michigan State University, 1980.

Lieven E. Language development in young children. Unpublished doctoral dissertation. Cambridge University, 1980.

Leonard L, Schwartz R, Folger M, et al. Children's imitations of lexical items. Child Dev 1979;59:19–27.

Leonard L, Newhoff M, Masalem L. Individual differences in early childhood phonology. Appl Psycholinguist 1980;1:7–30.

Maxwell E, Rockman B. Procedures of linguistic analysis of misarticulated speech. In: Elbert M, Dinnsen D, Weismer G, eds. Phonological theory and the misarticulating child. ASHA monograph No. 22, Rockville, MD: American Speech-Language-Hearing Association, 1984.

Miller J, Chapman R. The relation between age and mean length of utterance in morphemes. J Speech Hear Res 1981;24:154–161.

Muma J. Language assessment: some underlying assumptions. J Am Speech Hear Assoc 1973;15:331–338.

Muma J. Language acquisition: a functionalistic perspective. Austin, TX: Pro-Ed, 1986.

Nelson K. Structure and strategy in learning to talk. Monogr Soc Res Child Dev 1973;38:Serial No. 143.

Nelson K. Individual differences in language development: implications for development and language. Dev Psychol 1981;17:170–187.

Nelson K. The nominal shift in semantic-syntactic development. Cognit Psychol 1975;7:461–479.

Nelson KE, Baker N, Denninger M, et al. "Cookie" versus "do it again." Imitative-referential and personal-social-syntactic-initiating styles in young children. Linguistics 1985;23:433–454.

Nelson KE, Bonvillian J. Concepts and words in the two-year-old: acquisition of concept names under controlled conditions. In: Nelson KE, ed. Children's language. Vol. 1. New York: Gardner Press, 1978.

Panagos J, Quine H, Klich P. Syntactic and phonological influences in children's articulations. J Speech Hear Res 1979;22:841–848.

Paul R, Jennings P. Phonological behavior in toddlers with slow expressive language development. JSHR 1994;37:157–170.

Peters A. Language learning strategies: does the whole equal the sum of the parts? Language 1977; 53:560–573.

Ramer A. Syntactic styles in emerging language. J Child Lang 1976;3:49–62.

Rescorlta L, Gossens M. Symbolic play development in toddlers with expressive specific language impairment. JSHR 1992;35:1290–1302.

Rosenblatt D. Developmental trends in infant play. In: Tezard B, Harvey D, eds. Biology of play. London: William Heinemann Medical Books, 1977.

Ross G, Nelson K, Wetstone H, Tanouye E. Concept acquisition at 20 months. Manuscript, Graduate Center of the City University of New York. Cited in K. Nelson (1981). Individual differences in language development. Dev Psychol 1980;17: 170–187.

Snyder L, Bates E, Bretherton I. Content and context in early lexical development. J Child Lang 1981;8:565–582.

Starr S. The relationship of single words to two-word sentences. Child Dev 1975;46:701–708.

Thal D, Tobias S. Communicative gestures in children with delayed onset of oral expressive vocabulary. JSHR 1992;35:1281–1289.

Thal D, Tobias, S. Relationships between language and gesture in normally developing and late talking toddlers. JSHR 1994;37:157–170.

Weiner F. Systematic sound preference as a characteristic of phonological disability. J Speech Hear Res 1981;46:281–285.

Weismer S, Murray-Brand J, and Miller J. A prospective longitudinal study of language development in late talkers. JSHR 1994;37: 852–867.

Weiss A, Leonard L, Rowan L, Chapman K. Linguistic and nonlinguistic features of style in normal and language-impaired children. J Speech Hear Disord 1983;48:154–163.

Wells G. Variation in child language. In: Fletcher P, Garman M, eds. Language acquisition: studies in first language development. Cambridge: Cambridge University Press, 1986.

Wolf D, Gardner H. Style and sequence in symbolic play. In: Franklin M, Smith N, eds. Early symbolization. Hillsdale, NJ: Erlbaum, 1979.

Zachman L, Huisingh R, Jorgensen C, Barrett M. Oral language sentence imitation test. Moline, IL: LinguaSystems, 1978.

Author Index

Subject Index

Page numbers followed by t and f denote tables and figures, respectively.

A

Abstraction, 316, 319t
Accommodation
  in cognitive development, 106, 107
Activity
  nonliteral in play, 137
ADHD. *See* Attention deficit/hyperactivity disorder (ADHD)
Adverbial clauses, 300
Affective interactions
  caregiver contributions to
    baby talk, 175
    facial expressions, 174–175
    mainstream caregivers, 174–175
    turn-taking conversation, 175
    variations in, 175–176
    view of infants as intentional, 175
    view of infants as nonintentional, 176
  child's contributions to
    infant engagement tools, 169, 172–173
    mastery motivation, 174
    perceptual and motor abilities, 168–169
    temperament, 173–174
African-American children
  bidialectical diversity in, 366, 369–370
  communication development in
    first lexicon in, 371–372
    phonology in, 373
    pragmatics in, 373–374
    semantic relations in, 372
    syntax/morphology in, 372–373
  contrasts between Black and Standard English and
    grammatical, 368t–369t
    phonemic, 367t
  culture of, 369–370
  distribution of, 369
  language acquisition by
    research in, 370

AGS Early Screening Profiles (ESP), 71
Articles
  in creation of context, 296
  in expression of complex ideas, 291
  naming function of, 275
  for objects, people, and their properties
    in creation of possibilities, 285
  in specification of meaning, 268
  in subject and object position, 280
Artificial intelligence, 21–22
  in connectionism
    operation of, 21–22
    versus traditional, 22
Assimilation
  in cognitive development, 106, 107
Associative play, 142
Asymmetry
  electroencephalographic, 34
  hemispheric, 34
  studies of
    dichotic listening, 37
    electroencephalography, 38
    evoked potentials, 38–39
    invasive, 35–37
    lateral motor task, 38
    lesion data in, 35
    noninvasive, 37–39
    regional cerebral blood flow, 36–37
    sodium Amytal, 36
    split-brain, 35–36
    tachistoscopic tasks, 37–38
Attachment theory
  in communication development, 76–77
Attention deficit/hyperactivity disorder (ADHD)
  metacognitive deficits in, 341–342
  oral interactive discourse deficits in, 338–339
Attentional interactions
  definition of, 180
  goal and behaviors in, 178t
Attentional mechanisms
  in information processing, 43–44